"When it comes to the increasingly treacherous landscape of the American supermarket, with its marketing hype and competing health claims, Marion Nestle is an absolutely indispensable guide; knowledgeable, eminently sane—and wonderful company, too."

—Michael Pollan, author of *The Omnivore's Dilemma*

"The industry wants you to believe there are no good foods or bad foods. Well, that's not true. And I can't think of anyone who knows the difference better than Marion Nestle."

—Eric Schlosser, author of *Fast Food Nation*

"Meticulously researched, thorough, and indispensable—Marion Nestle's *What to Eat* delivers on its title. It's a reliable, riveting guide to the amazing truth about what we're sold by the American food distribution system. Refreshingly rigorous and fun to read."

—Alice Waters, founder and proprietor of Chez Panisse
and author of *Chez Panisse Café Cookbook*

"Accessible, reliable and comprehensive."

—Judith Weinraub, *The Washington Post*

"[This] book is for anyone who has read a food label; been annoyed at how often their children nag them for certain cereals; wondered about the difference between natural and organic; or questioned who is minding the store when it comes to nutrition and food safety."

—Marian Burros, *The New York Times*

"Easily digestible . . . Nestle is simply one of the nation's smartest and most influential authorities on nutrition and food policy."

—Carol Ness, *San Francisco Chronicle*

"The most comprehensive guide to the political and nutritional choices we make shopping for food." —Susan Salter Reynolds, *Los Angeles Times*

"Marion Nestle's *What to Eat* is the perfect guidebook to help navigate through the confusion of which foods are good for us, what labels we can believe and, most important, which are the foods to avoid . . . [This] book is both an everyday reference and political statement."
—Phil Lempert, *USA Today*

"Part muckraking journalism, part reference book and part consumer guide." —Steve Weinberg, *The Denver Post*

"In a field full of crackpots and food loathers and obfuscators, [Marion Nestle] stands out as a levelheaded, clear-thinking person who actually enjoys food (in moderation, of course, as Julia used to say) . . . She really is a treasure." —R. W. Apple, Jr.

"Includes practical advice and answers to everything you ever wanted to know about food . . . Dive in where you're most curious."
—Anna Lappé, *San Francisco Chronicle*

"Help[s] to clear the air." —Owen Dugan, *Wine Spectator*

"Develops your cart smarts by tackling the conventional wisdom about healthy eating." —Ericka Sóuter, *People*

"Cuts through the marketing claims and maze of offerings in today's supermarkets to provide advice for making healthy choices."
—*BusinessWeek*

"[Nestle's] research will permit you to make informed decisions about everything you eat, whether at home or out."
—Robin Mather Jenkins, *Chicago Tribune*

Marion Nestle

What to EAT

Useful information at your fingertips . . .

Expert understanding of the latest news and developments . . .

Discussions . . . updates . . . reference materials . . . community . . . and more . . .

www.whattoeatbook.com

At the companion website to *What to Eat*, you'll find Marion Nestle's insights on food, health, and nutrition issues that are in the news. You'll be able to exchange opinions and advice. And you'll be able to access *on your cellphone or handheld* specific information to guide you while shopping. It's easy. All you need to do is log on and become a registered user at www.whattoeatbook.com.

What to EAT

Marion Nestle

North Point Press

A division of Farrar, Straus and Giroux

New York

North Point Press
A division of Farrar, Straus and Giroux
18 West 18th Street, New York 10011

Copyright © 2006 by Marion Nestle
All rights reserved
Distributed in Canada by Douglas & McIntyre Ltd.
Printed in the United States of America
Published in 2006 by North Point Press
First paperback edition, 2007

The Library of Congress has cataloged the hardcover edition as follows:
Nestle, Marion.
      What to eat / Marion Nestle. — 1st ed.
          p.   cm.
      Includes index.
      ISBN-13: 978-0-86547-704-9 (hardcover : alk. paper).
      ISBN-10: 0-86547-704-3 (hardcover : alk. paper).
      1. Nutrition — Popular works.   2. Diet — Popular works.
      3. Health — Popular works.   I. Title.

      RA784.N46   2006
      613.2 — dc22

                                                        2006007886

Paperback ISBN-13: 978-0-86547-738-4
Paperback ISBN-10: 0-86547-738-8

Designed by Cassandra J. Pappas

www.fsgbooks.com

      13 14 15 16 17 18 19 20

To Mal

Contents

THE SPECIAL SECTIONS

What to
EAT

Introduction

I am a nutrition professor, and as soon as people find out what I do, they ask: Why is nutrition so confusing? Why is it so hard to know which foods are good for me? Why don't you nutritionists figure out what's right and make it simple for the rest of us to understand? Why can't you help me know what to eat?

Questions like these come up every time I give a talk, teach a class, or go out to dinner. For a long time, they puzzled me. I thought: Doesn't everyone know what a healthy diet is? And why are people so worried about what they eat? I just didn't get it. For me, food is one of life's greatest pleasures, and I have been teaching, writing, and talking about the joys of eating as well as the more cultural and scientific aspects of food for nearly thirty years. My work at a university means that I do research as well as teach, and for the past decade or so I have been studying the marketing of food and its effects on health. Everyone eats. This turns the growing, shipping, preparing, and serving of food into a business of titanic proportions, worth close to a trillion dollars a year in the United States alone. I wrote about the health consequences of the business of food—unintended as those consequences may be—in two books: *Food Politics: How the Food Industry Influences Nutrition and Health* and *Safe Food: Bacteria, Biotechnology, and Bioterrorism*.

Since writing them, I have spent much of my professional and social life talking to students, health professionals, academics, government officials, journalists, community organizers, farmers, school officials, and business leaders—as well as friends and colleagues—about the social and political aspects of food and nutrition. It hardly matters who I am talking to. Everyone goes right to what affects *them*. Their questions are *personal*. Everyone wants to know what the politics of food mean for what they personally should eat. Should they be worried about hormones, pesticides, antibiotics, mercury, or bacteria in foods? Is it acceptable to eat sugars, artificial sweeteners, or *trans* fats, and, if so, how much? What about foods that are raw, canned, irradiated, or genetically engineered? Do I recommend calcium or any other supplement? Which is the best choice of vegetables, yogurt, meat, or bread?

Eventually I came to realize that, for many people, food feels nothing at all like a source of pleasure; it feels more like a minefield. For one thing, there are far too many choices; about 320,000 food and beverage products are available in the United States, and an average supermarket carries 30,000 to 40,000 of them. As the social theorist Barry Schwartz explains in *The Paradox of Choice*, this volume of products turns supermarket and other kinds of shopping into "a complex decision in which [you] are forced to invest time, energy, and no small amount of self-doubt, anxiety, and dread." Bombarded with too many choices and conflicting messages, as everyone is, many people long for reassurance that they can ignore the "noise" and just go back to enjoying the food they eat. I began paying closer attention to hints of such longings in what people were telling me. I started asking my friends how they felt about food. Their responses were similar. Eating, they told me, feels nothing less than hazardous. And, they said, *you* need to do something about this. One after another told me things like this:

- You seem to think we have the information we need, but a lot of us are clueless and have no idea of how to eat.
- When I go into a supermarket, I feel like a deer caught in headlights. Tell me what I need to know so I can make reasonable choices, and quickly.
- I do not feel confident that I know what to eat. It's all so confusing.

- *You* tell me how to do this. I don't believe all those other people. They all seem to have axes to grind.
- Tell us how *you* eat.

The more I thought about what audiences and friends were telling me, the more I realized that changes in society and in the competitiveness of food companies had made the question of what to eat incredibly complicated for most people, and that while I had noticed some of the effects of such changes, I had missed others that were quite important. Years ago, I regularly shopped in suburban supermarkets in California and Massachusetts while cooking for my growing family, but that era in my life is long past. Besides, the whole shopping experience is different now. Today, too, I live in Manhattan. For reasons of space and real estate costs, Manhattan does not have enormous supermarkets like the ones in suburbs or in most cities in the United States. I live within easy walking distance of ten or fifteen grocery stores, but these are small—sometimes tiny—by national standards. Only recently have larger stores like Whole Foods come into the city. And I do much less food shopping than many people. My children are now adults and live on the other side of the continent. More than that, my job requires me to eat out a lot. Because I do not own a car I either have to walk home carrying what I buy, or arrange to have food delivered. It became clear to me that if I really wanted to understand how food marketing affects health, I needed to find out a lot more about what you and everyone else are up against when you shop for food—and the sooner the better. So I did, and this book is the result.

I began my research (and that is just what it was) by visiting supermarkets of all kinds and taking notes on what they were selling, section by section, aisle by aisle. I looked at the products on those shelves just as any shopper might, and tried to figure out which ones made the most sense to buy for reasons of taste, health, economy, or any number of social issues that might be of concern. Doing this turned out to be more complicated than I could have imagined. For one thing, it required careful reading of food labels, which, I can assure you, is hard work even for nutritionists. Science and politics make food labels exceptionally complicated, and they often appear in very small print. I found it impossible to do any kind of comparative shopping without putting on reading glasses, I frequently had to use a calculator, and I often wished I had a scale handy so I could weigh things.

Supermarkets turn out to be deeply fascinating, not least because even the smallest ones sell thousands of products. Much about these stores made me intensely curious. Why, I wondered, do they sell this and not that? Why are entire aisles devoted to soft drinks and snack foods? What do the pricing signs mean, and how do they work? Why is it so hard to find some things, but not others? Are there any genetically modified or irradiated foods among the fruits and vegetables? What does "Certified Organic" mean, can it be trusted, and is it worth the higher price? Is soy milk healthier than cow's milk? If an egg is "United Egg Producers Certified," is it better? Is it safe to eat farmed fish or, for that matter, any fish at all? Is it safe to eat take-out foods? If a sugary cereal sports a label saying it is whole grain, is it better for you? Does it make any real nutritional difference whether you buy white or whole wheat bread?

The answers to these questions might seem obvious, but I did not find them so. To arrive at decisions, I measured, counted, weighed, and calculated, and read the tiniest print on product labels. When I still did not understand something, I talked to section managers and store clerks. When they asked why I wanted to know (which they often did), I explained what I was doing and gave them my business card. If they could not answer my questions, I called the consumer affairs numbers on product labels, and sometimes talked to regional or national managers. I talked to farmers, farmers' market managers, product makers, food company executives, agriculture specialists, organic inspectors, fish inspectors, trade organization representatives, and university scientists. I went on field trips to places that roast coffee, bake bread, and package groceries for delivery. And I spent months searching the Internet and reading books, unearthing articles in my files, and examining trade and professional publications.

I tell you this not so much to impress you with the extent of the research as to explain that this is the kind of effort it took *me* to figure out what was going on, and I am supposed to know about such things. If you have trouble dealing with supermarkets, it is for a good reason. You need to know an amazing amount about our food system and about nutrition to make intelligent choices, but most of this information is anything but obvious. It is not *supposed* to be obvious. Supermarkets have one purpose and one purpose only: to sell food and make a profit, and as large a profit as possible. Your goals are more complicated: you want foods that are good for your health, but you also want them to taste good, to be affordable, to be convenient to eat, and to reflect social values that you might care about. In theory, your goals could overlap with the normal business interests of supermarkets. After all, they do sell plenty of inexpensive, convenient, tasty foods that are good for you. But in practice, you and the supermarket are likely to be at cross-purposes. The foods that sell best and bring in the most profits are not necessarily the ones that are best for your health, and the conflict between health and business goals is at the root of public confusion about food choices.

This conflict begins with dietary advice, much of which is hard to interpret. What, for example, does it really mean to "Consume a variety of nutrient-dense foods and beverages within and among the basic food groups" as advised by the *Dietary Guidelines for Americans* issued in 2005? Or to "know your fats" as advised by the 2005 version of the pyramid food guide? As I explained in *Food Politics*, government agencies cannot issue unambiguous dietary advice to eat this but not that without offending powerful industries. This is too bad, because nutrition is not "mission impossible." Its basic principles are simple. You need enough energy (measured in calories) and nutrients, but not too much of either. The range of healthful nutrient intake is broad, and foods from the earth, tree, or animal can be combined in a seemingly infinite number of ways to create diets that meet health goals. Think, for example, of how different the traditional diets are from Italy (pasta based, higher fat) and Japan (rice based, low fat), yet both are as healthful as can be.

Where diets get confusing is in the details: so many nutrients, so many foods, so many diseases, and so many conflicting research studies about one or another of them. The attention paid to single nutrients, to

> The foods that sell best and bring in the most profits are not necessarily the ones that are best for your health, and the conflict between health and business goals is at the root of public confusion about food choices.

individual foods, and to particular diseases distracts from the basic principles of diet and health, but is understandable. You choose foods one by one, and those diseases affect *you*. Single nutrients and foods are easier to talk about than messy dietary patterns. And they are much easier to study. But you are better off paying attention to your overall dietary pattern than worrying about whether any one single food is better for you than another.

THE BASICS OF DIET AND HEALTH

The basic principles of good diets are so simple that I can summarize them in just ten words: *eat less, move more, eat lots of fruits and vegetables.* For additional clarification, a five-word modifier helps: *go easy on junk foods.* Follow these precepts and you will go a long way toward preventing the major diseases of our overfed society—coronary heart disease, certain cancers, diabetes, stroke, osteoporosis, and a host of others. By keeping your weight down—an increasingly important concern in our increasingly overweight society—you will also reduce several "risk factors" for these diseases: obesity, high blood pressure, high blood cholesterol, and high blood sugar. These precepts constitute the bottom line of what seem to be the far more complicated dietary recommendations of many health organizations and national and international governments—the forty-one "key recommendations" of the 2005 *Dietary Guidelines*, for example. The guidelines also tend to deal with single nutrients or foods, not dietary patterns. Although you may feel as though advice about nutrition is constantly changing, the basic ideas behind my four precepts have not changed in half a century. And they leave plenty of room for enjoying the pleasures of food. To take them one by one:

Eat less means eating fewer calories. This, in turn, means not overeating fat (which is high in calories) or sugars (which have calories but no nutrients), avoiding between-meal snacks, and eating smaller por-

> The basic principles of good diets are so simple that I can summarize them in just ten words: *eat less, move more, eat lots of fruits and vegetables.* For additional clarification, a five-word modifier helps: *go easy on junk foods.*

tions. It is, of course, one thing to hear this advice and quite another to follow it, not least because advice to eat less is hugely controversial. Eating less is bad for business—very bad for business. If you eat less, it means that you are personally taking action to oppose the goals of food marketers

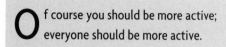

Of course you should be more active; everyone should be more active.

whose entire purpose is to get you to eat more of their products, not less.

Move more or, more elegantly, *be more active*, is the flip side of the body-weight equation. How much you weigh depends on the balance between the calories you eat and the ones you use up. Of course you should be more active; everyone should be more active. Being active uses more calories, builds muscle and bones, and regulates metabolism. Advice to move more is a no-brainer, and causes no political trouble. That is why food companies and government agencies place so much emphasis on exercise as a weight-loss strategy. It becomes *your* responsibility to move more, no matter how hard it is to find the time and place to do so.

Eat lots of fruits and vegetables means just that. It also means substituting these foods for those that are higher in calories and have fewer nutrients. Fruits and vegetables are the one point of consensus—an oasis—in arguments about what to eat. Everyone agrees that eating more of them is a good idea. But nobody does much to make it easier to follow the advice. The produce industry does not advertise fruits and vegetables much because its profit margins are low and its constituents are fragmented and competitive: broccoli growers versus carrot farmers, for example, or producers of peaches in Georgia versus apple growers in Washington State. This industry also cannot easily "add value" (as they put it) to fresh produce to command higher prices, the way food product makers add value so they can increase the price of inexpensive ingredients in junk food with additives, shapes, and packaging. The government does not subsidize fruit and vegetable production the way it supports corn, soybeans, sugarcane, and sugar beets. All of this may make fruits and vegetables appear to be expensive, in part because they don't give you many calories for the amount of money you spend. Fewer calories is a good reason to eat more produce, but the lack of profit means that less effort goes into making sure these foods are as fresh, tasty, well prepared, and easy to use as they might be.

Go easy on junk foods is an ungracious way of characterizing foods like soft drinks, candy, and snack foods that are low in nutrients but high in calories, fats, sugars, and noncaloric additives like salt and artificial flavors, colors, and sweeteners. Soft drinks are the prototypical junk food; they contain sugars—and, therefore, calories—but nothing else of nutritional value. The calories in junk foods add up fast and can displace more nutritious calories in the diet. Avoiding them, however, takes effort, as they are designed to be convenient, ubiquitous, inexpensive, and easy to eat. It is no coincidence that they are the most heavily promoted of all processed foods.

If you follow these four precepts—eat less, move more, eat lots of fruits and vegetables, and go easy on junk foods—the question of what to eat becomes much easier to answer. Once you balance calories from food against activity levels, and make sure that enough calories come from fruits and vegetables but not too many come from junk foods, other aspects of your diet matter much less. You can eat what you like as long as you don't eat too much. This approach to overall diets, by the way, has not changed in ages. Listen to this 1959 advice from the late cardiologist Ancel Keys (who died at the age of 100 in 2004) and his wife, Margaret: "Do not get fat; if you are fat, reduce. Favor fresh vegetables and fruits. Avoid heavy use of salt and refined sugar. Get plenty of exercise and outdoor recreation. See your doctor regularly, and do not worry"—advice as good today as it was then.

If you find it hard to view dietary advice as unchanging, it is surely because the research breakthroughs and seemingly contradictory findings about one or another nutrient, food, or diet plan are taken out of context. Nutrition arguments are almost invariably about single nutrients taken out of their food context, single foods taken out of their dietary context, or single risk factors and diseases taken out of their lifestyle context. Single-nutrient arguments are "reductive" in that they reduce diets and food choices to one simple decision: eat this or avoid that, and all problems will be solved. Food companies love this approach because they can use it to say that their particular products have special health benefits. But few issues in nutrition are that simple.

As you will see from this book, the choice of any one food over another is going to have only a small effect on your health, at best. Eating a food with sugar or *trans* fat is not going to kill you on the spot. Eating a particular fruit or vegetable is not going to provide lifetime protection against heart disease or cancer. It's what you habitually eat—and how much—that matters. Diets that typically balance calories by including fruits and vegetables and minimizing junk foods are better for you than the opposite, but the impact of any one food or food product is going to be small. Food marketers work hard to convince you that eating their particular products will make a big difference in your health. That might help, but only as part of a diet that is healthful to begin with.

MAKING INFORMED FOOD CHOICES

Even if you know what is good for you, you are likely to have a hard time putting principles into practice. For one thing, in America today—and practically everywhere else in the world—it is very, very hard not to overeat. Just about everything in the food scene is set up to encourage us to eat more food, not less. Why? Consider this question: What industry or professional organization might benefit if you ate more healthfully? Try as hard as I can, I cannot think of a single one (well, organic food producers, maybe). You might think that the health insurance industry would profit from better health, but not necessarily. It costs more to provide preventive services for an entire population than to pay for the treatment of the smaller number of people who become ill—or so some economists say. Phrasing the question the opposite way yields an even more disheartening answer: What industry or group benefits from public confusion about nutrition and health? Here the list is long and includes the food, restaurant, fast-food, diet, health club, drug, and health care industries, among many others.

Much of the pressure to eat more comes as a consequence of normal business practices. The deep dark secret of American agriculture (revealed only by agricultural economists behind closed doors) is that there is far too much food available—3,900 calories per day for every man, woman, and child in the country, whereas the average adult needs only a bit more than half that amount, and children much less. The 3,900 calorie figure is at the high end of the amount available in the food supply of industrialized countries. Even though these are the available calories (the number produced in the United States, minus exports, plus imports) and not necessarily the amount you actually eat, they reflect substantial excess.

Overabundance leaves food companies with three options. They can make fewer products or smaller portions and raise prices (a risky business strategy); they can entice you to buy their products instead of those of their competitors (hence: advertising); or they can get you to eat more of what they sell. This last option requires not only advertising but also more subtle methods for selling food that have had profound consequences for the way we eat in America. In the not so old days, to take just one example, we ate most meals at home, where calories are easier to control. Today, nearly half the typical family's food budget goes for foods prepared and eaten outside the home, where businesses with motives having nothing to do with health are in control of content and amounts. Competition for your food dollars has led food companies to develop marketing strategies that help them to sell more food and encourage you to eat more. Consider what the research says about strategies that encourage you to eat more food and more calories, whether or not you need them:

> Today, nearly half the typical family's food budget goes for foods prepared and eaten outside the home, where businesses with motives having nothing to do with health are in control of content and amounts.

- **Convenience:** if a food is easier to take with you and eat, you will eat more
- **Ubiquity:** the more places food is available, the more food you will eat
- **Proximity:** if a food is close at hand, you will eat more of it than if it is harder to get to
- **Frequency:** the more times a day you eat, the more food you will eat
- **Variety:** the more foods that are available, the more you will eat (the "buffet syndrome")
- **Larger portions:** the more food in front of you, the more you will eat
- **Low prices:** the cheaper the food, the more you will eat

Do not misunderstand me. I am not arguing against convenience, variety, or low prices, any of which might make your life easier or more pleasant. And I am fully aware that the industry has brought us a food supply of astonishing variety and abundance, independent of season and geography. I am simply pointing out that the food industry's normal methods of doing business encourage you to eat more, not less. Mind you, I do not for a minute think that corporate executives are sitting around a conference table saying, "How can we make our customers fat?" No, they are simply asking, "How can we sell *our* foods in this impossibly competitive environment?" As publicly traded corporations, most food companies must file quarterly reports with Wall Street. Investment analysts not only demand profits, they demand growth. It is not enough for Kraft Foods to generate $32 billion in sales in 2004. If that company wants its stock prices to rise, it has to increase sales by a sizable percentage every ninety days. Companies must sell more, and then more, and even more. In this kind of investment economy, weight gain is just collateral damage.

But obesity is not the only collateral result of pressures for corporate growth. Food marketing strategies have changed social patterns. It is now socially acceptable to eat more food, more often, in more places. Without provoking social disapproval, you can snack all day instead of eating meals, consume gigantic amounts of food at a sitting, and eat in formerly forbidden places like clothing stores, bookstores, and libraries. It has become socially acceptable for children to consume soft drinks all day long in school, and to decide for themselves what to eat at home. These are recent changes. They happened within my lifetime and, in fact, just since the early 1980s—exactly in parallel with rising rates of obesity. If you did not notice the changes in societal norms, or indeed welcomed them, it is because you are human. It is human nature to eat when presented with food, and to eat more when presented with more food, more often. You are not supposed to have noticed the changes. Marketing methods are meant to be invisible—"to slip below the radar of critical thinking"—and for the most part they do just that. Once you start noticing such things, the food scene looks quite different and making choices becomes easier. Your choice becomes *informed*.

I emphasize "informed" because debates about our increasingly overweight society (in which an astonishing 60 percent or more of adults weigh more than is considered healthy) tend to focus on who is to blame—you, the food industry, or the government—as well as on what should be done to fix the problem. If dietary choices are solely about personal responsibility, then it is entirely up to you to do the right thing. An alternative approach is to change the social and business environment so that it becomes easier for you to make better choices. Food companies are unlikely to change marketing practices on their own, however, so changing the social environment requires discussion of government regulations, lawsuits, taxes, new labeling requirements, or outright bans on junk foods. While waiting for the arguments about such measures to be resolved, you are on your own. You still have to eat. But once you recognize the vested interests behind food marketing, your choices become real: you can decide for yourself whether to accept, ignore, or oppose what marketers are trying to get you to do.

> This book is about how to think about the food you eat.

This book is about how to think about the food you eat. By the time you finish it, you should be able to walk into a supermarket, a restaurant, a fast-food outlet, or any other place that sells food and know why the foods are there, what they are, and whether they are worth buying.

At this point, I need to be clear about what this book is *not* about. This book is not going to tell you to choose one kind of vegetable over another, but it will explain how to think about such decisions. It will not tell you which food product is more nutritious than the next, but it will explain what you need to know in order to answer this question for yourself. This book will not take you through detailed explanations of the nutrients in food, but you should pick up a considerable amount of information about such things by the time you are done. I am not going to tell you how to lose weight or whether one diet plan is better than another, but instead I will argue that calories are the key factor in managing weight, and I will show you where the calories are in foods. I also will point out how you can stay focused on calories when food marketers try to distract you by talking about vitamins, omega-3 fats, *trans* fats, or low-carbohydrate diets, or by tempting you with larger portions.

The American food scene is vast and encompasses hundreds of thousands of products and places to sell them: convenience stores, grocery stores, supermarkets, retail warehouses, restaurants, fast-food and snack outlets, and, increasingly, Internet sites. But the things you need to think about when you buy foods from any source anywhere in the country (or throughout the world, for that matter) are much the same from place to place.

Because about 40 percent of food purchases still occur in supermarkets, and because such places are laid out systematically, they make a convenient organizing device for this discussion. So I begin the book with an account of what supermarkets are and how they work, and then move on through the supermarket just as you might wander through one with a shopping cart. Most supermarkets place fruits and vegetables at the front, so I begin with that section and work my way around the periphery, into the center aisles, and, eventually, to the specialty bakery and takeout sections. Along the way, I let curiosity flourish and look for answers to the questions that you or anyone else might have about the foods on supermarket shelves.

To avoid repetition, I tried to deal with these questions only once in detail. While reading about produce, for example, you might be curious about how safety inspections work, but I think that this question is more germane to take-out food, so I deal with it in that later chapter. Omega-3 fats come up in the eggs, fats, bread, and baby food chapters, but I put the more detailed discussion in the earlier chapters on fish, their greatest source. Reading ingredient lists on package labels is a critically important skill in choosing any food, but the topic comes up most prominently in the chapters on frozen foods, so that is where I put it. Health claims on package labels are a constant theme. The FDA requires claims that are not supported by much in the way of science to be "qualified" and placed in the context of daily diets. My favorite example is the qualified claim for green tea and cancer prevention, so I put it in the chapter on coffees and teas. Portion sizes are the key to controlling calorie intake, so much so that this relationship constitutes the Law of Portion Size: the more food you have, the more of it you will eat. Look for that discussion in the chapter on prepared foods. You may need and want to consult the index to find what you are looking for. The Notes identify sources, of course, but also contain definitions, explanations, comments, and digressions that I could not bear to leave out. If something in the book sparks your curiosity (as I hope it will), check the Notes.

I added two appendixes to the book. Reading labels requires familiarity with units of measurement, and supermarkets love to use as many different kinds as possible. Appendix 1 explains how you get from one kind to another. And because so many terms are used to describe the fats in foods, I've used Appendix 2 to explain what they mean for the kinds of issues discussed in this book.

Nutrition topics are often controversial, and here is the short reason why: the science is complicated. Complicated science is subject to interpretation, and interpretation depends on point of view. And point of view can reflect vested interests. That is why sources of information take on greater importance than they might in other fields. Throughout this book, I refer to books, studies, documents, and Web sites, and I often use direct quotations. I also have listed the sources for all of these citations in the Notes at the end of the book.

Nutrition topics are often controversial, and here is the short reason why: the science is complicated.

With these details out of the way, we are ready to enter the supermarket and ask the question: What to eat?

But first, a final comment: I cannot begin to tell you how much fun this book has been to research and write. It turned out to be as challenging a project as any I have ever undertaken, but also a lot more entertaining. Every time I walked into a supermarket, I discovered something new, and often unsuspected. The most seemingly mundane products (eggs! bottled water!) led me to discoveries I had not even imagined possible. I found something astonishing—and often quite amusing—in every section of the store. I hope that you are just as amazed and amused reading this book as I was while writing it. I also hope that you put it to immediate use. Enjoy, eat well, and change the world (for the better, of course).

The Supermarket:
Prime Real Estate

A visit to a large supermarket can be a daunting experience: so many aisles, so many brands and varieties, so many prices to keep track of and labels to read, so many choices to make. No wonder. To repeat: An astonishing 320,000 edible products are for sale in the United States, and any large supermarket might display as many as 40,000 of them. You are supposed to feel daunted—bewildered by all the choices and forced to wander through the aisles in search of the items you came to buy. The big companies that own most supermarkets want you to do as much searching as you can tolerate. It is no coincidence that one super-market is laid out much like another: breathtaking amounts of research have gone into designing these places. There are precise reasons why milk is at the back of the store and the center aisles are so long. You are forced to go past thousands of other products on your way to get what you need.

Supermarkets say they are in the business of offering "choice." Per-haps, but they do everything possible to make the choice theirs, not yours. Supermarkets are not social service agencies providing food for the hungry. Their job is to sell food, and more of it. From their perspec-tive, it is *your* problem if what you buy makes you eat more food than you need, and more of the wrong kinds of foods in particular.

And supermarket retailers know more than you could possibly imagine about how to push your "buy" buttons. Half a century ago, Vance Packard revealed their secrets in his book *The Hidden Persuaders*. His most shocking revelation? Corporations were hiring social scientists to study unconscious human emotions, not for the good of humanity but to help companies manipulate people into buying products. Packard's chapter on supermarket shopping, "Babes in Consumerland," is as good a guide as anything that has been written since to methods for getting you—and your children—to "reach out, hypnotically . . . and grab boxes of cookies, candies, dog food, and everything else that delights or interests [you]."

At the supermarket, you exercise freedom of choice and personal responsibility every time you put an item in your shopping cart, but massive efforts have gone into making it more convenient and desirable for you to choose some products rather than others.

More recent research on consumer behavior not only confirms his observations but continues to be awe-inspiring in its meticulous attention to detail. Your local library has entire textbooks and academic journals devoted to investigations of consumer behavior and ways to use the results of that research to sell products. Researchers are constantly interviewing shoppers and listening carefully to what they are told. Because of scanners, supermarkets can now track your purchases and compare what you tell researchers to what you actually buy. If you belong to a supermarket discount "shoppers club," the store gains your loyalty but gets to track your personal buying habits in exchange. This research tells food retailers how to lay out the stores, where to put specific products, how to position products on shelves, and how to set prices and advertise products. At the supermarket, you exercise freedom of choice and personal responsibility every time you put an item in your shopping cart, but massive efforts have gone into making it more convenient and desirable for you to choose some products rather than others.

As basic marketing textbooks explain, the object of the game is to "maximize sales and profit consistent with customer convenience." Translated, this means that supermarkets want to expose you to the largest possible number of items that you can stand to see, without annoying you so much that you run screaming from the store. This strategy is based on research proving that "the rate of exposure is directly related to the rate of sale of merchandise." In other words, the more you see, the more you buy. Supermarkets dearly wish they could expose you to every single item they carry, every time you shop. Terrific as that might be for your walking regimen, you are unlikely to endure having to trek through interminable aisles to find the few items you came in for—and retailers know it. This conflict creates a serious dilemma for the stores. They have to figure out how to get you to walk up and down those aisles for as long as possible, but not so long that you get frustrated. To resolve the dilemma, the stores make some compromises—but as few as possible. Overall, supermarket design follows fundamental rules, all of them based firmly on extensive research.

- Place the highest-selling food departments in the parts of the store that get the greatest flow of traffic—the periphery. Perishables—meat, produce, dairy, and frozen foods—generate the most sales, so put them against the back and side walls.

- Use the aisle nearest the entrance for items that sell especially well on impulse or look or smell enticing—produce, flowers, or freshly baked bread, for example. These must be the first things customers see in front or immediately to the left or right (the direction, according to researchers, doesn't matter).

- Use displays at the ends of aisles for high-profit, heavily advertised items likely to be bought on impulse.

- Place high-profit, center-aisle food items sixty inches above the floor where they are easily seen by adults, with or without eyeglasses.

- Devote as much shelf space as possible to brands that generate frequent sales; the more shelf space they occupy, the better they sell.

- Place store brands immediately to the right of those high-traffic items (people read from left to right), so that the name brands attract shoppers to the store brands too.

- Avoid using "islands." These make people bump into each other and want to move on. Keep the traffic moving, but slowly.

- Do not create gaps in the aisles that allow customers to cross over to the next one unless the aisles are so long that shoppers complain. If shoppers can escape mid-aisle, they will miss seeing half the products along that route.

Additional principles, equally well researched, guide every other aspect of supermarket design: product selection, placement on shelves, and display. The guiding principle of supermarket layout is the same: products seen most sell best. Think of the supermarket as a particularly intense real estate market in which every product competes fiercely against every other for precious space. Because you can see products most easily at eye level, at the ends of aisles, and at the checkout counters, these areas are prime real estate. Which products get the prime space? The obvious answer: the ones most profitable for the store.

> The guiding principle of supermarket layout is the same: products seen most sell best.

But store profitability is not simply a matter of the price charged for a product compared to its costs. Stores also collect revenue by "renting" real estate to the companies whose products they sell. Product placement depends on a system of "incentives" that sometimes sound suspiciously like bribes. Food companies pay supermarkets "slotting fees" for the shelf space they occupy. The rates are highest for premium, high-traffic space, such as the shelves near cash registers. Supermarkets demand and get additional sources of revenue from food companies in "trade allowances," guarantees that companies will buy local advertising for the products for which they pay slotting fees. The local advertising, of course, helps to make sure that products in prime real estate sell quickly.

This unsavory system puts retail food stores in firm control of the marketplace. They make the decisions about which products to sell and, therefore, which products you buy. This system goes beyond a simple matter of supply and demand. The stores *create* demand by putting some products where you cannot miss them. These are often "junk" foods full of cheap, shelf-stable ingredients like hydrogenated oils and corn sweeteners, made and promoted by giant food companies that can afford slotting fees, trade allowances, and advertising. This is why entire aisles of prime supermarket real estate are devoted to soft drinks, salty snacks, and sweetened breakfast cereals, and why you can always find candy next to cash registers. Any new product that comes into a store must come with guaranteed advertising, coupons, discounts, slotting fees, and other such incentives.

Slotting fees emerged in the 1980s as a way for stores to cover the added costs of dealing with new products: shelving, tracking inventory, and removing products that do not sell. But the system is so corrupt and so secret that Congress held hearings about it in 1999. The industry people who testified at those hearings were so afraid of retribution that they wore hoods and used gadgets to prevent voice recognition. The General Accounting Office, the congressional watchdog agency (now called the Government Accountability Office), was asked to do its own investigation but got nowhere because the retail food industry refused to cooperate.

The defense of the current system by both the retailers who demand the fees and the companies that agree to pay them comes at a high cost—out of your pocket. You pay for this system in at least three ways: higher prices at the supermarket; taxes that in part compensate for business tax deductions that food companies are allowed to take for slotting fees and advertising; and the costs of treating illnesses that might result from consuming more profitable but less healthful food products.

In 2005, supermarkets sold more than $350 billion worth of food in the United States, but this level of sales does not stop them from complaining about low after-tax profit margins—just 1 to 3 percent of sales. One percent of $350 billion is $3.5 billion, of course, but by some corporate standards that amount is too little to count. In any case, corporations have to grow to stay viable, so corporate pressures on supermarkets to increase sales are unrelenting. The best way to expand sales, say researchers, is to increase the size of the selling area and the number of items offered. Supermarkets do both. In the last decade, mergers and acquisitions have turned the top-ranking supermarkets—Kroger, Albertsons, and Safeway—into companies with annual sales of $56, $40, and $36 billion, respectively. Small chains, like Whole Foods and Wegmans, have sales in the range of just $4 billion a year.

But sales brought in by these small chains are peanuts compared to those of the store that now dominates the entire retail food marketplace: Wal-Mart. Wal-Mart sold $284 billion worth of goods in 2005. Groceries accounted for about one-quarter of that amount, but that meant $64 billion, and rising. Many food companies do a third of their business with this one retailer. Wal-Mart does not have to demand slotting fees. If a food company wants its products to be in Wal-Mart, it has to offer rock-bottom prices. Low prices sound good for people without much money, but nutritionally, there's a catch. Low prices encourage everyone to buy more food in bigger packages. If you buy more, you are quite likely to eat more. And if you eat more, you are more likely to gain weight and become less healthy.

Food retailers argue that if you eat too much it is your problem, not theirs. But they are in the business of encouraging you to buy more food, not less. Take the matter of package size and price. I often talk to business groups about such matters and at a program for food executives at Cornell University, I received a barrage of questions about where personal responsibility fits into this picture. One supermarket manager insisted that his store does not force customers to buy Pepsi in big bottles. He also offers Pepsi in 8-ounce cans. The sizes and prices are best shown in a Table.

> Low prices sound good for people without much money, but nutritionally, there's a catch. Low prices encourage everyone to buy more food in bigger packages. If you buy more, you are quite likely to eat more.

Price of Pepsi-Cola, P&C Market, Ithaca, New York, July 2005

CONTAINER SIZE	TOTAL OUNCES	PRICE	PRICE PER QUART
2-liter bottle	67	$1.49	$0.71
24-ounce bottles (6-pack)	144	$3.00*	$0.67
16-ounce bottles (6-pack)	96	$2.99	$1.00
12-ounce cans (12-pack)	144	$4.49	$1.00
8-ounce cans (6-pack)	48	$2.25	$1.50

*This is with a P&C store membership "Wild Card."

In this store, the 2-liter container and the special-for-members 6-pack of 24-ounce bottles were less than half the cost of the equivalent volume in 8-ounce cans. Supermarket managers tell me that this kind of pricing is not the store's problem. If you want smaller sizes, you should be willing to pay more for them. But if you care about how much you get for a price, you are likely to pick the larger sizes. And if you buy the larger sizes, you are likely to drink more Pepsi and take in more calories; the 8-ounce cans of Pepsi contain 100 calories each, but the 2-liter bottle holds 800 calories.

Sodas of any size are cheap because they are mostly water and corn sweeteners—water is practically free, and your taxes pay to subsidize corn production. This makes the cost of the ingredients trivial compared to labor and packaging, so the larger sizes are more profitable to the manufacturer and to the stores. The choice is yours, but anyone would have a hard time choosing a more expensive version of a product when a cheaper one is right there. Indeed, you have to be strong and courageous to hold out for healthier choices in the supermarket system as it currently exists.

You could, of course, bring a shopping list, but good luck sticking to it. Research says that about 70 percent of shoppers bring lists into supermarkets, but only about 10 percent adhere to them. Even with a list, most shoppers pick up two additional items for every item on it. The additions are "in-store decisions," or impulse buys. Stores directly appeal to your senses to distract you from worrying about lists. They hope you will:

- Listen to the background music. The slower the beat, the longer you will tarry.

- Search for the "loss leaders" (the items you always need, like meat, coffee, or bananas, that are offered at or below their actual cost). The longer you search, the more products you will see.

- Go to the bakery, prepared foods, and deli sections; the sights and good smells will keep you lingering and encourage sales.

- Taste the samples that companies are giving away. If you like what you taste, you are likely to buy it.

- Put your kids in the play areas; the longer they play there, the more time you have to walk those tempting aisles.

If you find yourself in a supermarket buying on impulse and not minding it a bit, you are behaving exactly the way store managers want you to. You will be buying the products they have worked long and hard to make most attractive and convenient for you—and most profitable for them.

But, you may ask, what about all those beautiful fruits and vegetables? Aren't you supposed to eat more of them? Isn't the produce section the one place in the supermarket where the store's goal to sell more is exactly the same as the goals of healthy eating? Perhaps, but nothing in a supermarket is that simple. Collect a shopping cart, turn right or left at the entrance to the store, and let's take a look at the produce section.

pers, eleven
exotic ro

Fruits and Vegetables:
The Price of Fresh

A couple of years ago I was spending some time in upstate New York and went to the Wegmans supermarket in Ithaca. I had read a Harvard Business School case study about Wegmans, a chain of seventy or so stores in the northeast region known for its unusual attention to quality, responsiveness to customers' concerns about health and social issues, and active commitment to "Making a Difference in Our Community." Because Wegmans is family owned, privately held, and not traded on the stock market, the company has more flexibility than publicly traded chains to offer services that do not immediately increase sales or profits.

When you enter the Ithaca Wegmans, you find yourself in a huge produce section, larger than the size of a basketball court. You can easily imagine that you are in a farmers' market in the south of France or in Italy; the only things missing are the hot sun and the sellers at the individual stalls. You see stacks of gleaming fruits and vegetables. You hear the spray misting the salad greens. It smells good in there. You want to sneak tastes of everything you see. And the variety is extraordinary. One late-spring day I counted nine kinds of melons, five kinds of sweet pep-

kinds of potatoes, five kinds of onions, and eight varieties of
ot vegetables, among them taro, yautia, and namé.

e variety can make the choices overwhelming, even if you are
oking for something as simple as lettuce. This produce section puts
lettuce in four places—in areas marked "homegrown," "salad greens,"
and "organic," and in a thirty-foot-long refrigerated case of bagged items.
These lettuces, you might suspect, are likely to differ in freshness, taste,
nutritional quality, and maybe even safety. They were produced using
methods that might bear on environmental matters or labor practices
you care about. And they most definitely differ in price.

You have only just arrived in the store and already you are confronted with the issues that come up in any produce section, wherever
you may shop: Are the differences in
freshness, taste, nutritional quality, or
production methods worth the differences in price? Questions like this one,
it turns out, are not so easy to answer.
Comparing the advantages of differ-
ent fruits and vegetables takes work, and lots of it. Even if you decide to
choose fruits and vegetables by price alone, you will need to read labels
carefully and you had best bring along a calculator.

> Even if you decide to choose fruits and vegetables by price alone, you will need to read labels carefully and you had best bring along a calculator.

Let's consider the issues one at a time, beginning with what supermarkets mean, exactly, when they call something "fresh."

FRESHNESS: A MATTER OF DEGREE

First, consider ancient history. Papyrus scrolls, excavated oil jars, and
other kinds of archaeological evidence prove that foods have always
been traded across long distances. To be traded, foods had to be preserved in some way or they would spoil. Bacteria and molds do not grow
well on salt cod or dried biscuits. But they flourish on fruits and vegetables, and these spoil quickly if not soaked in sugar (hence: jams and jel-
lies) or salt (pickles), or cooked in jars or cans, or, these days, frozen.
Citrus fruits have thick skins that spoil more slowly, which is why seafar-
ers carried lemons on long voyages to prevent scurvy, but even lemons
get moldy if not kept cold.

The spoilage problem explains why the produce sections of super-markets used to be limited in variety to whatever was in season, grown locally, or brought in from places no more than a few days away. The invention of trains, trucks, and airplanes lengthened the distances that foods could travel. Refrigeration changed everything. The ability to keep fruits and vegetables cold from the instant they are picked to the moment you put them in your shopping cart—what the industry calls the "cold chain"—means that produce sections are no longer constrained by growing location or season. You expect to be able to buy strawberries whenever you want them, and you can.

I first realized the significance of the cold chain a few years ago during a food conference in the Salinas region of northern California. The conference held a splendid lunch for participants in, of all places, a warehouse in the middle of a broccoli farm. The outside temperature was over 100 degrees that day, but I was sorry I hadn't brought a sweater. The warehouse was chilly. We ate at tables surrounded by high stacks of boxes filled with broccoli ready to be shipped across the country. This was so tempting that I had to pinch a piece. The broccoli was crisp and delicately flavored, and nothing at all like the limp and bitter stuff I was accustomed to buying at stores in New York City. This broccoli was *fresh*. It had been picked early that morning and had been immediately boxed and parked in the cool warehouse.

I spent the rest of lunch mulling over how long it would take to get those boxes to Manhattan. Supermarket produce managers are reluctant to provide such details, and I can understand why. With some gentle prodding, the manager of the largest store in my downtown neighborhood told me that perishable items like herbs that don't weigh much might come by air freight, but just about everything else gets trucked across the country. For a large supermarket chain with its own distribution system, that broccoli undergoes a journey like this: farm, local warehouse, regional distribution center, refrigerated truck, regional distribution center at destination, another truck, local supermarket, back-room stocking area, floor, and, finally, shelf. All of this can take a week, but ten days would not be unusual. Even if the broccoli is kept cold throughout this odyssey (something hardly likely with all those transfers in and out of trucks and warehouses), it isn't going to be my idea of fresh by the time I buy it, and it will be even less so by the time I actually get around to eating it.

But maintaining the cold chain is not the only factor that affects the quality of fruits and vegetables. Even "fresh" produce is often subjected to processing before it reaches a supermarket shelf. To allow them to endure transportation, bananas and tomatoes are picked while still green, then chilled, warmed, and treated with gases to make them ripen. Bagged vegetables and salads have been washed and cut, subjected to "modified-atmosphere packaging" (which changes the proportions of oxygen and carbon dioxide to delay spoilage), and sometimes treated with preservatives. Those munchy and convenient "baby" carrots are ordinary carrots which have been cut into small pieces and shaped to look like small whole carrots, then bagged and shipped.

> In supermarket terms, "fresh" refers to foods that spoil faster than others. It does not mean that foods were picked earlier that day, or even that week.

The conclusion: fresh is relative. The Food and Drug Administration says "fresh" foods have to be raw, never frozen or heated, and with no added preservatives. But even "fresh" fruits and vegetables are often subjected to processing before they reach a supermarket shelf. In supermarket terms, "fresh" refers to foods that spoil faster than others. It does not mean that foods were picked earlier that day, or even that week.

THE DISTANCE TRAVELED: "FOOD MILES" AND COUNTRY-OF-ORIGIN LABELING

The more time it takes to move a food from where it is grown to where you can buy it, the more the meaning of "fresh" gets stretched. If you demand strawberries in winter, you pay more for them not only in transportation costs (and a higher price per quart) but in lag time: they will be less fresh. You also pay in other ways that do not show up on your grocery bill. Food ecologists, who look closely at the social and environmental costs of commercial food production—in pollution of farmland or water supplies, in health care for farmworkers, or in depletion of world supplies of fuel oil, for example—refer to such distances as "food miles." That Salinas broccoli had to endure about 3,000 food miles getting from California to New York.

I can think of good nutritional reasons to have even not-so-fresh broccoli available, but sometimes the travel distances seem ridiculous. In London, I once was served bottled water from Australia. London water is quite drinkable, but those Australian bottles had been transported 12,000 miles at substantial cost in nonrenewable fuel energy. At a nutrition meeting in Norway, McDonald's was promoting its new lines of salads and vegetable snacks by giving out samples of baby carrots from Bakersfield, California, 7,000 food miles away. A few months later, I saw Bakersfield baby carrots on the fabulous food floor of the KaDeWe department store in Berlin. They can't grow carrots anyplace closer? Unless the cold chain is working perfectly and the travel time is short, the trade-off will be in freshness and taste.

Under rules passed by the European Union, the McDonald's carrots in Norway were labeled so I could see where they were from, but such labels are much less common in the United States. In 2002, Congress passed a law requiring country-of-origin labeling (the apt acronym is COOL) that was to take effect in 2004. Later, under pressure from food industries, Congress postponed the deadline until 2005 for fish, but until 2006 and, later, 2008 for other foods.

It is indeed "cool" to know where supermarket produce comes from. Knowing this lets you make some guesses about freshness, taste, and nutritional value. For several summers, I was the outside examiner for a culinary arts program at the Dublin Institute of Technology, and between sessions of reading examination papers I often dropped by the Marks & Spencer food hall near the hotel where I was staying. It was interesting to note that hardly any of the beautifully packaged fruits and vegetables came from Ireland—just berries, usually—but the store carried bananas from Ecuador, grapes from Chile, green peppers and string beans from Zimbabwe, apples from South Africa, and onions from New Zealand. Onions from New Zealand? The only explanation must be that it is cheaper for Marks & Spencer, a U.K. chain, to buy onions from remnants of the far-flung British Empire halfway around the world than it is to get them from nearby producers in the European Union.

In America, food industry opposition to COOL is just about universal. The industry complains that tracking the origin of foods is difficult, but also would prefer that you not know how far food has traveled before it gets to you. The Grocery Manufacturers of America, an especially vigilant trade advocacy group, called the 2002 bill "a nasty, snarly beast of a bill," but even stronger opposition came from the meat industry. Its lobbyists argued that COOL would be "extraordinarily costly with no discernible benefit," but their real objection was that meat producers would have to track where animals and products come from—another sensible idea that they have long resisted.

You might think that COOL would benefit American fruit and vegetable growers ("Buy American!"), but only producers in Florida and Western states were for it and even they soon joined the opposition (too complicated, too costly, too revealing). As the original deadline for implementation in 2004 drew closer, food industry lobbyists went to work to try to repeal COOL, remove its "regulatory teeth," and make it voluntary. At least ten trade associations, among them the United Fresh Fruit and Vegetable Association and the Produce Marketing Association, asked for relief from this "undue burden," which, they said, would produce "no meaningful benefit to any sector in the U.S. or abroad while increasing costs for everyone from the farmer to the consumer." Instead, they lobbied Congress to introduce legislation, the Food Promotion Act of 2004, that would make COOL entirely voluntary. This too had an apt acronym: VCOOL. Although this legislation did not pass, Congress delayed COOL implementation until October 2006 and then again until October 2008.

Anyone browsing in a European supermarket—or for that matter in Whole Foods supermarkets, which have voluntarily labeled the origins of fruits and vegetables for years—would have a hard time understanding what this fuss is about. What could possibly be wrong with letting customers know where food comes from? I like having this information and you might too. But food suppliers must think that COOL will hurt their profits by forcing them to track the source of their foods, keep foods from different locations separated, and label the foods accordingly. They also must be worrying that you might reject foods from places you distrust for reasons of safety or politics. Food suppliers do not want you to know how commonly food from different places is commingled. The foods in any one bin might come from anywhere. So the industry wants COOL to be voluntary—so they can voluntarily decline to put COOL labels on their products.

A glance in most American markets in 2004 and 2005 (Whole Foods was the great exception) made it clear that voluntary COOL was not working. The mangoes, melons, onions, and potatoes in the Ithaca Wegmans, for example, were handsome, but of unknown origin. The produce manager did not know where they came from because they arrived from the chain's central distribution system. The one unambiguous exception was Wegmans "homegrown" section, which features locally grown produce labeled by farm and location. Wegmans defines homegrown as from anywhere in New York State, but on one of the days I visited, all of the foods in that section came from nearby farms between Ithaca and Syracuse, no more than an hour away by truck.

That day, the store was not carrying any homegrown raspberries or blueberries, although these were available on a pick-your-own basis not ten miles away at Grisamore Farms. There, the berries—acres of them— were so ripe and so abundant that it took just minutes to fill a bucket. Grisamore charged pick-it-yourselfers by the pound: $2.70 for raspberries. Wegmans, however, sold berries from Driscoll in Watsonville, California. The Driscoll berries cost $2.50 for a six-ounce box ($6.67 per pound), but these were a bargain compared to Manhattan, where I saw the same company's berries priced at $3.99 ($10.64 per pound) a week later. Most of the time, it is easier, more reliable, and cheaper for the store (although not for you) to get raspberries from California than from down the road. None of this makes intuitive sense, but such are the economics of the retail food business.

> Most of the time, it is easier, more reliable, and cheaper for the store (although not for you) to get raspberries from California than from down the road.

A few days later, I went to Wegmans again and saw blueberries from Grisamore Farms prominently displayed on a front counter right next to blueberries from two other sources, all priced equally at $2.50 a box. The boxes, however, were different sizes. Following what comes next is easier with a Table.

Three Kinds of Blueberries, Ithaca, New York, July 2004

TYPE	PRICE PER BOX	BOX WEIGHT	PRICE PER POUND
Locally grown (Grisamore Farms)	$2.50	14 ounces	$2.86
California (Driscoll)	$2.50	11 ounces	$3.64
Organic (origin not given)	$2.50	4 ounces	$10.00

As part of its efforts to accommodate customers, Wegmans provides a scale in the produce section. Without it, I would never have been able to figure out the comparative costs, especially since the 11- and 14-ounce sizes were both packed in identical pint cartons. Wegmans' customers know a good thing when they see one and were grabbing the Grisamore blueberries as fast as they could be stocked. On that day, the Grisamore berries were an easy choice compared to the commercial California berries—in cost and in taste. Supermarket prices are remarkably fluid, however, and within a day or two Wegmans priced the Driscoll berries at three boxes for $5.00 ($1.67 per box) but kept Grisamore's at $2.50. Now the California berries were less expensive—but, of course, less fresh.

The organic blueberries require their own discussion, but that comes later. In the meantime, COOL is a great step forward in letting you in on some interesting secrets about our food supply. If you see how far foods travel before getting to you, you can make some guesses about freshness and taste. Locally grown foods are fresher. Because they are fresher, they should taste better. And that brings us to the matter of taste.

> Locally grown foods are fresher. Because they are fresher, they should taste better.

A QUESTION OF TASTE

Taste is a highly personal matter, of course, and you and I may not like the same things, but I feel safe in assuming that if you are not growing your own, you have no idea what fresh fruits and vegetables actually taste like. I certainly didn't. I grew up in New York City not exactly loving canned peas and corn, and was clueless about the real flavor of such things until I was sent off to a summer camp on a Vermont farm. The owners had a large vegetable garden, and tangles of blackberries grew wild on a hill above the property. If we were especially good, we got to pick berries for pancakes or vegetables for dinner. As we picked, we sampled. The taste of freshly picked blackberries, beans, or sweet corn, still warm from the sun, was a revelation.

Years later, I was working in Thailand during the summer fruit season and ate fresh lychees. These were an entirely different experience from the canned varieties served at Chinese restaurants or even the frozen or somewhat fresh ones you can find occasionally in supermarkets in the United States. In Hawaii, fresh mangoes taste like perfume; the ones I get in Manhattan look like mangoes but taste nothing like the ones I ate on the Big Island. Food writers mourn the disappearance of heirloom apples and disdain the flavor of tomatoes or strawberries bred for storage capacity rather than taste.

The flavor of fruits and vegetables certainly depends on freshness, but it also depends on the variety and the production methods. Supermarket raspberries are a case in point. At Grisamore Farms, the pick-it-yourself varieties burst with flavor but also burst when picked, and my picking fingers were stained with juice. The California Driscoll raspberries like those I find at my local markets are bred for "perfect berry architecture" and the ability to withstand thousands of food miles, and they are picked before they are fully ripe. They look like raspberries and they taste something like them, but the flavor lacks the intensity and complexity that makes eating "real" raspberries such an extraordinary experience. The same is true of strawberries. The more intensely flavored varieties tend to be small, soft, and delicate, and they do not travel well. But commercial growers consider taste as only one desirable characteristic among many others, such as size, shape, firmness, color, and resistance to pests.

The gain from commercial production of fruits and vegetables is a wonderfully abundant, varied, and inexpensive supply that is independent of season, weather, or geography, but these benefits come at a price. The cost is in loss of flavor, texture, and, perhaps, nutritional value, along with the loss of biodiversity and community. Growing fruits and vegetables on local farms has intangible values that are worth a lot to people who care about such things. But from the standpoint of the supermarket business, price has to be the dominant consideration. If stores can keep prices low, yours will also seem low, and you will be more likely to buy their products. Even the best stores play tricks to make prices seem lower than they are. The tricks show up in the produce section, as well as everywhere else.

THE PRICE YOU PAY

Supermarket prices are not a simple matter of cost plus markup, with the markup covering the cost of whatever needs to be done to get products on the shelves and make a small profit. The markup on produce is said to be especially high because of the special handling that is needed to refrigerate, stack, mist, rearrange picked-over items, discard outer lettuce leaves and spoiled fruit, keep the floor clean of debris, and so forth. Even so, the pricing of fruits and vegetables must be an arcane art because I certainly do not find much consistency. Shelf labels for packaged foods tell you the price and cost per weight or volume. But when it comes to produce, you practically have to do a cost-benefit analysis before you can buy something as simple as a head of lettuce. On the days I visited Wegmans, for example, the store offered a bewildering seven choices of romaine lettuce: whole or in bags; as heads, hearts, or chopped; in five different package sizes; and at six different prices. It took me several visits to figure out what they had and at what cost, and what it all meant, and it takes a Table to explain what I discovered.

If what you care about is price, your choice is relatively easy. You would choose either the locally grown or the conventional commercially grown lettuce at just under $1.00 per pound. The homegrown romaine came from Syracuse, but where the others were from was a mystery; the shelf label didn't say. I could not tell whether there was any difference in quality just by looking at them. I

> I would cast my vote for the homegrown lettuce. It is likely to be fresher and buying it gives me a chance to support local farming in New York State.

Romaine Lettuces Available in a Supermarket Produce Section, July 20

SECTION	WEIGHT IN OUNCES*	PRICE	
Loose		*Per head*	*Per pound*
Homegrown			$0.99
Conventional (not organic)			$0.99
Organic	11	$1.99	$2.89
Bagged		*Per bag*	*Per pound*
Hearts, Wegmans, conventional	16	$2.50	$2.50
Hearts, Dole, conventional	18	$2.99	$2.66
Hearts, organic	12	$2.99	$3.99
Precut for salad, conventional	10	$2.50	$4.00

*A pound is 16 ounces.

would cast my vote for the homegrown lettuce. It is likely to be fresher and buying it gives me a chance to support local farming in New York State.

There are reasons why organic foods are more expensive than their nonorganic counterparts, but supermarkets sometimes fix the weights and prices to make the bite appear less painful than it actually is. The organic romaine was twice the cost of homegrown or conventional, but per head, not per pound. I weighed several of the organic heads, and they all seemed to be about 11 ounces. This made the per pound comparative cost ($2.89) considerably higher than the price listed on the label ($1.99), but I had to use a calculator to figure that out.

The other romaine options trade convenience for price. To create romaine hearts, the packers pull off the outside leaves, wash the hearts, and bag them. You open the bag, chop the romaine hearts, and your salad is ready—and you didn't have to throw any leaves away. That's convenience. How much extra you are paying for this convenience is also not easy to figure out. The bags are all priced similarly, so you have to

hts. The shelf labels do the calculations for you, but the
t is in tiny print compared to the price per bag. On a per-
ie precut salads cost four times as much as the intact
nvenience of not having to clean and chop lettuce worth
ybe, but it would be nice to know the actual cost before

Wegmans prices its bags of romaine hearts 49 cents lower than the
competing Dole brand, but Dole's package weighs 2 ounces more. This
brings the real difference down to just 16 cents per pound—what retailers call the "brand tax," the extra price you pay for national brands. The
49-cent differential surely acts as an incentive to buy the Wegmans
brand, but Wegmans has unusually loyal customers who would choose it
anyway. Even if Dole's lettuce hearts
are better than Wegmans', is the supposed difference in quality worth the
brand tax? That would be hard to figure out unless you knew something
about where the two brands' hearts
came from, which you don't. People in the business tell me that the
quality of national and store-brand produce is usually similar. If so, the
store brand is likely to be a better buy.

> **P**eople in the business tell me that the quality of national and store-brand produce is usually similar. If so, the store brand is likely to be a better buy.

3

Organics: Hype or Hope

In 2003, I was invited to Austin, Texas, to give a talk at the annual meeting of a group I had never heard of called the Organic Trade Association (OTA). With "organic" in the name, I assumed that I would be talking to a friendly bunch of counterculture farmers in overalls and Birkenstocks. I could not have been more mistaken. I quickly discovered my error when my talk was introduced by a vice president of General Mills. This was corporate America, big-time agriculture, and suits. Later that year, I went with a group of journalists to a small organic farm overlooking a coastal inlet in Bolinas, California. This farm grew an astonishing variety of specialty vegetables for Bay Area restaurants, any kind you could possibly think of—except carrots. The owner had given up on carrots because he had no way to compete on price; a single company in California now produces the majority of organic carrots grown in America. Carrots and all else: organic foods are big business.

How big a business is a matter of debate, but by some estimates sales of organic foods brought in $20 billion in 2004 and might exceed $30 billion in 2007. Never mind the exact numbers. What makes food corporations so intensely interested in the organic business is the pace at which the market for these foods is growing. The overabundance of food in the United States limits the growth of the so-called "conventional" food producers (those who typically use pesticides and chemical fertilizers) to 1 or 2 percent a year. Organics, in contrast, are booming. Since 1990, sales have increased by about 20 percent annually—a phenomenal rate by industry standards. Organics may amount to only a small fraction of total food sales—estimates range from 1 to 10 percent—but the percentage is rising. The most attractive feature of organics to the food industry is this: customers are willing to pay more for organic foods. It is easy to understand why any big food company would want to get into this business.

The emergence of this new "organic-industrial complex" explains a lot about what you find in today's supermarkets. About three-fourths of American grocery stores now carry some organic foods. You can pick out the ones in produce sections by their labels, "Certified Organic," and by their PLU (Product Look-Up) codes—the numbers on those annoying little stickers that are so hard to get off your pears and tomatoes. The PLU codes on organic foods all start with a 9 in front of the next four numbers. The Certified Organic seal tells you many things about the food. Whatever the food is, it had to be grown according to principles established by the Organic Foods Production Act of 1990 and by USDA Organic Standards established twelve years later. Yes, it took the reluctant USDA twelve years to figure out how to define organics and to set the rules for their production. The standards are complicated; they divide organics into four categories, as shown in the Table on the facing page.

Fruits and vegetables are either grown organically or not, so the organic ones fall neatly into the 100 percent category, and organic greens are unlikely to be mixed with conventional greens in bagged salads. Meats and milk also are 100 percent organic if they are organic at all. The other three classifications apply to the ingredients in cereals, sodas, and other processed foods and food mixtures, but let's leave those for later discussion.

The Certified Organic seal conveys one other critically important piece of information. It tells you the grower has been inspected. This means three things: an inspector has verified that the producer of the food actually followed the Organic Standards; the inspector works for a state or private agency accredited by the USDA; and all inspectors hold food producers to the same set of production standards set by the USDA's National Organic Program.

Categories of USDA Certified Organic Foods

CONTENT OF ORGANIC INGREDIENTS	CERTIFIED ORGANIC SEAL ON LABEL?	LABEL STATEMENT PERMITTED*
100%	Yes	"100% Organic"
95 to 99%	Yes	"Organic"
74 to 94%	No	"Made with organic ingredients" (can list up to three such ingredients on front)
73% or less	No	Can list organic ingredients only on information panel

*These USDA label standards were established in 2002. See the National Organic Program at www.ams.usda.gov/nop.

To return to produce: a search for organic foods in my local Morton Williams Associated Supermarket one summer day turned up just three products: USDA Certified Organic carrots, California Certified Organic celery, and Colorado Certified Organic romaine lettuce. Even though this was the height of the growing season, and nearby farmers' markets had several stalls full of produce from organic farmers in New Jersey, Long Island, and upstate New York, this store carried no organic produce from closer than 2,000 food miles away. A food may be Certified Organic, but it is not necessarily locally grown.

> A food may be Certified Organic, but it is not necessarily locally grown.

Looking for a wider selection of organic fruits and vegetables sent me to explore Whole Foods, which calls itself "America's first national Certified Organic grocer." In February 2004, Whole Foods opened the largest supermarket in Manhattan—nearly 58,000 square feet—in the basement of the glittery new Time Warner Center at Columbus Circle. As you take the escalator down to that level, the flower section is right at your feet, adhering to the supermarket principles that place flowers or produce immediately at the front. In this store, you turn left to get to the produce area. Whole Foods carries both organic and conventional produce but makes it easy to tell which is which. The shelf labels for organics are bright yellow while the labels for industrially produced foods—"conventionals"—are purple. Well before country-of-origin labeling was to go into effect in October 2006, Whole Foods voluntarily provided origin labeling for every fruit and vegetable it carried, so I could tell right away where everything came from, organic or not.

One day in late July 2004, the store carried a large mix of organic and conventional produce. It had organic squash, corn, radishes, and blueberries, mostly from California. It carried conventionally grown papayas from Belize, pineapples and bananas from Costa Rica, pears from Argentina, plums from Chile, eggplant from Holland, and peppers from Canada. It sold organic apples from New Zealand and Argentina and conventional apples from New York and Washington States. If I wanted tomatoes, I could get organics from Holland, Canada, or Mexico, or conventionals from Florida or New Jersey.

But first I had to deal with the day's obvious loss leader: strawberries. Boxes of perfectly beautiful organic strawberries—California Driscoll's, of course—were on display at the entrance to the produce section. They were $2.98 per pound. Right next to them were equally beautiful Driscoll nonorganic strawberries, also $2.98 per pound. The organics were a bargain, and I could not imagine why anyone would buy the conventional ones, particularly because some of the berries hidden below the top layers in the boxes of conventionals were moldy (the bottom ones bruise and mold more easily—always a hazard when buying berries). Whole Foods usually charges a premium for organic produce, but not an especially large one, in part because the store's mission is to encourage consumers to try the organics. California cauliflower, for example, cost $2.49 for the organic as compared to $1.98 for the conventional. Ginger was an unusual exception: a pound cost $7.98 for the organic and $3.98 for the conventional; both had traveled 6,000 or so food miles from Hawaii.

Whole Foods started out in 1980 as a small supplier of organics in Austin, Texas, but it has grown over the years into a good-size player—tiny by the standards of Wal-Mart or Kroger, but big by the standards of the local food co-op. In 2005, Whole Foods ran nearly 170 stores in the United States and Great Britain, and I could see several under construction in Manhattan. Its 2004 revenues were $3.9 billion. The company's particular niche in the supermarket world is decidedly upscale. You will not find the usual commercial brands of margarine, salad oil, cereals, or sodas in its stores, but you will find a huge variety of high-quality—and high-price—ingredients and prepared foods. This may be why critics like to call it "Whole Paycheck," but if the checkout lines are any indication, lots of people must be delighted to trade price for quality and the ability to get what they want when they want it, organic and not. On that July afternoon, fifty-three customers were ahead of me in the checkout line waiting for the twenty-two customers who were already at open cash registers to finish. This felt like going through airport security at JFK.

Lines like this make it easy to understand how an average Whole Foods took in $482,000 per week in 2004 (and collects the reported $1 million per week at the Time Warner location). Although the Whole Foods slogan is "whole foods, whole people, whole planet," and its stated commitment is to promote sustainable agriculture (which uses environmentally friendly production methods), the company went public in 1992. This means that its business model is like that of any other publicly traded corporation: Whole Foods is required to place profits above values, expand rapidly, and keep costs down. Basic business imperatives explain the company's opposition to employee unionization and raise troubling questions about whether it can continue to maintain high quality standards in the face of relentless pressures to expand.

The contradiction between the company's original values and its need for corporate growth explains some of the idiosyncrasies of the Whole Foods produce section. The shelf labels are interspersed with photographs and descriptions of local organic farmers in New Jersey, Rhode Island, Pennsylvania, and New York, yet finding locally grown produce requires some label searching. I found peaches, corn, and tomatoes from New Jersey, and apples from New York, but all were conventionally grown. I looked hard for local organic foods but found only one (some red cabbage from New York State), unless you consider organic corn and tomatoes from Vermont as "local." On that particular midsummer day, hardly any of the produce was grown locally, and hardly any of the local produce was

> Organic produce is scarce because the organics business, like any other business, is as much about politics as it is about farming practices.

Certified Organic. This is a supply-chain problem that could change if more farmers went into the organics business. Organic produce is scarce because the organics business, like any other business, is as much about politics as it is about farming practices.

THE POLITICS OF ORGANICS

The organic seal tells you that the producers of the foods followed a long list of rules: they did not use any synthetic pesticides, herbicides, or fertilizers; they did not plant genetically modified seeds, use fertilizer derived from sewage sludge, or treat the seeds or foods with irradiation; and they kept records of everything they did and showed the paperwork and everything on their farms to inspectors from a USDA-accredited state or private certification agency any time they were asked to, announced in advance or not. The Organic Standards—the rules about what organic farmers can and cannot use—take up hundreds of pages in the *Federal Register* and do not make for light reading. Like any rules, they require interpretation.

The need for interpretation puts the USDA, the agency that runs the National Organic Program, in flagrant conflict of interest; its principal mandate from Congress is to promote conventional agriculture. Conventional growers are eager to make sure that nothing about organic foods even slightly suggests that organics might be better. This helps to explain why the USDA is so grudging about organics: "USDA makes no claims that organically produced food is safer or more nutritious than conventionally produced food. Organic food differs from conventionally grown food in the way it is grown, handled, and processed." This statement makes it sound as if such differences do not matter much, if at all. But I think they do.

Opponents of organics—and there are many—work hard to make you doubt the reliability of organic certification, to weaken the Organic Standards (so you really will have something to doubt), and to make you wonder whether organics are any better than conventionally grown foods. Let's consider these in order, starting with the issue of trust.

I cannot count the number of times that I have been asked whether the Certified Organic seal really means anything. It most definitely does.

I blame the question on how effectively the critics of organics have sown seeds of suspicion, as well as on the higher prices usually charged for foods grown this way. Nevertheless, the question deserves an answer. The Organic Standards call for hefty fines for violators, but my usual source for this sort of thing, *Food Chemical News*, has not reported any since the standards went into effect in 2002. Its editor suggested a call to Fred Ehlert at Quality Assurance International, one of the largest companies doing USDA-accredited organic certifications. Ehlert was hard-pressed to think of any serious violations among the more than 500 certifications he had done both before and after 2002. He could recall only a few minor infractions, but attributed these to understandable misinterpretations of the rules rather than to anything more sinister. He visits farms and suppliers; reviews records of purchases, crop rotations, and sales; and inspects the facilities, soils, supplies, and crops. Cheating may occur, he says, but if it does, it is rare because "the only thing we are selling is credibility." In his experience, organic producers care about what they are doing and go to substantial trouble and expense to grow foods without pesticides, to keep records, and to pay for inspections and certification. My guess is that they also keep a close eye on each other. Everyone I have talked to about the trust question—inspectors, produce managers, and the farmers themselves—thinks that the Certified Organic seal means that growers are following the rules and that the seal can be taken at face value.

But as for attempts to weaken the rules, think "relentless." Political appointees at USDA are always looking for loopholes that might favor conventional growers. Just before issuing the Organic Standards, for example, the USDA said it would be fine for farmers to use genetically modified seeds, irradiation, and sewage sludge, and still call their crops organic. After a barrage of 275,000 outraged letters, the agency backed off this peculiar idea. In 2004, the USDA—without consulting its own organics advisory board—ruled that organic farmers could use pesticides that might contain ingredients prohibited by the Environmental Protection Agency. Under protest, the USDA again backed down. My interpretation: if the Organic Standards require this level of vigilance, they must be doing something right. And by and large they are.

Whether they can remain this way is another matter. In 2005, a federal court in Maine ruled in favor of protecting the standards. It refused to allow use of nonorganic ingredients when organic ingredients were not available, unless those ingredients had been approved by the National Organic Board. It also denied exceptions to rules for converting dairy herds to organic production. Under pressure from large corporate producers of organic foods (Big Organics), the Organic Trade Association induced Republican leaders of Congress to attach a rider to the 2006 Agricultural Appropriations bill that would cancel the court decision. Despite more than 300,000 letters and phone calls from consumers who objected to this "profoundly undemocratic sneak attack" on the integrity of the Organic Standards, the rider remained. If such attacks continue, Certified Organic will lose its meaning—and its ability to command a premium price.

ARE ORGANICS BETTER?

Given the potential size of the organic market, you can understand why the idea that these foods might be better for you or for the planet so annoys critics. One is Dennis Avery of the Hudson Institute, a conservative Washington, D.C., think tank that receives funding from, among other sources, agribusiness corporations like Archer Daniels Midland, Cargill, ConAgra, Monsanto, and the National Agricultural Chemicals Association. No wonder these groups fund the institute's work. Mr. Avery argues that organic methods are so unreliable that they reduce productivity, cause higher prices, and, therefore, threaten the food security of the world's most vulnerable populations. Organic farming, he says, is an environmental disaster, an imminent danger to wildlife, and a hazard to the health of its own consumers. Strong words, indeed.

Consider first what is at stake. If farmers switched to organics, the makers of chemical fertilizers, herbicides, and pesticides would suffer. If you decided to buy organics, you would buy fewer conventionally grown foods. And if more of your friends bought organic foods, you all might go so far as to demand government subsidies for organics rather than for conventionally grown corn and soybeans. Research on the kinds of issues Avery raises also cannot help but have political biases. As is so often the case with food issues, the few studies that do get done are limited in scope and subject to interpretation. Interpretation depends on point of view, and viewpoints are subject to influence.

Fortunately, some questions about organics have been researched and do have clear answers. One such question is about productivity. As early as the mid-1970s, studies began to question the idea that agricultural efficiency necessarily depends on fertilizers and pesticides. In 1981, a review of such studies came to surprising conclusions: farmers who converted from conventional to organic methods reported only small declines in yields, but the loss in income was offset by lower fuel costs. The study found that the farms were equally profitable, but that organic production kept the soil in much better shape. More recent studies confirm these results. Overall they show that organic farms are nearly as productive, leave the soils healthier, and use energy more efficiently. The productivity issue seems settled. There is a difference, but it is small.

If crops are grown without pesticides, it seems self-evident that fewer pesticides will get into the soil and water, foods will contain less of them, and people who eat organic foods will have lower levels of pesticides in their bodies. Plenty of research confirms these obvious connections. Organically grown foods do have lower levels of pesticides, and children and adults who eat them have lower levels in their bodies. Avery and his fellow critics say: "So what? Pesticides are safe." As evidence, they say that nobody has ever died from eating the small amounts of pesticide residues on food. Oh, please. Pesticides are demonstrably harmful to farmworkers and to "nontarget" wildlife, and they accumulate in soils for ages. If they kill pests, can they be good for you? If they really were all that benign, there would be no reason for the government to bother to regulate them, but it does. Scientists may not be able to quantify the degree of harm they cause, but that does not mean that pesticides are safe for you. This is also a settled issue. Pesticide-free produce may not look as pretty, but if you want fewer pesticides in your body and in the bodies of your children, buy organics. If you want fewer pesticides in soil and water, organics are also a good idea. Questions about safety and nutritional value come next.

> **P**esticide-free produce may not look as pretty, but if you want fewer pesticides in your body and in the bodies of your children, buy organics.

4

Produce: Safe at Any Price

ealth officials say that in the United States alone bacteria, viruses, and parasites in foods cause 76 million cases of illness, 325,000 hospitalizations, and 5,000 deaths, and do so every year. This seems like a huge burden of disease, especially if you are one of the people who gets sick. But the numbers don't seem quite so big if you do the math and add up all of the foods everyone eats on an annual basis. Consider that there are nearly 300 million people who eat multiple foods several times a day 365 days a year—these come to hundreds of trillions of food exposures.

Mind you, nobody in government is really paying close attention to food safety or figuring out which foods cause what illnesses. In the United States food safety oversight is largely shared by two agencies: the Food and Drug Administration (FDA) and the U.S. Department of Agriculture (USDA). The FDA is under siege by Congress, which has given it too much to do and not nearly enough money to do it with. And the USDA is in constant conflict of interest: its primary mission is to promote sales of American agricultural products, and public health is decidedly secondary to these agribusiness interests. Given the lack of real government

Food can never be perfectly safe, but it can be safe enough when everyone involved—from farmer to consumer— does the right thing.

leadership, the food safety system relies largely on faith that food producers, processors, and handlers do not want to make anyone sick and are doing what they can to prevent illnesses transmitted by food. Food can never be perfectly safe, but it can be safe enough when everyone involved—from farmer to consumer—does the right thing. Mostly everyone does, which is why supermarket produce, no matter where it comes from, rarely causes problems.

But produce seems especially worrisome because fruits and vegetables are grown in what the FDA charmingly refers to as "non-sterile environments" (translation: in contact with animal manure), and because they are so often eaten raw. Fruits and vegetables are loaded with microbes, but even the ones acquired from feces are mostly harmless. Washing and cooking take care of most microbes on or in food, and any others are usually killed by stomach acid or blocked from doing harm by the immune system. That leaves just the few bad ones—the toxic kinds of *Salmonella* and *E. coli* (especially O157:H7), or hepatitis virus, for example—that make headlines when they harm people who innocently eat them.

Because the government doesn't track food safety very carefully, the Washington, D.C.–based advocacy group Center for Science in the Public Interest (CSPI) steps in to fill one of the gaps by issuing periodic reports about outbreaks—episodes in which more than one person gets sick from eating the same food. By its counts, fresh produce ranks as the number-two cause of outbreaks (but the number-one cause of individual cases of illness), just behind seafood. Between 1990 and 2003, CSPI recorded 554 outbreaks caused by eating produce, an average of 42 per year. These amounted to 12 percent of total outbreaks, but 20 percent of individual cases and more than 28,000 illnesses. Could some of these illnesses have been prevented by better federal regulation? I think so.

Fruits and vegetables come under the regulatory umbrella of the FDA, which has never had enough money

If problems arise, fruit and vegetable companies are subject to fines, confiscations, and the like, but the reality is that the safety of produce depends on the honor system.

or staff to do what it is required to—even before Congress, under pressure from tobacco and drug companies, started slashing its funding and, therefore, its regulatory ability in the 1990s. In 1998, the FDA issued guidelines for the safe handling of produce. These rely on Good Agricultural Practices (GAPs)—methods that food producers can use to protect fruits and vegetables from contamination with microbes coming from water, manure, or sick food handlers. They also rely on Good Manufacturing Practices (GMPs)—methods that food handlers can use to prevent contamination from microbes coming from trucks, storage facilities, equipment, packing materials, or the workers who deal with such things. The GAPs and GMPs, however, are just guidelines. In FDA-speak: "The produce guide is guidance and it is not a regulation." This means that food producers and handlers are not actually required to follow the guidelines. If problems arise, fruit and vegetable companies are subject to fines, confiscations, and the like, but the reality is that the safety of produce depends on the honor system.

Much of the produce sold in American supermarkets comes from developing countries where sanitation conditions are such that you shouldn't even be brushing your teeth with tap water, much less washing your food with it. I learned about the dangers of eating uncooked vegetables in such places when I was in public health school. Fieldwork is a big part of public health training, and part of mine was to study nutrition programs in urban areas of Thailand and Indonesia. Along with weeks of immunizations came firm instructions: do not drink tap water or put ice in drinks; do not eat salads; eat vegetables only if they are cooked and piping hot; and do not eat fruit unless you peel it yourself. Fortunately, it was the height of summer, and I had plenty of exotic tropical fruits to peel—fresh lychees, mangosteens, rambutans, longans, and other marvels I had never tasted before.

The FDA oversees imported produce by inspecting samples—about 2 percent of the total—and rarely is the agency able to dig deeper. In 1999, in one such instance, it tested 1,000 samples of fresh produce imported from 21 countries. About 4 percent of the samples turned out to have fecal microbes, fortunately none toxic. The following year, the FDA did a similar survey of domestic produce, which it usually does not inspect at all. Just 1 percent of the samples were found contaminated with fecal microorganisms, also none toxic. The agency followed up the "violative samples" by sending its agents to visit farms, offering advice about GAPs, and conducting later visits to see if the practices had improved. They had. The low level of contamination is reassuring, as is the attention to problems, but it would be even more reassuring if the FDA had the ability to do more than occasional spot-checks and could act more rapidly. In October 2005, for example, the FDA issued a warning about possible *E. coli* O157:H7 contamination of prepackaged Dole salads a week *after* the "best-if-used-by" dates on the packages. These packages were likely to have already been sold.

Prewashed and precut salads and vegetables go through many hands, and you would expect them to be especially vulnerable to microbial growth, particularly as time gets closer to the "sell by" date—the date voluntarily stamped on most bags to indicate how long the products can be considered "fresh." Processors know this, so they use "modified-atmosphere packaging" and, sometimes, preservatives, to inhibit microbial growth and extend shelf life. But I am less concerned about precut vegetables now than I used to be since I took a side trip to a processing plant after giving a lecture at the Steinbeck Center in Salinas. On the day of my visit, I watched this plant process broccoli and cauliflower heads for use in packages with dips. The freshly picked heads went through repeated washings before machines cleaved them into neat wedges and packed them into plastic containers. The wash water, like all United States public water supplies, is chlorinated to kill microbes, and nobody touches the vegetables once they get on the carrier belt. This process looked just fine to me—as long as the packages are kept cold during shipping.

Even so, I would wash those broccoli wedges again before eating them, especially if they have been sitting on shelves in the produce section getting misted at regular intervals. Some supermarkets keep produce looking fresh by storing it on chilled shelves. The cooling compressors blow a lot of cool air around, and lettuces are particularly prone to drying out if not kept moist. That is why some stores mist the open vegetables so they look dewy at all times. It is best not to look too closely at the misting devices, however. In some of the stores in my neighborhood, the misting gadgets are covered with green algae or encrusted with mold. So wash those lettuces! Washing cannot remove all of the microbes that might be harmful, but it takes care of most of them.

As for that suspicious wax on fruits and vegetables: last winter I bought a box of "candy sweet, easy to peel" clementines from Spain, covered in wax. The label explained: "coated with food-grade, vegetable, beeswax, and/or shellac-based wax or resin, to maintain freshness." It is common to wax citrus fruits like these—or apples, peppers, cucumbers, and other such fruits and vegetables—to replace the natural waxes that get washed off in processing. One type of wax is carnauba from the leaves of palm trees, which its producers describe as "a superior natural wax emulsion with a high gloss, long shelf life and superior drying characteristics," just exactly what you might want for polishing cars or furniture, its more familiar use. Wax retains the water in fruits and vegetables in the same way that moisturizers do for the skin after bathing. Wax also protects against bruising, prevents the growth of molds, and extends the time the fruits and vegetables last on the shelf without spoiling. Best of all—from the point of view of the supermarket—the high shine from the wax makes produce look fresh and attractive.

> So wash those lettuces! Washing cannot remove all of the microbes that might be harmful, but it takes care of most of them.

But is it safe? I have no problem with the waxes on clementines, avocados, cantaloupes, or pumpkins, because I am not going to eat the skin anyway. But I would rather not have it on apples or green peppers. For one thing, forget about washing it off. It adheres firmly to remaining traces of the natural waxes. For another, I cannot help but think the foods must be old. Why would they need wax if they were fresh?

These concerns are about aesthetics, not safety. Waxes are fats, but such big ones that you cannot easily absorb them; they usually slide right through the digestive tract. One gallon of wax is said to be enough to cover 12,000 pounds of fruit, so any one apple is not going to have much. At some point, food toxicologists tested fruit waxes in rats and beagle dogs, but found no effects on metabolism or cancer risk even when the animals were eating 10 percent of their diet as wax—which you would never do. Waxes are a nuisance, not a health problem. I buy unwaxed fruits and vegetables if I like eating their peels. Otherwise, I try to rinse off whatever I can, and save the worrying for more important issues.

The CSPI outbreak reports on produce do not say whether the safety problems were caused by organic or conventionally grown produce. "Conventional" means grown with pesticides; pesticides may kill insects, but they do not kill harmful bacteria or viruses. Because most produce is still conventionally grown you would, on the basis of quantity alone, expect this kind to cause most outbreaks, unless there is some reason why organic methods pose special risks. Critics say they do. They argue that because organic production uses composted manure instead of chemical fertilizers, organic foods are exposed to more potentially dangerous microbes and are riskier. But this argument does not really hold. In order to obtain organic certification, farmers have to follow strict rules about the use of manure to make sure that harmful microbes are destroyed, and they are inspected to make sure they do. Growers of conventional produce do not have to follow such rules.

It would be nice to know more about the comparative safety of organic and conventional produce, but research on this question is minimal. In the first study to directly compare farming practices, University of Minnesota scientists tested for harmless forms of *Salmonella* and *E. coli*, as well as for the deadly *E. coli* O157:H7, on vegetables grown on farms using three methods: conventional, Certified Organic, and supposedly following the organic rules but not certified. All three of the farms used aged or composted manure as fertilizer, but none of the vegetables had any *E. coli* O157:H7, no matter how they were grown. The investigators did find the harmless fecal bacteria on 2 percent of the conventionally grown produce, 4 percent of the Certified Organic, and 11 percent of the noncertified organic. These results require some interpretation. The Certified Organic vegetables seem to have had twice as much contamination as the conventional

> I n order to obtain organic certification, farmers have to follow strict rules about the use of manure to make sure that harmful microbes are destroyed, and they are inspected to make sure they do. Growers of conventional produce do not have to follow such rules.

ones, but the numbers were too small to reach statistical significance—meaning that the difference could have occurred by chance. When you allow for the usual margin of error, the Certified Organic produce was found to be about as safe as conventionally grown produce. The much higher level of contaminants in the noncertified organic vegetables did reach statistical significance, and confirms the notion that Certified Organic farms—which follow organic rules and are inspected to make sure they do—grow safer produce. So could any farm that firmly adhered to organic rules. But without inspection, you have to take what they say on trust. Because conventional food producers are not subject to such rules or inspections, it is difficult to assess the comparative safety of what they grow.

NUTRITIONAL VALUE: ORGANIC VERSUS CONVENTIONAL PRODUCE

So Certified Organic produce appears to be at least as safe as conventional produce. But this says nothing about whether organic production methods make organic fruits and vegetables more nutritious. Here is the deal: if you eat any fruits and vegetables at all, you get nutrients you cannot get as easily from other foods. These foods are loaded with substances that do good things for health. Fruits and vegetables are the main or only sources of vitamin C, folate (the vitamin called folic acid on food labels), and beta-carotene (a precursor of vitamin A), and they provide half the fiber in American diets (the other half comes from grains). They also contain varying combinations of phytonutrients, the chemicals in plants that singly and together protect against disease. These nutrients are all good reasons for eating fruits and vegetables.

If organic foods are grown in better soils, you would expect them to be more nutritious, and you would be right. This is easy to demonstrate for minerals; the mineral content of a plant food depends on how much is in the soil. But differences in the vitamin or phytonutrient content of a food plant are more likely to be due to its genetic strain or to how it is treated after harvest. The postharvest effects on nutrient values especially affect certain vitamins, but I'll defer discussion of the nutritional effects of time, temperature, light, and air for a later discussion of food processing.

Right now, the idea that organic soils yield food that is more nutritious has much appeal, and organic producers would dearly love to prove it. The Organic Trade Association has organized a center to promote research with a "singular focus — the universal benefits of organic production." Consumers, it says, "are looking for scientific justification of their largely intuitive feeling that organic products are safer and more beneficial to human health . . . [such as] Do organic farming methods have an important effect on the nutritional quality of food?"

If they ask me, I say: Don't go there. I can't think of any reason why organically grown foods would have fewer nutrients than conventionally grown foods, and I have no trouble thinking of several reasons why they might have more, but so what? I doubt the slight increase would be enough to make any measurable difference to health. Just as people differ, carrots or heads of cauliflower differ, and the differences in the nutrient content of one carrot or cauliflower and the next can be substantial.

Consider what you have to do to test for nutritional differences in organic versus conventional carrots. You start with identical carrot seeds and plant some in an organic plot and some in a conventional plot. The plots have to be identical in climate and geography, but will differ in soil quality (because more nutrient-rich soil is one of the underpinnings of organics). You treat the conventional carrots with pesticides but use biological pest control methods for the organic carrots. Once harvested, you perform the same set of nutrient analyses on both samples. Suppose you find differences. You must then ask: Do they mean anything for your health? To find out, you need to feed the carrots to animals or people. But because animals and people eat so many different foods, even a measurable difference in the nutrient content of carrots alone is unlikely to produce a measurable health benefit. Overall, such studies are hard to do, expensive, and difficult to interpret.

Nevertheless, a few intrepid souls have tried the agricultural parts of such studies (the only clinical studies I know about are the ones that demonstrate reassuringly lower levels of pesticides in the bodies of people who eat organics). These show, as expected, that organic foods grown in richer soils have more minerals than conventional foods grown in poorer soils. They also show that organic peaches and pears have somewhat higher levels of vitamins C and E, and organic berries and corn have higher levels of protective antioxidant substances. In general, the studies all point to slightly higher levels of nutrients in organically grown foods, as compared to those that were conventionally grown.

But organic foods, like all foods, are just that: foods. Some will have more of one kind of nutrient, and others will have more of another. Phytochemicals are a case in point. Broccoli is famous for its content of sulforaphane, shown in laboratory studies to protect against cancer. Tomatoes have lycopenes. Onions and garlic have allium compounds. Soybeans have flavonoids. My office file of studies extolling the special nutrient content or health benefits of one or another fruit or vegetable includes work on apples, avocados, broccoli, blueberries, cherries, cranberries, garlic, grapefruit, grapes, onions, pomegranates, raisins, spinach, strawberries, and tomatoes, among others. I conclude from this that *all* fruits and vegetables have something good about them, even though some have more of one good thing and others have more of another. That is why we nutritionists are always telling you to eat a variety of foods. It's the mix that is most beneficial and most protective.

Surely the best reason to eat blueberries is that they are delicious in season.

That all fruits and vegetables have much to offer is also why I don't think it makes much sense to push one over another. Yes, it's great to eat lettuce, but surely not for the reasons given by Wegmans on a shelf label: "High in vitamin A and a good source of folate." I like lettuce, but it is mostly water, and almost all richly colored vegetables—spinach or red peppers, for example—are better sources of folate (folic acid) and of beta-carotene, the vitamin A precursor.

Surely the best reason to eat blueberries is that they are delicious in season. Wegmans, however, undoubtedly sells more of them by displaying them in front of labels saying "A half-cup doubles the antioxidants most people get in a day according to the USDA lab at Tufts University." Other fruits also have antioxidants—and different ones—that may be equally important. Eating fruits and vegetables is a good thing to do for health, and eating a variety of them does even more good.

So: Are fruits and vegetables better if they are organic? Of course they are, but not necessarily for nutritional reasons. In this matter, I defer to Joan Gussow, the former head of the nutrition department at Columbia University, whose thinking about matters of agriculture and health I especially admire. She asks:

> shouldn't we hope that people will choose organic foods on grounds more reliable than whether they contain a little more carotene or zinc? Isn't the most important story that organic production conserves natural resources, solves rather than creates environmental problems, and reduces the pollution of air, water, soil . . . and food?

I like the way she keeps attention focused on these critically important environmental issues. My guess is that researchers will eventually be able to prove organic foods marginally more nutritious than those grown conventionally, and that such findings will make it easier to sell organic foods to a much larger number of people. In the meantime, there are loads of other good reasons to buy organics, and I do.

So: Are fruits and vegetables better if they are organic? Of course they are, but not necessarily for nutritional reasons.

5

Genetically Modified,
Irradiated, and Politicized

T he produce sections of supermarkets inspire no end of questions. One that particularly interests me, for example, is whether supermarkets are selling genetically modified (GM) fresh fruits and vegetables, those whose genes have been deliberately manipulated to give the plants some desirable trait—resistance to insects or viruses, for example. Tinkering with plant genes sometimes generates issues about safety and other matters, but when I asked produce managers if their stores carried GM foods, they looked puzzled and said they really didn't know. GM foods are supposed to be labeled voluntarily with PLU (Product Look-Up) codes that begin with 8, but I never have been able to find one. Once, I was intrigued to see a PLU code beginning with an 8 on a honeydew melon at a Costco in New Jersey, but I knew that the FDA had not permitted GM honeydews to be marketed. I called the grower, who told me that the melons were not, in fact, genetically engineered; instead, Costco uses its own coding system.

I did score the opposite, though. In the Hong Kong Supermarket in Manhattan's Chinatown I found a papaya with a label saying "no GMO, no irradiation, no hot water treatment, 100% natural tree-ripened" (no GMO stands for "no genetically modified organisms"). The papaya, however, was anything but ripe and I had no immediate way to evaluate the accuracy of the other statements.

Under our current system of food regulation, GM foods do not have to be labeled as such. Why not? In 1994, when the first GM foods were ready to be marketed, biotechnology companies argued that because genetic engineering methods were fundamentally identical to those used in conventional plant breeding, labeling would mislead you into thinking GM foods were different and somehow inferior. For reasons that were in part scientific and in part a response to industry pressures, the FDA agreed with the companies' interpretation of the science, and ruled that labeling was unnecessary. In *Safe Food*, I discussed whether GM techniques really do differ in any meaningful way from traditional methods, especially when they introduce "foreign" genes from one species into an entirely different species. My conclusion? This is a matter of judgment. Whether you view GM manipulations and traditional genetic techniques as the same or different depends on point of view, and, therefore, on politics. Scientifically based or not, the motivation of biotechnology companies for opposing labeling is obvious: if the foods are labeled as GM, you might choose not to buy them.

S cientifically based or not, the motivation of biotechnology companies for opposing labeling is obvious: if the foods are labeled as GM, you might choose not to buy them.

In theory, some GM fruits or vegetables should be in supermarket produce sections because the FDA allows several kinds to be grown and marketed. The list is short because only a few have gone through the FDA's review processes. The FDA does not exactly "approve" GM foods for human consumption. Instead, it requires the companies planning to grow such foods to enter into a "consultation process." The FDA explains the process in its inimitable fashion:

> The FDA does not conduct a comprehensive scientific review of data generated by the developer. Instead, the FDA considers, based on agency scientists' evaluation of the available information, whether any unresolved issues exist regarding the food derived from the new plant variety that would necessitate legal action by the agency if the product were introduced into commerce. Examples of unresolved issues may include, but

are not limited to, significantly increased levels of plant toxicants or anti-nutrients, reduction of important nutrients, new allergens, or the presence in the food of an unapproved food additive. The FDA considers a consultation to be completed when all safety and regulatory issues are resolved.

Whatever. As of 2004, the FDA had completed consultations for several GM field crops: corn, rice, soybeans, sugar beets, canola, oilseed rape, and wheat. These commodities are mainly used for animal feed, although they also are used as ingredients in processed foods on supermarket shelves. The FDA also "resolved the regulatory issues" for several kinds of fruits and vegetables: tomatoes and cantaloupe with genes that delay ripening or inhibit softening, tomatoes and potatoes with genes for insect resistance, radicchio resistant to herbicides, and squash and papaya resistant to viruses. Because the FDA has cleared these GM fruits and vegetables for production, they could—in theory—be for sale in supermarket produce sections.

But are they? I asked supermarket customer relations representatives, advocacy groups critical of biotechnology (Greenpeace, Environmental Defense, Union of Concerned Scientists, Friends of the Earth), trade associations for the produce industry (United Fresh Fruit and Vegetable Association, Produce for Better Health Foundation), and experts working in various branches of the USDA and in universities. Nobody could say for sure. University and government scientists said that GM tomatoes and potatoes were around at some point, but that developers stopped growing them either because of problems with production or maintaining quality during transportation, or because retailers did not want to risk objections from customers opposed to such foods. Roughly 10 percent of squash grown in the United States in 2004 were genetically modified to resist viruses, but these look just like any other squash.

The one GM fruit that seems to have held its own is the papaya. About 80 percent of the papayas grown in Hawaii are genetically modified to resist the ringspot virus, which nearly destroyed the Hawaiian industry for this fruit a few years ago. The GM varieties are widely regarded as saving that industry. But if GM papayas are being sold in continental supermarkets, this has to be an exceedingly well-kept secret.

In Hawaii, however, the secret is out. In September 2004, the Hawaii Genetic Engineering Action Network announced that tests proved that pollen from GM papayas must have "drifted" and gotten into conventional papayas. This meant that the modified genes for resistance to ringspot were now appearing in supposedly non-GM papayas. I did not think this had safety implications (the fruit seems just fine to eat), but it did say something about the inability of biotechnology companies to keep their genes under control.

If GM papayas are grown in Hawaii, I wondered whether they were being sold in continental supermarkets. I contacted GeneticID, a company in Fairfield, Iowa, that tests for such things, and an official sent me some instructions for collecting papaya seeds and preparing them for genetic evaluation. This required help from my adult children in California, because Hawaiian papayas rarely get to the East Coast (the ones sold in the east most often come from Central and South America). The instructions said we were to scoop out the seeds, separate them as best we could from the stringy flesh, wash them, freeze them, and ship them off to Iowa via overnight mail. For the samples I managed to collect in Manhattan, this was a sticky job, and I am still finding tiny pieces of orange papaya stuck in odd places in my kitchen.

Together, we came up with three Hawaiian papayas from different producers. Scientist that I am, I also tossed in a couple of controls: a Hawaiian papaya labeled Certified Organic, and the non-GMO papaya from the Hong Kong market in Chinatown, which turned out to have come from Jamaica. These two would be expected to test negative. Furthermore, to make sure the tests were fair, I labeled the frozen seeds with the places where we bought the papayas, but did not tell GeneticID the grower's brand name, the place where the papayas had been grown, or the PLU codes on their stickers. The results follow on the next page.

> If you buy a papaya from Hawaii, there is a good chance it is genetically modified. If the label says "non-GMO," you can believe that claim as well. And, if the label says a food is organic, it is.

The results of even this small sample provide evidence for some clear conclusions. If you buy a papaya from Hawaii, there is a good

Are Papayas Genetically Modified?

PAPAYA BRAND AND PLU CODE	PLACE PURCHASED	GENETICALLY MODIFIED TO CONTAIN GENE FOR RESISTANCE TO RINGSPOT VIRUS?
Hawaii Pride (labeled as irradiated) #4394	Cala Foods, San Francisco	Yes
Hawaiian Premium Cole #4394	Vons, South Pasadena	Yes
Hawaiian Calavo Gold #4394	Gourmet Garage, Manhattan	Yes
Hawaii Organics (Certified Organic) #9-3111	Wholesome Market, Manhattan	No
Martha's Best (from Jamaica) #3111	Hong Kong Supermarket, Chinatown, Manhattan	No

chance it is genetically modified. If the label says "non-GMO," you can believe that claim as well. And, if the label says a food is organic, it most likely *is* organic. This last conclusion is yet another reason for confidence in the Certified Organic seal. And organic foods always should be GM-free.

FOOD IRRADIATION

The Hawaii Pride papaya was labeled as irradiated, and the irradiation story is also interesting, but for different reasons. Hawaiian tropical fruits that could be infested by exotic species of fruit fly are under quarantine and cannot be imported to the continent unless treated first to get rid of the flies and their eggs. This used to be done with toxic gases, but such gases are now considered environmental hazards. Heat treatment also worked, but it ruined the appearance of the fruit. "Electronic" irradiation solves those problems. This form of irradiation is not what you might think. It uses electricity—not radioactive isotopes—to kill the flies and eggs on the skin of the fruit. This should not matter because you do not eat the papaya peel anyway.

Hawaii Pride discloses its use of irradiation on papayas shipped to the West Coast on labels and on its Web site. My daughter, who lives in San Francisco, mailed me a PLU-code sticker from one of that company's papayas and I was surprised to see that the sticker was printed with an irradiation symbol. I rarely see that symbol on foods, even though fruits and vegetables were approved for irradiation in 1986, as were herbs and spices, and Hawaii Pride has been shipping irradiated papayas to the continental United States since 2000.

By law, irradiated foods are supposed to be labeled with a symbol (the "radura," which looks rather like a flower) and a statement like "treated with irradiation." But Congress specified that the print did not have to be very large, and the papaya growers happily took the hint. PLU-code stickers are small to begin with, and the radura and disclosure statement on that papaya—"Irradiated for safety with SureBeam"—were so tiny that I practically needed a magnifying glass to read them.

Unless their labels state otherwise, I assume that commercial dried herbs and spices have been irradiated electronically or with use of radioisotopes, even though I have never found a box of them bearing a radura label. I do not think that electronic or any other kind of irradiation of fruit and dried spices poses health problems. Irradiation of meat, however, raises different issues that I will get to in the chapter on meat safety.

I was surprised to see SureBeam mentioned on the sticker as the source of the irradiation because I had read that the company went bankrupt in January 2004. A spokesperson for Hawaii Pride explained that another company (Titan Corporation's Pulse Science Division) had taken over SureBeam's facilities without a break in irradiation service. I found no other brands of Hawaiian papayas with raduras, yet all must have been treated in some way to get rid of fruit flies. How they were treated is another secret, apparently.

I think you should have a right to know whether the foods you buy are genetically modified or irradiated, and that companies should fully disclose these processes—for reasons of consumer choice if nothing else.

The issues may not matter much in practice because so few treated foods are in supermarkets—Hawaiian papayas are a rare exception. At the moment, practically no other GM or irradiated foods are in the produce (as opposed to the processed food) sections of American supermarkets, or supermarkets anywhere else, and many retailers would prefer not to carry them. The stores have plenty of choices to offer you without getting into issues—some scientifically resolvable, some not—that might make you want to shop elsewhere.

THE POLITICS OF FRUITS AND VEGETABLES

Any government dietary guideline that suggests eating less of anything is bound to be controversial, not least because the companies that produce foods singled out for "eat less" messages are sure to complain that the government has no right to say so. Messages to "eat more," however, please everyone in the food business. The pleasure of having a positive message explains why one guideline consistently remains unchallenged: eat more fruits and vegetables. If you eat a variety of fruits and vegetables, you will have less of a chance of getting heart disease, certain cancers, and many other health problems. People who eat five or more servings of fruits and vegetables daily, for example, seem to have half the cancer risk of people who eat only two servings. Vegetarians have lower rates of heart disease and cancer, as do Asian and Mediterranean populations who traditionally eat diets based largely on fruits, vegetables, and grains. Fruits and vegetables contain protective vitamins and minerals, phytochemicals, and fiber, and they are low in calories—all good reasons for eating them.

> People who eat five or more servings of fruits and vegetables daily, for example, seem to have half the cancer risk of people who eat only two servings.

But most people do not. The USDA's pyramid food guide released in 2005 recommends four daily servings of fruit, and five servings of vegetables, which seem like a lot. But these are "standard" servings and in comparison to what you might consider a serving, they are minuscule— the equivalent of half a cup (exception: the portion size for salad greens is 1 cup). Eat a good-size orange or banana, and you have consumed two pyramid fruit servings, or come close to that amount. But for reasons of taste preference, inconvenience, or expense, you probably eat only half the recommended amount of fruit. Whether you meet the recommendations for vegetables depends on your definition of vegetable. Unbelievable as it may seem, one-third of all vegetables consumed in the United States come from just three sources: french fries, potato chips, and iceberg lettuce.

So why don't Americans eat more fruits and vegetables? Perhaps you simply do not like them. Perhaps you do not like peeling oranges or dealing with apple cores (but there are precut varieties, and fruit juices as well). Perhaps it is a matter of waste; you will have to throw away inedible pits, stems, and leaves. Or perhaps like many people you think they are too expensive (but you are probably willing to pay $3.50 for a pound of potato chips, which is what the cost of a small package works out to be, or $15 for a pound of chocolates). Or perhaps produce seems expensive in comparison to meat. If this is the case, it is not because produce is artificially expensive; it is because meat is artificially cheap. The government subsidizes its cost by supporting farmers who produce feed for animals.

> Unbelievable as it may seem, one-third of all vegetables consumed in the United States come from just three sources: french fries, potato chips, and iceberg lettuce.

Because surveys and other studies say that expense is a major barrier that keeps many people from eating fruits and vegetables, some USDA economists thought it might be useful to find out what such foods really cost. These particular economists work for the Economic Research Service, a low-profile unit of the USDA that quietly goes about its business of looking at practical questions like this one. In the late 1990s, they recorded the cost of more than fifty commonly consumed fruits and vegetables, accounted for waste, and figured out the actual cost per serving. Their stunning conclusion: you can eat the full daily complement of servings recommended at that time—three fruits and four vegetables— for just 64 cents (in 1999 dollars). This cost is so little that even people on very low incomes could afford it.

How, you ask, could this be remotely possible? The answer: portion size. They counted servings by USDA standards, and you can get a lot of half-cup servings out of a pound of fruits or vegetables.

I have to confess that I found this study so hard to believe that I went right out and repeated the experiment myself. I got a supermarket checker to weigh me out exactly one pound of green beans, for which I paid 99 cents (in midsummer 2004). I took the beans home, washed them, trimmed off the ends, tossed out all the parts that seemed inedible, and cut what was left into bite-size pieces. I took a half-cup measure and started counting. That pound of cut green beans filled the half-cup measure nine times—nine half-cup servings—and these were generous half-cups. At this rate, a standard serving of green beans cost only 11 cents. Even if a full cup of green beans is a more reasonable serving size for any normal person, that pound of beans could serve four at a cost of 25 cents per person—and each person would be eating two standard USDA vegetable servings. This USDA study produced one other intriguing result. After accounting for the parts that get thrown out, the economists reported that most of the fruits and vegetables they examined cost less fresh than they did either canned or frozen. You don't believe this? You can easily repeat the experiment at the supermarket and see for yourself.

If this study has merit, and I think it does, cost cannot really be the barrier that keeps people from eating fresh fruits and vegetables. Indeed, the studies show that it is not the absolute cost of produce that seems so high, but its cost per calorie. You get a lot more calories for the price of hamburgers and french fries than you do for carrots, not least because the government subsidizes the production of corn and soybeans, the basis of cheap corn sweeteners and vegetable oil. But I also think marketing is an important barrier. American food-and-beverage producers spend $36 billion annually to advertise and market their products, but practically none of this goes to promote fruits and vegetables—a few million dollars a year compared to the tens or hundreds of millions used to promote any single soft drink, candy bar, or breakfast cereal. Produce is just not profitable enough. The companies that grow fruits and vegetables get about 18 cents of every food dollar you spend on them. The other 82 cents goes to everyone else in this game: the companies that store, truck, package, display, promote, and sell produce. What's more, there is no easy way for the companies to add value to fruits and vegetables and so increase their profit margins. Tomatoes are tomatoes, no matter what their brand. Baby carrots, bagged salads, and organic production methods are among the very few ways to add value. And because produce is perishable, it is more expensive to handle and keep fresh than processed foods.

All of this means that fruit and vegetable growers do not have the kind of money to put into advertising that is available to the makers of sodas, breakfast cereals, and potato chips. Many of the produce companies are small and independent. Perhaps most important, the industry is not unified. Growers view each other as competitors—peaches versus pears, carrots versus cauliflower—rather than as part of an industry with common goals. In contrast, the meat and dairy industries sell one product and can more easily band together to market milk or beef collectively. Without much marketing, the strongest encouragement for you to buy fruits and vegetables is their appearance—how beautiful and tasty they look in the produce sections of supermarkets.

Yes, supermarkets make money on fruits and vegetables—they are in business to do so—but some of them make remarkable efforts to acquire a large variety of excellent produce and to maintain its quality. If you are fortunate enough to live near a market with a good produce section, go meet its manager and offer heartfelt thanks.

ON CHOICES IN THE PRODUCE SECTION

After all of my wanderings through supermarket produce sections, it came as a great relief to shop at the Wholesome Market, an all-organic grocery that used to be located not far from where I work (it closed in spring 2005, shortly after a Whole Foods moved into the neighborhood a couple of blocks away). Its produce section had bananas from Ecuador, cantaloupe from California, coconuts from Hawaii, mangoes from Mexico, squash from Colorado, and fresh herbs, salad greens, and all of the usual vegetables, every single one of them Certified Organic, and every one of them with a PLU-code sticker beginning with a 9. This made the choice so much easier: organic versus organic. Locally grown? Well, that may be asking too much. It took a long time to get organics into supermarkets. Locally grown is the wave of the future and its time will surely come.

> When you choose organics, you are voting with your fork for a planet with fewer pesticides, richer soil, and cleaner water supplies—all better in the long run. When you choose locally grown produce, you are voting for conservation of fuel resources and the economic viability of local communities, along with freshness and better taste.

From a health perspective, fruits and vegetables are good to eat, whether they are organic or not. If the price of organics is a barrier, go ahead and buy conventional produce instead. Conventionally grown fruits and vegetables confer plenty of health benefits to people, if not to the planet. Does price matter? Of course it does. I view the price of organics as a political choice. When you choose organics, you are voting with your fork for a planet with fewer pesticides, richer soil, and cleaner water supplies—all better in the long run. When you choose locally grown produce, you are voting for conservation of fuel resources and the economic viability of local communities, along with freshness and better taste. Once you consider such things, the choices in the produce section are much easier to make. Whenever I have the choice, here are my priorities in that section: (1) organic and locally grown, (2) organic, (3) conventional and locally grown, (4) conventional.

6

Milk and More Milk

It should be easy to pop into a supermarket and pick up a carton of milk, but I find it a nuisance. The dairy section is almost always hard to get to, and not accidentally. Because almost every shopper will buy some dairy products, stores usually put these foods in remote places against the back walls. This makes it easier for the employees to stock the refrigerated cases, but the more important reason is to force you to walk past shelves of other products on your way there—and to pick up a few impulse buys along the way. Some larger supermarkets now put small refrigerated cases filled with staples like milk or orange juice near the cash registers where you can get to them quickly if you are in a rush, but the stores in my neighborhood are too small to do that.

From a distance, the dairy section looks attractive and uncomplicated, stacked as it is with rows and rows of cheery cartons in neat arrays. It is only when you get close enough to the cartons to read their labels that you realize how complicated dairy foods—and all the issues they present—can be. Yes, you can buy plain ordinary milk, but you also have the choice of milk with extra protein, extra calcium, no lactose, no hormones, and no antibiotics, or milk that is organic, ultrapasteurized, chocolate flavored, or low carbohydrate. Not only that, but the stores offer all of these variations at four different levels of fat and at prices ranging more than twofold. And these choices do not even begin to account for the competition—the dairy-free and soy "milks" placed right next to the dairy milks in the same refrigerated cases.

Dairy foods are supposed to be good for you. The USDA says: "Dairy products make important contributions to the American diet. They provide high-quality protein and are good sources of vitamins A, D, and B-12, and also riboflavin, phosphorus, magnesium, potassium, zinc, and calcium." Indeed they are. They provide more than 70 percent of the calcium in American diets, and are fortified with vitamin D to prevent rickets. Years ago, studies proved that dairy foods promoted the growth of children. More recent studies suggest that dairy foods not only might build strong bones but also might protect against a plethora of diseases and conditions. When the government first began to offer dietary advice nearly a century ago, its nutritionists advised children to eat three servings of dairy foods a day for good health, and adults to eat two servings daily. They now advise adults as well as children to eat three servings.

As with all else about what we eat these days, much about this advice is questionable and questioned. Dairy milk is a complex product. It is produced by living cows as food for their young and contains hundreds of substances that are terrific for feeding baby calves. This means that milk raises two quite different sets of issues: the effects of its various components on your health, and the effects of methods of milk production on the cows themselves.

With regard to human health, dairy foods bring up any number of concerns. Cow's milk is indeed high in calcium, but whether a diet high in dairy calcium protects you against osteoporosis or any other disease is a matter of considerable debate. Milk is also high in fat, saturated fat, and cholesterol, substances that are best avoided in large amounts. It contains lactose, a sugar that many people over the age of five cannot easily digest. And it contains proteins to which some people are allergic or sensitive.

How dairy foods are produced these days also generates controversy. Like any other industry, the dairy industry is expected to grow and increase profits, and to do so it has had to become more efficient. The dairy industry achieved greater efficiency in the way such things are typically done—through consolidation of its operations to cut costs and increase production. Since 1970, U.S. dairy producers have reduced the number of dairy farms from 650,000 to 90,000; increased the average number of cows per dairy farm from 20 to 100; and increased total milk production from 120 million to 160 million pounds per year—at the same time that they reduced the overall number of dairy cows from 12 million to 9 million. The dairy industry accomplished these so-called miracles of efficiency by doubling the amount of milk obtained from each cow from 9,700 to 19,000 pounds per year—just since 1970.

The dairy industry accomplished these so-called miracles of efficiency by doubling the amount of milk obtained from each cow from 9,700 to 19,000 pounds per year—just since 1970.

The only way to get more milk out of fewer dairy farms and fewer cows is to push the cows to produce more. But the more milk a cow produces, the greater the chance that her udders can become infected and that she will need antibiotics. To stimulate greater milk production, dairy cows also are treated with hormones. One such hormone—a cow growth hormone known as bovine somatotropin (bST)—is genetically engineered, a process that some people find objectionable. The fivefold increase in the number of cows on a typical dairy farm means that they live under more crowded conditions. Their wastes are more concentrated, they can spread infections more easily, and they need to be treated with antibiotics more often. The antibiotics and hormones can get into the milk and, perhaps, affect human health, and the crowding, infections, and treatment of the cows raise issues of animal rights. Consolidation of the dairy industry by a few big companies raises concerns about corporate control of the food supply. For all of these reasons, and because there is something primal and biological about milk, dairy foods elicit strong feelings. More than most foods, dairy foods do have their critics.

THE POLITICS OF DAIRY FOODS

The scientific arguments about dairy foods are difficult to resolve for the usual reasons. Milk—the source of all dairy products—is just one food in the diet of people who eat many different foods and who also differ in genetic heritage, social background, living circumstances, and behavior. Sorting out the health effects of milk from those of its many individual nutrient components, or distinguishing the effects of diet from those of other behavioral characteristics—cigarette smoking or exercise, for example—is never easy to do.

But trying to study the effects of dairy foods on health is especially difficult for one additional reason: the dairy industry is large and united and is especially diligent in exerting influence over anything that might affect production, marketing, and sales. Most Americans eat dairy foods, and the industry sells $21 billion worth of milk a year. Furthermore, dairy farms are located in all fifty states, and every state has two senators who eagerly accept campaign contributions from dairy donors and can be expected to listen attentively when called upon for assistance. As a result, dairy producers are largely exempt from the usual free market rules of supply and demand. For decades dairy producers have been protected by a system of government price supports and marketing payments so entrenched and so incomprehensible to anyone other than a lobbyist that any attempt to get rid of this system is doomed from the start.

When you hear economists talk about "externalities," this is what they mean: no matter what you pay for dairy foods at the checkout counter, you pay for them again when you file your tax return.

The result is that as a consumer, you pay for dairy foods in at least three ways: directly at the supermarket, indirectly through taxes that support subsidies to farmers who raise dairy cows, and also indirectly through tax-supported subsidies to the producers of commodities like corn and soybeans that are used for cattle feed. When you hear economists talk about "externalities," this is what they mean: no matter what you pay for dairy foods at the checkout counter, you pay for them again when you file your tax return.

When the rules of supply and demand do apply to the dairy industry, it is invariably to the industry's benefit: prices go up. This became evident in the summer of 2004, when the cost of milk nearly doubled at the already overpriced convenience store in my Manhattan neighborhood. In Ithaca, the Wegmans supermarket posted notices explaining the complex politics behind its slightly less shocking version of the price increase: the cost of soybeans had gone up, so farmers substituted cheaper feed and cows produced less milk; the number of dairy farms and cows had declined; less bovine growth hormone was being produced, which also led to a drop in the milk supply; and replacement cows could no longer be brought in from Canada because a Canadian cow had been found to have mad cow disease.

I was not sure any of this made sense, and I was curious to know if there could be other reasons for the price increase. Back at home, I asked the National Dairy Council for further explanation. A spokeswoman confirmed that the milk supply had been falling for the past eight months, in part because the number of dairy cows had dropped by more than 100,000, just within the past year. This sharp acceleration in the long-term trend, it seemed, was a result of the rise in fuel costs resulting from the war in Iraq. Higher fuel costs meant higher feed costs, and that was just enough to put even more dairy farms out of business. And the Austrian maker of genetically modified cow growth hormone was indeed having production problems, but supply and demand for that hormone were soon expected to return to balance. Could you have guessed that the price of milk at the grocery store would be so sensitive to so many national and international developments?

The seemingly universal jump in milk prices as a result of these events illustrates another reason why the dairy industry is powerful—its unity. Milk is milk no matter what company produces it. Recognizing this, dairy producers band together to form what might be considered a "cartel" of sorts, similar to the one that unites oil producers under OPEC (the Organization of Petroleum Exporting Companies). In the United States, the dairy version of this cartel operates under government sponsorship. USDA-sponsored marketing orders and advertising campaigns benefit all dairy producers. The USDA requires dairy producers to contribute to a generic marketing program called a "checkoff," in which producers must pay—check off—a 15-cent contribution for every 100 pounds of milk they sell. In 2005, this program generated nearly $160 million for the industry to spend on public "education" and marketing, with the funds funneled through national or state dairy councils. Funds from the dairy checkoff pay for advertising campaigns that feature celebrities—and sometimes government officials—with "milk mustaches." They also fund campaigns like the one designed to address "America's Calcium Crisis," explained as "America finds itself in a calcium crisis because consumers aren't drinking enough milk."

Some of the checkoff money is also spent on people like me. I am personally indebted to the National Dairy Council for almost daily e-mail messages providing copies of the latest studies supporting the health benefits of dairy foods (although I have to go elsewhere to learn of studies with contrary results) and for immediate and helpful responses to queries. The council works hard to encourage nutritionists and federal agencies to take actions favorable to the industry. It supports advice to increase calcium intake. It supports efforts to encourage lactose-sensitive people to consume as much dairy food as they can tolerate. It opposes advice to restrict dietary fat (especially from animals). It strongly opposes advice to substitute soy products for milk in the diets of infants, children, or adults, and makes sure that I see every study that casts doubt on the benefits of soy foods. And, of course, it promotes advice to eat more dairy foods. Such efforts are often successful, particularly when it comes to federal recommendations about diet and health.

The USDA has long identified dairy foods as a distinct food group, and for many decades it recommended a not unreasonable (especially if low-fat) two servings a day for adults who like and can eat these foods. In 2004, the dietary guidelines advisory committee recommended three servings a day, thereby endorsing a 50 percent increase in milk consumption. An investigative report in *The Wall Street Journal* called this change "a major victory for the $50 billion U.S. dairy industry," and attributed it to a skillful lobbying campaign based on the results of research that had been funded by the Dairy Council, as well as to the financial ties of dairy groups to several members of the advisory committee.

Pressures to increase milk recommendations make obvious business sense, but whether they make scientific or nutritional sense is highly debatable. The issues are legion, but the big ones concern calcium, potassium, fat, lactose, proteins, and hormones. Among these, the debates about calcium and fat get the most attention.

THE CALCIUM DEBATE

Calcium is a principal constituent of bones, and dairy foods provide the majority of calcium in American diets. Your bones may seem hard and static, but they are actually highly dynamic; their mineral and other nutrient constituents are constantly dissolving out of bone and being re-placed. The constant movement of calcium in and out of bones is called "turnover." You need enough calcium in your body to balance the amount that is lost through normal calcium turnover. This means that to have strong bones as an adult, you need to have eaten enough calcium in early childhood, and to be eating enough throughout life to balance calcium losses. Otherwise you are at risk for getting osteoporosis, the fractures that occur when too much bone is lost with aging. To prevent osteoporosis, the government-sponsored institute that deals with such matters says that you must eat more than 1 gram (1,000 to 1,200 mil-ligrams) of calcium a day, an amount much greater than anyone is likely to get from food. To get that much calcium, you have to make special efforts: eat lots of dairy foods, eat foods fortified with calcium, or take calcium supplements.

The need for eating that much calcium—especially from dairy foods—seems questionable to me. For one thing, dairy foods are com-plex mixtures; they have some components that promote calcium reten-tion, but others that promote its excretion. For another, the amount of calcium needed to balance losses is hard to know. Bones are not just made of calcium; they are built on a protein scaffold and need practi-cally all of the other required nutrients. Calcium balance depends on getting enough of every one of the nutrients involved in building bones, and also depends on how active you are, whether you smoke cigarettes, and how much alcohol you drink. When studies examine the effects of one nutrient at a time, they show that some nutrients—magnesium, potassium, vitamin D, and lactose, for example—promote calcium re-tention. Others—like protein, phosphorus, and sodium—promote cal-cium excretion. So calcium retention and the strength of your bones may depend much more on everything else you are eating, and how active you are, than on how much calcium you take in.

The complexity of the calcium story is best illustrated by studies of people who live in countries other than the United States. In parts of the world where cow's milk is not a staple of the diet, people often have less osteoporosis and fewer bone fractures than we do; they maintain cal-cium balance perfectly well on less than half the calcium intake recom-mended for Americans. This surprising observation could result from

In parts of the world where cow's milk is not a staple of the diet, people often have less osteoporosis and fewer bone fractures than we do; they maintain calcium balance perfectly well on less than half the calcium intake recommended for Americans.

differences in diet. Perhaps people elsewhere eat less junk food than we do, less protein from meat and dairy foods, and less sodium from processed foods. Or perhaps their diets help them retain calcium better. The dependence of calcium balance on intake of other nutrients may explain why the highest rates of osteoporosis are seen in countries where people eat the most dairy foods. That too may be just a coincidence and the real reason might be that people who consume the most dairy foods are also inactive, smoke cigarettes, and drink too many soft drinks or too much alcohol (all of which are bad for bones). In response to this extraordinarily confusing situation, the Australian biochemist B. E. Christopher Nordin says: "The conclusion is inescapable that there is no single, universal calcium requirement, only a requirement linked to the intake of other nutrients."

Regardless, dairy foods are not a nutritional requirement. Think of cows. Cows don't drink milk after calfhood, but they grow bones that fully support 800-pound weights and more. They do this by eating grass. Grass has calcium, and so does every other food plant: fruits, vegetables, grains, beans, nuts. These foods may have small amounts of calcium in comparison to dairy products, but small amounts add up, and food plants have fewer substances that promote calcium losses. Overall, it may be a lot healthier for bones to get calcium from plant foods. The large amount of calcium recommended for Americans seems necessary only because we eat diets so high in protein and sodium, both of which accompany the calcium in dairy foods. People who eat a greater proportion of foods from plant sources may do just as well—or better—with less calcium in their diets from any source.

THE FAT DEBATE

Dairy foods provide 15 percent of the total fat in the American food supply, but nearly 30 percent of the saturated fat, the bad kind that raises the risk for heart disease. Nearly 60 percent of the fat in milk is saturated. Fat of any kind is a concentrated source of calories. One tablespoon of butter supplies about 100 calories, as compared to the 60 calories that come in a tablespoon of a food that is mostly protein or carbohydrate. Dairy fat clearly belongs in the "eat less" category.

But it is not easy to eat less of it. Production of dairy foods is increasing. From 1970 to 2002, the amounts available in the food supply rose from 540 pounds per person per year to 585. Within that 45-pound increase lie three confusingly inconsistent trends: less whole milk (good); more low-fat milk (good); but more high-fat dairy products such as triple-cream brie and super-premium ice cream (uh-oh). The peak year for whole-milk production was 1945, when 41 gallons were available for every American man, woman, and child. It has been downhill ever since. In 1970, there were 25 gallons produced per capita, but by 2002 there were just 8. Production of low-fat milk only partially compensated; it went from 6 gallons per capita to 15 during that period. These changes reflected public concerns about fat and calories (good), but also competition from soft drinks (not so good).

Also not so good are trends in the supply of high-fat dairy foods. From 1970 to 2002, production of cream rose from 10 to 17 pounds per capita, and the cheese supply nearly tripled—from 11 to 30 pounds. Both are concentrated sources of calories and of saturated fat. Driving this trend is the need to do something with the butterfat left over from milk production. Commercial milk does not come straight from the cow. It is pooled with milk from other cows, separated into cream and skim fractions, and then reconstituted into milks of differing fat content (which are then pasteurized, homogenized, and vitamin fortified). Dairy producers would like to sell that fat, and do—to producers of butter, cream, and cheese.

From the standpoint of health, however, the development of reduced-fat milk seems like a good idea, and that of nonfat milk even better. If you drink milk at all, the lower its fat content, the better its nutritional value. Nonfat milk retains most of the nutrients in whole milk, but hardly any of the calories or fat, as shown in the following Table.

The Fat and Calorie Content of an 8-Ounce Glass of Milk*

MILK (PERCENT FAT)	FAT (GRAMS)	SATURATED FAT (GRAMS)	CALORIES
Whole (3.25%)	8	5	150
Reduced fat (2%)	5	3	120
Low-fat (1%)	2.5	1.5	100
Nonfat	0.5	0.3	80

*Figures are from USDA tables of food composition at www.nal.usda.gov/fnic/foodcomp/search.

I did not bother to list other nutrients in this Table because their amounts are about the same in milks of any fat content. The protein, minerals, and most vitamins dissolve in the watery part of the milk (the whey or skim), and removing the fat does not reduce them by much. Only the fat-soluble nutrients disappear—vitamins A and D. By law, vitamin D gets added back. This is a good thing if you are not exposed enough to the sun. Sunlight converts a precursor of vitamin D in skin to the active vitamin in your body. Among its other actions, vitamin D helps get calcium and other minerals into bones. The vitamin A lost from whole milk is often added back as well, but there are many other dietary sources for this vitamin. Whole milk does not have much of the other two fat-soluble vitamins (vitamins K and E) to begin with, and they are not added back. Vitamin K is involved in bone strength but some of the friendly bacteria that normally live in your intestinal tract usually make all you need, and vitamin E comes mainly from other foods like salad oils and grains.

THE WEIGHT DEBATE

Although dairy foods contribute about 13 percent of the calories in the American food supply, they are advertised these days as weight-loss products. This percentage of calories is low compared to the 38 percent from grain products, but it is about the same as that from sugars and meats. So in the spring of 2004, I was surprised to see a box of General Mills' Total Corn Flakes with these statements on its front panel:

- Lose more weight (in big letters)
- With 100% daily value of calcium (in smaller letters)
- As part of a reduced calorie diet (in tiny print)

General Mills saw fit to advertise this breakfast cereal as a weight-loss product on the basis of a study that had just appeared. The study placed thirty-two obese adults on one of three low-calorie diets: low calcium, high calcium from supplements, and high calcium from dairy foods. All participants lost weight, but the ones taking the calcium supplements lost more, and those getting the calcium from dairy foods lost the most. The authors' explanation for these results is that calcium stimulates fat breakdown, and that dairy foods may contain some additional factor that aids this process. A more obvious explanation is that the people who ate dairy foods ate less in general. This study was funded by the National Dairy Council, which kindly sent me a copy. The Dairy Council also made sure that dietitians knew about it through a full-color advertisement in the July 2004 issue of the *Journal of the American Dietetics Association*: "Milk, cheese, and yogurt may help your patients lose weight." This advertisement, however, failed to mention the Dairy Council's financial investment in the research, the lead researcher's patent on calcium as a weight-loss strategy, or his exclusive arrangement to license use of the health claim to dairy food companies—eyebrow-raising developments referred to later by *Advertising Age* as "an unusual arrangement for a nutritionist . . . [and] a sign, no doubt, of things to come as the lines between science and marketing continue to blur for growth-desperate food marketers." Overall, these and many other studies, some sponsored and some not, show that people on low-calorie diets can lose weight while eating dairy products—as of course they can. If your diet is low enough in calories, you will lose weight no matter what you eat.

Thus the role of dairy trade associations in promoting the weight-loss benefits of dairy foods deserves scrutiny. The Dairy Council advertises the results of the studies it sponsors in full pages in *The New York Times*. One said: "Drink milk. Lose weight. Looking to drop a few pounds? . . .

> **A**lthough dairy foods contribute about 13 percent of the calories in the American food supply, they are advertised these days as weight-loss products.

emerging research suggests that drinking 3 glasses of milk daily when dieting may promote the loss of body fat . . ." In August 2004, a four-page spread in the trade magazine *Progressive Grocer* urged supermarkets to advertise dairy foods as a weight-loss strategy: "Milk your diet. Lose weight! 24 ounces/24 hours." This was followed in very small print by this explanation: "Including 24 ounces of lowfat or fat free milk every 24 hours in a reduced-calorie diet provides calcium and protein to support healthy weight loss." And it certainly should, if you eat less in general.

Perhaps there is something special about dairy foods that might help you lose weight, and the Dairy Council frequently sends me studies that set forth one or another hypothesis about how calcium or dairy foods might speed up metabolism (so you use up more calories) or prevent the storage of fat. But I remain skeptical, mainly because dairy foods are just one component of daily diets that contain so many other foods. Dairy foods—like other foods—contribute calories, and sometimes lots of calories such as those from butter, cheese, and ice cream. I am withholding judgment until I see what happens when investigators independent of the Dairy Council study the effects of dairy foods on the weight of much larger numbers of people over a much longer time period. Some other critics are more than skeptical. In June 2005, the Physicians Committee for Responsible Medicine, a vegetarian and animal rights group in Washington, D.C., filed a class action suit against dairy industry groups for "duping overweight Americans into believing that milk and other dairy [products] are the magic bullet to weight control . . . We are serving notice with these lawsuits that we will not continue to let these false health claims go unchallenged."

THE HEALTH DEBATES

In the meantime, the research on dairy foods and other aspects of health is so inconsistent that it is hard to figure out what it means. The content of fat and saturated fat suggests that dairy foods might raise the risk of heart disease or of cancers of the colon, prostate, ovary, or breast. My files are filled with published papers on these connections, and their results could not be more confusing. The studies hardly ever distinguish high- from low-fat options, or fat from the calcium, lactose, growth hormones, or other components in milk. The least confusing studies relate to heart disease; they sometimes associate dairy foods with a higher risk and sometimes with a lower risk. But no matter what the results are, the differences are small. Indeed, the research results are so underwhelming that it is safe to conclude that dairy foods have no special role in heart disease beyond their contribution to the overall intake of saturated fat.

The cancer studies are more difficult to interpret. So many components in dairy foods might affect cancer risk, and so many different types of cancer might be affected. To pick just one example: some studies associate fat with an increased risk of colon cancer while others associate vitamin D and calcium with a decreased risk. An enormous review of the science linking diet to cancer in 1997 concluded that milk and dairy products might "possibly" increase the risk of prostate and kidney cancer, but that information on other types of cancer was too limited or inconsistent to go even that far. Subsequent studies continue to suggest a "modest" increase in the risk of prostate cancer. It is difficult to know how to interpret words like "possibly" and "modest" or the advice given in 2002 by the American Institute for Cancer Research: "From a purely-scientific standpoint, it would be irresponsible to assert that drinking milk increases a person's risk for prostate cancer in particular . . . but it would be equally irresponsible to insist that the existence of such a link was impossible." Another review concludes that the evidence available "does not support a strong association between the consumption of milk or other dairy products and breast cancer risk." With statements like this, your interpretation has to depend on whether you are an optimist or pessimist. My

> It isn't necessary to get into as yet unanswerable questions of heart disease or cancer to decide what to do about dairy foods. The calories and saturated fat are reason enough to choose lower-fat options.

guess is that if dairy foods do pose a risk for prostate, breast, or any other type of cancer, the risk must be quite small.

It isn't necessary to get into as yet unanswerable questions of heart disease or cancer to decide what to do about dairy foods. The calories and saturated fat are reason enough to choose lower-fat options.

7

Milk: Subject to Debate

I can hardly think of anything about milk that elicits a ho-hum reaction. Critics and defenders alike appear to care deeply about every nutrient or factor in it, whether naturally occurring or added during production or processing. The most intense debates center on the health effects of three specific components of milk: lactose, proteins, and hormones. Because commercial interests are so entangled in these arguments, the science is often difficult to sort out. Let's take a look.

THE LACTOSE DEBATE

> *Your heart yearns. Your stomach aches. Imagine being able to dig in and enjoy a bowl of creamy, delicious ice cream, a plate of Fettuccine Alfredo with extra Parmesan, or a tall, cold glass of milk with fresh-baked cookies! . . . LACTAID® milk is real milk! Great-tasting, farm-fresh and 100% lactose free.*
>
> —Lactaid® Web site, August 2004

This ad fails to mention that lactose free is not necessarily low calorie or fat free. It is a dead giveaway that the purpose of Lactaid is to promote the sale of milk—not necessarily to promote health. If you remove the lactose from milk, you open up new markets for dairy products. You make it possible for people who are "lactose intolerant" to drink milk and not feel sick. This is a service to lactose-sensitive people who like dairy foods and miss eating them, but it is an even greater service to the dairy industry, which now has a new "value-added" product to sell—and at a premium price.

Lactose is the sugar in milk, and an 8-ounce glass of milk contains about a tablespoon of this substance. Lactose is a "double" (two-sugar) sugar made of the single sugars, glucose and galactose, linked together. Double sugars are too big to be absorbed into your body from the intestinal tract. To use lactose, your body has to split the linkage between glucose and galactose and release them as single sugars; these are easily absorbed. The enzyme that does the splitting is called lactase (note: enzyme names usually end with –ase; sugars end in –ose). Babies make lactase from birth. The sweet taste of lactose sugar in breast milk encourages them to nurse. Within a few years after weaning, say by the age of five, most children—but not all—stop making the lactose-splitting enzyme or do not make much of it. From an evolutionary perspective, the enzyme is no longer needed.

If your body does not make much lactase after childhood, any lactose you eat goes through your digestive tract intact as a double sugar. This sugar would just be excreted, except for one not-so-minor problem: intestinal bacteria. The human intestines are full of bacteria and many of them just love lactose. If you do not digest it into its single component sugars, the bacteria will, and when undigested lactose comes their way, they go right to work on it. Bacterial digestion produces gas and small molecules that attract water into the intestines. This can make you uncomfortable, to say the least.

Some adults, particularly those of northern European ancestry, continue to make enough lactase to split lactose and are able to eat dairy foods with impunity, but these are the exceptions. About 75 percent of the world's adults—and this means most Asians, Southeast Asians, Africans, Middle Easterners, and Native Americans—do not make much or any of the lactose-splitting enzyme. As a matter of aversive conditioning or cultural tradition, they eat few, if any, dairy foods. If you are among this majority, the amount of milk you can comfortably drink is an individual matter, one that depends on the amount of the enzyme you make and the kinds of bacteria you house in your intestines.

If you are extremely sensitive to lactose, even a hint of dairy foods may upset your digestive system, or give you headaches, muscle pain, or dizziness. This may make you sad not to be able to eat dairy foods. But problems with lactose are even sadder for the dairy industry, which would love to convince you that lactose sensitivity is no reason to stop eating those foods. The National Dairy Council has sponsored numerous studies expressly designed to prove this point. These always show that even people who are highly sensitive to lactose can find ways to eat at least some dairy products some of the time.

Nevertheless, the lactose issue galvanizes anti-dairy groups such as the Physicians Committee for Responsible Medicine (PCRM). In 2000, this group sued the government on the grounds of racial bias. It pointed out that while federal dietary guidelines advise everyone to eat dairy foods every day, most nonwhite people cannot digest them. The guidelines, they said, should cite dairy foods as optional rather than superior sources of calcium. They noted that several members of the scientific committee working on the guidelines had financial ties to the dairy industry. Although the suit was thrown out of court, it brought attention to the unusual status given to dairy foods in American diets. This remarkable status was further revealed in 2004 when an even more financially tied committee urged government agencies to increase the recommendation for daily intake of dairy foods from two to three servings a day, and the government did just that in the 2005 *Dietary Guidelines* and food pyramid.

My files contain papers examining one additional health issue related to lactose: the possibility that one of the components of this sugar might be involved in development of ovarian cancer. This alarming suggestion comes from epidemiological observations: populations that drink the most milk on average, and have the greatest persistence of the lactase enzyme into adulthood, turn out to exhibit the highest rates of this cancer. Although some people have attributed this observation to the supposedly toxic effects of the galactose part of lactose, studies of "galactose toxicity" do not confirm any relationship to ovarian cancer. If anything, most research on this point suggests linkages between intake of low-fat milk, calcium, and lactose and a small *reduction* in the risk of ovarian cancer. Regardless, suggestions that galactose might be bad for you make no sense. Unless you have a rare genetic inability to handle this sugar (which you would surely know by now), your liver immediately converts galactose to glucose, a necessary sugar for your blood.

If you enjoy eating dairy products but think you might be lactose intolerant, you can follow the advice of the National Dairy Council. Get a doctor to give you a breath test to see if you really do not make the enzyme. If you do not make lactase, you will breathe out some of the gas produced by bacterial digestion: the breath test measures that gas. Then, if you do turn out to be sensitive to lactose but want to eat dairy foods anyway, you can do some experimenting. Start with hard cheeses and yogurt; the "friendly" bacteria used to make these foods have already digested most of the lactose they contain. You can try eating small amounts of dairy foods, one at a time. You also can try Lactaid or other such products that have been pretreated with the lactase enzyme to split lactose into its single sugars, or you can take lactase supplements whenever you are eating dairy foods. If, on the other hand, you do not wish to eat dairy products, there is no reason why you have to. You can get calcium from plenty of other food sources or from supplements, if need be.

> If, on the other hand, you do not wish to eat dairy products, there is no reason why you have to. You can get calcium from plenty of other food sources or from supplements, if need be.

THE PROTEIN DEBATE

Breast milk is the perfect food for baby people, and cow's milk is the perfect food for baby cows. But cow's milk is too concentrated for human babies and has to be diluted and otherwise treated to make infant formula. Formulas can cause allergic reactions in some infants. Allergies are caused by proteins, and cow's milk contains at least five kinds of proteins that can cause allergic reactions in children and adults who are sensitive to them. Milk proteins seem to be especially allergenic, perhaps because they are the first "foreign" proteins to which children are exposed. Infants who are not breast-fed and who are sensitive to cow's milk proteins can be switched to soy or other formulas. As an adult, if you have allergic reactions to the proteins in cow's milk, you must avoid not only dairy foods but every other food product to which milk, cheese, or yogurt has been added. This requires careful reading of food labels as well as detailed interviewing of waiters in restaurants.

Even if milk proteins do not cause allergies, they could—in theory—cause problems of "cross-reactivity." This means that your body might have an immune reaction to milk proteins and you might make antibodies to these proteins that—by coincidence—could cross-react with your own body's proteins. This could cause you to develop an autoimmune disease of one kind or another. This idea came from observations of groups with autoimmune diseases. The longer people had been breast-fed as infants, the less their chance of developing autoimmune conditions later in life. These observations, in turn, led to the idea that children fed cow's milk formulas might be more likely to develop type 1 diabetes, the type that typically starts in childhood. Children with type 1 diabetes often have antibodies against cow's milk proteins and—we are still talking theory here—these might have cross-reacted and destroyed the cells in the pancreas that produce insulin.

> As an adult, if you have allergic reactions to the proteins in cow's milk, you must avoid not only dairy foods but every other food product to which milk, cheese, or yogurt has been added.

Careful examination of these possibilities suggests that the science is circumstantial. We all make antibodies to many kinds of proteins in foods, and a great many children have some antibodies to cow's milk proteins and do not develop diabetes. Furthermore, the evidence does not particularly point to antibodies to milk proteins as a cause of autoimmune diseases or childhood diabetes, as distinct from antibodies to any other food proteins. The causes of autoimmune diseases are still obscure. Breast-feeding usually avoids problems related to overly early exposure of infants to cow's milk proteins, but few studies ever mention breast-feeding. Instead, they invariably call for further research, not only to resolve scientific uncertainties but also because advising children to avoid cow's milk "would have a serious economic effect and a tremendous impact on the feeding of infants . . ." Indeed it would.

In part because of such concerns, the dairy industry sponsors research to demonstrate the benefits of cow's milk proteins. Look, for example, at a collection of research papers sponsored by the National Dairy Council, Kraft Foods, the Whey Protein Institute, and the U.S. Dairy Export Council. Its editors, all either employed by or receiving research funds from one or another of the sponsors, explain that milk is no mere food: "milk is an integrated food system of structure-specific proteins, lipids, and carbohydrates that confer physiological benefits beyond the content of essential vitamins, minerals, and macronutrients." The scientific papers review evidence that "bioactive" proteins in milk do much more than meet protein requirements. They also help regulate blood sugar levels, hunger and satiety, body weight, and blood pressure. They prevent tooth decay. They even can be used as sugar substitutes. The challenge, the editors say, will be to develop this research to the point where it can "demonstrate efficacy for improving human health" and can be used "to develop foods that deliver documented health benefits." Well, yes, but sometimes a food is just a food.

THE HORMONE DEBATE

Milk cartons from Farmland Dairy say: "*No hormones added, no antibiotics." Follow the asterisk and you find this on a side panel: "*Delicious 100% real milk produced from cows not treated with rbST or Beta-lactam antibiotics. The FDA has found no significant difference from milk derived from rbST treated cows and those not treated." This peculiarly inconsistent combination of statements—either cow growth hormone and antibiotics matter or they don't—has only one explanation: politics.

In contrast, the science is reasonably straightforward. Lactating cows secrete estrogens and other hormones into their milk (as do lactating human mothers), but the amounts are small and do not seem to affect infants, older children, or adults who drink cow's milk. Pressures for greater efficiency and greater profits, however, make dairy farmers want cows to produce more milk than they typically can do. Cows can be made to produce 10 to 20 percent more milk if they are injected every two weeks with cow growth hormone. The most commonly used hormone is a genetically engineered version made by Monsanto, a large agricultural products company. The hormone is officially known as recombinant bovine somatotropin (rbST). The FDA approved rbST for use in dairy cows in 1993. A decade later, U.S. dairy farmers were injecting about 22 percent of their cows with this hormone, which was generating an estimated $250 to $300 million in annual sales (a mere 5 percent or so of Monsanto's business, however). Right from the start, the use of rbST has been fiercely controversial, not only because of questions about its effect on human health but also because of its role in a range of issues having to do with milk production: the health of cows, the use of antibiotics, and the viability of family dairy farms.

> The Monsanto company invoked science to argue that labeling would mislead the public into thinking there might be something different about rbST milk. Labels might make people suspect—horrors—that untreated milk might be better.

These issues might not generate quite so much controversy if it were not for the labeling problem. For reasons of science and politics, milk from cows treated with rbST (shorthand: rbST milk) is not labeled as such, so you have no way of knowing whether the milk for sale in your local supermarket came from treated cows. Assume it does. In 1993, when the FDA was considering whether and how to approve rbST, Monsanto mounted the most heavy-handed industry lobbying campaign imaginable to get the FDA to approve the drug but not require rbST milk to be labeled. The Monsanto company invoked science to argue that labeling would mislead the public into thinking there might be something different about rbST milk. Labels might make people suspect—horrors—that untreated milk might be better. At the time, the FDA's analytical methods could not tell the difference between milk from treated and untreated cows. This inability is not as surprising as it sounds. Cows make their own natural form of bST (not recombinant) and the natural form is always present in their milk. Milk from treated cows, therefore, contains both the natural and the recombinant forms of bST, but these are very much alike in chemical structure.

Monsanto lobbyists argued that because the FDA could not tell the two forms of bST apart, milks from treated and untreated cows were identical. Therefore, putting a label on rbST milk would suggest that it was different (when a difference could not be detected), and that the untreated milk was better (when they are indistinguishable). If so, labeling would mislead the public into thinking there was a difference. The FDA agreed. The result: no special labeling of rbST milk.

Dairies that were not using rbST, however, thought the difference would indeed matter to some consumers and that the ruling was unfair. They started labeling their products "bST-free." Monsanto objected, and the FDA again agreed with the company. It ruled that any such statement had to be "truthful and not misleading" and that the label "bST-free" was neither. It was untruthful because all milk contains bST, and it was misleading because the difference is undetectable. Dairy companies, said the FDA, could use such terms only when they put them "in context." Hence, the statement—"The FDA has found no significant difference . . ."—and the asterisk on Farmland Dairy milk cartons.

Much of the controversy over FDA approval of rbST involved questions of safety. Monsanto said rbST was demonstrably safe for human health because the natural cow hormone caused no harm to human health and rbST and the natural cow hormone bST were indistinguishable. In this instance, that similarity is reassuring. Both bST and rbST are specific to cows. They cannot harm you. They differ in structure from your own growth hormones, are not active in your body, and will not make you grow. Furthermore, they are protein hormones; like most other proteins, they are largely inactivated by acid in your stomach and broken into their constituent amino acids by enzymes in your intestines. So the hormone itself ought not to affect human health.

But use of rbST raises safety issues for three other reasons: the effects of rbST on dairy cows; the effects of antibiotics on human health; and the effects on human health of a substance called insulin-like growth factor-1 (IGF-1). The effects on cows have to do with what happens to their skin at the site of the biweekly rbST injections, and to their udders when they are forced to produce more milk. Injections break the skin and can permit infections to develop. As for udders, the more milk a cow produces, the more likely she is to get an udder infection (mastitis).

That is where antibiotics come in. The more infections a cow develops, the more antibiotics she needs. Antibiotics get into the milk she produces and into your digestive system when you drink the milk. Another reason is theoretical: drinking milk that contains antibiotics could kill off friendly bacteria in your intestinal tract and encourage the proliferation of unfriendly bacteria that resist treatment with these drugs. Although this is still just a possibility, dairies are supposed to have safeguards in place to make sure that milk from antibiotic-treated cows stays out of the food supply, and that dairy milk is routinely tested for traces of a range of antibiotics (although undoubtedly not all of the ones currently in use).

The IGF-1 issue is more complicated. Treating cows with rbST increases the level of the insulin-like growth factor in their milk. Ordinarily this would not matter, but it happens that a cow's IGF-1 is identical to the human form of IGF-1. This means that if you drink milk from rbST-treated cows, the amount of IGF-1 in your blood might increase. Fortunately, IGF-1 is a protein, and like bST should be mostly destroyed by stomach acid and digestive enzymes. Sometimes, however, protein digestion does not work all that well, so there is always a possibility that some IGF-1 protein could be absorbed intact. This does matter because IGF-1 might affect health. Studies have linked high blood levels of IGF-1 to increases in the risk of cancers of the prostate in men and the breast in premenopausal women. As is so often true, the observed increases were "modest." Even so, it is not at all clear that a modest increase in the risk of these cancers has anything to do with drinking rbST milk. Blood IGF-1 levels are known to depend on body weight and physical fitness as well as on genetic factors, and any of these might be more important in determining how much is in your blood than the amount of IGF-1 in cow's milk. As with so many other such issues, this one leaves room for uncertainty and, therefore, for speculation and lingering doubts.

The lingering doubts are one reason why organic milk seems so appealing, and why the largest organic dairy, Horizon Organic, proclaims on its milk cartons, "Produced WITHOUT the use of ANTIBIOTICS, added GROWTH HORMONES and DANGEROUS PESTICIDES." Horizon's Web site similarly boasts that "Our cows are treated with respect and dignity, fed a certified organic, vegetarian diet and never given growth hormones or antibiotics . . . Together we change the world—one organic acre at a time." Advertising like this drives anti-organic critics into a frenzy, and they devote entire Web sites to refuting even the slightest suggestion that organic milk might be safer or in any way superior to conventional milk.

I particularly enjoy visiting the Web site www.stoplabelinglies.com, which is devoted exclusively to exposing "unscrupulous marketing campaigns" by organic dairies. This site lets you look up any dairy you like and see how Alex Avery (the son and collaborator of Dennis Avery, the prominant critic of organic farming methods) and his colleagues parse label statements. The Horizon statements, they explain, are misleading because no milk contains antibiotics or pesticides and those statements fail to include an asterisk to the required FDA disclaimer. The vehemence with which such critics complain about the "unscruples" of organic products can only be due to fears that you might actually prefer to buy them.

These particular critics of organics are associated with the Hudson Institute, a think tank sponsored by conservative foundations and agribusiness companies. It would be expected to support conventional over organic agricultural methods. Such critics have undoubtedly noticed that organic dairy foods are the fastest-growing segment of that industry. Although organic production comprises a measly 1 percent or so of dairy farms and cows in the United States—not enough to bother anyone, you might think—the organic dairy industry predicts a 15 percent annual growth rate through 2008. Growth figures like those are enough to make any conventional food producer take notice.

Looked at another way, the numbers of organically raised cows are rising rapidly. In the early 1990s, only 2,000 cows produced organic milk in the United States; a decade later, there were more than 50,000. Organic dairy foods brought in $1.4 billion in sales in 2003, but that figure was 20 percent higher than in the previous year. To obtain a Certified Organic seal, milk must be taken from cows that are given organic feed and allowed access to pasture, outdoor air and sunlight, shade, and shelter (the meaning of "access," however, is subject to interpretation). They cannot be given antibiotics except to treat disease, and rules govern how long organic dairies have to wait before allowing milk from antibiotic-treated cows back into the food supply. They also can never be treated with hormones, genetically engineered or otherwise. All Certified Organic milk must meet those rules, so it is easy to see why organic milk might seem preferable to conventional milk.

Overall, the fact that so much milk is produced, and by such a strong industry, cannot help but raise suspicions that commerce—rather than health—gets the last word in the dairy debates. My take on the current state of the science is that if milk does increase health risks, these have to be small. I think the science also suggests that if milk does have health benefits, these too are small. Milk is just a food. There is nothing special about it. Cow's milk is not necessary and it is not perfect (at least not for humans). But cow's milk also is not a poison.

Yes, milk is sometimes produced in ways that are hard on cows, using hormones and other substances that you would just as soon avoid. But the dairy industry has even found a way for you to deal with those unattractive production issues: buy organic.

Yes, it is high in fat, saturated fat, and calories, but there is an easy alternative: choose nonfat. Yes, it contains lactose, but solutions to that "problem" also are readily available. Yes, milk is sometimes produced in ways that are hard on cows, using hormones and other substances that you would just as soon avoid. But the dairy industry has even found a way for you to deal with those unattractive production issues: buy organic. You do not have to drink milk to be healthy, but if you like drinking it, you can do so and also stay healthy.

8

Dairy Foods:
The Raw and the Cooked

I am old enough to remember what milk was like before it was routinely homogenized. In the small Long Island town where my family lived, the local dairy delivered glass bottles of milk to our door a couple of times a week. By the time we woke up, the cream had risen to the top and could be poured off to use in coffee or on cereal. Winter mornings, if we didn't bring the bottles in right away, the milk froze, expanded, and pushed a two-inch tube of frozen cream straight out of the bottle top—instant ice cream (unsweetened, alas).

Since then, dairy foods have come a long way. Milk is now a processed food, routinely clarified, separated, reconstituted, homogenized, and pasteurized—a big change from the way things used to be. Mostly this change has been for the better, but like everything else about milk, the processing generates its own special criticisms and critics.

MILK PROCESSING: SEPARATION AND RECONSTITUTION

All milk these days is processed to separate the cream from the watery whey. The processors then add back just the right amount of cream to make 1 percent, 2 percent, and full-fat (whole) milks. The leftover cream is used for heavy cream, butter, cheese, and other such products.

Dairy products have so much fat and saturated fat that the amounts of these components can be measured by the tablespoon, as shown in the Table below. Fat is where the calories in any food are concentrated. The more fat a food contains, the higher its calories. Butter is almost pure fat. Heavy cream has more fat and calories than lighter creams or whole milk. But a tablespoon of skim milk has hardly any fat or calories worth mentioning—another good reason for choosing it.

Calories and Fat in One Tablespoon of Butter, Cream, and Milk*

PRODUCT	CALORIES	FAT (GRAMS)	SATURATED FAT (GRAMS)
Butter	100	11.5	7
Heavy cream	50	5	3
Light cream	30	2.5	1.5
Half & half	20	1.5	1
Whole milk	9	0.5	0.3
Nonfat milk	5	0	0

A tablespoon is about 15 grams.

HOMOGENIZATION AND PASTEURIZATION

From the point of view of a chemist, fresh milk is a suspension of drops of fat in water—floating cream thoroughly dispersed in skim milk (whey). Fat is lighter than water, so left to its own devices it will rise to the top as cream. Homogenization is just mechanical mixing strong enough to break the fat into droplets so small that they stay in suspension.

Pasteurization is the way dairy producers deal with microbial contaminants in milk—bacteria, protozoa, viruses, and the like (shorthand: bacteria)—that can make milk spoil. The udders of cows are anything but sterile, and even when they are washed and disinfected, bacteria still get into the milk. If you drink "raw" milk straight from the cow, you are drinking whatever bacteria fell into it.

The bacteria in dairy foods come in three categories: the beneficial ones that turn milk into cheese, yogurt, buttermilk, and other such things; the bad ones that turn milk sour and spoil it; and the even worse ones that can make you sick. Most bacteria of any type are killed by the strong acid in your stomach, and the survivors in the "worse" category are the only ones to worry about. In the past, cows were often infected with the germs for tuberculosis, brucellosis, typhoid fever, diphtheria, and other such dangerous diseases. These got into the milk and caused no end of public health woes. Pasteurization fixed those problems.

Pasteurization is a simple process. All it does is heat milk to a high enough temperature to kill most (but never all) bacteria. As a rule, the higher the temperature of pasteurization, the more bacteria are killed. But when dairy processors heat milk to a temperature high enough to sterilize it completely, the milk tastes just awful. So pasteurization is a compromise. Louis Pasteur's contribution was to find a temperature hot enough to kill a reasonable number of bacteria in a short enough time to preserve the taste. For example, pasteurization heats milk for, say, half an hour at 145°F (63°C), or for just 15 seconds at about 161°F (72°C). Both methods work well. Alternatively, processors can use "ultrapasteurization" and scald milk under pressure at an extremely high temperature—285°F (141°C)—but for only one or two seconds. So many bacteria are killed in that short time that the milk can stay unspoiled for weeks at a time.

But even that temperature is not held long enough to kill all the bacteria and more microbes get introduced during the bottling process. Bacteria grow much faster at warm temperatures, which is why I cringe when I see crates of milk sitting around on New York City sidewalks or on supermarket floors. New York City is tough on food. That explains why milk sold there is stamped with two sell-by dates. In June 2005, the stamp on a quart of skim milk in my refrigerator said:

As a rule, the higher the temperature of pasteurization, the more bacteria are killed. But when dairy processors heat milk to a temperature high enough to sterilize it completely, the milk tastes just awful. So pasteurization is a compromise.

SELL BY JUNE 25
IN NYC JUNE 19

The milk may have been produced under the most sanitary of conditions, but if it is sold in New York City it needs to be used days earlier than milk sold anywhere else. The New York City Health Department, which regulates these dates, knows that grocery stores do not have much storage space and that it is hopeless to expect stores and distributors to maintain the "cold chain" and keep milk continuously chilled as it gets moved from trucks to delivery sites.

The effect of warmth in stimulating the growth of bacteria is so predictable that dairy scientists can say practically to the minute how long milk will stay fresh after pasteurization and bottling if they know its storage temperature. Their slogan is, "life begins at 40"—meaning 40°F, the warmest temperature your refrigerator should ever be. The bacteria that spoil milk grow slowly in the refrigerator, but above 40°F, even the slightest warming makes microbes grow faster and milk spoil sooner. This is easily seen in a Table.

Higher Temperatures Make Milk Spoil Faster

TEMPERATURE	TIME BEFORE SPOILING
32°F (freezer)	3 to 4 weeks
33° to 40°F (refrigerator)	10 to 14 days
45° to 50°F (chilly)	3 to 5 days
60° to 70°F (room temperature)	Less than 1 day

Homogenization and pasteurization make milk safer and easier to store, but they turn out to be surprisingly contentious issues for people who believe that raw milk tastes better and is healthier, or that the process of mixing milk from hundreds of different cows, separating the components and putting them back together again, and then heating them all together destroys vital components of milk. The flavor argument has some merit. Raw milk from a single cow has a taste unique to that cow, and milk from cows fed on the same pasture will have a similar taste, but nuances in taste get lost when milk from hundreds of commercially fed cows is pooled for processing. Pasteurization makes all milk taste pretty much alike, and homogenization takes care of any variations in mouth feel.

But the loss of unique tastes is not matched by a loss in nutritional value, at least according to research on food composition. Pasteurization heats milk for so short a time that it only reduces the amounts of some of the more delicate vitamins, and only minimally at that. And it also minimally inactivates some of the proteins, but these would be inactivated by stomach acid and intestinal enzymes soon after you drank the milk anyway.

Although bacteria in milk are largely harmless, my personal preference is to have most of the ones in the milk I drink dead before they get in me. I am not opposed to raw milk on principle, and I believe that it is quite possible to consume it safely, especially when, as the more reasonable proponents of raw milk advise, you know the "animal care standards and sanitary practices of your milk producers." If knowing those things were even remotely possible for someone like me who hardly ever visits dairy farms, I might feel differently about this issue. If I could see for myself that a raw milk producer had a well-designed and well-monitored safety system in place and was testing regularly for harmful bacteria, I would worry less about drinking it. The FDA counts 200 to 300 illnesses a year from drinking raw milk and does not allow it to be sold across state lines. I would much rather avoid such illness, and I view pasteurization as a small price to pay for not having to worry about whether milk is safe to drink.

Cheeses made from raw milk are another matter and require a separate discussion, as do issues related to cheeses in general.

CHEESE

By some accounts cheese is the leading source of saturated fat in American diets (beef is second and milk third). The best-tasting cheeses are absurdly high in fat, saturated fat, and calories—all things I usually try to avoid—but if I am going to eat saturated fat once in a while, I prefer to get it from cheese. A truly great cheese is unique in flavor in a way that no meat or milk can ever be. I live near the extraordinary Murray's Cheese Shop on Bleecker Street, owned by Rob Kaufelt, and it is always an adventure to sample the treasures he finds on his worldwide jaunts.

> By some accounts cheese is the leading source of saturated fat in American diets (beef is second and milk third).

If you are a dairy producer, the best thing about cheese is that it uses up surplus milk. It takes about 10 pounds of whole milk to make a pound of cheese (as compared to the 21 pounds of milk it takes to make a pound of butter). Whole milk, of course, is a source of fat, and that fat—along with some of the protein—goes into any cheese made from it. Fat (and the calories and saturated fatty acids it provides) are the big issues related to cheese, and they deserve scrutiny.

But before we do the scrutiny, let's take a digression into cheese making. Cheese makers begin by curdling the milk so they can separate the fat and protein from the watery whey. They do this by adding rennet, a curdling enzyme, to the milk (which can be whole or reduced fat, raw or pasteurized). Rennet, however, only works if acids are present, so cheese makers add "friendly" bacteria that feed on the nutrients in the milk and produce acid as a by-product. By the time the bacteria have done their work, the milk proteins are coagulated and the fat is loaded with flavor. A hard cheese without much water left, one that is aged and dried—like a cheddar, for example—is likely to be one-third fat by weight, and nearly two-thirds of that fat will be the saturated kind. Eat an ounce of cheese—and that means just a slice or a couple of one-inch cubes—and you are getting 10 grams of fat (6 of them saturated) and 120 calories. Softer cheeses have more water and, therefore, fewer calories. Cottage cheese is a special case; it is mostly protein and has a mere 30 calories per ounce. But for most cheeses, you can figure that an ounce will cost you about 100 calories and 8 grams of fat, 5 of them saturated. For an average adult, this is one-quarter of the "Daily Value," the food label's allowance for saturated fat. This means that cheese is best eaten in tiny amounts—gratings, shavings, slivers, and light smears, not scarfed by the half-pound or slathered a half-inch high on pizza.

As for low-fat cheeses, a reduced-fat cheddar cuts the damage in half, and a low-fat muenster or skim-milk ricotta cuts the calories and the fat by one-third, but I say: Why bother? They do not taste nearly as good. I much prefer to save my calorie and fat budgets for really good cheeses and just not eat too much of them at any one time.

Rob Kaufelt of Murray's, who sells cheeses made from raw as well as pasteurized milks, can demonstrate in seconds that superb cheeses can be made from either. But either can also carry harmful bacteria. Cheese-borne illnesses can be troublesome or deadly when the cause is a toxic *Salmonella* or *Listeria*, especially if the bacteria turn out to be resistant to antibiotics and, therefore, hard to cure. Outbreaks of illness from eating cheese are rare; the Center for Science in the Public Interest lists just eight outbreaks from raw-milk cheeses during the eleven-year period from 1990 to 2001, and just three or four per year from any kind of cheese. That is not many, but people are not statistics; if someone you know or love were to die as a result of a cheese-borne illness, even numbers that low would seem unacceptable.

Cheese is a rare cause of food-borne illness because most types get dried and aged, and both of those processes inhibit bacterial growth. That is why the cheeses most likely to be harmful are the soft, fresh ones—the Mexican *queso fresco* made from raw milk, for example—but other kinds of cheeses, pasteurized and not, also have caused illnesses on occasion.

When a raw-milk cheese is implicated, it invariably causes food-safety experts to demand that all cheeses produced domestically be made from pasteurized milk, and that imports of unpasteurized cheeses made in other countries be severely restricted. Whether the government should require cheese makers to pasteurize the milk they use or to follow other special safety procedures are matters that depend on point of view. Surely the maker of every food should have well-designed safety procedures firmly in place and should follow those procedures to the letter—and that includes the makers of raw-milk cheeses. If they are doing what they are supposed to do to ensure safety, the risk is negligible. But without government supervision—and there really isn't much—you and I can have no idea whether cheese makers are adhering to the best safety practices.

Surely the maker of every food should have well-designed safety procedures firmly in place and should follow those procedures to the letter—and that includes the makers of raw-milk cheeses.

I believe that it is possible to produce raw-milk cheeses safely because I have seen it done. In the summer, my New York University department offers a course on food and culture based in Florence, and in 2002 I joined the class for a field trip to the largest producer of raw-milk pecorino and ricotta cheeses in Italy. Ricotta—a soft cheese meant to be eaten fresh—was in full production on the day we visited, and the employees were elbow deep in warm, raw sheep's milk. I was curious to know if anyone in charge was the least concerned about safety. When I asked, as politely as I could, the manager immediately trotted out his resident full-time microbiologist. She seemed surprised by the question. Of course they had a safety plan in place. Of course they tested every batch of cheese for every bacterial species I could think of, required their milk suppliers to do the same, and aged and dried the other kinds of cheeses they made for a period twice as long as required by the FDA. Would I eat raw-milk cheeses from this company? Of course I would. But if I am thinking of eating any other raw-milk cheeses, I have no choice but to rely on the sellers to make certain that their suppliers are just as careful.

Safety issues do not arise often with cheeses, even though they are loaded with bacteria. That is because most of the bacteria are friendly types that are added deliberately to ferment the milk, coagulate it into curds, and give it flavor. Fermentation is how yeast turns grapes to wine; this process also turns milk to cheese, yogurt, and other such bacterially enhanced dairy products. One of these, yogurt, comes next on our tour.

9

Yogurt: Health Food or Dessert

Yogurt is fermented milk. It has the nutrient value of milk. Like any other milk product, the calories in yogurt depend on how much fat it has and whatever else is added to it. Plain yogurt can be a nutritious and satisfying snack or accompaniment to meals, but it is easier to sell—and is more profitable—when it gets turned into a product of infinite variety and cloying sweetness. Beyond that, what truly sets yogurt apart from most other dairy foods is its health mystique. Yogurt has the aura of health. Whether it deserves this special reputation is a matter worth examining. Let's take a good look at each of yogurt's selling points—infinite variety, cloying sweetness, and health mystique—and see how they work in practice.

INFINITE VARIETY

If you are a dairy producer and want to sell your product in a crowded supermarket, you need shelf space—and the more the better. Even if you are paying slotting fees, a carton of milk or a little cup of yogurt does not take up enough room to attract much notice. But variations on a basic product theme—"line extensions"—do. Suddenly that case is overflowing with your products, stacked one on top of another in dozens of flavors, each available in whole, low-fat, and nonfat varieties, organic and not.

Nowhere are line extensions more evident than in the yogurt section of the refrigerated dairy cases. One afternoon in August 2004, I did some counting in a local Associated Supermarket, a medium-size store by national standards. I had to go back twice to check my counts because I could not believe the number of different kinds of yogurts stocked in this store — more than 400. But just try to find a plain, unflavored yogurt with nothing added except the bacterial cultures required to make it. I found a few eventually, but I had to look hard for them.

CLOYING SWEETNESS

Flavor, of course, is how yogurt makers vary their lines and take up shelf space. With yogurt, however, the predominant flavor is sweet. Sweet sells, and nearly all yogurts are sweetened. But yogurts are not just sweetened; they are sweetened in the most artfully imaginative ways: anything you could dream up, from piña colada and custard, to cotton candy and cheesecake. Yogurts are sweetened with added sugar, of course, but also with honey, molasses, lactose, fructose, fruit concentrates, corn syrup, corn syrup solids, fructose syrup, high fructose corn syrup, or, if you prefer, aspartame and other artificial sweeteners. As if sugar does not make yogurts sweet enough, their makers throw in sweet additions: candy sprinkles, M&M's, chocolate (black and white), and Oreo cookies. As part of the health theme, you can get yogurt sugared and flavored with every conceivable choice of fruit: cherries, peaches, pineapples, guava, and berries galore. Some fruit-flavored yogurts actually have fruit in them, but caveat emptor: most have more sugar than fruit, and many have no real fruit at all — just fruit juice concentrates, added colors to make them look fruitier, and thickeners (flour, corn starch, pectin, and carrageenan) to hold them together. The 6-ounce containers vary from 80 to 240 calories, and the ones that are

> Some fruit-flavored yogurts actually have fruit in them, but caveat emptor: most have more sugar than fruit, and many have no real fruit at all—just fruit juice concentrates, added colors to make them look fruitier, and thickeners (flour, corn starch, pectin, and carrageenan) to hold them together.

most caloric hold an entire ounce of sugars. Even the 4-ounce "baby" yogurts contain half an ounce of sugars. Only if you are a yogurt purist and look carefully are you likely to find "authentic" Greek or other un-flavored yogurts with "no artificial sweeteners or other yucky stuff," as the Stonyfield yogurt containers proclaim.

THE HEALTH MYSTIQUE: "FRIENDLY BACTERIA"

It is because of the health mystique that *Dairy Foods Magazine* calls yo-gurt "a world of opportunity" for dairy producers. And it is the health mystique that makes *Organic Style* say: "Loaded with calcium and pro-tein, yogurt may also boost your immune system, thanks to healthful bacteria called probiotics. And it tastes like dessert!" Of course it tastes like dessert; most yogurts *are* desserts. Yogurt, it seems, has performed a marketing miracle; it is a fast-selling dairy dessert with the aura of a health food.

When I was growing up, you could hardly get yogurt except in health food stores. It was considered an exotic foreign food, although even then yogurt was rumored to be responsible for the exceptional longevity of people living in remote regions of the Cau-casian Mountains of Central Asia. The rumors dated back to the early 1900s, when a distinguished Russian scientist, Elie Metchnikoff, had the idea that Bulgarians lived to be very old be-cause they ate yogurt. Like cheese, yogurt is the curdled result of the action of friendly bacteria on milk. Metchnikoff identified the particular kind of friendly bacteria in Bulgarian yogurts as *Lactobacillus bulgaricus*. He suggested that these bacteria might replace harmful bacteria in the large intestine, thereby prolonging life.

In 1973, Alexander Leaf, a respected Harvard cardiologist, published an article about these long-lived people in *National Geographic*. This was gorgeously illustrated with photographs of people in the Soviet Cau-casus who looked truly ancient but were still remarkably active and enjoy-ing life. Two years later, the Dannon company used the article as the basis for a commercial filmed in the mountains of Soviet Georgia. It

> Yogurt, it seems, has performed a marketing miracle; it is a fast-selling dairy dessert with the aura of a health food.

showed an active elderly man (said to be 89) and his equally active mother (said to be 114) happily eating Dannon yogurt. Later scrutiny by skeptical investigators revealed that the Georgians typically exaggerated their ages and said they did not particularly like yogurt or eat it regularly. Today, research on the health effects of yogurt also turns out to be uncertain and exaggerated. Despite all this, yogurt hangs on to its healthful mystique.

For Americans, unflavored yogurt is an acquired taste. It is, after all, sour milk. But once you get used to it, yogurt has a refreshingly tart flavor and a thick, creamy texture that many people find delicious. I certainly do. Oddly, yogurt's healthful mystique depends on its bacteria. For most foods, ensuring safety and palatability means getting rid of bad bacteria, but each of those little yogurt containers is supposed to have hundreds of millions of good bacteria, all of them alive, active, and ready to multiply as soon as the temperature warms up. The mere thought makes you want to add sugar.

The starting point for yogurt is milk—whole, low fat, or skim—that is first pasteurized to kill off unwanted bacteria. Into it go two or more kinds of friendly bacteria, typically *Lactobacillus bulgaricus* and *Streptococcus thermophilus*. Yogurt makers refer to these bacteria as "cultures" because they are cultured—cultivated, fed, and grown—on nutrients in the milk. Because these particular bacteria are rather delicate and are largely killed by the strong acids in your stomach, commercial yogurt producers often add hardier species such as *Lactobacillus acidophilus* or other *Lactobacillus* and *Bifidus* species. Whatever the type, all of these bacteria go to work fermenting (that is, digesting) the nutrients in milk while producing lactic acid and other substances that curdle and flavor it. Most of the lactose gets used up, which is why yogurt is tolerable to many people who otherwise cannot eat dairy products.

Lactobacilli and other yogurt bacteria are not only harmless; they also may replace harmful bacteria in the intestinal tract and, perhaps, do other good deeds. But this means they have to be alive and present in large enough quantities to survive digestion. Just about every supermarket yogurt carries a "Live & Active** Cultures" seal. The text following the asterisks tells you that the product meets certain criteria for yogurt cultures set by the National Yogurt Association, a trade group for this industry. The National Yogurt Association grants its "Live & Active Cultures" seal to yogurts that contain at least 100 million living *Lactobacillus* and *Streptococcus* bacteria per gram at the time they were made, as demonstrated by certified laboratory tests.

If you are squeamish, you had best skip the next sentence. One of those 6-ounce yogurt containers holds about 180 grams, so it had, or still has, about 18 *billion* live bacteria. How many bacteria are still alive and kicking at the time you open the container and start eating, however, is a mystery. The Yogurt Association does not test products at the retail level. Fortunately, *Consumer Reports* did. Most of the yogurts it tested had plenty of live and active bacteria—15 billion to 155 billion per serving. Supplements of bacteria in capsules, however, sometimes had much less (as little as 20 million per dose).

> The National Yogurt Association grants its "Live & Active Cultures" seal to yogurts that contain at least 100 million living *Lactobacillus* and *Streptococcus* bacteria per gram at the time they were made, as demonstrated by certified laboratory tests.

Consumer Reports did not test for the number of living bacteria in frozen yogurt. Frozen yogurt only has to have 10 million bacteria per gram at the time it was made, because it is more difficult for bacteria to survive when frozen. Some undoubtedly do, but unless manufacturers add *Lactobacillus acidophilus* and other hardy bacteria, assume that there will not be many. This is too bad, because if yogurt has benefits, these depend on the ability of bacteria to grow and multiply and to replace the bacteria in your body that may not be so friendly.

YOGURT: A "FUNCTIONAL" HEALTH FOOD?

A rather large body of research supports the idea that *acidophilus* and some other *Lactobacillus* and *Bifidus* bacteria do survive digestion, which is not surprising since these bacteria are normal inhabitants of the human intestinal tract. There also is no question that these bacteria consume the lactose in dairy products, making yogurt—frozen or not—more tolerable to people who cannot digest this sugar. Yogurt bacteria have one other benefit. If you give foods cultured with these bacteria or supplements of such bacteria to infants with diarrhea, the symptoms do not last quite as long and are a little less severe, although not by much.

Beyond that, the research is less certain. In 2004, a group of scientists wrote a long and comprehensive review of research examining the effects of yogurt on health (yes, such research exists, and there is lots of it). They found yogurt or supplements of its bacteria to show "promising health benefits," suggesting that either form might alleviate symptoms of constipation, inflammatory bowel disease, colon cancer, stomach ulcers, and allergies. This review, conveniently initiated and paid for by the National Yogurt Association, unsurprisingly concluded that "Patients with any of these conditions could *possibly benefit* from the consumption of yogurt" (my emphasis).

I am never sure how to interpret the meaning of "possibly benefit," but I have no trouble understanding why the National Yogurt Association would pay for such a review. Yogurt has been the fastest-growing dairy product in the United States for decades. As long ago as January 1978, *Consumer Reports* published an analysis of the yogurts then on the market, noting how quickly sales were growing. Since then, yogurt production in the United States has increased fivefold—from 570 million pounds to a breathtaking 2.5 billion pounds in 2003. Although the recent figure seems like a lot of yogurt, it works out to just 7 pounds or so per capita per year—meager by international standards. The Swedes, for example, consume 63 pounds each per year, which means there is ample room for American yogurt producers to expand the market for their products. Health is a great way to sell food products, which is why the yogurt mystique matters so much.

> Yogurt has been the fastest-growing dairy product in the United States for decades.

Marketing imperatives, not health, explain attempts to turn yogurt into a "functional" food, meaning one that has special nutritional benefits over and above its content of nutrients. In March 2001, *Food Technology* described the reinvention of yogurt into products filled with added "designer" bacteria, now given their own new name: "probiotics." If you have not seen this term before, you might make a note of it because you will certainly be seeing it again. Probiotics means the opposite of antibiotics. The idea is that the added probiotic bacteria will survive passage through the digestive tract and help prevent the diarrhea that sometimes comes with antibiotic treatment.

An entire science has grown up around probiotics and—another new term—"prebiotics." This one means food that especially stimulates the growth of probiotic bacteria. Foods with fiber—fruits, vegetables, and whole grains—contain carbohydrates that resist the action of human digestive enzymes but can be digested by bacteria in the large intestine, probiotics among them.

Companies with vested interests in promoting the health benefits of dairy foods sponsor scientific conferences on probiotics and prebiotics and reviews of favorable studies. Unfortunately for yogurt companies, the results continue to suggest nothing more than "possible" benefits. The trade journal *Food Technology* dryly summarizes this situation: "If a downside to the probiotic trend exists, it relates to its newness and the lack of scientific evidence to back some of the claims . . ."

YOGURT FOR KIDS

The idea that yogurt is especially healthful makes it an ideal product for the dairy industry to market to kids. Parents will urge their children to eat yogurt without thinking too much about what is actually in it. This marketing opportunity is so enticing that it has resulted in "yogurt wars" between Dannon (which is owned by Groupe Danone) and Yoplait (which is owned by General Mills). In 1995, Yoplait had just half the sales of Dannon. But Go-GURT, Yoplait's "kid-friendly slurpable yogurt in a tube," changed all that. Introduced nationally in 1999 with a $10 million advertising campaign specifically directed to children aged eight to twelve, Go-GURT increased its market share practically overnight. In retaliation, Dannon created a virtually identical product (except for the packaging), Danimals, and backed it with a $12 million advertising campaign.

As far as I can tell, the chief weapon in the yogurt battles is sugar.

Both brands are desserts. Sugars constitute 55 percent of the 80 calories in Go-GURT, 67 percent of the 90 calories in Danimals Drinkable, and 68 percent of the 170 calories in Danimals XL. Even in Stonyfield's YoBaby organic yogurts, marketed for infants and toddlers, 53 percent of the 120 calories come from added sugars. Some of Stonyfield's yogurts for older kids appear berry-flavored, but they have no fruit at all; their sweetness comes from juice concentrate and sugars, of course, and their color comes from beet juice. Stonyfield may be organic, but it is Big Yogurt; Groupe Danone owns 85 percent of the company.

So is yogurt a health food or not? It depends. Beyond the marketing hype, I think there may be something to the *acidophilus* story, and I like the idea that friendly bacteria replace the bad ones and do good things for health. Even if the evidence for special health benefits is not as compelling as advertised, eating yogurt for its friendly bacteria is attractive, worth trying, and can't hurt.

When it comes to what kind of yogurt, however, I am a purist. I favor the plain, unadorned kind, especially when it is made from organic milk. I choose the level of fat depending on how I intend to eat the yogurt. The nonfat version, for example, tastes just fine when mixed with foods of other flavors, raw or cooked. If I want fruit, I'll add my own, fresh or frozen, and avoid the heavy sugars, fruitless juice concentrates, and other "yucky stuff" that comes in most supermarket yogurts. If I want it sweeter, I'll toss in my own teaspoonful or two of sugar. No matter how much I add, it will be a lot less than what is added commercially. And I cannot help but get cranky about the amount of sugar that yogurt makers are putting into products for babies and older children. Surely it is a good idea to teach children to enjoy flavors other than sweet, and all those extra sugar and sweetener calories cannot possibly help the national weight problem.

> I f I want fruit, I'll add my own, fresh or frozen, and avoid the heavy sugars, fruitless juice concentrates, and other "yucky stuff" that comes in most supermarket yogurts.

With that said, I am going to leave the dairy aisles without discussing the other products made with bacterially fermented milk: *acidophilus* milk, sour cream, buttermilk, kefir, koumiss, and all the others. Many of these products have long traditions of use in one or another part of the

world and they vary greatly in flavor, texture, and components introduced during fermentation. They raise no nutritional issues beyond the
ones already covered, however. These products can be appreciated for
their taste, nutritional value, and low lactose content, and the best ones
have live cultures and the fewest sweeteners and other additives.

10

Margarine: Accept No Substitutes

Margarines, nondairy creamers, and soy products are packaged to look just like butter, cream, and milk, but they contain practically nothing that actually comes from a cow. If you cannot eat or do not like dairy foods, and you enjoy the taste of the "substitutes," you will be glad they exist and will be happy to buy them, especially because they almost always cost less than actual dairy foods (their ingredients are cheaper). But I do not care for their taste very much, and I find them nutritionally confusing. They are usually lower in undesirable saturated fat than their dairy counterparts, and are free of lactose and hormones that you might want to avoid. So far so good, but then they are loaded with additives—emulsifiers, gels, flavors, and colors—to disguise their true nature and I do not like much of anything artificial when it comes to food.

Nevertheless, supermarkets shelve the dairy substitutes right next to the dairy foods, where they are in direct competition. Beyond price, the chief weapons in this competition are claims for health benefits. Their marketers position dairy substitutes as healthier alternatives to dairy foods, and tout them as "functional" foods, meaning ones with special health benefits that no dairy food can provide. Margarines are prime examples of this strategy.

Margarines are no longer just butter substitutes. The sticks, tubs, sprays, and squeeze bottles that you find in supermarkets carry labels with statements like these: no lactose, no gluten, no GMOs, organic, 100% vegan, light, no *trans* fats, or low saturated fat. Most improbably, one even says "fat free." Some have extra calcium, vitamin E, or omega-3 fats. Some are made from olive or canola oils. The most expensive margarines put statements like these on their labels: "Help promote healthy cholesterol balance" (Smart Balance brand), "Proven to significantly lower cholesterol" (Take Control), or "Clinically proven to significantly reduce cholesterol" (Benecol). These health claims are the kind requiring FDA approval, which means that some research backs them up even if the cholesterol lowering is small unless you eat large amounts. But however small the improvement, claims for health benefits help sell food products, and health claims on margarines especially help sell margarines.

> **N**o matter what their labels say, all margarines are basically the same—mixtures of soybean oil and food additives. Everything else is theater and greasepaint.

What I find most surprising about margarines is their similarity. No matter what their labels say, all margarines are basically the same—mixtures of soybean oil and food additives. Everything else is theater and greasepaint. The label of ConAgra's "cholesterol-free" Parkay says, "The flavor says BUTTER." But its list of ingredients says:

Liquid soybean oil, partially hydrogenated soybean oil, whey, water, salt, vegetable mono- and diglycerides and soy lecithin (emulsifiers), sodium benzoate (to preserve freshness), artificial flavor, phosphoric acid (acidulant), vitamin A palmitate, colored with beta carotene (source of vitamin A)

Translation: soy oil and additives. Soy oil may be a perfectly reasonable cooking and salad oil on its own, but margarine makers expect you to like what they have done to it and believe it is good for you.

Even the most elaborate margarines are soy oil and additives. The label of Smart Balance Omega-3 type (from GFA Brands) may say "New! No *trans*-fatty acids. Now with plant sterols & omega-3 from the sea," but it still has soy oil, in this case from a "Natural Oil Blend" of palm fruit, soy, canola, organic menhaden, and olive oils. This margarine has some additives that can lower blood cholesterol under certain circumstances, but the others are theater and greasepaint—cosmetics that thicken, flavor, and color the margarine to give it the feel, taste, and look of butter. Olive oil margarines contain soy oil. The Olivio brand from Lee Iacocca and Unilever may advertise its Mediterranean origins and "rich buttery taste," but that taste comes from a blend of liquid canola oil, partially hydrogenated soy oil, and third and last on the list (meaning its amount is smallest), extra light olive oil. If a margarine label says "vegetable oil," it means soy oil. There are rare exceptions like Canoleo margarine made from liquid and partially hydrogenated canola (rapeseed) oil, but that difference will cost you more money.

Margarines compete with butter on price, and are usually much cheaper. Nevertheless, margarines pose at least four difficult marketing challenges: (1) they are fats and, therefore, high in calories; (2) they require food additives to disguise their industrial origins and mask their unpleasant taste; and (3) their soy oil base is liquid, not solid, and it has to be hydrogenated to harden it—and this introduces unnatural and unhealthful *trans* fats. One further issue concerns some people: (4) unless the margarine is labeled as organic, you have to assume it was made from genetically modified (GM) soybeans or, occasionally, rapeseed. The industry's response to concerns about calories, taste, *trans* fats, and genetic modification has been to get you to ignore them by marketing margarine as healthier than butter or as a "functional" food.

The industry's response to concerns about calories, taste, *trans* fats, and genetic modification has been to get you to ignore them by marketing margarine as healthier than butter or as a "functional" food.

Of the challenges, the trickiest is the one involving hydrogenation and its consequences. Soy oil is a liquid at room temperature, but margarines are supposed to be solid yet soft enough to be spreadable and melt in your mouth. Getting margarine to be both at the same time is a triumph of food technology—in this case, accomplished through hydrogenation. To make margarine, food chemists purify soy oil and force just enough hydrogen through it to give the resulting mixture of fatty acids the precise degree of hardness required.

A quick word about fatty acids. Fatty acids are the building blocks of fats (solids) and oils (liquids). Fatty acids come in three types: saturated (fully hydrogenated), unsaturated (incompletely hydrogenated), and polyunsaturated (more incompletely hydrogenated). Adding hydrogen to soy oil has two consequences, neither of them good. Hydrogenation increases the proportion of saturated fatty acids, the type that tends to raise blood cholesterol levels and the risk for coronary heart disease. Hydrogenation also creates *trans*-fatty acids, which also raise heart disease risk. I will have more to say about the health aspects of fats and oils in the chapter devoted to that topic, but for the moment, let's take a detour into the making of margarine.

MARGARINE AS A FAT

The fats in soybeans, like the fats in all other foods, are *mixtures* of saturated, monounsaturated, and polyunsaturated fatty acids. No food fat is exclusively one or the other; it is the proportions that differ. Food fats that are largely saturated tend to be solid at room temperature—beef fat, for example. In contrast, soy fat, which is largely polyunsaturated, is a liquid oil and rather unstable. If left around long enough, polyunsaturated oils become rancid, and smell and taste bad. Hydrogenation fixes those problems; it makes the fat more solid and resistant to chemical damage. Soy oil naturally contains enough saturated fatty acids to require only a little hydrogenation to convert it to a solid and stable margarine.

But margarine never gets fully (100 percent) saturated because that would make it much too hard to spread. Instead, it is partially hydrogenated. What the partial hydrogenation of soy oil does to the mix of fatty acids in margarine is shown on the next page.

If margarine were 100 percent saturated (which it never is), no polyunsaturated or monounsaturated fatty acids would be left and the Table

Americans readily accepted margarine as a substitute for butter during the war out of a sense of patriotic duty and because of its cheap cost. It also was (and still is) a source of vitamin A. For this, thank food technology again. Soy oil has no vitamin A (vitamin A is found only in foods of animal origin). But in the years just before the war, in response to complaints that margarine had no nutritional value, margarine manufacturers lobbied for permission to add vitamin A (and sometimes vitamin D). Once they got that permission, they lobbied further for a federal standard that recognized margarine as nutritious. They drew support from food retailers who sold margarine, trade associations for soybeans and cottonseeds, and agricultural experts promoting greater use of American farm products. They won the standard in 1941. Together, these groups were able to bring about an end to taxes on margarine in 1950 and to get most states to allow sales of artificially colored margarine. Wisconsin was the last hold-out. In trying to protect its dairy interests, it managed to keep butter-colored margarine off supermarket shelves until 1967.

MARGARINE AND HEALTH

From the start, margarine was sold as a cheap substitute for butter. The idea that margarine was healthier than butter came up only after World War II and, as far as I can determine, as a result of a misleading interpretation of dietary advice. Right after the war, cardiologists noted a sharp increase in cases of coronary heart disease. They attributed the increase to changes in diet and activity patterns that had occurred as unforeseen consequences of rising prosperity. They soon figured out that diets high in saturated fatty acids raised blood cholesterol levels, and that these in turn increased the risk of coronary heart disease. Saturated fatty acids are more common in meat and dairy foods: more than 50 percent of the fatty acids in butter are saturated. In contrast, the hardest partially hydrogenated margarines are only about 20 percent saturated. Nobody knew anything about the *trans*-fat problem in the 1950s, so with less than half the saturated fatty acids of butter, margarine seemed healthier.

I often hear margarine used as a prime example of how nutrition advice changes all the time. First it was supposed to be good for you, then bad, and now it is supposed to be good for you again. But a careful reading of cardiologists' advice over the years gives a more consistent story. For more than forty years, the American Heart Association has issued cautious and nuanced advice about margarine. It has always put hard margarines in the same category as butter. As early as 1958, its nutrition advisers were saying that avoiding butter was a good way to reduce intake of saturated fat, but so was "avoiding oleomargarine, hydrogenated shortenings . . . and foods made from them." Without knowing anything about *trans* fat, they saw that hydrogenation made fats more saturated. In 1959, the cardiologist Ancel Keys and his wife, Margaret, published a cookbook with dietary guidelines in which they advised readers to "restrict saturated fats, the fats in . . . margarine, solid shortenings . . ." In 1968, the American Heart Association noted that heavily hydrogenated margarines "are ineffective in lowering the serum cholesterol" and the next year suggested replacing butter with polyunsaturated margarines (these are the softer ones that come in tubs; they have less saturated fat and also less *trans* fat). The American Heart Association continued to advise substituting soft margarines for butter until 2000, when it finally—and rather late in the game—recommended limits on anything containing *trans* fats.

For more than forty years, the American Heart Association has issued cautious and nuanced advice about margarine. It has always put hard margarines in the same category as butter.

GETTING RID OF *TRANS* FATS

More recent health concerns about *trans* fat put margarine makers in a quandary. There is no simple, inexpensive substitute for hydrogenated soy oil. The most obvious is palm fruit oil, which comes 50 percent saturated straight from the tree and, like butter, is solid at room temperature (this oil differs from palm kernel oil, which is at least 80 percent saturated). This alternative makes the margarine industry's quandary especially ironic. In the late 1980s, soybean lobbying groups did everything they could to get competing palm oils out of the food supply, but now they want them back as a substitute for *trans* fats. Most of the saturated fat in palm fruit oil is palmitic acid, a fat especially adept at raising cholesterol levels. In that sense—and because cultivation of palm oil trees in Indonesia and Malaysia destroys tropical rain forests and threatens endangered species of land mammals and birds—palm oils are decidedly worse than butter. You would never know this, however, from reading palm oil industry materials such as those I picked up at a nutrition meeting in Durban, South Africa, in 2005. Pamphlets and fliers extol the virtues of palm oil, among them "no cholesterol, no *trans* fat, no GMO, no sodium, 100 percent vegan, and attractive natural color"—all true of any vegetable oil, of course. Palm oil companies dispense with the troublesome palmitic acid problem by emphasizing the positive: half the fatty acids are unsaturated, after all.

Companies have taken steps to reduce *trans* fats, mainly by diluting them with water or air, but they still comprise 15 percent or more of the fat in hydrogenated margarines. A look at the Nutrition Facts label of ConAgra's Parkay margarine, for example, illustrates the problem. It lists 10 grams of total fat per tablespoon, but the grams of saturated, monounsaturated, and polyunsaturated fats add up to only 7.5 grams.

> One way margarine companies deal with the *trans* fat problem is to deny that it is a problem at all and, instead, put a favorable spin on the science.

The remaining 2.5 grams are mostly *trans* (unlabeled until 2006). The dilemma: if margarine makers do not hydrogenate, they have soy oil, not margarine. If they substitute palm oil, they get margarine but increase saturated fats. Their only alternative is to turn to complicated and expensive food technology to thicken the oil without hydrogenating it, but this will raise the price of margarine and make it less competitive with butter.

One way margarine companies deal with the *trans* fat problem is to deny that it is a problem at all and, instead, put a favorable spin on the science. To that end, the United Soybean Board and National Association of Margarine Manufacturers funded a study designed to produce data supporting the health "benefits" of margarine. Participants in the study used either butter or a margarine that had been specially formulated to be low in both saturated and *trans* fat. The investigators reported that soft margarines reduced cholesterol levels, and that any cholesterol-raising effect attributed to margarine must be due to genetics rather than to *trans* fats. The sponsors announced the results in full-page newspaper advertisements: "[This] groundbreaking study . . . proves that using margarine instead of butter *significantly lowers cholesterol.*" Of course it does—under these particular study conditions. The study unsurprisingly confirmed the already well-known advantage of replacing saturated with unsaturated fat in daily diets. The other claims made for the health benefits of margarine also must be interpreted in context, as I explain next.

11

Margarine: You *Can* Believe It's Not Butter

argarines may be cheaper than butter, but their prices range widely and roughly in proportion to the size of their health claims. The more extravagant the health claims, the more extravagant the price. The cheapest ones just say "no cholesterol." But you pay a higher price for margarines that are free of lactose, gluten, genetic modification (GM), or *trans* fat; the ones that are organic or vegan; and those that are "light"—low in calories, fat, or saturated fat, or with no fat at all. You pay more for margarines boosted with extra calcium, vitamin E, omega-3 fats, olive oil, or canola oil, and you pay much more for the ones that contain substances that really do lower your cholesterol, at least by a little.

Are the healthier margarines worth the higher cost? I am not convinced that they are. Some of the nutrition claims made for margarine are just silly—"no cholesterol," for example. Of course, margarines do not contain cholesterol. Soybeans are vegetables and cholesterol only comes from foods derived from animals: meat, dairy, eggs, and fish. For a similar reason, I would never expect these margarines to contain gluten; gluten comes from wheat and other grains and these are not typical margarine ingredients. Unless milk, whey, or the sugar from milk has been added, margarines would not have lactose—so margarine usually is "lactose free." The addition of healthier additives also makes little difference. Omega-3s, for example, are "good" fats that come mainly from fish oils. Margarine is an odd place for them, and researchers say you do not get enough omega-3s from this source to do much good.

The 100 percent vegan margarines also promise nutritional benefits that are not always specific to these products. The "natural buttery spreads" from Earth Balance are non-hydrogenated (good) and *trans* fat free (also good). These contain flavor additives "derived from corn, no MSG, no alcohol, no gluten"; lactic acid that is "nondairy, derived from sugar beets"; and annatto color rather than beta-carotene (but beta-carotene is also plant-derived). Margarines would not be expected to contain MSG (monosodium glutamate). Although the vegan margarines do not have dairy-derived whey, neither do most other kinds. Lactic acid is an isolated chemical no matter where it comes from. As far as I can tell, the various spreads from this company are much the same except for the one that is Certified Organic and another one that is Certified Kosher. All say they are made with "non-GMO" ingredients, meaning that the soybeans used to make the oil are not patented varieties genetically engineered to resist insects or pesticides. GMO or not, vegan or not, organic or not, margarines are concoctions of soy oil—fat and cosmetic additives. The health claims on these packages are there to distract you from remembering that margarine is a fat and has calories.

As for "light" margarines: these have fewer calories and less fat because their first ingredient is water. This type needs a greater range of emulsifier additives to keep the fat and water mixed, and these affect taste and cooking properties, not always happily.

That leaves the oxymoronic "no fat" margarine to be explained. The I Can't Believe It's Not Butter (Unilever/Bestfoods) brand includes a fat-free option with just 5 calories per tablespoon. The label for this particular miracle of food technology lists zeros for all possible sources

Some of the nutrition claims made for margarine are just silly—"no cholesterol," for example. Of course, margarines do not contain cholesterol. Soybeans are vegetables and cholesterol only comes from foods derived from animals: meat, dairy, eggs, and fish.

of those calories—fat, protein, and carbohydrate—meaning that the amounts of them in a serving have to be less than one-half gram each. So what *is* in this product? The first ingredient is water. Next come the additives, starting with mono- and diglycerides (emulsifiers), then salt and more emulsifiers and gels. These last include rice starch, gelatin, lecithin, and something called "vegetable Datem," which turns out to be yet another monoglyceride (fat) emulsifier. The product is sweetened with lactose and dolled up with color and flavor cosmetics. This "naturally cholesterol free," no-fat margarine looks like a tub margarine but tastes just the way you might expect of a mixture of water, salt, and plenty of food additives: smooth and spreadable, but salty and, well, chemical. Skeptic that I am, I certainly can believe it's not butter.

"No *trans* fat" also needs an explanation, not least because such margarines often list hydrogenated soy oil high up on their ingredient lists. This is a puzzle. If soy oil is hydrogenated, what happened to the *trans*-fatty acids? The answer: another miracle of food technology. This particular miracle depends on the fact that *trans*-fatty acids are unsaturated. Oil chemists add so much hydrogen to the soy oil that all of the fatty acids become completely saturated (and, therefore, free of the ones that are *trans*). Next, the chemists mix the fully hydrogenated solid fat with unhydrogenated liquid oil (which is also free of *trans*) until the combined fat spreads like butter. This clever trick is one way to eliminate *trans*-fatty acids, but it is much more difficult and expensive to do than partially hydrogenating the whole lot. That is why margarine manufacturers are engaged in an intense search for alternatives—the highly saturated palm oils among them.

> This "naturally cholesterol free," no-fat margarine looks like a tub margarine but tastes just the way you might expect of a mixture of water, salt, and plenty of food additives: smooth and spreadable, but salty and, well, chemical.

Margarine makers also are searching for additives that will reduce blood cholesterol levels. Such additives—like the plant sterols derived from wood pulp or vegetable oil that I will now discuss—instantly turn margarine from a low-cost spread into a high-end "functional" food, one that can boast of its special health benefits as well as command premium prices.

One Sunday morning, as I was browsing through the mess of fliers that routinely come with the weekend *New York Times*, an ad for Smart Balance Omega Plus margarine caught my eye: "Surprise yourself with the taste of real butter. No cholesterol. No hydrogenation. No *trans*-fatty acids. Helps promote healthy cholesterol balance"—this last statement followed by an asterisk. I love asterisks in food advertisements because they sometimes lead to wonderfully convoluted qualifying statements. This one did not disappoint:

> *The Smart Balance© patented natural vegetable oils can increase HDL "good" cholesterol and improve the ratio of HDL to LDL "bad" cholesterol in the blood. Total intake of this right balance of fats must equal at least two-thirds of the fat intake with total fat intake limited to about 30% of calories consumed and saturated fats to 10%. Avoid foods with partially hydrogenated oil to eliminate *trans* fatty acids. Regular exercise is important.

Regular exercise is very important but what are you to make of the rest of these mind-boggling statements? They no doubt meet the FDA's rule that cholesterol-lowering health claims have to be put in context, but nobody must be expecting you to read them. If you did read them, you might figure out what they really mean: that the other things you eat are more important for reducing your cholesterol level than margarine, and that margarine will help lower your cholesterol if—and only if— everything else you eat is low in saturated and *trans* fats, *and* you get plenty of exercise.

Smart Balance Omega Plus margarine contains 450 milligrams of phytosterols in 1 tablespoon. Phytosterols are chemicals in plants with a shape that resembles that of cholesterol, so they block its action in the body. Since 1999, the FDA has allowed a cholesterol-lowering claim for foods containing these chemicals when they are consumed as part of an otherwise healthy diet and lifestyle. The FDA gave its blessing to phytosterols as a result of petitions by Johnson and Johnson/McNeil Consumer Healthcare and Unilever/Lipton, the makers of Benecol and Take

Control margarines, respectively, for approved health claims they could use on product labels. At the time, the petition seemed surprising, since the companies knew perfectly well that margarine is a high fat table spread that adds calories and, sometimes, *trans* fats to diets.

The claim still seems strange, even though phytosterol-containing margarines are tub types, relatively low in calories, and *trans* fat free. The cholesterol-lowering phytosterols in Benecol come from pine-tree pulp or canola oil (from oilseed rape, a plant in the broccoli and cabbage family), and those in Take Control come from soybeans. Industry-sponsored research in Finland and Canada showed that these chemicals block the absorption of about half of any cholesterol present in the intestine, and can help reduce blood cholesterol levels by about 10 percent in people who eat low-fat diets *and* substitute these margarines for other spreads. Ten percent may not seem like much, but it can mean 20 or 30 points if your cholesterol is 200 or 300. If you are following these rules *and* taking cholesterol-lowering drugs, your blood cholesterol is likely to drop even more. But you have to eat three tablespoons a day of Benecol or two of Take Control or Smart Balance to make the whole scheme work. That is an ounce or more of fat and about 240 calories, which although slightly less than the 300 calories you would get from that amount of butter, is still about 10% of your daily calories.

Price is also an issue. The "functional" margarines cost a lot less than cholesterol-lowering medications, but they are not as effective as those drugs and they are much more expensive than "nonfunctional" margarines. In summer 2004, the cheapest margarine in a supermarket near where I live was the store brand priced at $1.19 per pound. In comparison, a pound of Smart Balance cost $5.58 and a pound of Take Control $8.78. Benecol was $11.98 per pound—ten times as much as the store brand. The high cost—and, perhaps, the not-so-buttery taste—help explain why the sales of these products have never reached the expectations of their manufacturers.

> The "functional" margarines cost a lot less than cholesterol-lowering medications, but they are not as effective as those drugs and they are much more expensive than "nonfunctional" margarines.

In 2003, I gave a talk on the politics of food at a meeting in Lisbon to executives of the Bunge company, the world's largest soybean processor — $22 billion in sales that year. I had been invited to talk about consumer perceptions of *trans* fats. I did not have reassuring news for this group. *Trans* fats, I said, were a no-brainer. They are bad for health — they raise the risk of heart disease — their risks have been known for at least thirty years, and companies should have figured out how to get them out of the food supply a long time ago.

Bunge was particularly interested in this issue at that time because after years of lobbying by nutrition groups on one side and the food industry on the other, the FDA had just ruled that the label of every packaged food would have to disclose its *trans* fat content, starting in 2006. The industry had balked at disclosure for three reasons. First, *trans*-fatty acids are so demonstrably bad for health that disclosure might depress sales. Second, removing *trans*-fatty acids raises costs and can reduce profits. Companies wanted to continue to use partially hydrogenated soy oil as an ingredient because of its perfect consistency, low production costs, and shelf stability. Third, as discussed in the previous chapter, no healthier alternative was available at the low cost of hydrogenated soy oil.

Although plenty of *trans* fat–free margarines were already in supermarkets at the time of the FDA decision in 2003, the Bunge executives in Lisbon explained to me why making such products is a challenge for their industry. About 2.5 billion pounds of margarine are available in the U.S. food supply every year. If *trans* types amount to just 15 percent of the fatty acids in margarine, nearly half a billion pounds of them would have to be replaced. During the 1990s, margarine makers were able to achieve about a 50 percent reduction in *trans* fats (roughly a quarter of a billion pounds), just by blending fully hydrogenated fats with liquid oils and water to produce softer tub margarines. But taking further steps to take *trans* fats out of the food supply would be very expensive. While margarine is one of the major sources of *trans* fats, partially hydrogenated soy oil is an ingredient in cookies, crackers, breakfast cereals, breads, and many other products shelved in supermarket center aisles, as well as in foods fried in such oil. Using oils free of *trans* fats would raise the prices of margarines and snack foods, which no food company ever wants to do.

Having gone through all this, I cannot say with complete confidence just how much you should be worried about *trans* fats. On their own, they are unlikely to be good for you. But neither are saturated fatty acids—and most people eat much more saturated than *trans*-fatty acids. Dietary intake of *trans*-fatty acids seems to average about 3 percent of total calories and as much as 8 percent of calories from fat. In contrast, the average intake of saturated fatty acids from meat and dairy foods is at least three times higher (about 11 percent of total calories and 33 percent of calories from fat) and would be expected to pose a greater risk.

U sing oils free of *trans* fats would raise the prices of margarines and snack foods, which no food company ever wants to do.

Again, while margarine is a major source of *trans*-fatty acids, partially hydrogenated soy oil is an ingredient in a great many foods shelved in supermarket center aisles, and it is also used for frying foods in restaurants and fast-food outlets. If you eat a lot of snack and fried foods, your intake of *trans*-fatty acids will be well above average. Nevertheless, companies selling foods with *trans*-fatty acids argue that you really do not need to worry much about them as the science is incomplete. Like pretty much all science related to diet and health, research on the health effects of *trans*-fatty acids indeed is incomplete.

Evidence from population surveys about the harm caused by *trans* fats in margarine, for example, is difficult to interpret. Heart disease rates in the United States reached their highest levels in the early 1960s and have declined steadily ever since. As the rates were falling, margarine production increased to an all-time high in 1976 of 12 pounds per capita. This looks like heart disease rates fell in parallel with an *increase* in margarine production, suggesting the possibility that eating margarine is a good thing to do. Since then, heart disease rates have continued to fall but so has margarine production; production is now a bit more than 8 pounds per capita per year, roughly twice that of butter. Now it looks like falling rates of heart disease are associated with a *decrease* in margarine production, so it is better to eat less margarine. These are associations and do not necessarily mean that margarine has anything to do with heart disease risk. It is not always easy to make sense of the research on *trans* fats but here's the short answer: if you can avoid *trans* fats, you should. These fatty acids may be only a small part of your total dietary fat, but small changes in your diet can add up to significant health benefits, and this is one change that is well worth making.

> It is not always easy to make sense of the research on *trans* fats but here's the short answer: if you can avoid *trans* fats, you should. These fatty acids may be only a small part of your total dietary fat, but small changes in your diet can add up to significant health benefits, and this is one change that is well worth making.

THE OTHER NONDAIRY SUBSTITUTES

I am not going to say much about nondairy creamers, mainly because the less said about them the better. From a nutritional standpoint, these products do not have much worth recommending. These are food-science concoctions of hydrogenated oils, sugars, and additives, usually with casein. Casein is a milk protein, which might make you wonder why these products are called "nondairy," but that oxymoron is a consequence of FDA rule making. One way to view nondairy creamers is as nothing more than white, sweet, liquid margarines. The fat-free varieties substitute milk solids for fat. The low-carbohydrate versions replace sugars with artificial sweeteners. The chocolate, mocha, and berry flavors mask the taste of the other additives.

> One way to view nondairy creamers is as nothing more than white, sweet, liquid margarines.

The ingredients are cheap and have a long shelf life so food-service companies love to use these products whenever they can get away with it. They package the products to look exactly like milk shakes, yogurt smoothies, and soy-milk drinks, but with a 1-tablespoon, 40-calorie serving size, just like the dry powder original. This may not sound like much but a 16-ounce bottle of Nestlé's Chocolate-Raspberry Coffee-Mate will set you back 1,280 calories. Its calories and high price tell you that you are supposed to use this like cream, and not drink it straight. The equally oxymoronic "Fat-free Half and Half" at least begins with real food. Nonfat milk is its starting ingredient, but the rest are the usual sugars and additives. Despite the milk, my local stores shelve it with the nondairy creamers.

These products—and the *trans* fat–free soft margarines (the ones in the tubs)—not only sell but also have their fans. A quick browse of the Internet shows that practically every brand of dairy substitutes has passionate devotees who write enthusiastic testimonials about how much they love the products. I am not one of them. Taste is a personal matter, and I am perfectly willing to believe that lots of people enjoy eating margarine or nondairy creamers. But I do not care for their taste. No matter what their labels say, to me they taste like the somewhat bitter mixtures of oil and chemicals that they are.

But if you do like margarines, you might as well choose the more nutritious ones. These are usually the softer and more expensive kinds with less saturated fat and *trans* fat (but more additives). So which butter substitute would I recommend? None of the above, really. I prefer butter. A good butter is a wonderful treat, and a little goes a long way. I buy the best butter I can find, store it well wrapped in the freezer, and use it sparingly.

12

Soy Milk: Panacea, or Just Another Food

f you do not like to eat dairy foods because of lactose intolerance, allergies, health concerns, vegetarian preferences, or any other reason, the soy foods—right there in the dairy section—look like good alternatives. But are they? If you are uncertain about whether soy dairy and other soy foods are good for you or not, you have plenty of company. To put the matter another way: if you are *not* confused about soy foods, you must not be reading the newspapers. These are filled with endlessly contradictory accounts of the latest research study on the effects of eating soy foods on one or another aspect of health. But for every research study in my files that promotes the health benefits of soy foods, I can find another that disputes those benefits.

Enthusiasts for soy foods call them "the shining star of the health-food firmament." Soybeans are high in good-quality protein (meaning that their proteins are similar in proportions of amino acids to those of meat and dairy foods), contain a good balance of carbohydrate and fat, and are loaded with minerals. Eat soy foods, say enthusiasts, and you will be protected against a wide array of illnesses: heart disease, cancers (stomach, colon, breast, and prostate), menopausal hot flashes, bone loss, cataracts, immune function disorders, muscle damage, kidney disease, memory loss, weight gain, and, praise be, anxiety. This seems like a lot to ask of any one food.

While plenty of research can be found to support these claims, I find the science to be painfully inconsistent. Some studies find no special effects of soy on health, while others actually suggest that soy foods might *cause* the very health problems they are believed to prevent. And soybeans contain two factors that might specifically affect health: proteins and isoflavones. Soy proteins have been found to reduce blood cholesterol levels and the risk of heart disease. Soybeans also contain unique phytochemicals called isoflavones that behave in the body like weak cousins of the female hormone, estrogen, so they are called "phytoestrogens." Although isoflavones work with soy proteins to reduce blood cholesterol levels, they also act like estrogens—and estrogens are known to increase the risk of breast and other cancers in women. This raises the uncomfortable possibility that soy isoflavones might increase cancer risks, and make you wonder whether infants fed on soy formulas might be exposed to harm from the estrogenic effects of isoflavones.

As I will explain, research about the health aspects of soy foods—pro and con—is so contradictory that it is difficult to draw firm conclusions. At the moment, I find it impossible to make sense of the health debates about soy foods, not least because so much of the research is sponsored by industries with a vested interest in its outcome. These industries include soy producers, processors, product makers, and marketers, all actively promoting the benefits of their products.

THE COMMODITY ISSUES

Soy is so heavily promoted as a health food that you can easily lose sight of its agricultural origins. Soybeans have been grown and consumed as part of traditional diets in China and other Asian countries for millennia, but they did not reach Europe until the seventeenth century and the Americas until even later. In the United States, soybeans were used for animal fodder, and Americans did not really

In the United States, soybeans were used for animal fodder, and Americans did not really begin to eat soy products until 1915 or so, when boll weevils destroyed the supply of cottonseeds.

begin to eat soy products until 1915 or so, when boll weevils destroyed the supply of cottonseeds used to make cooking oil. As a result, cottonseed processing plants went idle until processors figured out that soybeans would be a good substitute. The USDA soon began to promote the production of soybeans with complicated systems of guaranteed prices, tariffs, and subsidies that linger in one form or another to this day. For years, American soybean farmers produced about a third of the soybeans grown throughout the world—34 percent in 2003—but countries like Brazil and Argentina are rapidly catching up, and federal supports are not enough to offset the lower production costs in those countries. Big soy producers like Cargill and Archer Daniels Midland play both sides of the agricultural support game. They lobby for higher subsidies on the one hand, and move production operations to South America on the other.

In 2003, American farmers harvested about 145 billion pounds of soybeans, and it is interesting to see what happened to them. Forty percent got exported, leaving 87 billion pounds for domestic processing, meaning crushing the beans and separating the protein and carbohydrate solids (meal) from the fat (oil). The solids ended up as 70 billion pounds of soy meal, nearly all—90 percent—used to feed chickens, pigs, and other livestock. The remaining 10 percent (a mere 7 billion pounds) went to soy meal for human use. The fat became 18 billion pounds of oil, nearly all processed into margarine, salad oil, and cooking oil. Together, the meal and the oil created 25 billion pounds of soy-food ingredients in search of a market. To summarize the soy-food situation: soy companies produce about 25 billion pounds of meal and oil every year for your use,

> **B**ig soy producers like Cargill and Archer Daniels Midland play both sides of the agricultural support game. They lobby for higher subsidies on the one hand, and move production operations to South America on the other.

much of it federally subsidized, that they are eager to get you to buy. The federal government helps with this task, as well. Since 1991, a USDA-sponsored soybean checkoff program has generated about $45 million annually for "research and education"—meaning marketing—to promote the health benefits of soybeans to consumers.

But soy foods are a hard sell. They are still a relatively new food for most Americans, and we do not take easily to their taste. I, for example, like the fresh soybeans cooked and salted in their pods and served in Japanese restaurants (look for *edamame* on the menu), and I also like soybean curd (tofu) when it is stir-fried with vegetables in a ginger sauce. But I find the flavors and aftertaste of processed soy foods—soy milks, cultured soy, soy cereals, and power bars—unpleasantly bitter (from the soybeans) and "chemical" (from the additives used to mask the soy taste), and I am not alone in this view.

The soy-food industry is all too aware of the taste barrier, and puts much effort into trying to improve public attitudes about eating its products. One way it does this is through research, and soy companies and trade associations sponsor at least three kinds: (1) food science and technology research designed to develop new soy products, to remove their "beany" taste, or to mask the bitter taste with flavor additives; (2) consumer market research designed to encourage favorable attitudes toward soy foods so you will be willing to try them; and (3) basic and clinical research designed to convince you that soy is not only a health food, but a superior health food.

Much such research takes place at the University of Illinois, and not coincidentally. More soybeans are produced in Illinois than in any other state—22 billion pounds worth nearly $3 billion in sales in 2003, and this university is a land-grant institution established in part to promote local agriculture. The university's industry-supported National Soybean Research Laboratory, for example, defines its mission as "expanding the size, scope, and profitability of the U.S. soybean industry." The laboratory's research agenda is to find ways to increase soy production for animal use, but also to develop new foods and identify methods for selling them. The university's corporate-sponsored Illinois Center for Soy Foods conducts research and provides information about how schools can introduce more soy into their lunch programs, and how you might incorporate more soy foods into your daily diet. University Web sites offer online forums to answer your questions about why and how to use soy. For some years, the university housed a research program on functional foods, soy among them, but the "industry-based funding model" that paid for program activities did not generate enough revenue and it closed in 2004. In this case, the soy industry was willing to support favorable university research—but only up to a point.

Food technology research, university or private, often confronts the taste problem head-on. An advertisement to the soy-food trade from Butter Buds (an ingredient company) says: "Who was that masked flavor? No one will ever know, Kimosabe . . . Is added soy contributing off-flavors? Butter Buds will mask them." One from Nutrient (another ingredient company) says: "Too often, soy's mega-healthy benefits come with the baggage of tasting 'earthy' or 'grassy.' Until now . . . Finally, a company that not only provides you with the nutritional ingredients you need, but also the taste and flavors that you crave. *Ahhh*." And Cargill's Soy Protein Solutions advertises that it can "give your customers the great taste and added nutritional benefits they are looking for . . . And open your door to whole new marketing opportunities."

Soy foods have spawned an entire genre of cookbooks devoted to teaching you how to disguise or eliminate the off flavors and turn soybeans into something that you and your family will tolerate or even enjoy. A quick Internet search on Amazon.com for "soy cookbooks" turns up *New Soy, Whole Soy, Complete Soy, Indian Soy, Soy Sauce, Soy Miracle, Soy Health, Soy City,* and *Soy Virtues,* along with *Super Foods, Miracle Foods,* and 3,800 others with soy recipes for vegetarian and vegan diets or diets designed to prevent any number of diseases. Implicitly or explicitly, these books assume that you do not naturally take to soy, will have to work hard to like it, but should find trying to adjust to soy foods to be worth the trouble because they are so good for you.

> Soy foods have spawned an entire genre of cookbooks devoted to teaching you how to disguise or eliminate the off flavors and turn soybeans into something that you and your family will tolerate or even enjoy.

The "so good for you" is the principal selling point, and soybeans offer plenty to work with. To begin with, they contain the nutrients that you would expect to get from any legume, whether pea or bean. As shown in the Table, soybeans are higher in calories, protein, and fat than kidney beans, but lower in carbohydrate and fiber. Both beans are derived from plants so neither has cholesterol and their fats are largely unsaturated.

Composition of Soybeans and Kidney Beans (One-half Cup)*

NUTRIENT	SOYBEANS	KIDNEY BEANS
Calories	400	300
Protein (grams)	34	22
Fat (grams)	19	1
Carbohydrate (grams)	28	55
Fiber (grams)	9	23

*Source: USDA Nutrient Data at www.nal.usda.gov/fnic/foodcomp/search.

Soybeans, as I mentioned earlier, naturally contain isoflavones that are structurally similar to estrogen, and they behave weakly like estrogens in the body. In theory, eating soy foods could help protect women against heart disease and osteoporosis as well as hot flashes and other annoying symptoms of menopause. This idea is especially attractive because soy isoflavones are not real estrogens and real estrogens have their downside. Estrogens used as part of hormone replacement therapy (HRT), for example, have been shown to increase the risk of breast and other kinds of cancer. As a result, HRT is no longer considered advisable as a first-line preventive or treatment measure for health problems in women. Thus, the Solbar Plant Extracts company advertises a soy isoflavone ingredient as "Clearly a healthy solution . . . Nature's remedy to HRT."

Soy foods may be used as a natural remedy for hot flashes but despite vast amounts of research, it is unclear how effective they are for treatment or prevention of this or any other condition. Soy companies and trade associations—the USDA-sponsored United Soybean Board and Illinois Soybean Checkoff Board, Dr. Chung's Food Company, Archer Daniels Midland, and many others—sponsor research studies and conferences. Much of this research is designed to "prove" the health benefits of eating soy foods, soy proteins, or soy isoflavones. Despite cautionary comments by leading soy researchers about how difficult it is to design, conduct, and interpret studies of the health effects of any single food or ingredient—soy or its isoflavone components—many investigators imply or state explicitly that it is imperative "to introduce and to improve the consumption of soy and related products . . . not just as an alternative to animal protein foods but as a normal component of the diet." Researchers sponsored by soy companies almost always say that even though their studies are unable to prove that soy has special health benefits, you should eat soy foods anyway.

Sponsored or not, some researchers urge caution before recommending soy foods as natural remedies. This is in part because of concerns that soy or its components could be harmful. Isoflavones could be acting like estrogen in the body in situations where extra estrogen is not desirable—as in feeding infants, for example, or in women at risk for breast cancer. But, as I discuss in the chapter on baby foods, infants who have been fed soy formulas seem to do just fine and present no evidence of health problems related to excess estrogen. As for the effects of soy and its isoflavones on breast cancer, endometrial cancer, prostate cancer, hot flashes, and osteoporosis, all I can conclude is that the research is contradictory and difficult to interpret. Some studies show that eating soy foods protects against these conditions; some show no effect at all; and some show an increased risk.

> Researchers sponsored by soy companies almost always say that even though their studies are unable to prove that soy has special health benefits, you should eat soy foods anyway.

All this means that the degree of benefit or harm from soy must be too small to make much difference to health. At the moment, it is not possible to prove that soy has any special health benefits beyond minor effects on cholesterol lowering. It also is not possible to prove that soy is perfectly safe. This should not be surprising. Researchers have a hard time distinguishing the effects of any one food in your diet—in this case soy—from everything else you eat or do. Soy is just one food. If you eat soy because you think it is healthful, you probably also follow other good health habits. If you follow other good health habits and do not eat soy, this omission is unlikely to make a difference. And eating soy is unlikely to compensate for whatever unhealthy habits you might practice.

THE MARKETING ISSUES: HEALTH CLAIMS

Despite the inconclusive research, soy marketers particularly want to attract health-conscious consumers, and as many as they can. The thousands of soy foods now available can be understood as the result of a marketing opportunity, and one that has largely succeeded. The dairy sections of my local supermarkets sell several brands of soy milk and cultured soy intermingled with the dairy milks and yogurts. Soy foods are now a mainstream alternative or complement to dairy. This surprising development (in light of the great power of the dairy industry) occurred as a result of a brilliant move by the soy industry. In 1999, after an intense lobbying effort, soy companies won FDA approval for a health claim that could be used on labels and in advertisements: that soy proteins in soy milk and other foods reduce cholesterol. Today, this claim appears on most soy products in the United States and has been freely adapted for international use. In 2004, I saw this advertisement for So Good soy milk in England:

> Did you know that, unlike dairy milk, So Good actively lowers cholesterol? Sorry cows, I'm afraid it's true. So Good uses only the purest non-GM soya, which (when consumed as part of a healthy diet) has been shown to lower your LDL (bad) cholesterol levels . . . Decide for yourself—give dairy-free a try.

The "non-GM," of course, signals that the soybeans were not genetically modified. Most soy milks and cultured soy nondairy products in North America are Certified Organic non-GM and, therefore, consistent with their marketing as health foods. But how the soy industry convinced the FDA that soy proteins—more than proteins from any other vegetable—lower cholesterol and prevent heart disease is an example of even more sophisticated marketing at work.

The idea that eating soy might prevent heart disease or any other condition is based on wonderfully reductive logic:

- Asians have low rates of heart disease (or menopausal or other health problems).
- Asians eat soybeans.
- Soybeans contain proteins, fiber, and isoflavones.
- Soy proteins, fiber, or isoflavones must be responsible for the good health of Asians.

Never mind that there are billions of people who might be called Asians, with widely varying diets and ways of life, or that Asians share many characteristics other than the amount of soy they eat—any of which might better explain their low rates of heart disease. Reductive logic finds it attractive to attribute a lower risk for coronary disease to just one food associated with Asian diets. Attributing the benefits of eating soy to just one of its hundreds of components also seems attractive, especially to companies with vested interests in that particular component. In 1998, in what was hardly a coincidence, a division of DuPont that makes soy protein ingredients, Protein Technologies International, petitioned the FDA to allow a health claim linking soy protein to prevention of heart disease. As evidence, the company cited research indicating that if you have a high blood cholesterol level, substituting an ounce or two a day of soy protein for animal protein in your diet might reduce your cholesterol by as much as 10 percent.

Skeptics urged caution in interpreting that research. The Center for Science in the Public Interest warned its *Nutrition Action Healthletter* readers to be wary of health claims emanating from the marketing departments of soy-food companies. Other research by independent investigators suggested that isoflavones, the combination of isoflavones and proteins, or the entire soybean might be responsible for the benefit, and that the amount of cholesterol reduction was too small to have any real significance for health. But the FDA was under pressure from food companies and their friends in Congress to approve a wider range of health claims and to do so quickly. It rather uncritically allowed soy protein—independent of its isoflavone or other contents—to qualify for the carefully worded health claim now found on many soy products: "25 grams of soy protein, combined with a diet low in saturated fat and cholesterol, may reduce the risk of coronary heart disease." The claim refers only to the *protein* component of soybeans, and not to the whole beans or to the foods made from them.

> The FDA decision requires foods bearing the soy claim to contain 6.25 grams of soy protein—a heaping teaspoonful—per serving, meaning that you need to eat four such servings (say, four 8-ounce glasses of soy milk) to reap the daily benefit.

The FDA decision requires foods bearing the soy claim to contain 6.25 grams of soy protein—a heaping teaspoonful—per serving, meaning that you need to eat four such servings (say, four 8-ounce glasses of soy milk) to reap the daily benefit. This is a great marketing incentive to eat soy products but, as *Nutrition Action Healthletter* pointed out in 2002, not even Asians eat that much soy every day. Subsequent research provides further grounds for skepticism. Some studies find no change in cholesterol from substituting soy for animal proteins. Others find a "modest" benefit, in the range of 3 to 6 percent. Even a benefit this small can be helpful when added to other cholesterol-lowering strategies, but in the end the decision as to whether it is large enough to induce you to eat four servings of soy foods a day should depend on how much you like eating such foods.

SOY FOODS: THE CHOICES

If the science behind the health benefits of soy foods is not particularly compelling, neither is the science suggesting that there is harm in eating reasonable amounts of them. Indeed, the research on soy and cancer is

so uncertain that even soy industry publications print articles concluding that "at this point, the evidence in both directions is too speculative
for this area of research to form a basis for a decision about consuming
soy foods." So how can you make sense of this situation? Here is my approach. Soy formulas are valuable for infants allergic to cow's milk. Soy
foods are a good substitute for dairy foods (if you want or need to find
substitutes for them), a good source of protein for vegetarians and vegans, and a good source of nutrients for everyone who likes eating them.
Small improvements in blood cholesterol can be helpful, particularly in
combination with other heart-healthy strategies. I have no doubt that
many women find soy products to give some relief from menopausal
symptoms, and that this relief is helpful even if it is just a placebo effect.

But soy products are not essential, any more than dairy foods are essential. They are just a food, one that you can choose to eat or not as a
matter of personal preference. Soybeans and the minimally processed
foods made from them make sense to eat but the principal result of the
approval of the soy health claim has been the massive proliferation of
processed soy products that can be labeled with that claim. You now can
buy thousands of processed foods made with soy: dairy substitutes,
breads, cereals, power bars, drinks, and snack foods. These range from
reasonable products to what have to be viewed as soy-supplemented
"junk foods." Are the better soy foods worth the premium price you pay?
Yes—but only if you enjoy eating them.

13

A Range of Meaty Issues

Americans are meat eaters. We like meat, and lots of it. And we *have* lots of it. The numbers are staggering. For starters, we share this country with nearly 100 million cattle. We slaughter 35 million of them each year to produce 26 billion pounds of steaks, hamburgers, and ground taco filling. But beef is nothing compared to chicken. Each year about 8 billion chickens get turned into 43 billion pounds of breasts, Buffalo wings, and Chicken McNuggets. And then there are the 96 million pigs slaughtered for fresh pork, ham, or bacon, and a few million each of calves (veal) and lamb. We do not lack for meat.

Whether we personally choose to eat meat is another matter. The neat, plastic-wrapped chilled meats that appear in grocery stores are far removed from the crowded, hot, smelly, and dangerous feedlots, confinement barns, batteries, and slaughterhouses from which they come. If you think too much about what is involved in the raising and killing of animals, you may find meat hard to eat. If you eat meat at all, you are happy to have someone else take care of its unsavory aspects and relieved that you do not have to watch. So we turn the dirty work of slaughter over to the meat companies and avert our eyes when this industry grows huge and monopolistic. We allow Tyson Foods to control one-fourth of the entire United States market for chicken, beef, and pork, and we do not object when just four meat processing firms slaughter 80 percent of all beef cattle and 50 percent of the hogs.

But concentration and power in the meat industry should make you think of many issues related to the realities of meat production. One is the issue of humane treatment of people as well as animals. Workers in this industry are hired at minimum wages and perform their duties under difficult and often dangerous conditions. Feedlots, batteries, and barns are large and dirty, and animals are confined and crowded into small spaces for virtually their entire lives. Another issue has to do with the environment and the use of natural resources. Raising cattle is a good way to turn grasses that we humans cannot use as food into high-quality meat protein, but feedlots instead use enormous quantities of perfectly edible corn and soybeans to feed animals, not people. Raising cattle also consumes vast amounts of nonrenewable energy. According to figures in the June 2004 *National Geographic*, it takes more than 200 gallons of fuel oil to raise a 1,200 pound steer on a feedlot. The cost of feed, fertilizers, and machinery, and the fuel to produce or run them, get factored into the price of meat, but the "externalities"—the costs of cleaning up animal wastes and pollutants in air, land, and water—do not. You pay the costs of loss of environmental quality in taxes, not at the grocery store.

> We allow Tyson Foods to control one-fourth of the entire United States market for chicken, beef, and pork, and we do not object when just four meat processing firms slaughter 80 percent of all beef cattle and 50 percent of the hogs.

For these reasons and others, the matter of whether to eat meat, and if so how much and what kind, taps into deep emotions. I saw these emotions in action at a 2002 conference at Yale University on, of all things, chickens. The Yale Program in Agrarian Studies convened sociologists, medieval scholars, nutritionists, and other professorial types to talk about chickens from their particular perspectives, but this unusually inclusive conference also featured talks by union organizers, workers in chicken plants, and animal welfare advocates. The academic participants could not help but be drawn into fierce debates about chicken eating. Most confessed that they ate chicken unthinkingly, but soon had to deal with charges from defenders of the welfare of chickens that it is only acceptable to eat birds that are raised humanely, or that it is immoral to eat any living creature, or that eating industrially raised chickens is so deeply immoral that advocates are justified in "liberating" birds from their cages.

Meat also taps into deep emotions for reasons of health. Meat eating, argue its critics, elevates blood cholesterol levels and is responsible for heart disease, cancer, diabetes, autoimmune diseases, and diseases of the kidneys, bones, eyes, and brain. We eat meat, they say, at our peril. I will deal with these concerns later on, but in the meantime, I must point out that meat is also a commodity competing for sales. The meat industry badly wants to overcome your worries about cholesterol and cancer, your queasiness about eating animal flesh, your qualms about how food animals are raised, and your suspicions about what meat might have in it—and to keep production costs low enough so you will not be deterred by its price. Meat industries are especially skilled at keeping costs down by encouraging the production of cheap feed, avoiding responsibility for cleaning up pollution, hiring low-wage workers, and cutting corners on food safety. These industries are also infamous for promoting meat not only as good for health but as essential. And they have a long history of employing lobbyists whose job is to minimize health risks and make sure that no government agency ever says, "Eat less meat."

> M eat industries are especially skilled at keeping costs down by encouraging the production of cheap feed, avoiding responsibility for cleaning up pollution, hiring low-wage workers, and cutting corners on food safety.

THE MEAT MARKETING ISSUES

The meat you see in the supermarket is usually more or less ready to cook: refrigerated cases of prepackaged steaks, chops, and hamburger; chickens whole and separated; pork chops, bacon, lunch meats, and a miscellaneous collection of ready-to-cook breaded and sauced animal parts. Custom, convenience, taste, and price—not nutrition—are the main selling points.

The meat industry would like you to believe that you are supposed to buy meat and put it at the center of the plate at every meal. And Americans do eat meat, more and more of it every year. It is just the mix of meat that changes. We used to eat mainly pork, but beef beat out pork in the 1950s, and chicken beat out beef in the 1980s. Today, the per capita annual share of meat available for consumption in the United States is about 102 pounds of chicken, 98 pounds of beef, 67 pounds of pork, 17 pounds of turkey, and 2 or 3 pounds of lamb and veal (these figures are based on the amounts produced, plus imports, less exports, divided by the total population—they are not necessarily what the average person actually eats). If you are a baby eating only a little meat or a vegetarian eating none at all, you are just leaving more for everyone else. Even so, beef producers mourn their declining market share, and everyone in this business wishes that you would eat more—and preferably lots more—of the meat they produce.

To encourage Americans to eat more meat, the beef and pork industries have long relied on mandatory "checkoff" marketing programs. These programs, which are managed—and strongly defended—by the USDA, tax producers according to the number or weight of their animals; for example, $1 for each head of cattle (hence: checkoff). Checkoff assessments collect tens of millions of dollars yearly for generic marketing campaigns. In *Food Politics*, I explained how the programs are run by boards that do "education." They are not supposed to do any lobbying, but the line between education and lobbying of public officials and nutritionists is exceedingly fine. The education campaigns of the Cattlemen's Beef Board are "directed to nutrition professionals and aim to increase consumer recognition of beef as lower in fat, higher in essential nutrients and lower in calories and cholesterol" than chicken or pork—as in its highly visible "Beef. It's What's for Dinner" advertisements. The Beef Board's mission statement could not be more explicit: "improving producer profitability, expanding consumer demand for beef, and strengthening beef's position in the marketplace."

Despite the reach of such campaigns, not all meat producers appreciate the checkoff programs and some have sued the courts for the right to opt out of them on First Amendment (free speech) grounds. Starting in 2002, for example, dissident beef producers got their lawsuit as far as the U.S. Court of Appeals, which declared the beef checkoff unconstitutional because it forced producers to pay for advertising messages even if they did not want to. In 2005, however, the Supreme Court overturned that decision. It ruled that the USDA had every right to compel food producers to contribute to checkoff funds because such programs represent "government speech" and, therefore, cannot be subject to First Amendment challenges. This decision means that the USDA is more responsible than the relevant industries for maintaining the milk, beef, and other checkoff-funded marketing campaigns.

A year or so before this decision, pork producers held an election and voted to end their checkoff program but were overturned by their deeply entrenched National Pork Board. These matters were still under litigation in 2004 when the Pork Board ran a trendy educational campaign: "Counting carbs? Pork's a perfect source of protein." Its Web site explained how people with diabetes and high blood pressure can incorporate pork into their diets, and provided a "Porkfolio" of recipes. The board pushes pork as leaner than other meats, and it can be if you choose carefully. A Master Choice–brand pork tenderloin, for example, is so low in fat (just 3 grams in a 4-ounce portion) that it qualifies for an American Heart Association seal of endorsement, presumably justifying its price, which is twice as high as most other cuts. In a Vons supermarket in California, I saw Farmer John ground pork advertised as a "lean alternative to ground beef." It also had an American Heart Association seal, testimony to its low fat and cholesterol. Pigs that produce this pork are indeed raised to be leaner, but many chefs and pork aficionados decry the loss of succulence and flavor that disappeared with the fat.

Tyson Foods may own 25 percent of the country's meat supply, but still wants a greater market share. In 2004, the company paid $75 million to no less than six advertising and public relations agencies to convince you to demand meats with Tyson's red oval logo. Some of the money went for strategic analyses of the responses of ninety focus groups, many of them made up of black and Hispanic consumers. The result: online and retail promotions based on the theme "protein provides energy, and energy provides power" and the slogan "Have you had your protein today?" From a nutritional standpoint, the focus on protein is silly—Americans are anything but protein deficient—but the campaign distracts attention from the high-fat and saturated-fat content of meat, and from other issues of health and safety that result from production and handling methods. Let's take a look at the nutrition issues now, and defer the safety concerns for the next chapter.

The industry's nutritional mantra is that meat is so good for you that you should not think twice about eating it. Beef is the leading source of protein in American diets, and meat in general provides lots of vitamins — especially vitamin B_{12} — and minerals. But again, protein is not exactly lacking in American diets. To meet nutritional requirements, you only need to eat about half a gram of protein each day for every pound you weigh, which works out to 55 grams (just under two ounces) for a 120-pound woman and 65 grams (just over two ounces) for a 180-pound man. Note: these are ounces of *protein*, not meat; meat has other components like fat and water that contribute to its weight. Even so, 4 ounces of cooked beef, poultry, or pork can easily provide 20 or 30 grams of protein (and so can beans). On surveys of daily dietary intake, women report eating an average of 70 grams of protein, and men 100 grams, and respondents to these kinds of surveys typically underestimate actual intake by as much as one-third. Even if you are a vegan and eat no animal products at all, you almost certainly get more than enough protein from the grains, beans, and vegetables you eat.

Indeed, unless your diet is unusually restrictive, you will get enough protein as long as you get enough calories. If you think about it, the diets of entire civilizations — in ancient Egypt, China, and Mexico, for example — have been based on wheat, rice, beans, or corn as sources of protein. Nutritionists used to worry that you had to be careful about combining plant foods to get the right proportion of amino acids — like mixing beans with rice or corn, for example — but we know now that variety and calories take care of that. A little meat (or dairy, fish, or eggs) also helps with vitamin B_{12} and some of the scarcer minerals, but you can do fine without animal-based foods if you get those nutrients from other sources.

It does not take much meat to improve the nutritional quality of diets that need improving. But if you eat more than a little meat, you come up against the fat problem. Meat, like all foods from animals, is high in saturated fat, the kind that raises blood cholesterol levels and the risk of coronary heart disease. Meat also may have something to do with development of certain kinds of cancers. Meat marketers emphasize the nutritional benefits of eating meat and do not want you to think about health risks. My local supermarket carries "zero carb" roast beef and smoked turkey, and Oscar Meyer labels its bacon "o grams total carbs" and "70 calories per serving." These are correct, but designed to take your mind off the real issues. Even the richest, most succulent piece of meat does not ever have carbohydrates unless it is breaded. Two see-through-thin slices of bacon amount to only 70 calories, but you have to read the Nutrition Facts label to see that nearly 90 percent of those calories come from fat, and one-third of that fat is saturated. The fats in bacon are either a little or a lot depending on how much of it you eat and what else you eat with it.

Health authorities say that 20 grams of saturated fat a day—a heaping tablespoon—is more than enough, but it is not so easy to figure out how much saturated fat there is in the food you eat. You have to make educated guesses. All fats contain some saturated fat, but animal fats have more than vegetable fats. If you eat meat, the saturated fat adds up quickly. According to the nutrition information provided by McDonald's, one of its hamburgers has 3.5 grams of saturated fat, and a Quarter Pounder has 7. Splurge on a 22-ounce T-bone steak at a Ruth's Chris Steak House, and you will pay not only its $40 cost but also the consequences of its 48 grams of saturated fat (more than a two-day allotment) and 1,750 calories. That steak is best shared with friends, and as many as possible.

> Skinless chicken has hardly any saturated fat, but the minute it is breaded and fried the grams go up. If you eat the skin, you might as well be eating a hamburger.

Chicken is leaner, of course. Skinless chicken has hardly any saturated fat, but the minute it is breaded and fried the grams go up. If you eat the skin, you might as well be eating a hamburger. But just try to figure this out. Restaurants don't tell you these things, nor do supermarkets; neither is required to provide nutrition labels on "fresh" meats.

THE LABELING ISSUES

Although some meat packages are labeled with nutrition messages— "30% less fat," "only 70 calories per serving," "o grams *trans* fat"—you will not easily find out the amount of saturated fat in the meat you buy.

Some packages have Nutrition Facts labels, but many do not. The USDA makes the labeling of fresh meat voluntary. This is because the meat industry does not want compulsory labeling, ostensibly because it would be too difficult and expensive, but mostly because this industry just does not like being told what to do. *The Washington Post* once quoted a former Secretary of Agriculture, Clayton Yeutter, equating nutrition labels on meat "to restrictions imposed by the former totalitarian governments of Eastern Europe." Nevertheless, the USDA proposed to require nutrition labels for processed (meaning cooked) meat—but not fresh (meaning raw) meat—in 1991 and those rules went into effect in 1994. This distinction might also seem like splitting hairs since "fresh" as applied to meat often involves considerable processing (chickens are eviscerated, chilled, cut, and sometimes boned; beef is aged and dried). Whatever. Prepackaged lunch meats now must—and do—have Nutrition Facts labels. Some national brands such as Hormel and Perdue label their prepackaged fresh meats, proving that it can be done, but the other fresh meats are a nutritional mystery. You don't like this? Write your congressional representative.

Here is another one: hamburger meats can be especially fatty but the USDA gave the industry a big concession in 2001 and said that ground meats could be labeled by percent "lean" rather than percent fat. Your local store probably offers fresh ground beef and more expensive ground chuck, ground round, or ground sirloin; these can range from 70 to 95 percent lean.

Suppose a meat is 80 percent lean. That means it is actually 20 percent fat, by weight, and this fat makes up more than two-thirds of its calories.

Meat managers tell me that their suppliers test to make sure the percentages are labeled correctly, but here's how this system works. Suppose a meat is 80 percent lean. That means it is actually 20 percent fat, by weight, and this fat makes up more than two-thirds of its calories. But beef is never really a low-fat food; even 95 percent lean ground beef has one-third of its calories from fat. Meats other than ground beef need to be less than 3 percent fat by weight to qualify as "lean," but that's politics for you.

The latest labeling fuss is over country-of-origin labeling (COOL). After years of industry opposition, the rules were to go into effect in

October 2004, but Congress postponed implementation until October 2006, allowing the industry time to press for voluntary labeling. In 2005, the advocacy group Public Citizen charged agribusiness companies and trade associations with spending nearly $13 million on campaign contributions and lobbying activities to delay or repeal mandatory COOL. This worked. Toward the end of that year, in what such groups termed "a travesty" and an "utterly corrupt" process, a House-Senate conference committee—deliberating behind closed doors—approved an additional two-year delay in implementation of COOL for meat, fresh produce, and peanuts, until October 2008. This delay meant that the original enacting legislation would expire before the new due date and remove any threat that COOL might be implemented. If COOL survives the opposition, you will be able to tell whether meat comes from Argentina or some other faraway place. You can imagine that COOL labeling might encourage people to buy American meat, on the logic that meat butchered closer to home will be cleaner and taste the way you like it, but the meat industry does not see it that way. Instead, the National Livestock Producers Association thinks COOL will have the opposite effect: "When a foreign source produces a product that surpasses quality . . . consumers will become motivated to prefer the product . . . The automobile and electronics industries stand as examples that illustrate this concern." This may seem like an astonishing admission, but American meat producers must believe that if you eat meat from Argentina or New Zealand, you will like it better and, perhaps, think it is produced under conditions more favorable to the health of animals and the people who eat them. You think COOL is a good idea? Take the matter up with your representative in Congress.

THE HEALTH ISSUES

The meat industry's big public relations problem is that vegetarians are demonstrably healthier than meat eaters. If you do not eat beef, pork, lamb, or even chicken, your risk of heart disease and certain cancers is likely to be lower than that of the average meat-eating American. And as long as you eat any other animal product at all—dairy, fish, or eggs—you can avoid eating meat without affecting the nutritional quality of your diet. The only vegetarians who need to do anything special to prevent nutrient deficiencies are vegans, who eat no animal products whatsoever. If you follow vegan practices, you need to be sure to eat a variety of grains and beans (to get enough protein), to take in enough calories (so you don't lose weight), and to find an alternative source for vitamin B_{12} (the one vitamin that is found only in foods from animal sources).

Worldwide, meat intake varies from practically nothing among the poorest people in agrarian societies in Africa, for example, to 20 percent or more of calories in the United States and Europe. Poor populations subsisting mainly on a single plant crop like corn or rice are healthier when they get a little meat in their diets. Eating a lot of meat, however, is not so healthy for anyone. As poor people begin to prosper, they eat more meat. This takes care of their nutrient deficiencies, but also adds fat, saturated fat, and calories. This sudden change toward Western-style eating patterns—and toward Western-style disease patterns—happens so fast and is so common that it has its own name: the "nutrition transition." Meat is not the only food that counts in that transition (sugars and processed foods are also high on the list), but it is the one that is most evident.

Why meat might increase heart disease or cancer risk is a matter of much conjecture. Scientists began to link red meat to the risk of cancer in the 1970s, but even after several decades of subsequent research cannot say whether the culprit is fat, saturated fat, protein, carcinogens induced when meat is cooked at high temperature, or some other component. Eating meat might stimulate the growth of intestinal bacteria that produce carcinogenic or other toxic chemicals, or some other as yet unknown mechanism might be at work. By the late 1990s, the best the experts could say is that red meat "probably" increases the risk of colon and rectal cancers, and "possibly" increases the risk of cancers of the pancreas, breast, prostate, and kidney. As always, it is hard to interpret what such conditional words mean in this context, but one point is clear: vegetarians and near-vegetarians display lower rates of those cancers. That is why the American Cancer Society says that if you do eat red meat, you can lower your cancer risk by selecting leaner cuts, eating smaller portions, or choosing chicken, fish, or beans as alternatives. All of this seems like sensible advice. Government dietary advice, however, minimizes or obscures health concerns about eating meat, and does so for reasons of politics—not health.

THE ADVICE ISSUES

Many areas of dietary advice are subject to industry meddling, and the meat industry's meddling started early. Until the 1950s or so, when nutrient deficiencies more or less disappeared as public health problems, everybody agreed that eating more meat would make people healthier. But soon after World War II, Americans began to have more money and started buying more expensive foods, meat among them. Cardiologists, alarmed at a sharp rise in heart attacks, thought the saturated fat in meat might be one cause. Heart disease, they knew, had multiple causes, and one of them was a high level of cholesterol in the blood. Animal fats, which are highly saturated, raise blood cholesterol levels. The obvious solution was to advise people to eat less meat or to substitute leaner meat, fish, poultry, and animal products for fatty beef. In 1959, as I mentioned earlier, Ancel and Margaret Keys published a cookbook, *Eat Well and Stay Well*, with advice to help people prevent heart disease. Among their recommendations was one that said "Restrict saturated fats, the fats in beef, pork, lamb sausages . . ." By 1961, the American Heart Association also was advising doctors to tell their patients to eat less saturated fat and its dietary sources, meat prominently among them.

The U.S. government, however, did not say anything about meat and heart disease until 1977 when the Senate Select Committee on Nutrition and Human Needs (chaired by George McGovern, a Democrat from South Dakota), issued a report, "Dietary Goals for the United States." This committee made a huge political mistake. It said: "reduce consumption of meat." Protests from beef producers were immediate and vehement. In *Food Politics*, I described the ensuing furor and its long-lasting consequences: The committee backed down and rephrased the offending statement to "Choose meats, poultry, and fish which will reduce saturated fat intake" (as if you would have any idea how to do that).

Since then, under pressure from beef industry lobbying groups, government agencies have issued increasingly euphemistic advice. The direct statement "eat less meat" morphed into the self-canceling "choose lean meats" or the more convoluted "limit use of animal fats." In 2004, the committee advising the government about how to revise the *Dietary Guidelines for Americans* pointed to links between eating meat and cancers of the colon and rectum, and between animal fat and prostate cancer. The committee said: "Limit one's intake of animal fats, among them fatty meat; bacon and sausage; and poultry skin and fat." But the government agencies (the USDA and Department of Health and Human Services) must have found even this mild advice to be too focused on eating less meat. Their final guidelines in 2005 said: "When selecting and preparing meat . . . make choices that are lean, low-fat, or fat-free."

The guidelines are supposed to be a set of "science-based" dietary principles to be applied by policymakers and nutrition and health professionals. In contrast, the Pyramid food guide, issued solely by the USDA, is meant to help you put those principles into practice. Later in 2005, the USDA issued its MyPyramid guide to food choices. The USDA, an agency with primary responsibility for promoting sales of American food commodities, is hardly likely to issue advice—to eat less meat, for example—that conflicts with its assigned mission. As it has in the past, the USDA lumped meat into a category that also includes poultry, fish, dry beans, eggs, and nuts. But the USDA's key statement about meat in the new pyramid breaks new ground in euphemism: "Meat & Beans: Go lean on protein." So now you are supposed to eat less meat—and fewer beans—

> The USDA, an agency with primary responsibility for promoting sales of American food commodities, is hardly likely to issue advice—to eat less meat, for example—that conflicts with its assigned mission.

because of their *protein* content? Since when did protein (and especially protein from beans) become a problem in American diets? We may eat more protein than we need, but what happened to saturated fat and cholesterol? Beans, of course, have hardly any saturated fat and no cholesterol at all, but you will have to scroll patiently through much of the pyramid Web site (www.mypyramid.gov) before you get to advice to "Choose low-fat or lean meats and poultry."

For years, the meat guideline has been a prime example of food politics in action. The result: you are on your own to interpret government advice and figure out for yourself that you would be healthier if you ate less meat. The 2005 *Dietary Guidelines*, however, do have much to say about food safety and your role in it: "Consumers can take simple measures to reduce their risk of foodborne illness, especially in the home." But, as I explain in the next chapter, they say not a word about the need for the industry to produce safer meat.

14

Meat: Questions of Safety

Meat safety should be a major concern for reasons of health—
and politics. Politics enters into just about every aspect of the
safety of meat, starting with the glaring observation that the
government does not have a national system in place for tracking episodes
of food poisoning—outbreaks—in which more than one person gets sick
from eating the same food. To fill this gap, the consumer advocacy
group Center for Science in the Public Interest (CSPI) does its best to
keep track of outbreaks caused by one food or another. Since 1990, CSPI
has counted more than 900 outbreaks affecting 30,000 or so people who
had inadvertently eaten beef, pork, or poultry contaminated with dangerous bacteria. Some of the meats might have become contaminated
after they were purchased and taken home, but most episodes of food
poisoning are caused by bacteria that did their contaminating long before the meats arrived on supermarket shelves.

The outbreak information tells you that the meat safety problem is
one that needs to be solved *before* you buy the meats, and that means on
the farm and in meatpacking plants. In the mid-1990s, the USDA issued
regulations that required meatpacking companies to institute safety
plans and to test for hazardous bacteria. But these rules, relentlessly opposed by meat producers and processors, ended up with gaps, disincen-

tives, and loopholes. One gap is that the rules begin at the slaughter-house and do not apply to production methods on the farm or feedlot. One disincentive is this: the more carefully meat companies and the USDA test for harmful bacteria, the more they are likely to find—and if meat is contaminated, it cannot be sold. One loophole allows tested meat to go out into the food supply before the test results are known, and another prohibits the USDA from recalling meat that tests positive for harmful bacteria. The rules only permit the USDA to ask companies to recall contaminated meat voluntarily. Companies do comply, but grudgingly.

The USDA posts recall requests on its Web site (www.fsis.usda.gov), and its correspondence with the companies makes interesting reading. The agency requests dozens of voluntary recalls every year, most of which involve unpleasant or deadly variants of common bacteria that usually do no harm: *E. coli* O157:H7 (a toxic form of the common intestinal bacteria), *Listeria*, and *Salmonella*. In 2004, among more than fifty such examples, a Wisconsin company recalled 59,000 pounds of ground beef because a sample tested positive for *E. coli* O157:H7; a North Carolina company recalled more than 400,000 pounds of frozen, fully cooked chicken products testing positive for *Listeria*; and an Illinois company recalled nearly 25,000 pounds of pork rinds found contaminated with *Salmonella*. Two years earlier, in one of the more impressive incidents, ConAgra (in Colorado) recalled 19 million pounds of fresh and frozen ground beef products because tests for *E. coli* O157:H7 had come back positive. In these and most other recalls, the test samples had been taken two weeks earlier, the meat had already been sold and eaten, and only a tiny fraction could be recovered. How could something like this happen? Easily, as it turns out.

MEAT SAFETY: THE POLITICS

Never mind that the meat you buy might be loaded with bad bacteria. It is *your* responsibility to deal with the problem. Look carefully at any package of meat in the United States and you will find a "Safe Handling" label that explains the problem, although in print so small that you may need eyeglasses to read it:

This product was prepared from inspected and passed meat and/or poultry. Some food products may contain bacteria that could cause illness if the product is mishandled or cooked improperly. For your protection, follow the safe handling instructions.

The instructions, also in tiny print, come with icons:

- [Refrigerator] Keep refrigerated or frozen. Thaw in refrigerator or microwave.
- [Faucet] Keep raw meat and poultry separate from other foods. Wash working surfaces (including cutting boards), utensils, and hands after touching raw meat or poultry.
- [Frying Pan] Keep hot foods hot.
- [Thermometer] Refrigerate leftovers immediately or discard. Cook thoroughly.

These labels illustrate the four basic rules for keeping food safe: chill, clean, separate, cook. It is a really good idea to pay close attention to these rules. Just because meat is stamped "USDA Inspected" does not mean that it is free of harmful bacteria. Even if you buy products from companies like Coleman's Natural Foods, which makes safety a point of pride as well as of added value (meaning you pay more for its products), you have to handle uncooked and previously cooked meat with care. Meat producers like it that way. They can cut corners in processing and testing and shift most of the burden of ensuring meat safety to you.

They can do this, in part, because of the long history of cozy relations among meat producers, congressional agriculture committees, and the USDA—the government agency responsible both for promoting meat and poultry production and for regulating its safety. As I discussed in my book *Safe Food*, cozy relations and conflicts of interest explain why our current food safety system is so firmly locked in rules established at the time Upton Sinclair wrote his muckraking book *The Jungle* in 1906, decades before anyone had a clue about the dangers of bacteria in meat.

The USDA was founded in 1862 for the express purpose of encouraging development of agriculture, including meat production. In the early

1900s, one way it did so was to advise Americans to eat foods from a variety of groups—an "eat more" strategy. In the 1970s, Congress gave the USDA "lead agency" responsibility for educating the public about diet and health, which increasingly meant advice to "eat less." When these purposes came into conflict, which they frequently did, the USDA's default position was to support the industry it regulates. On occasion, the USDA's actions are so egregiously in favor of industry that they cause public uproar. When this happens, the USDA sometimes reverses its decisions. In one such instance, the USDA wanted to allow Certified Organic foods to be genetically modified, irradiated, and fertilized with sewage sludge, but had to back down when hundreds of thousands of citizens complained. History demonstrates that, at best, the USDA acts grudgingly in the public interest if there is any chance that doing so might cause problems for the meat industry. The unfortunate result is that you are almost entirely responsible for the safety of the food you eat. It is your responsibility to make sure that the meat you buy gets cooked properly and does not cross-contaminate anything else in your kitchen with dangerous bacteria. And you cannot count on the government to demand that meat companies produce safe meat to begin with.

> History demonstrates that, at best, the USDA acts grudgingly in the public interest if there is any chance that doing so might cause problems for the meat industry.

UNSAFE MEAT: BACTERIA

Animals are not sterile, and neither are we. They carry many different kinds of bacteria in unimaginably large numbers (we do too). Fortunately, most bacteria are harmless, but some, like that especially nasty form of *E. coli*, are deadly. Toxic bacteria often do not make the animals sick, but they can make you sick—and sometimes kill you—if you eat meat from animals that carry them.

How bacteria of any kind get into the meat you buy in supermarkets is not a pretty story. Like all animals, food animals excrete bacteria in their wastes, and these bacteria spread quickly under the crowded conditions in feedlots, batteries, and slaughterhouses. Bacteria also spread from one animal to another during slaughter and when meat is cut and ground. Bacteria usually only contaminate the outer surfaces of whole cuts of meat like roasts, steaks, or chops; if you sear pieces of meat like these, you kill the bacteria on their surfaces. Bacteria cannot easily get into the inside of a steak, for example, unless it has been pierced, cut, or ground. That is why hamburger poses safety problems; once ground, the bacteria on its surface can mix into its interior. Meat packers make commercial hamburger from the parts of a large number (sometimes hundreds) of beef cattle, so if just one animal is contaminated with harmful bacteria, the entire batch of hamburger can make people ill. That is also why it makes sense to cook commercial hamburger thoroughly, so you kill bacteria throughout the mix. Meat will never be completely free of bacteria, but you have every right to wonder why producers are not doing a better job of keeping their meats free of harmful ones.

> **M**eat will never be completely free of bacteria, but you have every right to wonder why producers are not doing a better job of keeping their meats free of harmful ones.

PREVENTING UNSAFE MEAT: HACCP

The most frustrating aspect of problems with meat safety is that everyone involved knows how to produce safe meat; they just are not doing it as diligently as they should. In the mid-1990s, after years of meat-industry opposition and political dithering, Congress finally authorized the USDA to issue regulations to establish safety systems for meat and poultry. These systems are known collectively by the off-putting acronym HACCP (pronounced "hass-ip"), which stands for the equally unhelpful Hazard Analysis and Critical Control Point, and includes pathogen reduction. In translation, HACCP makes perfect sense. It simply requires meat processors and packers to examine their production processes to see where harmful bacteria might get into meat (the hazard analysis), put methods in place to stop contamination at those places (the critical control points), and monitor the processes and test for bacteria to make sure the system is working properly (the pathogen reduction).

HACCP systems originated in the late 1950s as a side benefit of space travel. The National Aeronautics and Space Administration (NASA) was eager to make sure that astronauts never got food poisoning or its accompanying nausea, vomiting, or diarrhea, especially under (horrible thought) conditions of zero gravity. The system created for this agency by the Pillsbury baking company, no less, worked beautifully. The astronauts ate whatever they had on board and did not get sick. HACCP plans—when thoughtfully and diligently designed, followed, and monitored—should work just as well on Earth as they do in outer space. But they are expensive for companies to follow, and meat packers like to keep costs down, so they sometimes cut corners on compliance. Hence: recalls.

No question, producing safer meat costs more, which is one of the reasons why "natural" and organic meats are priced so high (I will have more to say about these kinds in the next chapter). The Coleman Natural Meat Company, for example, which sells meats packaged as "Purely Natural," advertises on its Web site that it follows a HACCP plan. All packing companies must have such plans, of course, but Coleman says it goes beyond those requirements. The company trims the meat to remove surface bacteria before grinding it into hamburger (a good idea), and tests ground meat for bacteria every hour—a sensible practice, but one that is voluntary (HACCP, in contrast, only requires spot-checks). These practices should work and the company says they do. In 2004, it reported never having found the toxic forms of *E. coli* or *Salmonella* in its meat.

PREVENTING UNSAFE MEAT: IRRADIATION

Luckily, cooking takes care of most bacteria, harmful or not. Outbreaks of food poisoning happen when the "chill, clean, separate, cook" rules get broken in some way, at home or, more commonly, where food is served. The meat industry wishes its products could just be irradiated to stop such problems. In the frozen food section of a Tops Market in Ithaca, New York, I came across some Huisken beef patties with labels indicating that they had been zapped with "electron beam irradiation." The label explained: "This safe process helps eliminate food-borne pathogens." Despite such reassurances, irradiation has yet to overcome consumer resistance, and you will have to search hard to find irradiated meats in supermarkets. I do not find this resistance particularly tragic.

The meat industry would do better if it did everything it could to produce safe meat from the get-go, so irradiation would not be needed.

Instead, meat companies wish that toxic bacteria would just go away; they resent having to worry about them, test for them, and recall meat containing them. They think the problem is your fault. If you would just learn to cook your food properly, meat safety would not be an issue. But since you are evidently unteachable, the next-best approach is to kill off the bacteria before they get to you. And that is where irradiation enters the picture. Irradiation would allow meat producers to rid meat of harmful bacteria in the package, and otherwise go on and conduct business as usual. Government food safety officials also think irradiation would solve food safety problems, and have approved its use on meat and poultry. They say that if meat packers irradiated just half the supply of meat and poultry, they would save more than 300 lives and prevent more than 900,000 cases of illness each year. They also say that irradiation is safe, so safe that irradiated ground beef can be served to children in school.

Nevertheless, irradiation continues to generate controversy about the technology itself, its effects on food, and whether it really does keep meat safe. The process involves bombarding food with high-energy gamma rays, X-rays, or, as is most common these days, electron beams. Whatever their source, the rays kill bacteria. The more intense the rays, the more bacteria they kill. Irradiation does not make foods radioactive. It has only small effects on nutritional values; it destroys vitamin C and other delicate vitamins, but not by much. But more intense "doses" of radiation induce off tastes and smells, particularly in fatty meats. Critics charge that irradiation creates toxic chemicals in foods. This may be true, but it is not clear that these chemicals are any different from those caused by frying, baking, or any other cooking method, or whether they cause harm when you eat them.

> Critics charge that irradiation creates toxic chemicals in foods. This may be true, but it is not clear that these chemicals are any different from those caused by frying, baking, or any other cooking method, or whether they cause harm when you eat them.

Irradiation has been used on dried spices for years, but its use on fresh meat is recent. In the late 1990s, a company based in San Diego, SureBeam, built electronic-beam irradiation facilities for use on meat and Hawaiian tropical fruits (see Chapter 5). By 2003, it had irradiated 20 million pounds of foods, had obtained contracts from meat suppliers that would fill 85 percent of its ground-beef irradiating capacity, and was looking forward to increasing its production of irradiated meat by at least 30 percent a year. The company based this projection on its own expectations of consumer demand, which apparently failed to consider the long history of consumer resistance to irradiation. Such optimistic projections might be thought delusional and, indeed, SureBeam never showed a profit.

In January 2004, SureBeam unexpectedly filed for bankruptcy and sold off its assets to pay creditors. Later that year when I saw the Huisken meat patties, I wondered where they had been irradiated. A call to the company's San Diego offices, which were still open, identified a surprising source: Texas A&M University. A year or so earlier, SureBeam had donated $10 million to Texas A&M to establish an Electron Beam Food Research Facility. This university-based facility picked up where Sure-Beam left off and now works with meat companies like Huisken to perform what it euphemistically calls "food pasteurization."

The idea that irradiation would even be needed points out weaknesses in the food safety system. Meat should be free of harmful bacteria to begin with. Irradiation makes sense for killing fruit flies on the skin of Hawaiian papayas—we don't want those flies on the continent and we do not eat papaya skins—but meat is different. Irradiation is done late in the process of producing meat. It allows companies to produce dirty meat and fix it later. Because irradiation changes the taste of meat, it cannot be done intensely enough to kill all of the bacteria. This means that the survivors of irradiation can multiply and the meat can be recontaminated, in turn meaning that irradiated meat still needs to be cooked and handled properly. You might as well buy meat that has not been irradiated. Still worried? Read the Safe Handling rules and follow them to the letter—and then write your congressional representatives and demand that they pass laws that require HACCP plans at every stage of meat production, from farm to table.

> The idea that irradiation would even be needed points out weaknesses in the food safety system. Meat should be free of harmful bacteria to begin with.

Irradiation is imperfectly protective for another reason: it does not protect you against the small, but finite, risk of mad cow disease. This disease, formally known as bovine spongiform encephalopathy (BSE), caused the destruction of hundreds of thousands of cows in Great Britain during the early 1990s, but also killed about 150 people believed unlucky enough to have eaten meat from sick cows. If any meat risk is invisible, uncertain, and frightening, this one surely is. It is invariably fatal. Labels of meat packages that say "all vegetable diet," "no animal by-products," or "no animal cannibalism" were put there to reassure you that the animals were never exposed to mad cow disease, and that you will not be exposed to it either.

If you were to eat meat from cattle afflicted with BSE, you might run a slight risk of contracting the human form of this disease, but the science of everything about the disease—except its fatality—is uncertain, incomplete, and quite unusual. Unlike any other disease, BSE (and similar diseases in other animals and in humans) seems to be caused by proteins that are "folded" wrong. These proteins are called "prions" (pronounced pree-ons). In the brain, misfolded prion proteins act like dominoes; they cause normal prion proteins to misfold, one after another. This destroys brain tissues (hence: encephalopathy) and leaves gaping holes (hence: spongiform).

The prion disease in cattle—steers as well as cows—is called BSE. The related human disease is called variant Creutzfeldt-Jacob disease (vCJD). Prion diseases also occur in many other animals; in sheep, for example, it is called "scrapie." These diseases occur spontaneously—with no apparent cause—in older animals or humans. How they arise and spread is not really known, but one scenario to explain the epidemic in Great Britain seems most plausible: the British cattle got mad cow disease because they were fed brains from sheep that had scrapie, and people

> Labels of meat packages that say "all vegetable diet," "no animal by-products," or "no animal cannibalism" were put there to reassure you that the animals were never exposed to mad cow disease, and that you will not be exposed to it either.

got the human variant of the disease because they ate meat from cows that had BSE. If this scenario turns out to be true, it would be good to know that animals are free of BSE before eating meat that comes from them.

As a result of the British experience, scientists know how to keep cattle free of BSE. The guidelines are quite straightforward.

- Do not ever feed meat-and-bone meal made from parts of the brain, nervous system, or other organs ("by-products") of animals that could have prion diseases to cows.

- Test older cows for BSE (because these diseases take a long time to develop) before slaughtering the animals.

- Do not allow meat from tested animals into the food supply until the test results prove negative.

- Kill and destroy any animal that tests positive for BSE and make sure its meat never gets into the food supply.

These measures were well understood by the time the British epidemic of mad cow disease reached its peak in 1993. But most countries, the United States among them, delayed putting such rules in place (or applied them only casually) until several years later.

If a delay of any length seems inexplicable, consider this logistical problem: What is to be done with the offal—the bones, intestines, ears, brains, and other inedible parts—of the 35 million cattle slaughtered each year in the United States? Assume that an animal weighs 1,000 pounds at slaughter, and the bones and other offal amount to one-third of its weight; if so, the leftover parts add up to more than 12 billion pounds annually. What are meat producers to do with these parts? Burn them? Bury them? Needless to say, the meat industry prefers an alternative solution: make some money from them. So for decades, meat companies have cooked the offal—rendered them—into an unappetizing but highly nutritious meat-and-bone meal, which can be sold either for industrial uses (cosmetics, gelatin, and the like) or for animal feed. Unfortunately, as the British found out, cooking and rendering do not get rid of misfolded prions. The result was a catastrophe for the diseased cattle, the British beef industry, and the unfortunate people who died years after eating meat from those cattle.

Nevertheless, Canada and the United States took the position that "it can't happen here." They did not take even the most basic preventive step—a ban on the use of meat-and-bone meal as feed for cattle—until 1997. It took three more years, until 2000, for the United States to ban imports of meat-and-bone meal from countries that had not been testing their cattle for BSE. In 2003, when one cow in Canada and another in the United States were found to have mad cow disease, Japan and numerous other countries immediately banned imports of beef from both countries. Early in 2004, to protect the beef export market, the USDA finally required beef producers to take some of the additional precautionary measures that seemed so obvious to scientists and food safety advocates.

During 2004, the USDA increased the number of animals it tested from 20,000 to more than 165,000 (out of 35 million) and, despite some apparently false alarms, happily reported finding none with BSE. Overall, it acted as if BSE were no threat. Its weirdest decision was to block a private meatpacking company, Creekstone Farms Premium Beef, from doing its own BSE testing. Creekstone used to have a lively market in Japan, but was losing about $200,000 a day in export sales due to the Japanese ban on American beef. In the hope of reopening this market, the company built a laboratory to test *all* of its cattle scheduled for slaughter, whether young or old. The USDA refused to allow the company to use the laboratory for this purpose. Private testing, the USDA said, would confuse customers because it would imply that untested beef might not be safe.

Could the National Cattlemen's Beef Association, a lobbying group for 27,000 cattle ranchers, have had anything to do with this decision? A spokesman for the association said that testing younger animals (under age three, for example) for BSE was absurd, "like testing kindergartners for Alzheimer's." If the USDA allowed one company to test for BSE, said the association, other companies also would have to, and at considerable expense. Later the USDA refused to allow its own inspectors to decide whether "downer" (collapsed) cattle should be tested for BSE. It also backed off from a decision to allow untested beef products to be imported from Canada only when threatened with a lawsuit from a cattle ranchers' association, "dedicated to ensuring the continued profitability and viability of independent U.S. cattle producers" through legal action on trade and marketing issues.

The USDA's reluctance to take vigorous action to protect the public from the threat of BSE must be understood in the context of its historically close relationship with the industry it regulates. Cattle and meatpacking companies routinely oppose regulations that might increase production costs or suggest that meat is unsafe. They expect the USDA to back them up, and the USDA usually does. In a crisis, such as that brought on by mad cow disease, the USDA sometimes manages to find ways to do the right thing—but only when pushed.

> The USDA's reluctance to take vigorous action to protect the public from the threat of BSE must be understood in the context of its historically close relationship with the industry it regulates.

If you are statistically inclined, you will not worry much about the chance that mad cow disease will affect you. Although a huge number of cows had the disease, the number of human cases was relatively small and does not seem to be increasing much over time. This is a good sign that control measures for BSE must be working. The numbers loom large, however, if one of those human cases is you or someone you know.

In 2004, Canada found two cases of BSE, and another two cases turned up in 2005—all in older cows. The USDA said that none of the cattle it tested in 2004 had BSE, but this reassuring statement turned out to be based on relatively insensitive testing procedures. In June 2005, the USDA disclosed that an "experimental" test in November 2004 had identified a case of BSE in a sick cow, but that the laboratory had failed to report the result to USDA officials. When the USDA's inspector general insisted that tissue samples from this cow be sent to England to be tested using more sensitive methods, the tests confirmed that the cow had BSE. Fortunately, meat from that cow did not get into the food supply—this time. Early in 2006, more than thirty-five countries, among them Japan, South Korea, Russia, and China, were still refusing to import American beef because of what they perceived as inadequate testing for BSE.

The effect of this ban on American meat exports is striking. In 1999, the United States produced 19 percent of world beef exports, but that percentage fell to 3 percent in 2004. You might guess that the beef industry would be desperate to put the tightest possible controls in place, but you would be wrong. This industry continues to argue that American beef is "very, very safe" and that countries are using the threat of BSE as an excuse to protect their own beef industries.

How you should interpret the BSE situation depends on your point of view. From a statistical standpoint, the chance of your getting the human form of the disease from eating meat is very small. But it is not zero. If you are an optimist, you will not give the matter another thought. If you are a pessimist, you will want the risk to be closer to zero than it now is and will want to know that everything possible is being done to keep BSE out of cows and cows with BSE out of the meat supply. You will worry that the more than 500,000 cattle tested in 2005 amount to less than two-tenths of a percent of those killed for food.

I fall somewhere in between. I think the risk is low and that the rules now in place, if diligently followed, should keep cattle free of BSE, but I am troubled by errors in compliance and the loopholes that remain: meat-and-bone meal from pigs and chickens (which, as far as we know, do not get prion diseases) can still be fed to cattle as can blood (to calves) and chicken wastes and feathers, and the remains of visibly sick "downer" animals are still allowed to be fed to chickens, pigs, farmed fish, and your favorite pets. In 2004, the FDA (which, in the peculiar division of federal responsibility for food safety, is in charge of assuring the safety of animal feed) proposed to close most of these loopholes, but was delayed in doing so by White House officials in the Bush administration, reportedly under heavy lobbying from the beef and cattle feed industries. Soon after the delay was announced, beef lobbying groups broke a long tradition of nonpartisanship and endorsed President Bush for re-election. In 2005, the FDA again proposed loophole-closing rules, this time much weaker than those initiated in previous years, undoubtedly in response to continued pressure from the meat and rendering industries.

The industry's compliance with the feed rules is also a concern. Early in 2005, while the FDA was still attempting to close the loopholes, the Government Accountability Office (GAO) issued a report accusing this agency of overstating industry compliance with the ban on feeding leftover cow parts to cows. Weaknesses in the FDA's policies and programs, said GAO investigators, "limit the effectiveness of the ban and place U.S. cattle at risk of spreading BSE." What findings like these make me fear is not so much the immediate risk of BSE, but the much longer term and more pervasive risks to the safety of the food supply from this kind of politics—politics that place industry profits above public health.

Fortunately, this is one situation in which you have a real choice. If you are worried about mad cow disease, if you are concerned about what food animals are fed, or if you just want to vote with your fork and register an objection to the lack of firm government oversight of the meat industry, you can buy meat from animals raised on an "all vegetable diet" with "no animal by-products" and "no animal cannibalism." The threat of mad cow disease, remote as it may be, is an excellent reason to buy Certified Organic meats, as I do whenever I can. But even if you are willing to pay the premium prices they command, you might have difficulty finding organic meats in your neighborhood grocery store, and may have to settle for the "near-organic" and "natural" alternatives, as I explain next.

15

Meat: Organic Versus "Natural"

I f you want to reduce the risk of mad cow disease to as close to zero as possible, organic meats offer a real choice. The rules for organic meat production expressly forbid feeding animal by-products to other animals. They also forbid the use of antibiotics and hormones and require animals and birds to be raised under conditions that appear more humane than those typical of commercial feedlots and batteries. These are good reasons to choose organic meats. So when I set out to look for organic beef, pork, and chicken in supermarkets, I thought these meats would be easy to find. Not so. If the stores sold any organic meats at all, they offered only a few kinds. Instead, I found meats labeled "natural." Natural? If the word "lean" on hamburger is a signal that you better pay attention to the fat content, the word "natural" on meat is a sure sign that you need to start asking questions.

To give one example: just about any supermarket sells chicken parts from huge corporate producers like Perdue or Tyson Foods labeled "All Natural.*" Follow the asterisk to "*Minimally processed, no artificial ingredients, all vegetable diet, no animal by-products." Such statements describe *any* chicken, and these particular chickens were undoubtedly produced by typical industrial methods—confined under crowded conditions in batteries of thousands, treated with antibiotics to keep diseases from spreading, and slaughtered under hot and dirty factory conditions.

In contrast, companies like Coleman Natural Products produce meat labeled "no antibiotics, no added hormones, no animal by-products in feed, and grass fed." These are practices designed to improve the health and safety of the animals you eat, and they are required for meats labeled organic. But meats from such companies do not carry the Certified Organic seal. Instead, they are just what the company's name implies; they are "natural." They are not organic. The statements tell you that the meats come from animals that may have been treated better than conventionally raised animals, but the missing organic seal is a sign that the animals were not necessarily raised according to the more rigorous standards set by the USDA's National Organic Program. No rules require "natural" animals to be fed organically grown grain; to be allowed freedom of movement and access to the outdoors; to be raised without using antibiotics, hormones, or other animal drugs; or to be inspected for adherence to such practices. If the producers of "natural" meats follow such practices, they do so voluntarily.

The blurred distinction between organic and "natural" is the result of some USDA history. The USDA permits the producers of conventionally raised animals and birds to label their meat as "natural" as long as they define the term truthfully. The statement "no added hormones" on packages of "natural" chicken is a good example of how this system works. The statement is truthful, but so what? Hormones are never used in raising chickens (this is like saying vegetable oils have "no cholesterol"). "No added hormones" on beef, however, does mean something. Beef producers use hormones to promote more rapid growth in cattle and sheep in the United States, and the U.S. government says these drugs are safe. In contrast, the European Union has concluded that animal hormones are bad for human health, forbids their use in European-raised beef, and refuses to allow hormone-treated American beef to be sold in its member countries. U.S. officials argue that this ban is not about health but really is designed to protect the European beef industry from American competition. Research cannot yet settle the issue of hormone safety, so you can argue the situation either way.

Buying organic meat should resolve uneasiness about hormones and mad cow disease, but finding organic chicken or beef in grocery stores is a challenge. One summer day, I went to the Columbus Circle outpost of the decidedly pro-organic supermarket, Whole Foods. A brochure in the store describes its meats as "beyond natural" and says the animals from which they come are raised according to "stringent quality standards . . . [that] help ensure the meat we sell is not at risk from Mad Cow Disease." Meats at Whole Foods may be beyond natural, but on that day the selection of meats labeled Certified Organic was limited to one line of organic turkey bacon and chicken hot dogs, some fresh organic chickens, and a few kinds of organic beef (85 percent lean ground round, marrow bones, and suet). These packages all carried the Certified Organic seal, indicating that production methods had been verified by an inspector working for an independent certifying group accredited by a federal or state agency. Companies are not allowed to use the word "organic" on package labels unless their production methods meet such requirements.

Back in my neighborhood, one supermarket had some organic hot dogs made with turkey or chicken, but that was all. The Florence Meat Market, a tiny, nostalgia-inducing, sawdust-on-the-floor butcher shop in Greenwich Village, had organic chicken but no beef. The upscale Citarella market had free-range, organic chicken from D'Artagnan, the specialty meat company, but also had no beef. Later, at the Saturday farmers' market in Union Square, Hawthorne Valley Farms was selling Certified Organic beef and pork, "grass fed and free range." Next I tried the Internet. FreshDirect, the online grocery, had just started selling organic and antibiotic-free beef and chicken. Its chicken was Certified Organic. The beef was antibiotic free but not organic. Only the organic food store on University Place, Wholesome Market, had a good selection of Certified Organic beef as well as poultry (but that store went out of business just a few months later). I thought it would be easier to find organic meats in California where so many people are interested in how food is produced. Wrong again. The Vons supermarket in

South Pasadena carried Coastal Range Organics frozen chicken breasts, and the nearby Trader Joe's carried its own brand of "Organic Drumettes" ("organic free-range chicken, sustainably farmed"), but even this environmentally friendly purveyor had no organic beef on the day I visited.

The limited selection seemed puzzling, and I could not figure out whether this was a matter of low supply, low demand, or prohibitively high prices, and I began searching for an explanation. I soon gave up trying to ask supermarket meat managers why they did not have a wider choice of Certified Organic meats. Most thought their meat *was* organic. They pointed to packages of beef and cut-up chickens labeled "all natural, no antibiotics, no hormones, grass-fed"—again "natural," but not organic. I heard about a small specialty butcher in Manhattan advertised as selling 100 percent organic meats. When I visited, the butcher said all the meats in the store were organic ("organic suckling pig"), but I did not find a Certified Organic seal on any of the packaged meats on display. This place, like meat markets everywhere I looked, sold meats labeled "all natural." Whole Foods sold its own line of "our natural" beef and chicken ("no antibiotics ever, vegetarian diet") and lunch meats made with pork ("never administered any antibiotics . . . no nitrites added"). The Trader Joe's in South Pasadena even had its own "New Naturally Raised Beef Program." A handwritten sign posted on top of the meat shelves said:

- Raised from birth without the use of antibiotics or growth hormones
- Sustainably farmed
- Free-range
- Never given any animal by-products
- All vegetable fed
- Pretty darn tasty

These practices sound so much better than conventional practices that you might think the meats must be organic, but none of their packages had the organic seal. If you set out to look for organic meats, you may feel just as bewildered as I did. Does "natural" mean nonorganic, near organic, fully organic, or none of the above? And does it matter? Before I was able to answer these questions, I had to talk to meat managers, inspectors, trade associations, producers,

> **D**oes "natural" mean nonorganic, near organic, fully organic, or none of the above? And does it matter?

and purveyors, and to take a short but enlightening detour into the truly strange world of the rules for certifying meat as organic.

ORGANIC MEATS: THE SAGA

To understand why Certified Organic meats are scarce, and why many supermarket meat managers do not seem to know the difference between "natural" and organic, you have to delve into some arcane aspects of USDA history. The USDA is a large and complicated agency, so much so that it is not at all unusual for its different units to work at cross-purposes. In developing standards for certifying meats as organic, for example, one unit of the USDA followed an entirely different pathway than the unit responsible for certifying organic fruits and vegetables. These differences became apparent soon after Congress passed the Organic Foods Production Act of 1990.

That act required the USDA to appoint an advisory committee—the National Organic Standards Board—to define standards for production practices that would qualify for organic certification. During the twelve years (1990 to 2002) that it took the board to develop the standards, the USDA unit that deals with fruits and vegetables allowed producers who did not use pesticides or chemical fertilizers to market their products as organic. But the USDA unit that deals with meat and poultry, the Food Safety and Inspection Service (FSIS), followed a quite different course. This particular section of the USDA has an unusually long and deep history of entrenched "partnership" with the industries it regulates. The FSIS listens carefully when meat industry lobbyists speak. Meat industry officials firmly opposed the idea of labeling any meat as organic. Use of the "O word," they said, might make people think that meats without the organic label were not as safe or healthy. They convinced the FSIS (and, therefore, the USDA) to decide that no meat company could use the term "organic" in its name, in descriptions of its production practices, or on its product labels.

Instead, the FSIS said that meat companies could use the word "natural" when it was appropriate to do so. Meat industry lobbying groups had no objections to this word (no surprise). The appropriate use of "natural," said the FSIS, applied to all fresh meat with only three restrictions: (1) the meat must have no artificial flavors, colors, or preservatives; (2) the meat must be processed only minimally (ground, but not cooked, for example); and (3) the companies had to define what they meant by "natural" on the package labels (hence: "no antibiotics, no hormones"). The USDA requires these terms to be truthful, but does not monitor them. It just trusts meat companies to use the word "natural" appropriately, even if the word gives the impression that it means organic—and you pay more for meat as a result.

> **M**eat industry officials firmly opposed the idea of labeling any meat as organic. Use of the "O word," they said, might make people think that meats without the organic label were not as safe or healthy.

During the years that the USDA's board was developing the standards, organic foods emerged as a small but rapidly growing segment of the food industry. Producers of organic fruits and vegetables pressed the board to develop uniform rules for the produce industry. But once developed, organic standards would apply to *all* foods—including meat—and there was little that the producers of conventional meats could do to stop this from happening. In 1999, realizing that organic standards for meat were inevitably on the way, the USDA began to allow meat producers to use "organic" as a descriptive term. But by that time, the producers of "natural" meats knew that their customers interpreted the term and its definitions—"no antibiotics," "no hormones," and "grass fed"—as practices equivalent to organic. Producers no longer needed to obtain organic certification to convince consumers (or, so it seems, managers of supermarket meat sections) that their meats were of higher quality and worth premium prices. "Natural" would do just as well.

But even the best "natural" meat is not the same as organic meat. Producers who want their meats certified as organic have to adhere to stringent criteria that producers of "natural" meats do not. "Natural" meat producers can pick and choose among desirable raising practices, but organic meat producers must adhere to *all* of them. Organic producers cannot feed parts of any other animal to their cattle or chickens ("no animal by-products or animal cannibalism"). They must never use drugs to make the animals grow faster ("no antibiotics, no hormones"). They must allow their livestock to have fresh air, sunlight, freedom of movement, and access to pasture ("grass fed"). They also must use 100 percent organic grain as feed—grain grown without the use of pesticides or artificial fertilizers (and, therefore, more expensive). And—the most critical difference—their adherence to these practices must be verified by inspectors who are certified by state or federally accredited agencies. Producers of "natural" meats do not have to follow the same rigorous practices that organic producers do in raising their animals, and they are not subject to anywhere near the same level of accountability. In return, Certified Organic meat and poultry command higher prices.

> Producers of "natural" meats do not have to follow the same rigorous practices that organic producers do in raising their animals, and they are not subject to anywhere near the same level of accountability.

The differences in the means of production and in the prices charged for organic meats explain why the distinction between "natural" and organic matters. Organic meats may be hard to find, may represent an infinitesimally small fraction of total meat sales, and may amount to only 1 percent or so of all organic products, but their sales are increasing rapidly. Sales in 2003 were just $75 million, but that was double the amount in 2002. This sharp increase gives the organic industry high hopes for growth. Industry analysts expect sales of organic meat and poultry to increase by 30 percent or more a year through 2008—faster than for any other organic food. To achieve such growth, organic meats must be clearly distinguished from "natural" meats, but doing so will not be easy. The Table explains the differences.

A Quick Comparison of Conventional, "Natural," and Organic Meats

PRODUCTION PRACTICE	CONVENTIONAL	NATURAL	ORGANIC
Animals can be fed only Certified Organic feed	No	No	Yes
Feed grains can be grown using chemical pesticides and fertilizers; can be genetically engineered, irradiated, or fertilized with sewage sludge	Yes	Yes	No
Animals can be treated with antibiotics or hormones	Yes	Yes*	No
Animals can be fed the by-products of other animals	Yes	Yes*	No
Animals may be routinely confined	Yes	Yes*	No
Animals must be treated in ways that reduce stress	No	No*	Yes
Animals must have access to outdoors, exercise areas, sunlight	No	No*	Yes
Cattle must have access to pasture ("grass fed" or "grass finished")	No	No*	Yes
Farms must be inspected for compliance by a qualified person certified by a federal or state agency	No	No (although some have their own inspectors)	Yes

* Unless otherwise stated on the product label or in advertising

"Natural" meats may follow some or all of the organic practices, but they do not have to. "Natural" is on the honor system. Some producers of "natural" meats may be honorable, but you have to take what they say on faith. The Niman Ranch, for example, says it produces the finest tasting meat in the world by adhering to a strict code of husbandry principles: our livestock are humanely treated, fed the finest natural feeds, never given growth-promoting hormones or antibiotics, and are raised on land that is cared for as a sustainable resource.

This and other such ranches have developed their own systems for inspecting and keeping track of their animals. If you have met Bill Niman, as I have, you have good reason to think that his company does precisely as advertised. But if you do not know how companies raise their meat, how can you know whether or not to believe what they say? It is hard to know what to make of the practices of a company like B3R All Natural Beef (now owned by a company that also owns Coleman) when its slogan until 2005 was "Helping cattlemen merchandise maximum dollars from their cow herd." Maybe such companies follow organic principles in letter and in spirit, but I would feel more confident that they did so if I knew that a qualified certifying inspector checked up on them at regular intervals and was holding them accountable.

> "Natural" meats may follow some or all of the organic practices, but they do not have to. "Natural" is on the honor system.

CERTIFIED MEATS: ALTERNATIVES

I am also unsure how to interpret alternative systems of certification. At my nearby Wholesome Market, I found Murray's chicken labeled as "Certified Humane." The label said the chickens met Humane Farm Animal Care Standards, including the usual "all natural" prohibitions—no antibiotics, hormones, by-products, or confinement—along with one I hadn't seen before: the "ability to engage in natural behaviors" (these were not specified). These methods sound promising, but unless you take the trouble to go to the Web site and see that this is a program of the American Society for the Prevention of Cruelty to Animals and various humane societies—groups you may feel you can trust—you would have no way of knowing whether this kind of certification has any real meaning.

All of this made me want to know: If natural and humane producers like Coleman, Niman, and Murray's are doing such a good job of raising their animals, why aren't their meats Certified Organic? I asked this question of everyone I could. The reasons given by these producers and others are complicated, and sometimes troubling. Some told me they intend to become certified but are still in the process; the rules only went into effect in October 2002, after all, and obtaining certification can take several years. Others, particularly small ranchers, said it was just too time-consuming and expensive to do what was needed to obtain certification. A spokesman for the Coleman ranch, however, gave a more practical reason: the company was unable to require all of its suppliers to graze their animals on organic pasture or feed them Certified Organic grain (as required by the organic standards) because it would be too expensive for the ranchers to do so. Still others told me that their herds are small and if they had to cull animals that had been treated with antibiotics (as is also required by the standards), they would lose too much money.

Ranching is a business and there is no question that it costs more—sometimes a lot more—to raise organic beef or poultry than it does to raise conventional or "natural" meat. A representative of the Niman Ranch, Frankie Whitman, explained that the cost of organic feed is the main reason why the company had decided not to seek organic certification. For that company, the cost of organic feed makes it impossible to price its humanely and sustainably raised meat at a level that consumers would be willing to pay. Its ranchers feed lambs on alfalfa, which does not grow well without pesticides. They feed soy meal to pigs, but soy processors who make the meal have no simple or inexpensive method for keeping organic soybeans separate from those that are genetically engineered. These factors increase the cost of producing organic feed to a level that companies view as prohibitive. The Niman Ranch would have to pass those costs along to consumers. This would make its meats too much more expensive than either conventional or "natural" meats.

These reasons, if unfortunate, are understandable enough. But I cannot accept one additional argument that I often hear from meat producers. They tell me they do not like having to deal with government bureaucracy. They do not trust government in general, and they particularly distrust the USDA's commitment to organics. There may well be good reasons for this view—some parts of the USDA are much less consumer-friendly than others—but they take the argument one step further. These meat producers say they are refusing to seek certification because the USDA's Organic Standards are "too easy," whereas they are raising animals under conditions that go "beyond organic" and exceed USDA requirements. This contention is unverifiable, however, since their ranches are not subject to inspection. If, as they say, it were easy to become certified, the process should be a slam-dunk and I think they should do it. By not obtaining organic certification, "natural" meat companies raise questions about their own credibility.

The best evidence that Organic Standards really do mean something—and are not so easy to achieve—comes from the unrelenting efforts to weaken them from Big Meat, Big Organics, the USDA itself, and now Congress.

The history of these efforts is sobering. Soon after the standards went into effect, a commercial poultry producer in Georgia got his local congressman to sneak a clause into a federal spending bill just as it was about to be passed. The clause would allow him to feed nonorganic grain to his "organic" chickens any time the cost of

> The best evidence that Organic Standards really do mean something—and are not so easy to achieve—comes from the unrelenting efforts to weaken them.

100 percent organic feed went up to twice the cost of conventional feed. Congress eventually undid this mistake, but only after an uproar spearheaded by, among others, the Organic Trade Association (which, because it represents large as well as small producers, has clout with Congress). The USDA also ignored its own Organic Standards Board and overruled a decision by one of its accredited certifying agencies to refuse to certify eggs as organic from chickens denied access to the outdoors. Large producers of eggs successfully argued that chickens would be healthier and safer if kept indoors. In a concession to large meat producers interested in reducing feed costs, the USDA said it would allow organic ranchers to feed nonorganic fish meal to their livestock and to keep antibiotic-treated dairy cows in their organic herds. Organic producers and their constituents again went into an uproar, and the USDA again backed down and withdrew the proposals. In 2005, the Organic Standards Board recommended that dairy cows producing

organic milk be allowed access to pasture during summer months; USDA officials sent the recommendation back to the board for reconsideration.

This repeated pattern—the USDA proposes weakening the rules, sees how much fuss its proposal causes, and backs down if it causes too much—is a clear indication that the Organic Standards are meaningful and worth fighting for. It is also worth fighting some of the lobbying actions of the "Big Organic" Trade Association and the stealth attacks on the Organic Standards by Congress that I discussed in Chapter 3. The standards have to be set high to maintain their credibility as well as to convince you that paying more for organic meats is worth it—for the animals, the environment, and yourself.

ANIMALS: "GRASS FED" AND "GRASS FINISHED"

The Trader Joe's in South Pasadena carries its own brand of Grassfed Angus Ground Beef—"always grassfed, always natural." "Grass fed" is a healthier alternative to conventional feeding (in which cattle eat more concentrated calories from soybeans and corn to fatten them up as quickly as possible). The "grass-fed" alternative sounds bucolic, but you have no easy way of knowing what it really means, because when it comes to grass feeding, even the Organic Standards are ambiguous—they simply require cattle to have access to the outdoors, sunlight, exercise areas, and pasture. "Access to pasture" may suggest that the animals are outside grazing on grass, but grass feeding is not a requirement for organic certification. The animals just have to be allowed out (but do not have to *be* out), and can be fed corn and soybeans as long as the feed is organic. When meat is advertised as "grass fed," the labels never say how long the animals are allowed to graze or how much of their diet they get from grass. And cattle advertised as "grass fed" do not have to be exclusively grass fed. Nor do they have to be "grass finished," which means fed exclusively on grass in the weeks just before slaughter. ·

In other words, grass feeding and finishing are open to interpretation, and neither is subject to inspection. This is too bad because grass feeding improves the safety and the nutritional quality of meat. The digestive systems of cows and sheep are set up to handle grass. The rumen stomach works like a fermentation vat; it contains vast numbers of bacteria that convert chewed-up grass and hay into nutrients (something we cannot do). The animals use these nutrients to grow and make meat. Ruminants are not well designed to handle the more concentrated fats, proteins, and carbohydrates in soybeans and corn. Eating concentrated feed made from corn and soybeans makes cattle grow faster and fatter, but it alters the mix of bacteria in their rumens. This gives them the equivalent of cow indigestion; the animals are not as healthy and need antibiotic treatment more frequently. The concentrated feed also encourages the growth of harmful kinds of bacteria; these do not bother the animals but can make you sick if you are exposed to them. Researchers who have looked at the comparative safety and nutritional value of beef fed grain or grass declare grass fed the winner, and here is why:

- Pasture-fed cattle have lower levels of harmful *Campylobacter* and *E. coli* O157:H7 than those raised in feedlots.

- Calves raised on pasture have less *E. coli* O157:H7 than calves raised in barns.

- Grass-finished cattle excrete fewer dangerous bacteria in their feces; this reduces the spread of such bacteria onto meat in slaughterhouses.

- Grass-fed cattle get sick less often and need fewer treatments with antibiotics.

All this makes perfect sense. Cows are *supposed* to eat grass, so it should come as no surprise to learn that grass feeding affects the nutritional composition of meat. The adage "you are what you eat" applies to cows as well as to people. The purpose of feedlots is to fatten up animals in a hurry. In contrast, access to pasture allows the cattle to graze on low-calorie grass while using up energy as they move around. The result: meat with less fat and fewer calories. Grass feeding also affects the type of fat in the meat. Grass-fed beef is still high in saturated fat (the bad kind), but it has more of some good fats—omega-3s—because these are prevalent in grass. And this kind of meat is also higher in vitamin E and other vitamins present in grass.

But grass feeding tends to be a big selling point for one other nutritional reason: an obscure group of fatty acids called conjugated linoleic acids, or CLAs. Because some researchers think CLAs confer special health benefits, it is worth taking a look at what those might be. CLAs are found in tiny amounts in all animals and their milk, but ruminants (cows and the like) have more. CLAs are more plentiful in ruminants because rumens house bacteria that convert some of the fatty acids in grass—particularly linoleic acid—to CLAs. Ruminants fed on grass have twice as many CLAs as those fed concentrated grains (1 percent of fat as opposed to 0.5 percent). You might not think of grass as a good source of fat, and of course it is not. But because cows eat such a huge volume of grass, the rumen bacteria have plenty of fat to work with. And what they do to grass fats is almost the same as what food chemists do to soy oil to make margarine: rumen bacteria add hydrogen. But in this case, hydrogenation may do some good as well as bad.

Bacterial hydrogenation works much like the hydrogenation of margarine in three ways. First, the bad: bacterial hydrogenation makes the grass fats more saturated. This is why the fats in the meat and milk of ruminant animals are twice as saturated as the fat from chickens—60 percent as compared to 30 percent. Chickens do not have rumens. Second, the good: like the hydrogenation of margarine, bacterial hydrogenation only partially hydrogenates the fat. But here is one important difference: bacteria partially hydrogenate linoleic acid to form a variety of unusual chemical variants referred to as "conjugated"—hence, conjugated linoleic acids. The third similarity is that bacterial hydrogenation creates *trans* fats in meat and milk. But here there is an important distinction: the effects of feeding *trans* CLAs to experimental animals are markedly different from the heart disease–raising effects of the *trans* fats in margarine. Indeed, they are so different that proponents of grass feeding and purveyors of CLA supplements talk about CLAs as nothing short of a new miracle "drug."

In rats and mice, the CLA "drug" appears to do wonders for preventing cancer, which is reason enough to attract interest. But in other animals, CLAs are also said to prevent or reduce symptoms of diabetes, heart disease, bone diseases, and immune system disorders. Any list of benefits this long should make you suspicious and, in this case, some skepticism is warranted. The results of animal studies are inconsistent and contradictory, and leave many questions unanswered. And when it comes to human health, the picture becomes even murkier. Because the levels of CLAs in milk and meat are so low, researchers study health effects by giving people CLA supplements—and in amounts much higher than those ever found in food. I am not aware of CLA studies involving cancer prevention (those would be difficult to do), but the few human studies of other conditions that have been done to date should not convince you that CLA supplements improve blood cholesterol levels, body weight, or immune function. Maybe the very low levels of CLAs in meat and milk improve health better than the higher-dose supplements, but it is too soon to tell. At the moment, CLAs are another issue for which "more research is needed," and are not yet a compelling reason to eat grass-fed beef.

Ah, but what about the taste of grass-fed beef? I like it. I find it more subtle than the taste of grain-fed beef, but such judgments are personal. The November 2002 issue of *Consumer Reports* gives the results of taste tests of strip steaks from animals fed on grass or grain. Its panelists judged grass-fed steaks as milder and less tender, but not really all that different. Whatever your feelings about leanness, nutritional benefits, or taste, there are many other good reasons for allowing cows out to pasture—humane treatment and meat safety among them.

MEAT: THE CHOICES

With so many issues to be evaluated and balanced against one another, the choice of meat and poultry seems especially complicated. When price is no object, my hierarchy of choices goes like this:

1. Certified Organic because the rules make sense and production is monitored by regular inspections that hold growers accountable for their practices

2. "Natural" when it is near organic, meaning "no antibiotics, no hormones, no animal by-products, humanely treated, and grass fed"

3. All the other kinds

I think it matters a lot that Certified Organic meat producers have to be inspected, and I wish that near-organic producers could solve their feed problems, become certified, and make organic meats more widely available. Perhaps the easiest way to support organic meat production would be to press for a reallocation of some of the $22 billion spent annually on farm subsidies. Instead of supporting the production of conventional oilseeds and grains, transfer the subsidies to the growers of organic feed. If you care about this issue, consider a letter-writing campaign to your congressional representatives.

In the meantime, you can help create a demand for organic meats. Talk to your meat department managers, and they may get the idea and start looking for sources. As Frankie Whitman of the Niman Ranch explained this company's dilemma, "We certainly support the organic industry and applaud organic producers, but it isn't part of our current business model right now. We believe economic sustainability is the key to agricultural sustainability. If we can't find a viable, consistent market willing to pay the price, we can't source the product."

If you want organic meats, ask for them and be willing to pay your small share of the costs of production. If you cannot find them in your local stores, try farmers' markets and the Internet. You will have to search for suppliers of Certified Organic meat and poultry, but they do exist, are increasing in number and strength, and deserve support.

16

Fish: Dilemmas and Quandaries

One Saturday morning in mid-October, I found a surprising item at the seafood counter of the Wegmans market in Ithaca. Ithaca is in central New York State, 250 miles or so from Long Island Sound, but there, laid out on an only slightly bloodied bed of ice, was an enormous mako shark—at least five feet long and, in answer to my immediate questions, 198 pounds and caught just a few days earlier in the North Atlantic. Customers could buy steaks cut from its underside, but mostly the shark was there to attract attention to the dozens of other iced, smoked, or cooked fish and shellfish on display, some whole, others cut into portion-size pieces. These had been carefully selected by the market's seafood manager, Chris Maxwell, whose enthusiastic interest in fish—from its supply to its nutritional value—borders on the encyclopedic. Wegmans, he told me, buys fish only from known suppliers, relies on just two sources of farmed fish, tests the fish for bacterial and chemical contaminants, visits suppliers to make sure they follow safety procedures, and generally takes care to offer its customers only the freshest and safest products. Knowing this, he explained, a Boston-based fishing crew had called him personally to offer its prize catch. On ice from the moment it was caught, this shark would be fully converted to steaks by the next day. In the meantime, Maxwell was showing it off with a small fish placed between its jaws, and not just for dramatic effect. He wanted to make sure that nobody on his staff got cut on the rows of razor-sharp teeth.

Those teeth pointed to the first of several troubling dilemmas and quandaries that come with eating fish. Shark meat is a rich source of omega-3 fats, the type said to do good things for human development and for the heart. But the teeth tell you that sharks are meat eaters near the very top of the food chain. Sharks feast on seals and whales (and, occasionally, people) whenever they can, but mostly they eat big fish which, in turn, eat successively smaller fish. Only the tiniest fish are omnivores; they eat plankton—microscopic plants and animals—at the bottom of the food chain. The position of a fish in the food chain matters because rivers and oceans are highly polluted with toxic chemicals that get into the water from industrial wastes and agricultural runoff. These become incorporated into the muscles and fat of small fish, and get passed up the food chain. Sharks do not come with Chemical Facts labels, and you have no way of knowing what toxins they may carry. That is why shark tops the list of fish that you should hardly ever eat—and should never give to young children or eat yourself if you are pregnant or even remotely likely to become pregnant. When you see a shark or any other predatory fish of impressive size, you have to assume that its meat is loaded with toxic chemicals. Shark is for adults only, and nonpregnant ones at that.

As Maxwell will be happy to discuss with you, seafood poses several such dilemmas, and these affect fish sellers as well as eaters. His job is to offer fresh, delicious, and safe seafood at a price you are willing to pay, but the minute he has to deal with problems related to health and safety, his costs go up. Your dilemmas go way beyond price. To make an intelligent choice of fish at a supermarket, you have to know more than you could possibly imagine about nutrition, fish toxicology, and the life cycle and ecology of fish—what kind of fish it is, what it eats, where it was caught, and whether it was farmed or wild. If you are at all concerned about environmental is-

W hen you see a shark or any other predatory fish of impressive size, you have to assume that its meat is loaded with toxic chemicals. Shark is for adults only, and nonpregnant ones at that.

sues, you will also want to know how it was caught and raised and whether its stocks are sustainable.

Short of gaining this level of expertise—which, I can assure you, is not easy to do—you have only two choices. You must buy your fish from someone you trust, or you must rely on a seafood advisory card produced by one or another advocacy group that ranks fish according to standards of safety and sustainability. As you might imagine, neither approach is entirely satisfactory. It is not always easy or possible to know whether your fishmonger is trustworthy, and the seafood cards, invaluable as they are, tend to focus more on environmental than on health issues. Hence: the dilemmas.

FISH DILEMMA #1: OMEGA-3 FATS VERSUS METHYLMERCURY

The most troubling health dilemma is the one posed by the Wegmans shark: balancing the health benefits of a fish against the harm that might be caused by its content of toxic chemicals—most of all, methylmercury.

As a group, fish are excellent sources of protein, vitamins, and minerals. Their fats are largely unsaturated and are especially rich in omega-3 fatty acids, particularly the ones abbreviated EPA and DHA. Because these omega-3s show up in the brain, they are believed critical to the normal development of the infant nervous system. Fish are the best source of omega-3 fatty acids, and practically all health authorities advise pregnant women to eat fish once or twice a week. More than that, some research suggests that EPA and DHA might prevent the blood clots and irregular heartbeats that often lead to heart attacks or strokes. Although the studies are neither consistent nor entirely compelling, the American Heart Association draws on them as evidence that *everyone* should eat fish twice a week.

In 2004, the scientific committee updating the *Dietary Guidelines for Americans* agreed with this advice and also recommended two servings of fish a week for most people. As part of its recommendation to "Choose fats wisely for good health," this committee laid out the dilemma faced by anyone who enjoys eating fish:

A reduced risk of both sudden death and CHD [coronary heart disease] death in adults is associated with the consumption of two servings (approximately eight ounces) per week of fish high in the [omega-3] fatty acids called eicosapentaenoic acid (EPA) and docosahexaenoic acid (DHA). To benefit from the potential cardioprotective effects of EPA and DHA, the weekly consumption of two servings of fish, particularly fish rich in EPA and DHA, is suggested. However, it is advisable for pregnant women, lactating women, and children to avoid eating fish with a high mercury content and to limit their consumption of fish with a moderate mercury content.

The committee did not say how you are supposed to know which fish are rich in EPA and DHA, nor did it offer much help with figuring out which fish are high or moderate in mercury: "Consulting current consumer advisories helps one know which species of fish to limit or avoid . . ." This, of course, requires that you identify and obtain a consumer advisory card that lists fish you can eat always, sometimes, or never. Perhaps for these reasons, the federal agencies involved in this process dropped this part of the discussion of fish from the published version of the guidelines and said only:

Limited evidence suggests an association between consumption of fatty acids in fish and reduced risks of mortality from cardiovascular disease for the general population. Other sources of EPA and DHA may provide similar benefits; however, more research is needed.

Here we see that "more research is needed" phrase again, a clear sign that the importance of fish to health is uncertain. I will have more to say about the consumer advisory cards toward the end of the fish section. But for now, let's examine the delicate problem of how to balance whatever the health benefits of fish might be against the hazards of high or moderate amounts of methylmercury.

The beneficial effects of omega-3 fats on heart disease risk have been of interest since the early 1970s. At that time, Danish researchers observed that indigenous people in Greenland had unusually few heart attacks even though they ate diets very high in fat. Because the fats came mainly from fish, seals, and whales, the researchers soon decided that the EPA and DHA in these marine animals must be protective. Much subsequent research supports the idea that eating fish is good for heart health. One potentially important effect of omega-3s is to reduce blood triglycerides (fats). In some studies, omega-3 fatty acids appear to protect against high blood pressure and irregular heartbeats (but other studies suggest that they make irregular heartbeats worse in some people). Most— but also not all—studies also find that omega-3s help prevent sudden death from heart disease.

Despite the inconsistencies in the research, many health authorities believe that omega-3s are good for your heart's health. Just how good, though, is one of the uncertainties. So is whether the evidence means that you must eat fish to get such benefits. Another question is whether fish oil supplements are as effective as fish. Supplements are often problematic because they are basically unregulated, but tests of omega-3 supplements indicate that most are fine and contain what they say they do. *Consumer Reports*, for example, evaluated omega-3 supplements in July 2003; all of the sixteen samples it tested contained about as much EPA and DHA as promised on their labels, and none had much in the way of toxins. In 2004, a private laboratory tested samples of EPA and DHA supplements and found most to be fresh (not rancid), to be free of detectable contaminants, and to contain the amounts listed on the package labels; just two of forty-one samples failed to meet one or another of these criteria.

OMEGA-3S: THE HEALTH CLAIMS

The quality and effectiveness of supplements are worth discussion because, like other foods, fish have an industry behind them eager to get you to eat more fish, more often. One way to convince people to eat more fish is to promote fish as the best (or only) source of omega-3s. Thus the fish industry lobbied vigorously and successfully to convince the FDA to approve a health claim for the benefits of omega-3 fatty acids in fish and fish oils.

To follow the story of the omega-3 health claim, we must go back to 1990, when Congress passed the Nutrition Labeling and Education Act.

This act required food companies to put Nutrition Facts labels on their products, something long opposed by the food industry. In 1990, to obtain industry support for requiring Nutrition Facts labels on food products, Congress granted a huge concession. For the first time, it allowed food companies to put claims about the health benefits of certain nutrients in their products on the package labels. To start the process, Congress ordered the FDA to review the scientific evidence for ten possible claims for health benefits, among them the claim that omega-3 fatty acids protect against heart disease. The FDA conducted that review but found the studies to be so limited and so contradictory that it refused to allow companies to use the claim. Seafood companies, said the FDA, could label their products "rich in omega-3," but could not say that eating fish protects against heart disease.

I n 1990, to obtain industry support for requiring Nutrition Facts labels on food products, Congress granted a huge concession. For the first time, it allowed food companies to put claims about the health benefits of certain nutrients in their products on the package labels.

More than a decade later, the science is still limited and contradictory, but the political environment has changed. In response to petitions and lawsuits from industry groups, the FDA has been forced to relax its scientific standards for health claims. It now permits health claims that do not meet rigorous scientific standards as long as the claims are "qualified" so they are not misleading. In 2000, as a result of a lawsuit, the FDA allowed a qualified health claim for dietary supplements of fish oils containing omega-3 fats. In 2004, in response to further petitions, the FDA said that conventional foods as well as omega-3 supplements could be labeled with this statement: "Supportive but *not conclusive* research shows that consumption of EPA and DHA omega-3 fatty acids *may* reduce the risk of coronary heart disease" (italics are mine).

Rosie Mestel, a reporter for the *Los Angeles Times*, guessed why food companies wanted to make this claim: "As Madison Avenue might prefer to put it," she said, "Fish oils! They're healthy! And they're not just for fish anymore!" Together, the claim and the advice about fish in the dietary guidelines were hailed as excellent news for the seafood industry. Linda Candler of the National Fisheries Institute, a trade association for this industry, told *SeaFood Business* magazine that the two government actions meant "Opportunity and more opportunity . . . We're thrilled to death with both because in combination this has the potential to really boost seafood consumption."

Evie Hansen, the owner of National Seafood Educators, a public relations arm of the seafood industry, noted that she would no longer "have to go into the health-claim info and pick apart EPA and DHA. We can now say to the consumer, 'Have you eaten seafood at least twice this week?'" Her company put a logo, "Seafood Twice-a-Week," on posters: "The American Heart Association recommends eating 2 weekly servings of fish, preferably fatty fish such as tuna and salmon." The poster, however, failed to include the rest of the American Heart Association's qualified advice: "the fish recommendations must be balanced with concerns about environmental pollutants, in particular PCB and methylmercury . . ." Concerns about PCBs are the basis of a second dilemma (a discussion that comes in a later chapter). In the meantime, we have methylmercury to consider.

THE METHYLMERCURY PROBLEM

Mercury is a naturally occurring heavy metal best known for its function in thermometers of the pre-digital era. If you are old enough, you may remember playing with little balls of mercury that rolled out of broken thermometers. The phrase "mad as a hatter" and the Mad Hatter of the *Alice in Wonderland* tea party refer to the severe damage to the brain and nervous system that resulted from constant exposure to the mercury used in making felt hats. Mercury is no longer used in that process. Instead, one of its major sources these days is emissions from coal-burning power plants. Because it is heavy, mercury falls from those emissions into nearby fields and waterways. By itself, mercury is not very toxic; if you eat it, you do not absorb much of it from your digestive tract. But when mercury gets into water, microorganisms

> If you are pregnant, methylmercury crosses the placenta and goes right to the brain and nervous system of your developing fetus, with potentially disastrous consequences.

"methylate" it and convert it to methylmercury, which you can absorb easily and quickly. If you are pregnant, methylmercury crosses the placenta and goes right to the brain and nervous system of your developing fetus, with potentially disastrous consequences.

You may have seen the poignant photographs of children who were poisoned by methylmercury in the town of Minamata, Japan. The most memorable of these images shows a mother tenderly bathing her emaciated, deformed, and twisted child—the result of the methylmercury unknowingly consumed during pregnancy. The Minamata tragedy began in the 1930s, when Chisso, a company that made fertilizer and plastics, began dumping industrial waste—including an estimated twenty-seven tons of mercury—into Minamata Bay. Mercury became methylmercury. Small fish took in methylmercury from the water as they fed on plankton, and the methylmercury stuck tightly to proteins in their muscles. Larger fish ate smaller fish, and methylmercury passed up the food chain. Pregnant Minamata women who ate larger fish passed the toxin to their developing fetuses. By the 1950s, thousands of children in the area around Minamata Bay were crippled by damage to their brains and nervous systems.

Although investigations soon revealed that Minamata waters had more than fifty times more methylmercury than anyone considered safe, Chisso continued dumping its wastes into the bay until 1968, and the Japanese government continued to allow people to fish there until 1976. The decades of delays are explained in part by ignorance, but even more by corporate greed and government collusion. Chisso did not have a low-cost alternative to mercury in its plastics-making process, the government did not want to shut down an industry that brought prosperity to the region, and local fishermen who opposed the dumping were silenced by company payoffs.

Minamata should have served as a worldwide warning that mercury industrial wastes must be kept out of waterways, but no such luck. Mercury may be heavy and stay near where it lands, but rivers, lakes, and oceans are full of small fish that grow up near mercury-laden industrial sites, swim away, and pass methylmercury up the food chain to fish that swim even longer distances.

In 1991, the Institute of Medicine (IOM), a prestigious think tank in Washington, D.C., that advises the U.S. government about health issues, identified methylmercury as a serious hazard for three groups of people: anyone who does recreational fishing, all children, and all pregnant women. The IOM pointed out that methylmercury is especially hard to deal with because its effects in adults "do not take the form of obvious, distinctive, and acute illnesses." Instead, symptoms start with numbness and tingling, and include such vague problems as muscle weakness, fatigue, headache, irritability, and an inability to concentrate, all of which could be due to any number of other causes. Nevertheless, the IOM warned that current actions to prevent mercury contamination were "too few and too permissive." Everyone, the IOM said, should avoid eating much of the fish that are highest in methylmercury—especially shark, swordfish, and tuna. Worse, it said pregnant women and young children should not eat such fish at all. This report should have set off immediate alarm bells, but it did not—for reasons of politics, of course.

17

Fish: The Methylmercury Dilemma

Here is a quick summary of the first of the fish dilemmas: fish are good to eat for their nutritional value, and especially for their content of omega-3 fats. But all seafood is contaminated with methylmercury, a toxic substance that is dangerous for a developing fetus—especially during the early months of pregnancy. The amounts of methylmercury in fish vary widely, and it is a good idea to avoid eating the most contaminated kinds. To do this, you need to know which fish have the most methylmercury. Avoiding it sounds simple enough, but like much else about fish, the methylmercury dilemma is inevitably complicated by politics.

This fish story starts in 1994, when the FDA issued its first "advisory" about methylmercury in seafood. Mercury, the FDA said, could be quite elevated in waters near industrial pollution. As a result, predatory fish like shark, swordfish, and albacore tuna (the expensive "white" tuna that you eat as steaks or from cans) could have amounts that exceed levels considered safe. For most adults, the FDA considered these fish "safe, provided they are eaten infrequently (no more than once a week) as part of a balanced diet." But because nobody really knows the amount that is safe to eat, the advice for pregnant women was more restrictive. The FDA said that pregnant women—and women who *might* become pregnant—should not eat shark or swordfish more than once a month.

The 1994 FDA advisory said not a word about restrictions on albacore tuna. This kind of tuna has less methylmercury than shark or swordfish, but three times more than the smaller and cheaper varieties— the "chunk light" tunas that you usually find in cans. But Americans eat more tuna than any other predatory fish. So the FDA's omission of an advisory for albacore tuna seemed an odd oversight. It is best explained by the FDA's regulatory mission, which is to balance health risks against cost considerations, among them costs to industry. Albacore tuna clearly belonged on the list of fish to avoid, but advice to restrict its consumption would surely affect the livelihoods of people who fish for, can, and sell tuna. Because hardly anyone knows the difference between one kind of tuna and another, fish companies worried that consumers would interpret advice to avoid albacore tuna as advice to avoid *all* tuna. Industry lobbyists urged the FDA to keep albacore tuna off the methylmercury advisory. Somehow, albacore tuna got left off.

B ecause hardly anyone knows the difference between one kind of tuna and another, fish companies worried that consumers would interpret advice to avoid albacore tuna as advice to avoid *all* tuna. Industry lobbyists urged the FDA to keep albacore tuna off the methylmercury advisory.

FEDERAL ADVISORIES: FDA AND EPA

At this point, another federal agency enters the picture—the Environmental Protection Agency (EPA). The EPA is responsible for protecting the health of the public against pollutants in air and water. Since toxic contaminants in water get incorporated into fish, the EPA issues advisories about which fish are safe to eat—particularly those caught for sport and private use. In 1999, Congress directed the EPA to commission a report from the National Research Council (NRC) about the toxic effects of methylmercury. The NRC often recruits scientists to write reports on matters that affect government policy, and Congress wanted it to help the EPA set safety standards for levels of methylmercury in the body.

The NRC produced its report in 2000. You can interpret the conclusions of this report as reassuring or not. The NRC said that if you eat an average amount of fish, you have a low risk of harm. But if you eat a lot of predatory fish, you "might have little or no margin of safety," meaning that your intake of methylmercury could be uncomfortably close to levels considered unsafe. Because methylmercury is most harmful during fetal development, the risks are highest for children born to women who eat a lot of seafood during pregnancy. The possibility of harm, said the NRC, is so great that it might increase

> the number of children who have to struggle to keep up in school and who might require remedial classes or special education. Because of the beneficial effects of fish consumption, the long-term goal needs to be a reduction in the concentrations of [methylmercury] in fish rather than replacement of fish in the diet by other foods.

Important as this goal might be, the NRC did not discuss what needed to be done to reach it. Instead, the NRC concluded that "In the interim, the best method of maintaining fish consumption and minimizing [mercury] exposure is the consumption of fish known to have lower [methylmercury] concentrations." The report also did not identify what those desirable fish might be.

In 2001, the FDA used this report as the basis for an update of its mercury advisory. Since the advice of the two agencies—EPA and FDA—can be hard to follow, I've summarized the progression of advice over time in the Table on the facing page.

In its 2001 advisory, the FDA warned pregnant women to avoid eating four kinds of fish—shark, swordfish, king mackerel, and tilefish—but said it was safe to continue eating all other fish twice a week as long as amounts did not exceed 12 ounces in total. Once again, the FDA said nothing about the danger of methylmercury in albacore tuna, which is eaten much more frequently than those other four fish.

Indeed, because so few people eat those fish regularly, this advisory did not get much attention—except from the Environmental Working Group (EWG). This "public interest watchdog" organization had a different interpretation of the data on methylmercury exposure than the FDA's. According to the EWG's analysis, if pregnant women ate other fish twice a week, especially albacore tuna, at least one quarter of them

Evolution of Government Advice to Pregnant Women (and Women Who Might Become Pregnant) About Methylmercury in Commercial Fish

ADVISORY	FISH HIGH IN METHYL-MERCURY	ADVISABLE TO EAT	ALBACORE TUNA	OTHER FISH
FDA, 1994	Shark Swordfish	Once a month	No limits	No limits
FDA, 2001	Shark Swordfish King Mackerel Tilefish	Never	No limits	Twice a week (12 ounces total)
FDA and EPA, 2004	Shark Swordfish King Mackerel Tilefish	Never	Once a week (6 ounces)	Twice a week (12 ounces, of which 6 ounces can be albacore tuna)

would be taking in levels of methylmercury that come uncomfortably close to unsafe. The FDA's weak advice, said the EWG, "fails to meet standards for accuracy and scientific integrity" and, if followed, would actually "increase the number of women of childbearing age with unsafe levels of mercury in their blood."

In response to this charge, the FDA explained that it could not issue more restrictive advice because the results of its focus-group testing indicated that women would misinterpret that kind of advice. If the FDA said to "limit" fish intake, women would think they should *never* eat fish. The EWG was not convinced by this explanation; it filed a Freedom of Information Act request for the documents related to the FDA's mercury advisory. These documents revealed that the FDA originally planned to include warnings about tuna steaks and canned tuna in its advisory, but dropped them after three meetings with representatives of the tuna industry. The documents also provided evidence for a different interpretation of the focus-group results. The EWG's interpretation was that most women understood quite well that they only needed to avoid fish high in methylmercury. The documents showed that FDA officials had met

These documents revealed that the FDA originally planned to include warnings about tuna steaks and canned tuna in its advisory, but dropped them after three meetings with representatives of the tuna industry.

with many groups that urged stricter standards for methylmercury, but only paid attention to advice from the tuna lobbyists. One tuna lobbyist told *The New York Times*, "I certainly hope we had an impact because we showed them the nutritional benefits of tuna."

Following these revelations, the FDA asked its Food Advisory Committee for help in dealing with the methylmercury problem. The committee honed in on the inconsistencies in the FDA and EPA standards for safe levels of mercury, especially as applied to tuna—the fish eaten most often by American women. These inconsistencies occur as a result of the different mandates of the advising agencies. The FDA regulates commercial seafood and considers the effects of harm to the industry as well as to human health. The EPA sets standards for fish caught by people who fish for sport or personal consumption, and only considers risks to the health of people who eat such fish; it is not supposed to consider risks to the industry. Because, as I will soon explain, virtually all waterways in the United States are heavily contaminated with methylmercury or other chemical pollutants, the EPA's safety limits are invariably stricter than those of the FDA. The NRC writes reports and is just advisory, but if the FDA did what the NRC suggested in 2000, it would have to tell pregnant women that they should never eat albacore tuna and should only eat the cheaper kinds of canned tuna once a month if at all.

The Food Advisory Committee urged the FDA and the EPA to get together and issue just one set of recommendations for methylmercury, and the two agencies did so in March 2004. Given the antiregulatory climate in Washington at the time, their joint advisory reflected the more relaxed standards used by the FDA in 2001. The advisory said that if you are in any of four categories—a woman who might become pregnant, a pregnant woman, a nursing mother, or a young child—you should avoid shark, swordfish, king mackerel, and tilefish altogether, but you can eat up to two meals (12 ounces total) a week of low-mercury seafood like canned light tuna, among others. Children should eat proportionately less. But, the agencies said, because albacore tuna has more mercury than canned light tuna, only one of those meals could be alba-core tuna.

The joint advice for eating sports fish said nothing about eating commercially caught types that are high in methylmercury, but did say you should eat fish caught by friends only once a week (friends don't let friends eat fish?). If you do eat fish caught for sport, said the FDA and the EPA, you should not eat any other fish that week, and you also should not let your kids eat much sports fish, if any.

Although federal advice was becoming a bit more restrictive, the Environmental Working Group thought it was still way too lax. By its analysis, the FDA and the EPA should have included albacore tuna in the "do not eat" category for pregnant women, along with a list of other kinds of commercial fish and sports fish that exceed standards for methylmercury. Because that list is so long (and, perhaps, because one fish seems much like another to most people) this advocacy group argued that the FDA and the EPA should have instructed pregnant women not to eat any other fish—except those lowest in methylmercury—more than once a month.

The tuna industry, however, was greatly relieved by the joint federal advisory. The Tuna Foundation placed a large advertisement in national newspapers headlined "Plain Talk About Canned Tuna, a Safe & Healthy Food for Everyone," with these facts, among others:

> Fact: The omega-3 fatty acids found in canned tuna are considered "wonder nutrients" for pregnant and nursing women . . . Fact: Canned light tuna has very low levels of mercury . . . Fact: FDA and EPA also make it clear that pregnant women can eat albacore, which is also low in mercury . . . So, follow the advice of FDA and EPA and nearly every other health organization in America, and make canned tuna an important part of your family's balanced diet.

Note that figuring out how to follow advice about methylmercury is *your* problem to solve. *You* have to remember which fish are high in methylmercury so you can avoid them. *You* have to keep track of the amounts of fish you eat in a week or a month. And *you* have to decide whose information is more believable—the FDA's, the EPA's, the Tuna Foundation's, or the Environmental Working Group's.

If anything, this task is likely to become more difficult, not less. In the year following the 2004 joint FDA and EPA advisory, sales of tuna in the United States fell by 10 percent. The tuna industry asked the USDA to sponsor a "checkoff" generic advertising program for tuna, similar to the programs in place for beef, pork, soybeans, and other commodities. The campaign would be called "Tuna—a Smart Catch," would attempt to convince the public that tuna is a "wonder food," and would emphasize tuna's health benefits: less fat than beef or pork, no carbohydrates, and omega-3s.

What I find astonishing about the methylmercury dilemma is that neither the government nor the fish industry is doing much to resolve it in the most obvious way—by dealing with its cause and keeping mercury from getting into fish in the first place. The reason? As always, politics.

THE POLITICS OF MERCURY EMISSIONS

The FDA and EPA advisory should have made everyone realize the importance of keeping mercury out of waterways, but the politics of methylmercury involve much more than the interests of the tuna industry. Mercury gets into water from two sources: natural (volcanos and the weathering of cinnabar-containing rock), and "anthropogenic," meaning the result of human activity—in this case, coal-fired power plants. In the United States, power plants are the leading source of mercury contamination and are responsible for about 40 percent of mercury emissions. In response to the 2004 advisory, the National Resources Defense Council, an environmental advocacy group, and MoveOn.org, a group organizing grassroots opposition to the administration of President George W. Bush, sponsored a joint advertisement headlined "First Arsenic, Now Mercury: George Bush's EPA and the Politics of Pollution." The ad went on to say:

America learned this week that tuna, and many other fish, can contain harmful levels of toxic mercury . . . So why is President Bush trying to weaken controls on mercury pollution? . . . Now, he wants the EPA to let coal-fired power plants treat their mercury pollution as "non-hazardous" even though mercury threatens pregnant women and children. The Bush administration's ploy would allow coal-fired power plants to put more mercury into the air, where it rains down on lakes and oceans, is swallowed by fish, and could wind up on your plate . . . Guess who is praising this scheme? Coal power companies, who are big mercury polluters and big political contributors, too.

Coal-burning power plants send forty or more tons of mercury into the atmosphere every year. During the 1990s, under the administration of President Bill Clinton, the EPA imposed rules that reduced mercury emissions from most other industries—except power plants. In 2000, with the environment-friendly vice president Al Gore running for president, the EPA decided to take on this last remaining source and ruled that power plant emissions violated the Clean Air Act. If coal-burning power plants cleaned up their emissions, they could achieve a 90 percent reduction in mercury by 2008. The EPA proposed to force them to do so. In 2003, however, Bush administration appointees at the EPA reversed that decision.

Whenever the EPA rules said something like "mercury poses confirmed hazards to public health," the White House changed it to something like "emissions of mercury warrant regulation."

Journalists who wondered how such a thing could happen soon found out that White House staff not only consulted lobbyists for the power industry but actually let the lobbyists "edit" the rules to minimize the emission hazards. Whenever the EPA rules said something like "mercury poses confirmed hazards to public health," the White House changed it to something like "emissions of mercury warrant regulation."

The editing imposed by the Bush administration also gave power companies an additional decade—until 2018—to reduce emissions by 70 percent rather than 90 percent, and allowed them to trade pollution rights among themselves (meaning a company with low methylmercury emissions could trade its allowances to a company that exceeded the emissions limits). White House staff did not allow EPA officials to comment on the changes and told those who disagreed with the changes not to press the matter. The edited rules were to go into effect in March 2005. As word of all this leaked out, complaints poured in and by June

2004 more than 600,000 letters had been sent to the EPA, mostly opposing the weakening of the rules. In 2005, nine states and several major health associations—like the American Public Health Association, the American Academy of Pediatrics, and the American Nurses Association—filed a lawsuit challenging the more permissive standards, but the Bush administration continued to argue that weaker standards were sufficient and to oppose all attempts to restore the stronger proposals.

You might think that the fish industry, eager to make sure that its products could be eaten safely by women and children as well as men, would be right at the vanguard of efforts to strengthen controls over mercury emissions, but not a chance. When I asked the most active seafood trade association, the National Fisheries Institute, if it had filed comments calling for stronger controls on mercury emissions and, if so, what the institute had said, its communications director wrote back: "This just in: we did not file comments." To my query "Why Not?," there was no response. Instead of doing everything possible to get emissions reduced, the fish industry takes the short-term tack and publicly ignores or tries to minimize methylmercury as a health problem.

As for recreational fishing, the EPA announced in August 2004 that virtually all sports fish are so contaminated with methylmercury that forty-eight states (exceptions: Wyoming and Alaska) have issued advisory warnings to residents not to eat fish from certain waters. Indeed, nineteen states have placed all of their lakes and rivers under advisories. The top EPA administrator, Michael Leavitt, told *The New York Times*, "Mercury is everywhere." He was not exaggerating. The EPA collects information about state fish advisories on its Web site. I looked up New York, my home state. Its advisory tells me that I am not to eat more than half a pound per week of fish caught in any freshwater stream or river, and I am allowed only one meal per month from the 90 lakes and streams contaminated beyond federal standards. If I am under age fifteen or pregnant, I must never eat fish from those waters. Even Idaho, famous for its pristine waters, has plenty of contaminated lakes. Its advisory says that if you catch fish from those lakes, you need to have them tested

> Instead of doing everything possible to get emissions reduced, the fish industry takes the short-term tack and publicly ignores or tries to minimize methylmercury as a health problem.

for mercury, and the Idaho site provides a list of laboratories that will do this for you for a fee. Here, too, the obvious implication is that protecting yourself against methylmercury poisoning is *your* responsibility—not that of the state or federal government.

CONFLICTING RECOMMENDATIONS: OMEGA-3S VERSUS METHYLMERCURY

The various stakeholders—fishers, fishmongers, the canning industry, environmental advocates, and government and private health agencies—are clearly at odds over what to tell you to do about eating fish. If you like eating fish, you have some hard choices to make without having anywhere near the amount of information you need to make those choices sensibly. My approach to this dilemma is to ask two questions.

First question: how important is it to eat omega-3 fatty acids from fish? Fish are the best sources of omega-3 fats, but the amounts of EPA and DHA in three ounces of fish vary from 0.1 gram in cod to a gram or more in fish like anchovies, herring, mackerel, tuna, and salmon. The richest source of omega-3s turns out to be caviar (5.5 grams) but you would have to be rich as well as greedy to eat three ounces; sturgeon eggs cost more than $50 per ounce and the higher quality Russian and Iranian caviars can run more than $150 per ounce. Most American fish are relatively low in omega-3s, but, fortunately, it only takes small amounts of EPA and DHA to produce benefits.

Fish are not the only sources of omega-3s. Chicken and eggs naturally have small amounts of EPA and DHA (and are commonly eaten so they are an important source). Plants also contain omega-3 fats, but in the form of alpha-linolenic acid. Your body slowly converts this fatty acid to EPA and DHA. All food plants—beans, nuts, and seeds, but also fruits and vegetables—contain alpha-linolenic acid, although in much smaller amounts than the EPA and DHA in fish. The better plant sources are cooking oils made from seeds like flax and canola (as I explain in the chapter devoted to fats and oils). You also can get omega-3s by taking fish oil supplements, although the thought of these reminds me too much of the cod liver oil I was forced to swallow as a kid. Happily, the supplements come in capsules these days so you don't have to taste them.

Finally, it helps to keep omega-3s and fish in perspective. Omega-3s may be good for the heart, but so are other nutrients—vitamins, minerals, phytochemicals, and fiber—in the vegetables, nuts, and seeds that also contain alpha-linolenic acid. Fish, as I pointed out earlier, are excellent sources of many nutrients, but you can also get those nutrients from other foods. Fish are not essential requirements of healthful diets, and there is no compelling nutritional reason to eat fish if you don't like to.

Second question: how dangerous is mercury at current levels of fish eating? It troubles me that so little information is available to answer this question. Fish are not routinely tested for levels of methylmercury, and tests done by federal agencies produce results that differ from those done by environmental advocacy groups. Neither you nor Wegmans knows how much methylmercury is in that mako shark on display and whether that shark should bear a warning label: "If you are pregnant (or likely to become pregnant), do not eat me." Recent information suggests that blood levels of methylmercury are low in American women and declining, but perhaps 8 percent of women are within striking distance of levels considered harmful. Studies of the effects of "moderate" methylmercury intake on child development give inconsistent results. The children of women in New Zealand, the Faroe Islands, and some other places where predatory fish are eaten regularly display more than the usual number of problems with memory, attention, and language. But studies of children in the Seychelles, where pregnant women frequently eat fish that are lower on the food chain, have not shown such effects. This apparently reassuring result (which suggests that eating small fish is not evidently harmful) leads some commentators to conclude that "For now there is no reason for pregnant women to reduce fish consumption below current levels, which are probably safe." *Probably* safe?

> R ecent information suggests that blood levels of methylmercury are low in American women and declining, but perhaps 8 percent of women are within striking distance of levels considered harmful.

Perhaps methylmercury has to be eaten at Minamata-like levels before it causes overt harm, but do we really know that? If it turns out that methylmercury is similar to lead in the way it causes problems in the body, no level of methylmercury intake can ever be considered safe. Some hopeful studies suggest that omega-3 fats cancel out the toxic effects of methylmercury, but others suggest that the reverse is also true: methylmercury blunts the protective action of omega-3s. The amounts of methylmercury in fish may not be demonstrably harmful, but there is no evidence whatsoever that methylmercury is good for you. That is why mercury emissions are such an important issue, remote as coal-burning power plants may seem from the fish you buy at supermarkets.

DEALING WITH THE METHYLMERCURY DILEMMA

How much of what kind of fish you can safely eat depends on what fish it is and who you are. Since you have no way of knowing the methylmercury content of a particular fish, the best you can do is guess. Methylmercury does not seem harmful for adults at current levels of intake, but it is demonstrably bad for early fetal development and if you are a woman it is best not to have much of this toxin in your body before you become pregnant. Methylmercury attaches to red blood cells and does not generally get into breast milk, but nursing infants readily absorb whatever is there. If you are pregnant, thinking (or not thinking but "at risk") of becoming pregnant, or nursing an infant, why take a chance? You will not eat shark, swordfish, tilefish, king mackerel, albacore tuna, or any other predatory fish at the top of the food chain; you will politely decline to eat fish caught by your friends or anyone else who fishes for fun; you will eat other fish in small amounts, if at all; and you will feed your children even smaller amounts (how much smaller, nobody knows, but caution suggests as little as possible). Even if you are not pregnant, and not likely to become pregnant, you should still say no to predatory fish and limit the amounts of other fish you say yes to.

At the moment, the only practical way to deal with the fish dilemma is to carry a seafood card from an advocacy group that lists the fish lowest in methylmercury. On the bright side, the safest tuna (canned chunk or light tuna that is not labeled "white") is likely to be the least expensive, and methylmercury, unlike lead, does not stay in the body for long. Its "half-life" is just two or three months, meaning that if you start now to reduce the amount of methylmercury you eat, half will be gone in a few months, half of what's left will disappear in another few months, and most will be gone in a year or so, along with any risks it might pose. That is why reducing mercury emissions now, rather than years from now, makes such good sense.

18

The Fish-Farming Dilemma

I f you are going to follow heart-healthy advice to eat two servings of fish a week, you will need to know more than you ever wanted to about the diets of fish, as well as your own. Did the fish eat smaller fish? If so, they might have not only methylmercury but also more than their share of other dilemma-inducing pollutants—PCBs (polychlorinated biphenyls) and related toxic chemicals. The PCBs in fish cause the same type of dilemma as the one involving omega-3s and methylmercury, but with one unpleasant addition: all fish have PCBs, but farmed fish—those fed fish meal and fish oils—have more. This is because farmed fish need proteins and fats to help them grow; they grow better when those nutrients come from fish meal and oils, but these feeds contain high concentrations of PCBs.

> The PCBs in fish cause the same type of dilemma as the one involving omega-3s and methylmercury, but with one unpleasant addition: all fish have PCBs, but farmed fish—those fed fish meal and fish oils—have more.

As I will soon explain, the number of fish in the ocean is declining rapidly. If you are going to continue to have fish to eat—and to contribute omega-3s to your diet—something has to be done to increase the fish supply. Fish farming seems like an obvious way to produce more fish. But if farmed fish are fed fish oils loaded with PCBs, you should not be eating much of them. And that is the second dilemma.

It is not so hard to avoid eating shark and swordfish if you want to avoid methylmercury, but all fish, small as well as large, are contaminated with PCBs and similar chemicals that are also best avoided. These chemicals are "organic hydrocarbons," usually with chlorine or bromine attached (the "polychlorinated" in PCBs). They include especially nasty agricultural pesticides like chlordane, dieldrin, and DDT, as well as PCBs and dioxins from industrial wastes and emissions. Although most of these chemicals have been discontinued or banned for years, they persist in the environment and thoroughly pollute streams, lakes, and oceans. PCBs cause the most concern so I will use this term as collective shorthand for the hundreds of such chemicals that contaminate commercial and sports fish.

PCBs—and their relatives—are not likely to be good for you. At high levels of exposure, such as those experienced by victims of industrial accidents, they cause severe problems with skin, reproduction, development, and behavior. The amounts you get from food are much lower and cause no demonstrable harm, but a safe level of intake is not really known. The amounts of PCBs in fish seem harmless, but the word most often used to describe their effects is "uncertain."

What is certain is that fish that eat other fish will have more PCBs than those that do not. Although the levels of PCBs (and those other chemicals) have been greatly reduced in the decades since the publication of Rachel Carson's *Silent Spring* in 1962, they are still with us and appear in most foods—as well as in fish—in low amounts. But unlike methylmercury, which is stored in the muscles of fish, PCBs preferentially accumulate in fatty tissues as they move up the food chain. All fish and shellfish carry them, but in amounts that vary widely depending on their species, how fat they are, where they grew, and what they ate. Fish from the most polluted waters have the most PCBs, and fattier fish have more PCBs than leaner fish. State fish advisories make it clear that many fish caught for sport have amounts of these chemicals so high that they are no longer safe to eat. To pick an entirely typical example: the Texas advisory tells you not to eat any fish from the Trinity River near Fort Worth because of PCBs and chlordane, and to eat fish from Llano Grande Lake no more than twice a month because of PCB-like agricultural pesticides that have leached into it over the years.

When you eat fatty fish such as albacore tuna, herring, or mackerel, precisely the ones that are among the highest in omega-3 fatty acids, you also get a relatively high dose of PCBs. Fish oil supplements—the kind you buy in supermarkets and health food stores—would have even higher amounts of PCBs if they were not first cleaned up (refined) but, fortunately, most are. You can remove the fatty skin from a fish and reduce its PCB level to some extent, but beyond that you are in a quandary. You cannot tell which fish have the most PCBs, so you can either act on faith and hope that the fish has been tested, buy only from purveyors you know test fish for PCBs, or trust a seafood advisory list to tell you which kinds are least likely to be contaminated. How fish are raised and whether they are tested are factors that especially bear on the safety of farmed fish, which brings us to a deeper discussion of this second dilemma.

FISH DILEMMA #2: NOT ENOUGH FISH VERSUS PCBs IN FARMED FISH

Fish biologists tell us that formerly abundant food fish are disappearing from the oceans. Mind you, this depletion of whole fish populations has happened just within my lifetime. While still in college, I lived for a year or so in Monterey, California, and woke up many mornings to the loud whistle of local sardine canneries calling employees to work. Even without that noise I could tell when the canneries were in operation from the smell of fish in the air. Those sardines and their smells are long gone from the California coast, and the canneries are now restaurants and shopping malls. Years later, at the Woods Hole Science Aquarium on Cape Cod, I pored over maps of the recent changes in catches of local fish. New England fishers used to bring in hundreds of thousands of tons of cod, flounder, and haddock every year. Now they have to go farther away and work harder to find such fish, and instead bring back odd things that used to be considered "bycatch" (unwanted fish inadvertently caught in nets): cusk, hake, pout—and even dogfish sharks like the ones I used as examples for teaching anatomy to premedical biology students at Brandeis University years ago.

Oceans are large and fish hard to count, but unless you believe that masses of fish are hidden away in the deepest oceanic recesses (a highly unlikely possibility), you have to recognize that natural populations of wild fish are in steep decline. By some estimates, the "biomass" of large predatory fish has declined by 90 percent since the preindustrial fishing era. This is not just a problem for oceans off the coasts of the United States. Most of the world's fishing zones are considered to be unsustainable, meaning that fish cannot reproduce fast enough to replace the ones that get taken. Some fish are even considered endangered, among them certain species of salmon, sturgeon, and trout. Just about everyone except the most diehard lobbyists for the fishing industry attributes this decline to overfishing—too many boats using too efficient methods to catch the too few fish that remain. Fish do not have a chance against modern catching methods: sonar, satellite communications, dragging nets, and lines dozens of miles long. Attempts to protect spawning grounds, to limit catches, or to enforce catching rules run smack up against business and government interests. Commercial fishers are as eager as any other kind of industry to maximize income while they can, and governments want to protect their own countries' fishing industries by letting their fishers take everything available while keeping other countries' fishers away. This approach is strictly short term: take every available fish while you can, make the money now, and let someone else worry about whether there will be fish to catch in the future. Commercial fishing is no longer a business that people expect to pass on to their children. They know that the fish will be gone from the sea and too few will be left for anyone to catch.

If getting commercial fishers to take fewer fish seems politically impossible, fish farming looks like the answer to the supply problem. On

> Commercial fishing is no longer a business that people expect to pass on to their children. They know that the fish will be gone from the sea and too few will be left for anyone to catch.

vacation in Norway, I saw fish farms along every fjord, and just about every country with a convenient coastline is encouraging this industry. Fish farming has its own agricultural designation—aquaculture—and this particular form of agribusiness is booming. Since 1980, the value of U.S. aquaculture alone has increased by 400 percent, with half the sales coming from catfish production in states such as Mississippi, Alabama, Arkansas, and Louisiana. U.S. companies produce fish not only for food but also for ornamental ponds, fishing bait, and—most troubling—feed for animals and other fish. They also produce crawfish, shrimp, abalone, oysters, clams, and mussels. Fish farms can be found in most states and along nearly every section of the U.S. coastline. Alaska is an exception; to protect its wild salmon industry, this state bans salmon farms.

In 2002, the USDA identified more than 6,600 aquatic farms in the United States, and these generated more than $1.1 billion in sales that year. But this is nothing—just a bit over 1 percent of the total—compared to the production of fish farmed in other countries. If you believe China's production figures (and not everyone does), that country accounted for a whopping 71 percent of the 112 billion pounds (51 million metric tons) of farmed seafood produced in 2002. Eight additional countries, six of them in Asia (the others are Norway and Chile), lead the U.S. in fish farming. Like other industries, aquaculture is becoming increasingly concentrated, and just three companies produce more than half of the farmed fish sold in North America. One of these companies, Marine Harvest, says it is "the world's leading fish farming company, and the leading producer and supplier of farmed salmon in the world." From its corporate base in the Netherlands, it farms ten species of fish in eight countries on five continents, and supplies fish to seventy countries.

In contrast to wild fish, which spawn, grow, and develop on their own without any human intervention, farmed fish are managed throughout life to produce as many fish as possible in the shortest possible time. Fish farming begins by selecting fish of the desired genetic strain (the "broodstock"), collecting eggs from the females and sperm from the males (an art in itself), fertilizing the eggs with the sperm, hatching the embryos, rearing the young, and gradually transferring the growing fish to larger and larger pens, a process that can take more than a year. A fish farm puts

50,000 or so maturing fish in netted pens, feeds them to size, collects them, and ships them off weeks or months later to market. Shrimp farms hold even greater numbers.

Fish farming generates all kinds of questions about what the fish are fed, how they are treated, and what these practices do to their nutritional value, to the local environment, and to local economies, particularly in developing countries. Environmental advocacy groups point out that many shrimp farmers, for example, use massive amounts of antibiotics, disinfectants, and pesticides, none of them good for human health, none of them strictly necessary, and some, like antibiotics, highly inappropriate.

FARMED SALMON: A CASE IN POINT

Even so, the farming of shellfish and other fish low on the food chain causes fewer problems than the farming of predatory fish like salmon. Indeed, salmon farming is so controversial that it has spawned its very own opposition groups. One, the Coastal Alliance for Aquaculture Reform, runs a "Farmed and Dangerous" campaign to encourage you to think twice before eating farm-raised salmon. Farmed salmon, this group says, are raised like cattle in feedlots. They are confined in pools of antibiotics, pesticides, chemicals, and wastes, which then spill the equivalent of raw sewage into local waters. If the fish escape—which millions invariably do every year—they can end up in the wrong ocean (Atlantic salmon in the Pacific Northwest, for example), compete for resources, and spread diseases like sea lice to wild fish, and, when they mate with wild fish, change the genetic basis of the population and reduce biodiversity. The Coastal Alliance (its Web site is www.farmedanddangerous.org) insists that you are much better off eating wild salmon for reasons of safety, health, and environmental protection.

Since farm-raised salmon constitute such a large part of the fish-farming industry in industrialized countries and in Chile, it is well

Indeed, salmon farming is so controversial that it has spawned its very own opposition groups. One, the Coastal Alliance for Aquaculture Reform, runs a "Farmed and Dangerous" campaign to encourage you to think twice before eating farm-raised salmon.

worth examining these charges. As it turns out, they are backed up by a good deal of evidence. In part because of what gets fed to farmed salmon and in part because farmed fish are less active, these fish have twice the fat and more than twice the saturated fat of their wild counterparts. Their omega-3 content depends entirely on what they are fed, and varies by species and by farm.

Adult salmon are carnivores. In the wild, newly hatched salmon start out eating microscopic plants and animals; as they get bigger and move from rivers to oceans, they eat tiny crustaceans (krill). Some kinds continue to eat krill throughout life, while others eat small fish and then increasingly larger fish. In captivity on fish farms, however, salmon eat the equivalent of dog food: first small and then larger pellets of fish meal and fish oil, soy protein, wheat (as a binder), and vitamins and minerals. The pellets also contain meat-and-bone meal made from the rendered leftover meat, blood, and bones of cows, pigs, and other animals (those very same by-products excluded from "natural" beef because of concerns about mad cow disease). The several billion chickens that get killed for food each year produce tons of feathers, many of which end up as feather meal in fish pellets.

None of that may sound appetizing, but safety, not taste, is the issue in this dilemma. The fish meal and fish oil in the feed are responsible for the PCB problem. Fish have short digestive tracts and the carnivorous types do not grow well or quickly enough unless their diets include fats and proteins from fish. Wild salmon get the nutrients they need by eating other fish; farm-raised salmon get their nutrients from fish-meal pellets. To make fish-meal and fish oil, you grind up wild "industrial" or forage fish—menhaden, anchovies, mackerel, and the like—that do not usually end up on dinner tables but are caught specifically for fish feeding. Many farmed fish need to eat four or five pounds of industrial fish to gain one pound of weight, and some (like farmed tuna) need twice that much or more.

This feeding system is not only inherently wasteful but also causes farm-raised fish to accumulate higher levels of PCBs than are found in fish that roam the oceans. This happens because fish farming reverses the food chain. Baby wild fish eat krill, which is low in PCBs. As they grow, some start to eat other fish but ones that are small and relatively low in chemical contaminants. But young farmed fish eat meal and oils from larger fish—those with concentrated PCBs—right from the start, so farmed fish accumulate PCBs throughout their entire lives.

Everyone wishes this system could change. Fish farmers would love to find a replacement for industrial fish because the supply is limited and they are expensive to catch. In theory, you could make feed pellets with proteins and oils from soybeans, corn, and cottonseeds, but these are low in omega-3s and they change the way fish taste. Also in theory, you could feed vegetable-based proteins and oils to farmed fish until they are nearly grown and then finish them off—feed them fish meal and oils until they mature—but this method is still experimental and is not yet widely used. Because the price of farm-raised fish depends so much on the cost of feed, there is much pressure to use the cheapest ingredients possible. It is difficult and expensive to treat fish meal and oil to remove PCBs, so cheap feed ingredients are likely to have loads of such contaminants.

SALMON: "FARMED AND DANGEROUS"

In 2002, three research groups published studies concluding that farm-raised salmon have higher levels of PCBs than wild salmon. All three groups attributed the difference to high levels of PCBs in the food pellets, and to the higher fat content—and, therefore, higher contaminant content—of farm-raised fish. The next year, the Environmental Working Group did its own testing and also reported more PCBs in farmed than wild salmon. Although the PCB levels were well below the cutoff level considered unsafe by the FDA, they were higher than the safety standard set by the EPA. Perhaps because these research studies were done on small samples of fish and appeared in relatively obscure scientific journals or as a report from an advocacy group, they did not get much attention. Even so, the discrepancy drew attention to the differing standards of the FDA and the EPA. Which is the correct standard, or does the difference even matter? Without studies to answer such questions, customers might exercise caution and decide not to eat farm-raised salmon.

To head off that possibility, supermarket chains like Wild Oats and

Whole Foods said they would buy farm-raised salmon only from companies whose farms use feed low in PCBs and whose fish tested low in such chemicals. The salmon-farmers' trade association, Salmon of the Americas (SOTA), took a different approach. It argued that such actions were completely unnecessary because the levels of PCBs in salmon were below the FDA standard: "When, and if, the F.D.A. changes its limits, we will be the first to comply."

In 2004, however, a group of researchers led by Ronald Hites of Indiana University took a large number of samples—700 or more—from tons of fish raised in farms or caught wild in many areas of the world, and published the results in one of the most prestigious journals in the United States, *Science*. The Hites group confirmed that PCBs, dioxins, and a dozen more such chemicals were higher in farm-raised than in wild salmon, but also found the levels to vary widely with geography. Salmon from fish farms in Europe had the most PCBs while those from farms in North and South America had the least. This, the researchers said, was because the fish meal used to feed European farmed salmon contained higher levels of PCBs than the feed used in salmon farms in North and South America, a difference they attributed to the greater contamination of forage fish in waters near industrialized coastal areas of Europe.

These observations caused the researchers to draw three riveting conclusions [numbers added]: "Although the risk/benefit computation is complicated," they said, "[1] consumption of farmed Atlantic salmon may pose risks that detract from the beneficial effects of fish consumption." Their study "also demonstrates [2] the importance of labeling salmon as farmed and [3] identifying the country of origin." If these conclusions were not inflammatory enough, one of the authors explained to *The New York Times* what all this meant in practice: "The vast majority of farm-raised Atlantic salmon should be consumed at one meal or less per month."

It is hard to know which of the three conclusions could have been worse news for the fish-farming industry. All meant that consumers who knew how and where the fish were raised might be likely to boycott them. For example, if you want to avoid PCBs, you will stop eating farmed salmon or eat less of it. If salmon are labeled as farmed, you will not buy them, and if you know that the salmon were farmed in Europe, you will especially avoid buying them.

Predictably, the Hites study got plenty of attention. Government and industry representatives rushed to reassure consumers. The FDA said: "We certainly don't think there's a public health concern here." A consultant for SOTA said: "I think it's unconscionable to direct pregnant women away from farmed salmon. Omega-3 fatty acids are important for brain development, and they may reduce the risk of preterm births and slightly increase a child's cognitive abilities."

Apparently, the Hites study sent SOTA into full damage control. It is worth examining some of the arguments set forth by this lobbying group. Here they are, with my responses to their charges in parentheses. SOTA says:

- Beef is a greater source of PCBs than salmon (yes, but only because most people eat beef more often than they eat salmon; on its own, a serving of beef is lower in PCBs than a serving of farm-raised salmon).

- Farmed Atlantic salmon "is the best source of omega-3 fatty acids of any available food" (not necessarily; plenty of other fatty fish—sardines and herring, for example—can have as much).

- Salmon, "because it has fewer calorie dense proteins than many other meat protein sources, may help fight obesity" (this one I do not understand; proteins have the same calories by weight—4 per gram—no matter where they come from).

- To date, "when valid studies are used there are no significant differences in PCB levels between wild and farmed salmon" (but SOTA's Web site fails to reference those "valid" studies).

- "SOTA members strictly comply with the FDA tolerance and believe that in light of the risk-benefit equation, it is adequate" (maybe, but there is that troubling matter of the more restrictive EPA standards).

Never mind. This trade association is hard at work for its industry. And SOTA needs to work especially hard these days because Professor Hites and his colleagues are keeping its public relations staff busy. In

August 2004, these researchers produced further evidence of organic hy-drocarbons in salmon (wild as well as farmed): this time brominated flame retardants called PBDEs (polybrominated diphenyl ethers). At the high levels used in studies on newborn rats and mice, these act as en-docrine disruptors and cause problems with behavior, learning, growth, and development. Their effects in humans have not been studied (it is hard to imagine how such studies could be done) but they are presumed to be similar to those of PCBs, and not good. Half of the PBDEs in the environment have leached out of polyurethane foam stuffing for furni-ture, a material now banned in Europe and slowly being phased out in the United States. As with PCBs, the Hites group found more PBDEs in farmed than wild salmon, and drew similar conclusions: "Our data indi-cate that frequent consumption of farmed salmon and wild Pacific Chi-nook salmon will increase dietary exposure to PBDEs much more so than consumption of most other wild Pacific salmon . . . This study demonstrates the importance of labeling salmon as farmed and identify-ing the country of origin."

This new study confronted the industry with the need to do even more damage control: a director of the Bromine Science and Environ-mental Forum, a trade association for the bromine industry (yes, even the makers of brominated flame retardants have their own lobbyists), told *Food Chemical News* that PBDE levels in fish were so low that a 150-pound person "would have to eat more than six tons of salmon each day before experiencing any related adverse effects on their health." SOTA said that the reported levels of PBDEs "do not present a health hazard" and urged consumers not to stop eating salmon. In making such state-ments, fish trade groups suggest that they view organic hydrocarbon chemicals as a problem of public relations, not public health. Rather than demanding actions to protect your health or the health of the envi-ronment—meaning preventing those chemicals from getting into fish in the first place—they pretend the problem does not exist.

Hiding the problem, however, will not be easy. In 2005, the same de-termined group of investigators examined the relative amounts of yet an-other toxic hydrocarbon—this time, dioxins—in farmed and wild salmon. Their conclusion: "Consumption of farmed salmon at relatively low frequencies results in elevated exposure to dioxins and dioxin-like compounds with commensurate elevations in estimate of health risks." These researchers warn that the increase in cancer risk caused by consuming farmed salmon may well outweigh the benefits of omega-3 fats, particularly among girls, young women who might eventually become pregnant, pregnant women who can pass the toxins to their developing fetuses, and nursing mothers. Farmed and dangerous, indeed.

FISH INDUSTRY PUBLIC RELATIONS

The most curious part of industry public relations efforts surely must be the outright attacks on the funder of the Hites studies, the Pew Charitable Trusts, and the other main funding source of fish advocacy, the David and Lucile Packard Foundation. Pew is a philanthropic foundation established by the family of the founders of Sun Oil; it spent about $177 million in 2005 on projects "supporting civic life," among them environmental programs focused on global warming, wilderness protection, and promotion of sustainable seafood policies. The Packard Foundation (of the Packard side of Hewlett-Packard) granted about $200 million in 2005 to groups focused on population, children, and communities and on conservation, with a special focus on northern California. In this last context, the foundation sponsors the Monterey Bay Aquarium's Seafood Watch program and other fish advocacy groups that encourage consumers to understand sustainability and safety issues and to make more thoughtful seafood choices.

Despite the obviously worthy goals of these groups, the fish industry says that they and their "multibillion-dollar" foundation funders do not really care about the public: "the PCB issue is not necessarily about public health . . . environmental groups are using food safety—specifically seafood safety—to garner public attention for environmental issues." The fish-farming industry views the foundations and the groups they fund as conspiratorially connected and part of a larger, sophisticated campaign to convert fishing and aquaculture into their vision of environmentally sustainable industries. Their real agenda, according to the industry, is to replace the more liberal FDA allowances for contaminants with the more restrictive levels set by the EPA, regardless of the harm done to consumers (in fear and in loss of omega-3s) or to fish farmers (in loss of livelihood). To such charges, the Packard Foundation responds: "The agenda is support for sustainable fisheries. If that's a conspiracy, it's a good one." Packard argues that its goal is not to reduce consumer demand for farm-raised salmon. Instead, it encourages companies to improve their farming practices so their fish will qualify for the "eat any time" sections of seafood advisory lists.

In October 2004, SOTA announced that it had done its own PCB tests and that these proved you can "ditch the pills, potions and diets, and eat salmon." The SOTA tests found the same amounts of PCBs in farmed salmon as in wild salmon. This, it said, "should put to rest any fears that arose from the notorious Hites study that appeared in the journal *Science* . . . The bottom line? The benefits of salmon far outweigh the risks." Maybe, but SOTA did not make the study available or publish it, so there is no way to compare its methods with those of the Hites research. Nor did SOTA disclose the number of salmon sampled (the more fish sampled, the more meaningful the results), or the part of the world its tested fish came from (a factor that has as much bearing on PCB levels as whether the fish were raised on a farm or grew wild).

So the fish industry fights the environmental groups, much to its own detriment. Although environmental sustainability ought to help—if not save—the fishing industry, SOTA's actions on behalf of salmon are understandable as a matter of narrow self-interest. You might think that sustainable fishing would be a terrific boost for the fishing industry, but sustainability is for the long term, and fishers and fish farmers want to make a living now. In October 2004, *SeaFood Business* reported that sales of farmed salmon dropped by 10 percent in the first half of that year—meaning a loss of 24 million pounds—from the same period a year earlier, and it attributed the drop to the bad press about PCBs.

MAKING SENSE OF THE PCB DILEMMA

Are PCBs a big or a trivial problem, and how can you possibly know? The PCB situation can be interpreted as farce or tragedy, but however you view it you have some choices to make. You can follow industry advice, ignore PCBs, and hope for the best. But that would not be my choice. The levels of PCBs (and their equally unpleasant relatives) in fish, farmed and otherwise, may not be high enough to do measurable harm, but these chemicals can hardly be good for you. It makes good sense to do everything possible to avoid them. Knowing what fish to eat, then, means knowing

- where the fish comes from
- whether it is farmed or wild
- where it is on the food chain
- whether it is listed in a state advisory
- how much fat it contains

Once you have this information, you can avoid the fish likely to be most heavily contaminated with PCBs. On this basis, you will want to avoid farm-raised fish from Europe, farmed fish fed lots of fish meal and fish oils, the ones listed on state advisories, and the larger and fattier species, such as those also highest in methylmercury. Even so, it will be difficult to keep up with changes in fish-farming methods. In June 2005, for example, *The Vancouver Sun* announced that secret government tests had found farmed salmon in British Columbia to contain six times the level of PCBs, dioxins, and other such chemicals as in wild Canadian salmon—although the higher levels were still below those considered unsafe. If you would rather not do the sleuthing necessary to answer questions about fish safety, you can hope to find a fish seller who buys only from farms providing fish that are low in PCBs and makes sure that those fish have been tested before they get to you. Such vendors exist, but you will need to ask that list of questions to find them.

If you care about this issue, you may find yourself wanting to join efforts to protect the safety of waterways and oceans so that fish have a healthier and more protected environment in which to grow and reproduce. Like methylmercury, PCBs and their cousins have no business being in the fish supply. In the years when they were routinely dumped out of factories, these toxins made their way into waters where they were eaten by fish; they also got into crops and animals fed to farmed fish. Resolving the PCB dilemma means making sure that no more PCBs get dumped, and that no PCB-laden forage fish and animal parts get fed to smaller fish. Shouldn't fish be safe for pregnant women, children, and everyone else to eat? I think so. If you do too, you might consider encouraging your fish seller to join with environmental groups that are trying to make fish healthier and safer for everyone.

In the meantime, you can—and should—ask whether fish are farmed or wild and what country they come from. The Center for Science in the Public Interest, the Washington, D.C.–based consumer advocacy group that deals so effectively with many such matters, says that if you have this information, the bottom line on farmed salmon is easy: You can safely eat farmed salmon from Chile and Washington State, but you should avoid farmed salmon if it comes from more polluted places like Scotland and the Faroe Islands. You can get rid of about half the PCBs in farmed salmon by following these steps: score the flesh; grill or broil the salmon until it reaches an internal temperature of 175°F and the juices run off; and remove the skin before eating. You don't want to bother with all that? Complain to your fishmonger—and to your congressional representatives.

19

The Fish-Labeling Quandaries

Just about any American supermarket has a fish counter offering fresh, frozen, whole, and filleted seafood, almost certain to be bewildering in variety, quality, and price. The signs that accompany the fish do not always help much. Like other fresh foods, fish do not come with Nutrition Facts labels, but sellers are supposed to tell you what species they are and whether they were previously frozen. Beginning in spring 2005, they also were supposed to tell you what country the fish came from and whether they were farmed. Late in fall 2004, before those rules were supposed to go into effect, I took inventory in several places, starting with Citarella, a decidedly upscale specialty market in New York City. On any given day, Citarella sells more than 100 kinds of fresh fish: cockles and mussels from New Zealand, salmon from Norway, mackerel from Spain, lobster tails from South Africa, sea bass and whiting from Chile, and nine different kinds of oysters from the United States, Canada, and New Zealand. If I wanted sea urchins or razor clams, Citarella had them. The origin of most of the seafood was not labeled, however, and it was hard to tell which ones were farmed or wild.

A nearby and decidedly less upscale Gristede's supermarket does not have a fish counter, but offered a refrigerator case packed with plastic-wrapped seafood: previously frozen fillets of tuna, tilapia, flounder, catfish, salmon, and shrimp, along with a large assortment of "artificial" products that looked like crab or lobster. Although the wrappings were clearly marked with the species, weight, and price, none said where or how the fish had been raised. In answer to a question about whether a piece of salmon was farm-raised or wild, a clerk replied, "I really have no idea where this thing comes from."

A few blocks away, the Wholesome Market, which used to carry mostly organic foods (but closed in 2005), carried salmon labeled "organic, color added." In Ithaca, a Tops Market offered fresh tuna, orange roughy, tilapia, swordfish, perch, scrod, flounder, catfish, and hake, all of unknown origin. A few signs did say something about origins and nutritional matters: "Iceland wild haddock," "color added farm-raised Atlantic salmon," and salmon heads "high in omega-3s."

How anyone can make a reasonable choice about which fish to buy on the basis of these seemingly arbitrary and confusing labels is a mystery to me. Better labeling would certainly help, particularly of the country of origin, but you might also want to know what the fish signs really mean when they tell you that seafood is "artificial," "color-added," "organic," or, for that matter, "not genetically modified." By this time, you can guess that each of these labeling terms takes you into matters that do not precisely qualify as fish dilemmas, but do present any number of what I think of as fish quandaries—puzzles you have to deal with when deciding what fish to buy.

LABEL QUANDARY #1: COUNTRY-OF-ORIGIN LABELING (COOL)

About 75 percent of the fish (and 90 percent of the shrimp) sold at supermarkets and restaurants in the United States is imported, and most comes from developing countries in Asia and Latin America. If fish from some parts of the world is likely to be fresher and less contaminated than fish from other parts, wouldn't it be helpful to know which country's waters that piece of fish comes from? Of course it would. And, amazingly enough, the U.S. Congress agreed.

> About 75 percent of the fish (and 90 percent of the shrimp) sold at supermarkets and restaurants in the United States is imported, and most comes from developing countries in Asia and Latin America.

In 2002, mainly because of concerns about mad cow disease in beef cattle, Congress directed the USDA to develop rules for mandatory country-of-origin labeling (COOL) for meats, produce, and peanuts, as well as for fish and shellfish. Congress also told the USDA to make sure that seafood would be labeled as to whether it was wild or farmed, and to start enforcing the new rules by October 2004. Before that could happen, however, politics intervened. In January 2004, nine months before the COOL rules were to go into effect, industry complaints (the difficulty! the cost!) induced Congress to give producers of meat, produce, and peanuts an additional two years — until October 2006 — to start labeling the origin of their products. At that point, some members of Congress introduced bills to block COOL requirements altogether, whereas others, particularly Senate Democratic majority leader Tom Daschle (South Dakota), introduced bills to reinstate the original September 2004 deadline. Those bills got nowhere, but indicated the ferocity of the debate about labeling the countries of origin of foods, a debate eventually leading Congress to delay COOL for produce, meat, and peanuts until October 2008.

But Congress continued to require fish and shellfish sellers to institute COOL by October 2004. The USDA then gave the industry a small break and allowed a delay in compliance until April 2005. After that, retailers and suppliers would have to disclose the country of origin of all farm-raised and wild fish and seafood ("including fillets, steaks, nuggets, and any other flesh"). They also would have to disclose whether the products were wild or farmed. Congress granted an exemption for processed seafood, saying that fish that had been breaded, sauced, cooked, canned, cured, or "restructured" did not need labels stating the country of origin. This meant that COOL rules would not apply to things like fish sticks, soups, patés, sushi, or canned tuna or salmon.

So from the start, seafood COOL, useful as it might be in theory, would have only a limited reach in practice. The rules for seafood COOL include one other odd feature. For farm-raised seafood to be labeled as coming from the United States, it must be hatched, raised, harvested, and processed in U.S. waters. But wild fish are labeled according to the origin of the fishing boat, not the location of the waters where the fish are actually caught. If wild fish are "harvested in the waters of the

United States or by a U.S. flagged vessel and processed in the United States or aboard a U.S. flagged vessel," they are of U.S. origin, even if that boat was catching fish off the polluted coast of northern Europe.

The USDA said that these rules would affect the 3,500 U.S. companies involved in fish farming as well as the more than 75,000 fishing firms, 8,000 intermediates, and 37,000 retailers who deal with nearly 8 billion pounds of seafood each year. As a whole, the U.S. seafood industry thinks COOL rules are costly and unnecessary, and wishes origin labeling could continue to be voluntary. It joins the rest of the food industry in this view. The Food Marketing Institute, which leads food-industry opposition to COOL, says the rules overlook "the lack of need for a mandatory country-of-origin labeling program of any kind. In fact, retailers and wholesalers are prepared to institute a voluntary labeling and marketing program that would benefit consumers and producers at a fraction of the cost." In October 2004, faced with the April 2005 deadline for labeling to begin, the National Fisheries Institute (NFI), the principal seafood lobbying group, somewhat grudgingly pointed out that the rules

> When I ask the managers of fish counters if they are complying with COOL, most have no idea what I am talking about.

did contain "dramatic improvements suggested by NFI, including product exemptions, delayed enforcement, and simplified record-keeping."

In November 2004, Daschle, the strongest proponent of COOL in the U.S. Senate, lost his bid for reelection, leaving the future of the rules in doubt. The new Republican majority immediately introduced bills to repeal COOL requirements outright or to make them voluntary. If these bills passed, seafood producers would not have to disclose the origin of fish and seafood after all. The bills did not pass, and seafood COOL went into effect on schedule in April 2005.

But you would never know this from looking at your local fish counter, at least not in my neighborhood. The labeling of country of origin continues to appear haphazard. Some fish seem to be labeled by origin, some not. When I ask the managers of fish counters if they are complying with COOL, most have no idea what I am talking about. Identifying the country of origin may be a necessary first step in figuring out whether seafood is low in PCBs and similar chemicals, but some stores will not use COOL labeling unless you demand it. Here is a situation in which asking ought to do some good. The more consumer-friendly stores should be happy to comply with the law if for no other reason than you might take your business elsewhere if they refuse.

This, of course, immediately raises the vexing question of whether you can believe what the signs say about fish origins. I am not aware of studies evaluating the accuracy of the country-of-origin labels, but Marian Burros, a veteran reporter for *The New York Times*, wanted to know whether fish stores were telling the truth about the other requirement of the COOL legislation—labeling fish as farmed. In March 2005, toward the end of the off-season for wild salmon (when they are out in the ocean and hard to catch), she bought salmon labeled "wild" from eight fish markets in New York City. She sent the fish to a laboratory and got them tested to see whether their salmon-pink color came from natural pigments (derived from eating krill) or from the dyes fed to farm-raised salmon. You probably cannot tell the colors apart by looking at them, but a laboratory can easily distinguish the krill pigment, astaxanthin, from a similar pigment that is also used to turn farmed salmon pink.

The results? Bad news. Only one of the eight stores, Eli's Manhattan, sold salmon that was really wild. One other, Whole Foods, sold a salmon that tested someplace in between wild and farmed, suggesting that the fish might have escaped from the farm into the ocean where it then ate krill. The other stores, however, were selling farm-raised salmon as wild—and at the much higher prices charged for wild salmon. Burros asked store managers to explain. One told her: "Our salmon is from Canada. All wild salmon in Canada is farm raised." This impossibly self-canceling answer makes me think that some of the labeling problems are simply due to ignorance, but Burros pointed out that farmed salmon was going for about $5 a pound, while the stores were charging $17 to $29 a pound for the "wild." The *Times* story appeared in April, just as COOL rules for fish were going into effect. In June, Eli's displayed a large blowup of the article in its window with a sign saying "only a sample from Eli's Manhattan was genuine." Whereas in April this store priced wild salmon at $22.99 a pound, it was charging $29.99 a pound in June. Honesty does have its rewards, sometimes.

The rules for COOL specifically exclude fish and shellfish that have been "restructured," meaning emulsified, extruded, compressed into blocks, or cut into portions. They most definitely do not apply to surimi, seafood made through a 900-year-old Japanese process for converting what were once real fish into fake crab meat, lobster, shrimp, scallops, and other such things. Surimi originated as a method for preserving fresh fish; these could be made to last longer when washed, salted, spiced, ground to a paste, and cooked by steaming or broiling. Modern surimi evolved into something much weirder. Suppose commercial fishing operations do not want to waste the less profitable fish in their harvest. They can do what the Japanese have done with cheap fish for centuries. They wash the flesh of a fish repeatedly until it loses all odor and color; drain it; add cornstarch, other binders, sugar, flavors, and maybe even real fish; shape it into blocks; form it into a paste that they can shape and paint to look like whatever they want it to; and freeze it. That is surimi.

The Japanese make more than 2,000 products using surimi and have turned the making of those products into somewhat of an art form. Never mind the 900-year cultural tradition. The point of surimi, most of which is made industrially in huge quantities, is to fool you into thinking you are eating expensive shellfish instead of the cheapest fish available. Much of the nutritional value has been washed out of the fish, and I find even the more expensive products to taste gelatinous and salty.

And yet the fish industry is allowed to pass off surimi as "real" seafood. It looks like fresh seafood, but it is practically impervious to decay and has a shelf life of three years. Here, too, the labels do not help much. The FDA has no established standards for surimi, but until 2006 required it to be labeled as "imitation" or "artificial," which it most certainly is. I've seen surimi imitation crab labeled as "Seafood for the low carb lifestyle . . . high in omega 3, less than 3 g [grams] net carbs . . . imitation crab meat." All seafood is low in carbohydrates, but surimi products often have added sugars, and you cannot easily convince me that added omega-3s will bring surimi to the nutritional level of real fish.

Only about 10 percent of U.S. households use these products (although they do so to the tune of about 200 million pounds annually), and business is relatively flat. Surimi companies worry about the gap in quality between the lowest and highest priced products, and they should; the content of fish and fillers varies widely. Surimi companies much prefer the Canadian

> When Canada allowed the labels of surimi products to say "crab-flavored fish" and "lobster-flavored fish" instead of "imitation," sales went up.

system. When Canada allowed the labels of surimi products to say "crab-flavored fish" and "lobster-flavored fish" instead of "imitation," sales went up. In 2006, the FDA gave up and allowed labels to say "made with surimi, a fully cooked fish protein."

The most common use of surimi is in seafood salads. You will find surimi in, for example, Subway's Seafood Sensation sandwich. This sandwich is filled with something that looks like crab but costs less than you might expect. If you wonder why, a brochure explains that the sandwich contains "a processed seafood and crab blend made with light mayonnaise." You have to go to the Web site to get the complete list of its thirty ingredients (most of them thickeners and flavor additives) and the nutrition information: 450 calories and more than a gram of sodium in the 6-inch sandwich. If you look in supermarkets, you also can find jars of imitation salmon roe made from seafood gelatin filled with salad oil. Just as surimi costs practically nothing compared to crab meat, these cost practically nothing compared to caviar. You get what you pay for. I prefer real fish.

LABEL QUANDARY #3: ARTIFICIAL COLOR

Wild salmon are a gorgeous salmon pink because the fish eat marine krill, tiny crustaceans loaded with pigments—mainly one called astaxanthin but also another called canthaxanthin. These get incorporated into the salmon's flesh and can be identified by testing laboratories like the one Marian Burros used to check the accuracy of "wild" labels. Farmed salmon, alas, are not fed krill. Instead they are fed pellets like the ones fed to cats or dogs. As a result, their flesh is an unattractive gray color. Research on the industry-important question of what best sells salmon demonstrates two things: the darker its pink color, the more likely you are to choose it over more lightly colored salmon; and if the salmon is gray, you will not buy it at all.

So salmon farmers resort to cosmetics. They add dyes to the feed pellets, knowing that the farmed salmon can easily absorb the color and that their flesh will turn as pink as that of wild salmon. This, as it turns out, can be done with amazing precision. In the same way you match paint to color chips at paint stores, salmon farmers can choose the color they want the salmon to be from a chart made by Hoffmann-La Roche, the company that makes synthetic astaxanthin and canthaxanthin. The intensity of color on the Hoffman-La Roche SalmoFan ranges from #20 (pale salmon pink) to #34 (bright orange-red). Focus group tests show that customers prefer the natural color of wild salmon (#33 on the SalmoFan) by a ratio of 2 to 1, equate that color with quality, and say they are willing to pay more for it. When farmed salmon comes in at a pinkish #27, customers reject it. You can bet that salmon farmers give their fish plenty of the dyes.

> Research on the industry-important question of what best sells salmon demonstrates two things: the darker its pink color, the more likely you are to choose it over more lightly colored salmon; and if the salmon is gray, you will not buy it at all.

FDA rules require disclosure of the added color, but most retailers used to ignore that requirement. In 2004, Smith & Lowney, a law firm specializing in public interest cases, filed class action suits against three large supermarket chains—Safeway, Albertsons, and Kroger—for failing to disclose the added color. This was misbranding, the firm argued, because by "imitating wild salmon, Defendant unfairly and deceptively dissociates its product from the real and/or perceived defects of farmed salmon." The purported defects, the lawyers said, are treatment with antibiotics or pesticides; fewer omega-3s; more fat, PCBs, and other dangerous chemicals; pollution of the surrounding seas; and the ability of farmed salmon to escape and spread diseases to wild salmon—a succinct summary of many of the dilemmas and quandaries that farm-raised fish present. These suits failed in the courts but did succeed in getting the grocery chains to "voluntarily" follow the existing law.

You can tell whether your retailer is following the law by looking at the labels alongside the farmed salmon at the fish counter. *All* farmed salmon contain added color, so all should be labeled "color added." Does this matter? I think it does. The absence of a "color added" label means that you cannot know all you might like to about a piece of fish you want to buy and eat tonight. Aside from fooling you into thinking you are getting wild salmon (and, in that case, paying a lot more than you should), the unlabeled color might lead you to think that coloring fish is perfectly harmless. But in this case, it may not be. Canthaxanthin is related to beta-carotene (a natural pigment in carrots and other fruits and vegetables), acts as an antioxidant, and may have other useful biological functions. But this pigment has been found to accumulate in the retina of the eye in much the same way that the carotene pigments in carrots show up in the palms of your hands after you eat a lot of them. Carotenes in the palm are considered harmless, but the health consequences of canthaxanthin accumulation in the eye are unknown. Without better safety information, the European Commission's Health and Consumer Protection agency is worried about what canthaxanthin might do to your eyes and has called for a sharp reduction in use of this pigment. Perhaps for this reason, Hoffman-La Roche promotes sales of its synthetic "nature-identical" astaxanthin for use in farmed salmon and trout.

> *All farmed salmon contain added color, so all should be labeled "color added."*

But farmed fish are not the only fish that get cosmetic treatment. Wild tuna steaks, which are naturally red, tend to turn brown when exposed to air or when frozen, so seafood companies spray them with carbon monoxide to keep this from happening. You probably prefer red tuna — it looks fresher. You will not be harmed by this treatment, but you might be tricked into thinking that the tuna is freshly caught when it may have been caught days ago (or weeks ago, if frozen). Japan, Canada, and the European Union do not allow carbon monoxide spraying. But in the United States, if tuna steaks are bright red, you have to assume that they were treated with carbon monoxide to maintain the color. The treatment is unlikely to be stated on labels because it does not have to be; if you want to know, you have to ask.

If you think that feeding synthetic canthaxanthin to fish is antithetical to organic principles (and you would be right), you might wonder how "organically" raised farmed salmon get so pink. As it turns out, "organic" salmon get their color in a different way—by eating a species of yeast called *Phaffia rhodozyma*, which naturally makes the same astaxanthin pigment as that found in krill. In response to a petition from Archer Daniels Midland, the company that makes this yeast, the FDA allows organic producers to add phaffia yeast to fish pellets. This makes "organic" farmed salmon look good enough to eat.

LABEL QUANDARY #4: "ORGANIC" FISH

I keep putting "organic" in quotation marks because it is hard to know what it would take to consider a fish organically raised or grown. The basis of organic food production is control over growing conditions. But big fish eat smaller fish and migrate thousands of miles over rivers and oceans. If they end up full of methylmercury and PCBs, how can they possibly be considered organic? Fish farming also seems anything but organic. Farm-raised fish are treated with pesticides to prevent lice, and they eat pellets containing artificial colors, parts of fish and other animals, and binders and thickeners made from soybeans that could be genetically modified. How, you might want to know, could any farmed fish be labeled organic?

Answering this question requires brief detours into the way the government regulates seafood and into the USDA's rules—the standards—for calling food organic. In the typical way the government does such things, the Department of Commerce's National Oceanic and Atmospheric Administration is in charge of promoting sustainable ocean fisheries, the FDA is in charge of fish and shellfish safety, and the USDA is in charge of aquaculture just as it oversees any other agricultural product. The USDA also houses the National Organic Program, so organic seafood necessarily comes under this agency's purview.

Because the life cycle of fish is so complicated and because nobody had ever produced or thought of fish as "organic," the USDA did not pay much attention to seafood during the twelve years (from 1990 to 2002) that it took its National Organic Standards Board to decide on standards for organic food production. Fish farming had not yet come into prominence, and the food industry was not much interested in going the organic route. Although the Organic Foods Production Act of 1990 included seafood, the USDA's final rules for the National Organic Program said nothing about what fish and shellfish producers would have to do to qualify for organic certification. Without defining standards, producers cannot be certified and the USDA Certified Organic seal cannot be used on any seafood product.

That is why I am astonished to see "organic" salmon and shrimp in supermarkets or available for order from FreshDirect. What does "organic" mean if there are no organic standards? FreshDirect explains that its Clare Island "organic" salmon come from a farm off the coast of Ireland where they are "hand-fed an entirely natural and organic diet with no synthetic colorants." If you want to know what this means, you can look up Clare Island Sea Farm on the Internet and discover that it is owned by Marine Harvest, the leading worldwide producer of farm-raised fish. The company states that Clare Island's practices meet four different sets of organic standards set by four different European certifying agencies, one of which (Naturland-Verband in Germany) is accredited by the USDA. But without standards for organic fish, those certifiers must be assuming that the organic standards for livestock production also apply to seafood, and you have to assume that they are interpreting the rules as best they can.

In August 2004, I received an e-mail message from Victoria Freeman, the manager of stockholder relations for OceanBoy Farms in Clewiston, Florida, who thought I might like to know that her company had just obtained organic certification for its farmed shrimp. I did indeed want to know this and could not wait to find out how its seafood could possibly have been certified as organic. The certifier turned out to be Quality Certification Services (QCS) of Florida, a private company accredited by the USDA for doing organic certifications. With no USDA rules to guide it, QCS developed its own standards based on those used for organic livestock and applied them to OceanBoy's shrimp-raising practices. This means that the "organic" shrimp are not treated with antibiotics or hormones (but shrimp do not get these treatments anyway). It also means that OceanBoy has to give the shrimp organic feed.

And how does the company manage this feat? The company solves the feed problem by operating an entirely separate fish farm where it raises "organic" tilapia to be used exclusively as a feed additive for the shrimp. I leave it to ecologists to figure out the environmental costs of raising a decent, if bland, fish that you might eat for dinner for the express purpose of feeding shrimp, but such are the ironic economic realities of modern seafood farming.

In 2001, a task force reporting to the USDA's National Organic Standards Board said that the USDA should develop organic standards for farmed fish, but not for wild fish. The Alaska salmon industry, however, badly wants to market wild salmon as organic or at least to be allowed to say something like "Sustainably raised and organically processed." The board agreed that this and other considerations required attention and forwarded the task force recommendations to the USDA where, late in 2005, they were still under consideration.

While the USDA was deciding what to do about organic seafood, QCS—the same private certifier that worked with OceanBoy—took it upon itself to grant organic certification to another company, Permian Sea Shrimp, also using livestock standards as guidelines. Several international certifying groups also began to issue organic certificates to farmers of salmon, shrimp, and other fish outside the United States, using standards that they developed themselves. In response to these confusing developments, the USDA said it would create its own agency committee to draft U.S. organic standards for seafood. When this happens, it will be the first step in a lengthy process that is certain to take years.

So for now, "organic" on seafood means much the same as "natural" does on meat—however the seller chooses to define it. Until the USDA issues organic seafood standards, there is no way for you to know for sure what the "organic" label on shrimp or fish really means. The USDA Certified Organic seal on livestock tells you that the rules for raising cattle have been followed and the ranch has been inspected to make sure it adheres to those rules. The USDA seal also tells you that no genetically modified

So for now, "organic" on seafood means much the same as "natural" does on meat—however the seller chooses to define it.

ingredients went into the feed. Without USDA certification, you cannot assume that such practices were followed. All you know is that the seafood was certified by a domestic or international certifier that applied standards of its own making. You cannot know whether those standards fit your own idea of what "organic" should mean. The result is that you had best ask fish sellers some tough questions before you fork over a premium price for fish and shellfish labeled "organic."

LABEL QUANDARY #5: NOT GENETICALLY MODIFIED

You will not find genetically modified (GM) fish in your supermarket—not yet, at least. This is not for lack of trying on the part of the seafood industry. Fish can be genetically modified to overcome their annoyingly unprofitable habit of only growing during certain seasons. Salmon, for example, produce growth hormone only during the summer months when they are returning to the coasts on their spawning runs (a time when they can be caught in large numbers). Wild salmon do not grow in the winter. Farm-raised salmon, however, can be grown and harvested throughout the year—a great benefit if you like eating salmon. Not only that, but with a bit of genetic engineering they can be induced to grow faster than wild salmon.

Researchers working for what is now called Aqua Bounty Technologies, a company that uses genetic engineering to develop farm-raised fish that grow bigger and faster, discovered that part of an "antifreeze" gene (one that keeps fish blood from freezing in very cold water) also stimulates production of growth hormone and keeps the fish growing year-round. The resulting "frankenfish," according to critics, grow five times faster in the first few months, and twice as fast overall, meaning that these fish can be ready to harvest in record time. In theory at least, if GM fish were allowed to be farmed, more fish could be produced and sold in a shorter time. This would do good things for people who like to eat fish as well as for people who make a living by selling fish. In practice, however, GM fish might not be so good for fish ecology, as I shall soon explain.

By the end of 2005, however, the FDA had not approved the production or sale of GM fish. Instead, the FDA decided to consider Aqua

Bounty's use of a modified gene for growth hormone under existing rules for new animal drugs, rather than considering it under the more liberal rules in place for GM foods. This meant that Aqua Bounty would have to prove that the GM farmed salmon really do grow faster and are safe to eat before the company would be allowed to license them to be grown commercially. Not to be deterred, the company tried another tack. It applied for approval to farm its GM fish in Canada. This application was still pending as this book went to press.

The Canadian application worries critics. Farmed salmon escape from pens in large numbers and can swim long distances. Because GM salmon grow faster and bigger than wild salmon, and so might outmate their competitors if they escaped into the wild, they generate additional concerns beyond the usual ones I discussed in my book *Safe Food*. For example, local governments and regulators are concerned that GM fish will irrevocably alter the existing populations of wild fish. The unknown effects of introducing such fish into the wild caused the state of Maryland to ban GM fish from its waterways in 2001. In 2003, the Pew Charitable Trusts warned that regulators did not seem to have "the tools they need to adequately evaluate these new products, and there is reason to wonder if innovation is getting ahead of our ability to manage it." Also in 2003, California banned the cultivation of GM fish in state waterways and ocean waters within three miles of the shore.

In 2005, despite strong opposition by the Biotechnology Industry Organization, a trade group, the Alaska legislature passed a law requiring GM fish and fish products to be labeled as such. Alaska legislators were concerned that Canada might allow GM fish to be farmed and that these fish might "pollute" or compete with the state's wild salmon. They also viewed "non-GM" and "natural" as excellent marketing tools for selling their state's wild fish and did not want the reputation of those fish sullied in any way.

Perhaps because state opposition is so evident, the FDA is taking a more cautious position on GM fish (and GM animals) than it did on foods derived from plants. It points out that "Development of a world market for a transgenic animal variety [fish, for example] is currently fraught with difficulties owing to the varying cultural views and governments." In this sense, the FDA recognizes public and international distaste for this kind of tampering with animals or fish. At the moment, it is uncertain when, if ever, GM fish for human consumption will be grown commercially in the United States. Late in 2003, however, pet stores announced that you could now buy GM pet fish for your home aquarium. The new glow-in-the-dark GloFish are zebra fish genetically engineered to contain a gene from sea coral that makes them fluoresce under ultraviolet light. The FDA claims jurisdiction over these fish, but decided not to regulate them because zebra fish are not food.

DEALING WITH THE QUANDARIES

Once you face the labeling quandaries, you will see that you can hardly avoid them if you like eating seafood. You also can see why I view fish as the Wild West of the food industry. Much of this industry acts like it is virtually unregulated and as if all it cares about is selling fish as quickly as possible at as high a price as the traffic will bear. Out of ignorance or, sometimes, unscrupulousness, the more profit-minded segments of this industry bend rules to their own advantage any time they can get away with it. No wonder "fishy" translates as "suspicious." If you want to buy fish, you need to watch out for labels that are sometimes untruthful and often misleading.

> You also can see why I view fish as the Wild West of the food industry. Much of this industry acts like it is virtually unregulated and as if all it cares about is selling fish as quickly as possible at as high a price as the traffic will bear.

Some of the quandaries are easier to manage than others. You do not need to make any decisions about genetically modified fish because none are marketed (not yet, anyway). Surimi is also easy; if you do not like the way it tastes, or dislike the idea on principle, you do not have to buy it. "Organic" may be a step in the right direction, but still lacks agreement as to what it means in practice, especially as applied to farmed fish. As for salmon, until farming methods improve there is only one choice—wild. Wild salmon tastes better than farmed salmon and is healthier for you and for the planet. Because wild salmon is so expensive, you have to buy it in small pieces and treasure every bite. Farmed salmon, "organic" or not, raises too many environmental questions to make me comfortable about buying it. As for all the other kinds of fish and shellfish, wild and farmed, I have to confess that I cannot keep them straight. I need help. The only way I can decide what to do about them is to use a fish advisory card prepared by groups that pay much closer attention to such things than I do. And that brings us at last to the fish lists.

20

More Seafood Dilemmas: Safety and Sustainability

You might think that seafood could not possibly command any further issues, but it does. We have two more fish dilemmas to deal with, one involving biological hazards that occur in nature or as a result of pollution or the mishandling of fish, and the other arising from questions about whether fish can be farmed in ways that conserve their nutritional benefits and also protect ocean ecosystems.

FISH DILEMMA #3: HEALTH BENEFITS VERSUS "BIOHAZARDS"

Until now, I haven't said anything about the safety issues raised by naturally occurring toxins or microbes that get into fish from polluted waters or from sloppy handling during processing, storage, and display. This is not because these biological hazards are trivial. Quite the contrary. Fish and shellfish are leading sources of food-borne illnesses in the United States, and the more of these foods you eat, the greater your chance of picking up something

> **F**ish and shellfish are leading sources of food-borne illnesses in the United States, and the more of these foods you eat, the greater your chance of picking up something from them that might make you sick.

from them that might make you sick. The exact number of people who get sick each year from eating seafood is not known, and guesses vary widely. Food-borne illnesses are hard to count. If you become sick from something you ate, you probably will not go to a doctor. Even if you did, your doctor probably would not bother to notify health authorities. This leaves health authorities with no reliable way to count cases, let alone verify them. Nevertheless, they believe that seafood safety is a serious problem.

The Center for Science in the Public Interest (CSPI), which fills the outbreak gap in federal oversight by tracking episodes of illnesses that occur in groups of people who ate the same food, says that seafood accounts for 20 percent of all such incidents. CSPI counted 899 outbreaks caused by seafood from 1990 to 2003, and these affected more than 9,000 people. The FDA's estimates of cases are 100 times higher—up to 60,000 a year. The Centers for Disease Control and Prevention (CDC), which guesses that there are 76 million annual cases of food-borne illness in the United States, also guesses that seafood accounts for 15 percent of those cases—that would be 11 million a year.

Whatever. Lots of people get sick from eating fish and shellfish, and you do not want to be one of them. The catalog of seafood biohazards is long and includes a host of especially unpleasant things like the naturally occurring toxins from "red tide" organisms that get into shellfish, and the toxin from reef fish called ciguatera. Other natural causes are histamines that develop in tuna and shark that have not been stored properly (these cause scombroid poisonings). Still others are bacteria such as *Vibrio* and *Listeria* and viruses of the Norwalk type and hepatitis, as well as Anisakis worms. Viruses are a frequent cause of illness from seafood. If you eat uncooked shellfish from American waters, for example, you have about a 1-in-100 chance of picking up a viral infection. Those odds may not sound too serious, but if you eat raw oysters once a week or so, sooner or later you are likely to pick up some virus that they carry, much to your regret.

To protect yourself against fish biohazards, the fish industry tells you to "buy only from reputable suppliers." As with most else having to do with fish, this advice suggests that it is your responsibility to figure out which dealers might fall into the "reputable" category, not the industry's to root out suppliers with poor safety practices. And, as with most fish issues, figuring out how to identify suppliers you can trust is a challenge, to say the least. Even investigators from *Consumer Reports* had problems finding dealers who met their idea of "reputable"—fish sellers who stored, displayed, tested, and labeled their seafood appropriately and safely.

In February 1992, that magazine published an account of a six-month investigation into the safety of fish and shellfish sold in American supermarkets. The results were disheartening, if not outright alarming. Nearly half the tested samples of salmon and whitefish contained PCBs (a percentage that seems low by current testing standards), and practically all—90 percent—of swordfish samples contained methylmercury. More than one-third of the fish samples were mislabeled as to species or origin, and more than 40 percent were contaminated by bacteria from human or animal feces—often massively. The investigators often observed seafood to be mishandled, stored at temperatures that were too warm, or displayed on ice that was dirty. They routinely found raw seafood placed right next to cooked seafood on ice, where melting water can cause cross-contamination. And they often saw frozen-and-thawed fish sold as fresh. As for the people behind the fish counters, the magazine reported: "When we asked questions, the answers were not reassuring and often wrong." For example, when the investigators asked where some scallops came from, a clerk answered, "the ocean."

That was then and this is now, but I am sorry to report that I do not see much improvement. Country-of-origin labels, which have been required since spring 2005, are still confusing or missing; farmed fish is not identified as such; thawed fish is still sold as fresh ("frozen fresh," "whole live lobster, previously frozen"), and the clerks are just as clueless. At the counter of a specialty fish store, I asked if anyone could tell me where some striped bass had been farmed. "We get them from the Fulton Fish Market" (New York City's wholesale distribution center until November 2005). The one visible sign of progress is the quality of the ice. Most stores in my neighborhood keep seafood packed in ice

> Most stores in my neighborhood keep seafood packed in ice and it mostly looks clean, although at least one store manager told me that it is changed only every other day.

and it mostly looks clean, although at least one store manager told me that it is changed only every other day.

And where is the government in all of this? Fish regulation is divided among at least four federal agencies. For the most part, the USDA is responsible for aquaculture marketing, the National Oceanic and Atmospheric Administration (NOAA) is responsible for ocean fisheries, and the Environmental Protection Agency deals with fish caught for sport and recreation. That leaves fish safety to the FDA, an agency with limited resources for doing everything it is required to, such as inspecting fish imports. Because most FDA funding is used for regulating pharmaceutical drugs and medical devices, food safety oversight gets shorter shrift than it should.

But soon after the *Consumer Reports* investigations, the FDA told fish processors and importers that they would have to start developing and using food safety plans of the HACCP (Hazard Analysis and Critical Control Point) type, like the ones I discussed in the chapter on meat safety. Doing so, said the FDA, would prevent 20,000 to 60,000 seafood poisonings a year from biological hazards (for reasons unexplained, a far more conservative estimate than that of the CDC). In the usual manner, HACCP for seafood requires fish processors to identify places in the production process where biological contamination might occur, take steps to prevent contamination at those places, and check and test to make sure the steps are routinely followed.

The FDA proposed Seafood HACCP in 1994, issued the rules in 1995, and required them to be followed in 1997. Since then, all processors of seafood sold in the United States—domestic and imported—are supposed to be producing fish according to HACCP plans. These require the processors to monitor the temperature and cleanliness of the water in which fish are held, the cleanliness of cutting surfaces and tools, the adequacy of hand-washing facilities, the health of employees, and the ability of the facility to exclude pests and contaminants. Seafood producers must demonstrate that they harvest shellfish only from approved waters—those that are not excessively polluted—and that the shellfish sent to market do not have dangerous levels of microbial contaminants, chemical contaminants, or natural toxins. Seafood importers are responsible for making sure that their suppliers outside the U.S. borders follow such rules.

All of that sounds great. Four years after the rules were made mandatory, however, the government watchdog agency, then called the General Accounting Office (GAO), issued two reports with titles that succinctly summarized the state of affairs: "Federal Oversight of Seafood Does Not Sufficiently Protect Consumers" (January 2001) and "Federal Oversight of Shellfish Safety Needs Improvement" (July 2001).

These depressing reports identified serious gaps in FDA oversight of seafood safety. Many fish firms were not using HACCP plans, particularly companies that processed fresh fish on ships on their way back to harbor (the usual practice). The FDA could not get adequate cooperation from international firms, enforce documentation requirements, follow up on violations, or keep pace with inspection demands. By 1999, only 44 percent of seafood processing firms had HACCP plans in place and the FDA was testing less than 1 percent of imported seafood. Furthermore, by 2001 it was evident that the shellfish industry's efforts to make you responsible for properly choosing, storing, and cooking its products were not working. The number of illnesses and deaths caused by eating raw oysters contaminated with *Vibrio*, for example, had not changed in years as far as anyone could tell. There is no national system for tracking *Vibrio* infections, so reporting is regional, but Southern states still were counting twenty to thirty cases a year. This is a small number, but the death rate from *Vibrio* infection exceeds 50 percent. This illness is something worth taking steps to prevent.

In response to the GAO findings, the FDA said it would increase its rate of inspection and would visit each processing firm once a year, but the message was clear: neither the FDA nor the industry was doing much about prevention of illnesses caused by contaminated seafood. A report from CSPI later in 2001 complained that virtually all shellfish harvested from the Gulf of Mexico carried dangerous *Vibrio* bacteria but that the FDA had ceded its oversight authority to state officials who are so heavily influenced by local fishing industries that they were doing practically nothing to protect public health. Instead, everyone was leaving prevention up to consumers. Seafood safety does not have to be this way. Seafood companies are perfectly capable of maintaining high safety standards, pleasing their customers, and making money at the same time.

Colleagues who knew I was writing about fish told me that Legal Sea Foods, the Boston-based "fish company in the restaurant business," had an amazing seafood safety program, so I called Stephen Martinello, the company's longtime director of quality control, to ask him about it. The program is more than amazing; it is inspiring. He told me that Legal Sea Foods has about thirty stores along the eastern seaboard from Massachusetts to Florida, runs a mail order business, serves fish to 70,000 people per week in its restaurants and catering operations, and does not want any of its customers ever to get sick. The company started testing for toxins and contaminants in shellfish in 1980 and introduced its own HACCP plan in 1990, long before the FDA required such plans.

Legal Sea Foods has its own laboratory. Its staff routinely sample shellfish for "fecal coliforms"; these are bacteria like *E. coli* that are not themselves harmful but indicate exposure to raw sewage, which could be loaded with pathogens. They hold shellfish in quarantine until the tests come back clean. They test crab and lobster for the usual suspects—*E. coli, Listeria,* and *Salmonella,* and others—and tuna and swordfish for scombroid. They test *every* large predatory fish for methylmercury, which means they are running twenty or thirty tests a day. Every store, Martinello said, is subjected to regular inspections by registered sanitarians. Most impressive, the results of those inspections directly affect the bonuses of managers: the safer the fish in the store, the higher the bonus. This should work, and apparently does. Considering the scale of its operations, the company seems remarkably free of food poisoning scandals, any of which would be sure to be covered by the press and investigated by the CDC. Would I buy fish at Legal Sea Foods? In a New York minute.

Other stores also tell me that they take extra care with seafood. A spokeswoman for Wegmans, the family-owned supermarket chain in the northeast, says they do in-house testing of fish samples for microbial levels and scombroid, and send other samples out for more complicated testing. They limit the number of suppliers they buy from, and send inspectors on personal visits to make sure the suppliers and processors are following good sanitation procedures. This level of diligence, however, is rare. Even the most "organic" of stores pay more attention to seafood sustainability than they do to safety. Whole Foods partners with the Marine Stewardship Council, and Tops Markets (owned by Ahold) partners with the New England Aquarium. But both companies generally outsource safety monitoring and depend on their suppliers to make sure that the fish they buy are not unduly contaminated. The seafood manager of one such chain told me that his company's fish meet the FDA's standards for allowable contaminants, and that he saw no reason why anything more would be needed. "We are not in the health-food business," he said. Maybe not, but I found that statement disappointing, if not alarming. It did not seem to reflect a genuine commitment to selling high-quality seafood. I buy fish elsewhere.

> **E**ven the most "organic" of stores pay more attention to seafood sustainability than they do to safety.

FISH DILEMMA #4: NUTRITIONAL BENEFITS VERSUS THE SUSTAINABILITY OF FARM-RAISED FISH

This last dilemma has to do with the environmental cost of obtaining the nutritional benefits of farmed fish. As the fish industry and many health authorities say again and again, fish are an excellent source of protein, vitamins, and minerals; are low in saturated fat; and are the best sources of the omega-3 fatty acids, EPA and DHA. But because these nutritional benefits can be offset by the harm caused by the methylmercury, PCBs, viruses, bacteria, and natural toxins in seafood, you and everyone else who eats fish has a stake in the environmental issues that affect seafood, wild as well as farmed. To repeat: farmed salmon are fattier than wild salmon because they are fed so much fish meal and fish oil. If you substitute soybeans, corn, or canola (rapeseed) for the "industrial" fish used to make feed pellets, you can reduce the PCBs but you also lower the omega-3s. If you eat fewer omega-3s, you do not get their health benefits. When people with heart disease eat fish fed on vegetable oils instead of fish oils, they do not accumulate much EPA and DHA in their blood. That is why it makes biological sense to add fish meal and fish oils to "finish off" the diets of farmed fish raised as vegetarians during the late stages of their growth.

The farming of salmon was once a relatively small-scale industry, but it has now grown to account for more than half of salmon sales. At the moment, you might as well assume that all shrimp and salmon are farmed, unless they are labeled (and labeled honestly) as wild. Fish farming requires consideration of environmental as well as safety issues. Farmed fish must eat pounds of wild fish for each pound they gain, they discharge nutrients and wastes into local waters, and they all too often escape into the wild—sometimes in places where their particular species never used to be. Even the argument that they increase the overall availability of edible fish is not simple. Although farming increases the overall supply of some kinds of fish, it depletes stocks of others. That is why advocacy groups are pushing hard for more sustainable management of fish farms. This means raising fish that do not require heavy feeding of "industrial" fish, minimizing the use of antibiotics and pesticides, preventing discharge of nutrients and chemicals into the surrounding seas, managing wastes, and considering environmental effects in all fish-farming practices. Farms raising fish that eat low on the food chain—shellfish, tilapia, carp, catfish, and the like—can do these things fairly easily. But farms that raise carnivorous fish like salmon do

> Although farming increases the overall supply of some kinds of fish, it depletes stocks of others.

not follow these practices, which is why farm-raised salmon invariably end up on the "Avoid" side of fish advisories. And this brings us, at last, to the use of seafood advisory cards—fish lists—as a short-term approach to solving the fish dilemmas.

THE IMMEDIATE SOLUTION: SEAFOOD CARDS (FISH LISTS)

Whenever you go to a seafood counter or order fish in a restaurant, you are faced with complicated choices that require decisions not only about what kind of fish you might enjoy eating but also about the nutritional, toxicological, and environmental dilemmas that come along as baggage. Consider what it means to choose a fish that does everything you might want it to: high omega-3s, low chemical and biological hazards, and environmental sustainability—and delicious taste as well. If you cannot figure out how to make that choice on your own, you are supposed to find yourself a reputable supplier and ask. Well, good luck finding one who understands all of those issues well enough to be of real help. Such people exist, but you have to ask a lot of hard questions to find them.

For these reasons, even I find seafood decisions overwhelming: too many kinds of fish, too many issues to track, and not nearly enough information about any of them. Among fish highest in omega-3s, for example, I see few choices that do not involve dilemmas. Albacore tuna has methylmercury. Farmed salmon has PCBs. Cod, halibut, and sea bass are overfished. Fortunately, seafood advocacy groups are well aware of this problem and have devised two ways to help: Seafood Safe labels, and fish advisory cards.

Seafood Safe labels identify fish that have been tested by independent laboratories for their content of mercury and PCBs. This program, launched in 2005, puts a large red number on a black-and-white label. This tells you the number of 4-ounce servings of that fish that are safe for women of childbearing age to eat per month (and, therefore, are surely safe for most other healthy people). Seafood Safe 10, for example, means that you can eat that fish ten times a month if the servings are 4 ounces, but just five times a month if you eat 8-ounce servings. The Seafood Safe program "strongly recommends" that you keep track of your cumulative fish consumption, especially if you are eating different kinds of fish. Its labels make it clear that you cannot consider fish an everyday food.

> The Seafood Safe program "strongly recommends" that you keep track of your cumulative fish consumption, especially if you are eating different kinds of fish. Its labels make it clear that you cannot consider fish an everyday food.

Fish advisory cards not only are helpful but are essential tools for anyone who likes eating fish. In the late 1990s, the Monterey Bay Aquarium and some other groups started producing wallet-card guides for the fish perplexed. The aquarium's first guide, for example, was designed to make it easy for you to choose fish based on environmental considerations. Its current Seafood Watch guides divide the kinds of fish you might eat into three categories: green ("Best Choices"), yellow ("Good Alternatives," formerly known as "Proceed with Caution"), and red ("Avoid"). The aquarium produces seafood cards specific to various regions of the country and updates the lists regularly on its Web site (www.mbayaq.org).

As you might imagine, the fishing industry hates the fish cards and lists. This industry recognizes that the advocacy groups have an overt agenda: to create market incentives that will force fish suppliers to raise and catch seafood in ways that are friendlier to the environment. But instead of embracing environmental advocates as partners in a long-term effort to maintain healthy fisheries, the industry and its lobbyists go on the attack. They criticize the fish lists for being scientifically unsound and inconsistent, for mistaking one kind of fish for another, and for over-simplifying complexities. My own concern about the earliest lists was that they focused exclusively on the health of the environment—fish and fisheries—but ignored the issues related to human health.

In recent years, fish advocacy groups have responded to such complaints. The groups now routinely update, correct, and refine their lists. They also identify fish that are most highly contaminated with toxic chemicals. Environmental Defense, for example, lists "eco-best" and "eco-worst" seafood choices on its Web site (www.environmentaldefense. org), and best and worst "eco-choices" on a handy Pocket Seafood Selector that folds to the size of a business card (available at www. oceansalive.org). The best eco-choices include fish farmed "in an ecologically responsible manner," such as catfish, which are raised in ponds that do not routinely discharge waste, are native to the areas in which they are farmed, and eat mostly vegetarian diets. Farmed abalone, clams, oysters, mussels, and bay scallops are also "eco-best" because they require no feed, filter plankton out of the water, and are grown on ropes, rafts, or other devices that allow harvesting without damage to the surroundings. The "eco-worst" list includes fish at risk of depletion, shrimp and fish farmed in ways that damage the environment, and those that are known to be highly contaminated (the contaminated ones are indicated in red on the pocket card).

A third seafood-card provider, the Blue Ocean Institute, "works to inspire a new relationship with the sea through science, art, and literature" (www.blueoceaninstitute.org). It publishes a "Miniguide to ocean friendly seafood" with a color-coded key ranging from green (abundant species, gentle methods) to yellow (some problems exist or not enough information is available) to red (problems: overfishing, bycatch, harmful farming methods). It has high praise for Alaska wild salmon, farmed mollusks, and Pacific halibut, but little good to say about eating Chilean sea bass (the fish formerly known as Patagonian toothfish), Atlantic cod, or, no surprise, farmed Atlantic salmon.

The fish cards from these three groups differ in the way they present the information, and the differences can make a confusing situation even more so. This is where a fourth organization used to come in: the Seafood Choices Alliance. This alliance functions something like a trade association for advocates of fish sustainability. The three fish-guide producers belong to the alliance, and so do a long list of other environmental and food-advocacy and professional associations (www.seafoodchoices.com). Under the auspices of the alliance, the three groups got together, reconciled the differences, and produced a single guide that addressed health as well as environmental concerns. They called the unified guide the Fish List. This guide simplified seafood choices into just two categories: green ("Enjoy!") and red ("Avoid!"). The "Enjoy" category included seafood that is uniformly "better for ocean ecosystems." The Fish List's "Avoid" category listed seafood choices "associated with ecological harm to our oceans."

Because the Monterey Bay Aquarium was doing such a good job of keeping up with rapidly changing information about seafood stocks and contamination levels, the Seafood Choices Alliance discontinued its Fish List in 2006. You can replace it with a constantly updated Seafood Watch Pocket Guide for your own region posted on the Monterey Bay Aquarium's Web site (www.mbayaq.org/cr/seafoodwatch.asp).

You can take the Guides with you to a supermarket or restaurant and order farmed catfish, tilapia, clams, and the other "Best Choices" with a clear conscience. The Guides make it easy for you to know that you should avoid shark, farmed salmon, and bluefin tuna because they are likely to be highly contaminated, or Atlantic cod and imported shrimp for ecological reasons. The Alliance and Aquarium sites offer easy links to detailed information about each fish or shellfish assigned to the three categories of the Guides.

THE LONG-TERM SOLUTION: ADVOCACY

As must be evident by now, supermarket seafood is a long and fishy story. What I find most striking is the repetitiveness of this story's main theme:

no matter what dilemma is under discussion, it is up to *you* to resolve it. It is your responsibility to learn which fish have omega-3s, which are too high in chemicals, which might be contaminated with biohazards, which you can safely eat or feed to your children, and how much and how often you can eat fish without harm. It is also your job to figure out which kinds of seafood are fished or farmed at high cost to the health of fisheries and the environment. For the most part, fish retailers cannot help you through the dilemmas; most of them know as little or less about these issues than you do. You cannot count on the government to protect you against unsafe fish, either. Oceans are too large, the issues are too complicated, and the dangers seem too remote to command the regulatory attention that seafood truly deserves.

Another theme: you cannot count on the fishing industry to look out for your interests. This industry is too small and dispersed among catchers of too many kinds of fish to have much clout with Congress, except in states that have large fisheries. Fishing and fish farming together supply about 16 pounds of seafood per capita per year in the United States, with revenues of about $60 billion in food service and retail—tiny in comparison to meat, dairy, or packaged foods.

C ommercial fishing companies behave like any other "extraction" industry (mining and timber, for example). They have seen the fisheries decline, see little future in the industry, and want to get from the ocean what they can while the fish are still there.

More than 8 of those 16 pounds come just from the top five market performers: shrimp, canned tuna, salmon, pollack, and catfish. The rest come from dozens of other kinds, and the fishers and sellers of all of these seafoods view each other as competitors (much like the growers of fruits and vegetables do). Despite—or perhaps because of—the complexity of the industry, I find its attitude to be remarkably shortsighted. You might think it would be in the fishing industry's self-interest to maintain wild fish stocks, protect the ocean environment, and farm fish in ways that do more good than harm. You also might think the industry would want to keep methylmercury and PCBs away from fish and would want every company dealing with fish to have a well-designed and diligently followed HACCP plan in place. But no. Commercial fishing companies behave like any other "extraction" industry (mining and timber, for example). They have seen the fisheries decline, see little future in the industry, and want to get from the ocean what they can while the fish are still there.

But I still find it hard to understand why fish trade groups do not use what lobbying power they have to argue for tighter controls over mercury and dioxin emissions and for HACCP requirements that cover a broader range of fishing activities. That the National Fisheries Institute did not weigh in on the Environmental Protection Agency's proposed standards for mercury emissions seems like a lost opportunity for the industry as well as for the fish-eating public. In contrast, the Pew Charitable Trusts led that lobbying effort. Industry leaders would be doing much more for their constituents if they worked side by side with such philanthropic groups instead of against them.

That you cannot safely eat as much fish as you want from local waters in your state is a national scandal. Once you understand this situation, you cannot help but become angry about how such high levels of contaminants were allowed to get into your local streams and lakes and why so little is being done to stop the continued pollution of our national waterways. That, of course, brings us to the role of government. The government's lack of commitment to making fish healthier to eat can only be understood as responding to the political clout of industrial polluters and commercial seafood producers. The 2005 proposal of the Bush administration to have NOAA, its oceans agency, allow fish farming beyond state waters to locations 200 miles offshore, to license the farming of a greater variety of predatory fish (which must be fed other fish), and to increase the production of farmed fish by fivefold in twenty years must be understood in that context. NOAA officials argue that the United States is falling behind other countries in fish farming, and that fish farming is the only way to compensate for the loss in natural fisheries. Strong sea currents, they say, will dilute wastes from the pens. But the proposed law says not one word about environmental requirements, and those farms will be in federal waters beyond the jurisdiction of states— like Alaska and California—that are demanding higher standards for environmental protection. If you want environmental issues to be considered in decisions about fish farming, you need to share your opinion with your congressional representatives. Like many food issues, sustainable fisheries require the exercise of democracy in action.

As an individual, you can also express your dismay about the current situation directly and forcefully by voting with your fork: use the Fish List every time you buy fish at a market or in a restaurant, tell your fish supplier you want the "Enjoy" fish in the store whenever they are in season, and inform store managers that you have no intention of ever buying fish on the "Avoid" list. If seafood managers get that message, they may demand more thoughtful action from their suppliers, suppliers may demand better support from their trade associations, and trade associations may demand more consumer-friendly policies from the government. For anyone who might like to become an advocate for healthier and more sustainable fish, the Web sites of the Seafood Choices Alliance and the Monterey Bay Aquarium (www.seafoodchoices.com, www.seafoodwatch.org) provide handy lists of members, partners, and ocean allies—groups that work for preservation of marine life, reduction of pollutants, and promotion of environmental rights in the United States and elsewhere.

21

Eggs: The "Incredible" Edibles

A s always bears repeating, supermarkets typically position the perishable foods that you have to buy every few days well away from the entrance and along the peripheral—the outside perimeter—aisles. That way, you have to walk by hundreds of feet of foods displayed in ways that tempt you to buy on impulse. On that basis, stores usually stock the dairy foods, meats, and fish along the perimeter, but they place other foods that need to be kept cold (to retard the growth of bacteria) wherever they can.

Our tour of the peripheral perishables now brings us to eggs. These often are stacked next to the dairy sections, but not always; sometimes you have to ask where a store has hidden them. In my neighborhood stores, eggs take up so few feet of shelf space that it is difficult to imagine that they might pose complicated choices. But they do.

> I n my neighborhood stores, eggs take up so few feet of shelf space that it is difficult to imagine that they might pose complicated choices. But they do.

In the old days, eggs were eggs and you only had to decide whether you wanted them with white or brown shells, or small, medium, or large. But today, eggs have emerged as a classic example of the ways "adding value" to foods makes customers willing to pay more—and sometimes much more—to obtain the purported advantages. You now have to decide whether it is worth a higher price to buy "designer" eggs—those marketed as healthier for you and for the environment—than it is to stick with less expensive eggs that are merely ordinary.

One afternoon, I went from store to store in my neighborhood, just to make a list of the claims written on egg cartons about how kindly the chickens are treated or how healthy their eggs are for you. Here are a few of the statements I jotted down about how the chickens are kept and fed:

- cage free: they roam where they please
- naturally healthy habitat
- raised on a farm, not in a factory
- sunlit barns and porches
- hens are not force-fed
- fed pure nutritional grains
- all-vegetable ration . . . without antibiotics, arsenicals, sulfa drugs, pesticides, or hormones
- no animal by-products

And here are some of the claims about how good eggs are for your health:

- naturally low carb
- naturally low fat
- selenium 10 mcg (micrograms)
- choline 215 mg (milligrams)
- six times more vitamin E
- lutein 345 mcg
- 310 mg omega-3s per egg
- supports a healthy pregnancy

Leaving the health and welfare of chickens aside for the moment, let's examine the statements that relate to *your* health, one by one. Statements like these, by the way, are the kind that make my nutritionist colleagues either laugh (because the claims seem funny to someone trained in this field) or get upset (because the claims seem so absurd). From the top: all eggs are naturally low in carbohydrate (they are mostly protein and fat). Eggs are naturally low in fat only if you look at grams—each has only about 5—but the fat grams account for 60 percent of an egg's calories, so by that criterion, eggs are not a low-fat food. All eggs contain selenium and choline in about the amounts stated in the claims; all eggs also contain vitamin E, but six times more vitamin E than what? Despite what the claims imply, there are plenty of other dietary sources for these nutrients—nuts, seeds, and meats for selenium and choline, for example; and nuts, seed, oils, and greens for vitamin E.

Lutein requires a digression. It is a plant pigment in the same chemical family as beta-carotene. Some research suggests that it might protect against eye diseases like macular degeneration and cataracts. Its main dietary sources are dark green leafy vegetables. Egg yolks have some too, which was all it took to get the Egg Nutrition Center, the educational arm of egg producers' trade associations, to fund a study—also paid for in part by the USDA and conducted by scientists working at a USDA-funded research center—to prove that you absorb more lutein from egg yolks than you do from an equal amount in spinach. Of course you absorb more lutein from eggs than from spinach. Lutein, like beta-carotene, is a fat-soluble nutrient, meaning that you need to eat it along with fat in order to absorb it. Put some olive oil on your spinach and its lutein will be absorbed just as well as the lutein from egg yolks. Besides, there are drawbacks to getting your lutein from eggs. An average egg contains 200 or so micrograms of lutein and the "designer" eggs in supermarkets may have 345, but it takes a mere half-cup of steamed spinach to give you 8,000. To get that amount of lutein from eggs, you would have to eat nearly two dozen, along with all the calories, saturated fat, and cholesterol they contain. USDA scientists should have known better than to get involved in this study; one can only hope that the Egg Nutrition Center's funding was generous.

As for omega-3s: putting them into eggs is a clever marketing strategy. An egg normally contains omega-3 fatty acids, perhaps as much as 40 milligrams each. Putting in five or ten times as much positions eggs alongside fish as a special food that can be recommended for pregnant women—and as a food able to command high prices. A manager of a D'Agostino supermarket near my home, visibly relieved that my note taking did not mean that I was either a competitor or a city inspector, assured me that eggs are eggs and the point of all this nutritional nonsense was to justify charging more for them. He was not kidding about charging more. The cheapest large eggs at that store that day were $1.79 a dozen, but I paid $3.49 for a half-dozen Certified Organic eggs with omega-3s. These came from Country Hen in an earthy-looking carton printed with a drawing of an adorable black hen with a bright-red heart to show how heart healthy they were. I paid the equivalent of $6.98 a dozen for that attractive package—nearly four times as much as ordinary eggs of comparable size.

Price is not the only reason egg producers are giving so much attention to nutritional claims. The more important reason is that they want to make you forget about the downside of eggs: cholesterol and *Salmonella*. Delicious as they may be, eggs are the number-one food source of cholesterol in American diets, and a common source of food-borne illness. Cholesterol and *Salmonella* may be health problems for you, but each constitutes a major headache for the egg industry in public relations.

THE POLITICS OF CHOLESTEROL

Let's consider the "C word" first. Eggs have more cholesterol than any other single food (all of it in the yolk—the white has none to speak of), and they account for 35 percent of the overall cholesterol intake in American diets (the rest comes from meat and dairy foods, of which we eat a lot more). Although saturated fat and *trans* fat raise blood cholesterol the most, eating foods with cholesterol can also raise your blood cholesterol level and, therefore, increase your risk for coronary heart disease. In 2004, the scientific committee advising the government about revisions to the *Dietary Guidelines for Americans* concluded that "Keeping intake of saturated fat, *trans* fat and cholesterol very low can help . . . reduce the risk of CHD [coronary heart disease]." The committee said that anyone trying to eat a heart-healthy diet should restrict cholesterol intake to 300 milligrams per day or less because "the relationship between cholesterol intake and . . . cholesterol concentrations is direct and progressive, increasing the risk of CHD." By this, the committee meant that the more cholesterol you eat, the more cholesterol you have in your blood and the greater your chance of getting heart disease. Since a large hen's egg contains about 215 milligrams of cholesterol, and "cholesterol intake should be kept as low as possible," the committee concluded: "To limit dietary intake of cholesterol, one needs to limit the intake of eggs . . ."

For any industry, these are fighting words, and egg producers are an industry unto themselves. And like all industries, the egg industry has trade associations whose job it is to spin the science so research results look like they support eating more eggs, not less. So meet the American Egg Board: "As the egg industry's promotion arm, [our] foremost challenge is to convince the American public that the egg is still one of nature's most nearly perfect foods." The Egg Board gets its mandate from a USDA-sponsored program that requires companies with more than 75,000 laying hens to contribute to a common fund— a "checkoff"—to be used for generic advertising and promotion around its catchy slogan: "The Incredible, Edible Egg." In 1984, the Egg Board and another trade association, the United Egg Producers, created the Egg Nutrition Center for the express purpose of dealing with the "complicated health issue" of cholesterol. If anything, these groups have made the issue more complicated, not less so. For years, egg trade groups have worked tirelessly to minimize cholesterol as a health problem, to fund research expressly designed to prove that eating eggs does not raise blood cholesterol levels, and to promote the supposedly extra-special nutritional value of eggs.

Knowing this, I can only guess what happened between August 2004, when the dietary guidelines advisory committee released its report, and January 2005, when federal agencies issued their final guidelines. Despite its seventy-page length, the guidelines report dropped that inflammatory remark about cholesterol in eggs, and simply said: "many

> So meet the American Egg Board: "As the egg industry's promotion arm, [our] foremost challenge is to convince the American public that the egg is still one of nature's most nearly perfect foods."

[Americans] need to decrease their dietary intake of cholesterol. Because men tend to have higher intakes of dietary cholesterol, it is especially important for them to meet this recommendation." Although the guidelines say virtually nothing about eggs (other than to urge you to cook them properly), the underlying recommendation remained the same: you should eat less than 300 milligrams of cholesterol a day. This means eating no more than the equivalent of one and one-half eggs per day from all sources—whole eggs, of course, but also those used in making egg noodles, cookies, and ice cream. The 300-milligram target figure also includes the cholesterol you might get from meat and dairy foods. A small hamburger can easily contribute 100 milligrams, and an 8-ounce glass of whole milk has 25. In translation, the guidelines are telling you not only to "eat fewer eggs" but also to eat less of all foods from animal sources. Still, eggs have more cholesterol than any other food, so the "eat less" advice hits eggs the hardest. Egg industry lobbyists have their work cut out for them.

It is not hard to understand why the egg industry frets about its image. Americans eat fewer eggs than in the past. From the early 1900s through the 1930s, the egg industry produced enough eggs to offer every American, from youngest to oldest, the equivalent of nearly one egg a day from all food sources (about 300 a year). In 1945, at the end of World War II, egg production soared to 420 per capita. Since then, consumption—and, therefore, production—has dwindled, in part because of the introduction of packaged breakfast cereals that replace eggs as the morning meal, but also because of public fears of cholesterol. By the early 1990s, per capita production had declined to just 230 eggs per year. A recent increase to just over 250 heartens egg producers, who would dearly love those numbers to rise to former heights. And they might, to the extent that the egg industry can convince you that cholesterol does not matter, eggs are a perfect food, and putting omega-3s into eggs brings them to an even higher level of perfection.

> It is not hard to understand why the egg industry frets about its image. Americans eat fewer eggs than in the past.

Cholesterol is a fatty substance related to steroid hormones. It is made only by animals, including you (foods derived from plants, even fatty ones like coconuts, avocados, nuts, olives, and salad oils, never have cholesterol). It is a normal component of every one of your cells, and your body makes all the cholesterol you need. That's the problem. Other animals make cholesterol too. If you eat meat from cows, pigs, chickens, or fish, or their products—milk, cheese, or eggs—you get some of their cholesterol as well as your own.

Years ago, scientists figured out that having too much cholesterol in your blood can make the inside of the arteries in your heart clog up. The higher your blood cholesterol, the more likely you are to have arteries clogged so badly that blood cannot get through and you have a heart attack. That is why doctors measure blood cholesterol levels and government programs urge you to have your blood cholesterol checked, to know your cholesterol number, and, if it is too high, to improve your diet or take cholesterol-lowering medications.

Scientists do not argue about whether dietary cholesterol raises blood cholesterol; it does. They also do not argue about whether a high level of cholesterol in blood raises the risk for heart disease; it does. But they do argue a lot about how dangerous the effects of high blood cholesterol might be, and about whether having high blood cholesterol is bad for everyone or only for those individuals who are especially sensitive to its effects for reasons of family history.

Cholesterol arguments also are noisy for other reasons. One is that the amount of cholesterol in your blood does not necessarily reflect the amount of cholesterol you are eating. To complicate matters, dietary factors other than cholesterol also affect your blood cholesterol level. Saturated fats and *trans* fats in foods raise blood cholesterol levels, and do so more effectively than the cholesterol in eggs or any other food. This means that if you eat potatoes fried in partially hydrogenated vegetable oil (which contains *trans* fats), your cholesterol might go up even though potatoes and vegetable oils are plant foods and do not contain cholesterol. And although palm oils come from a vegetable source, they can raise blood cholesterol levels because of their high content of saturated fatty acids.

To complicate matters even more, other dietary components—unsaturated oils, fruits and vegetables, and whole grains, for example—can help to reduce blood cholesterol levels. So when researchers study the effects of eggs on blood cholesterol, they have to account for everything else you eat that might affect the amount of cholesterol in your blood. This makes the studies difficult to design, conduct, and interpret. All of this means that the results of cholesterol studies often seem confusing, especially because you must pay close attention to whether the experiments are about the cholesterol in food or are about the cholesterol in blood. They are related, but not always directly.

EGGS AND BLOOD CHOLESTEROL

These research complications have enabled the egg industry to sow further confusion by challenging the obvious connection between eating eggs and the level of cholesterol in your blood. Since the 1970s, the American Egg Board and, later, its Egg Nutrition Center have funded investigators willing to do studies designed to prove that eating eggs has no effect on blood cholesterol levels. Typically such studies compare blood cholesterol levels in people who do or do not eat up to four eggs a day on top of their usual diets. These studies invariably show no increase in blood cholesterol levels during the egg-eating periods. In contrast, studies by independent investigators almost always show that eating four eggs a day makes blood cholesterol levels go up. The difference in study results could be due to any number of uncontrolled variables: for example, the effects of other foods that people are eating, or the characteristics of the particular groups of people studied.

Blood cholesterol levels vary widely among individuals and tend to increase with age, but the healthiest range is considered to include no more than 200 milligrams of cholesterol per 100 milliliters of blood, a cutoff point that applies to adults of any age. Lower blood levels may be somewhat better, but above the 200 milligram cutoff, the risk of heart disease definitely increases. Despite this association, it is clear that some people can eat all the cholesterol they like without increasing the amount of cholesterol in their blood. A few years ago, the *New England Journal of Medicine* ran a story about an eighty-eight-year-old man who ate twenty-five soft-boiled eggs every day and whose blood cholesterol level nevertheless remained well within the healthy range. The man appeared to have early Alzheimer's disease and could not remember most things he did during the day, but he felt compelled to keep a diary in which he carefully recorded every egg he ate. About this obsessive behavior, he said: "Eating these eggs ruins my life," he said, "but I can't help it."

People like that man can eat all the eggs they want without affecting their blood cholesterol levels. And people who already have high blood cholesterol do not experience much of a rise in blood cholesterol from eating eggs. Food cholesterol causes blood cholesterol to rise much more in people with low blood cholesterol than it does in people who have a high blood cholesterol to begin with. So if you typically eat a low-cholesterol diet, and then start eating a lot of eggs, you should not be surprised if your blood cholesterol rises rapidly. Furthermore, if you have diabetes or other such conditions, you are likely to be even more susceptible to the cholesterol-raising effects of eggs.

Egg trade associations, however, largely ignore such complexities. They follow up every study that appears to exonerate eggs with press releases, advertising campaigns, newsletters, and letters to nutrition and health professionals. I received an avalanche of such materials following the publication of an independent study by Harvard investigators who found that adding up to one egg a day (note: not four) to people's diets had no noticeable effect on their risk of heart disease or stroke if they were healthy to begin with. Study participants with diabetes, however, doubled their risk of heart disease if they were given one or more eggs per day, an inconvenient finding that somehow did not get mentioned in egg industry public relations materials. Instead, one of the industry's letters to me pointed out that "dietary cholesterol has little effect on blood cholesterol levels in most individuals" (which, of course, is true if your blood cholesterol is high to begin with and you do not have diabetes). "Rather, the interaction of dietary saturated fatty acids and one's genetic disposition seems to be more important . . ." (true, but the cholesterol in eggs still counts for most people). Egg industry advertisements also did not discuss that issue. Instead, they said: "Love eggs? Watching your cholesterol? You're in luck."

Following that study, the Egg Nutrition Center produced an egg-shaped flier giving twelve reasons to eat eggs, among them that eggs have nutrients, that they satisfy hunger, that they make convenient snacks, that they taste good, and that they don't cost much. Again all true, but as Bonnie Liebman explained in a 1997 article in *Nutrition Action Healthletter*, you could make exactly the same claims about "incredible, edible peas" or most other vegetables and fruits that provide similar benefits without all that cholesterol.

Reason #12 in the egg-shaped flier was this: "Eating 7 eggs a week does not increase heart disease risk." This research finding and others encouraged the American Heart Association to revise its dietary guidelines so as to permit people to "enjoy an egg everyday as part of an average daily cholesterol intake of 300 mg." Indeed, the American Heart Association no longer specifies a limit on the number of eggs. It does, however, continue to advise keeping dietary cholesterol below 300 milligrams a day. Furthermore, its position statement on eggs points out that "Extra-large and jumbo eggs contain . . . up to 93 percent of the daily limit . . . If you eat a whole egg, try to avoid or limit other sources of dietary cholesterol on that day. If you have coronary heart disease, diabetes, high LDL cholesterol or other cardiovascular disease, your daily cholesterol limit is less than 200 mg . . ."

The American Heart Association's limits come to this: you should eat no more than one egg a day, and if you do eat an egg, you should be careful to avoid eating other foods made with eggs during that day as well as to avoid meat or dairy foods high in cholesterol. You can, of course, eat more eggs if you only eat the whites (because cholesterol is confined to the yolks). Otherwise, unless you have the remarkable physical constitution of that eighty-eight-year-old man (and only your doctor can assure you of that), you had best keep a close eye on the cholesterol in your diet. He, as it turned out, did not absorb much of the cholesterol he ate, had double its usual rate of excretion, and compensated by not making so much in his own body. We should all be so lucky.

THE OMEGA-3 SOLUTION

That pricey carton of Country Hen omega-3 eggs included a nice note from the company's owner, George S. Bass, inviting letters and telephone calls, so I promptly took him up on his invitation. I was curious to know what he was feeding chickens to get 300 milligrams of omega-3s into each of their eggs, what kinds of omega-3s these were, and how he knew the omega-3 levels of his eggs. I tried to reach Bass himself, but he did not return my calls. Instead, I spoke with two of his employees. Both told me that the information I was asking for is so "super top secret" that they had been required to sign nondisclosure agreements when they started their jobs. They were sorry but there was no way they could answer my questions. The most they were allowed to say was that the feed given to the Country Hens contains soybeans (for protein and fats), oyster shells (for the calcium needed to make eggshells), and flaxseed (source of the omega-3s). Those ingredients are exactly what might be expected for organic chicken feed, and the only surprise here was the secrecy, which seemed unnecessary. Months later, a spokeswoman from the company admitted that one of their omega-3 sources is marine and that "we do use a processed fish meal in our feed."

I first ran into omega-3 eggs in American markets late in 2000, when I saw this statement on an egg carton: "Chickens produce more omega-3s when they eat a diet rich in flaxseed and fish oil. In addition, we boosted our chicken feed with vitamin E . . . so why bother with pills when you can enjoy the goodness of eggs!" Omega-3 eggs are now a worldwide phenomenon. In 2005, I bought a carton of "DHA omega-3 eggs," with "Health benefits approved by the M.O.H. [Ministry of Health] of the U.A.E. [United Arab Emirates]" that came from the Al Jazira Poultry Farm in Dubai.

I can see why feeding flaxseed and fish oil to chickens would make their eggs have more omega-3s. Chickens, like most animals, make body fat that closely reflects the composition of the fat in their diets (cows are an exception; their rumen bacteria make whatever fat they eat more saturated). So if producers want chickens to lay eggs containing higher-than-normal amounts of omega-3s, they feed them seeds or seed oils containing alpha-linolenic acid or fish oils containing EPA and DHA—all omega-3 fatty acids. But if hens eat too much fish oil, their eggs taste fishy, so that approach only works to a point. Fortunately, hens are good at converting alpha-linolenic acid to the more biologically active EPA and DHA, so flaxseed (which is high in the alpha-linolenic acid form of omega-3s) does the trick. The feed for these chickens also contains mixtures of vitamins and other minerals, extra amounts of whatever nutrients are advertised, and carotenes to make the egg yolks a bright yellow. In August 2004, *Consumer Reports*, which usually does a good job of such things, tested for omega-3s in eggs and reported that their amounts—and those of some other nutrients—were about what the package labels claimed. If the cartons say 200 or 300 milligrams of omega-3s, it looks like you can believe it.

Are omega-3 eggs worth the higher price charged for them? One study, of undisclosed funding source, compared volunteers who ate four eggs a day high in omega-3s to those who ate four regular eggs a day. The group eating the high omega-3 eggs did better on measures of blood cholesterol and blood pressure, and the investigators concluded that they were healthier as a result. A more recent research review, however, found little or no effect of omega-3s on most such measures of heart disease risk.

While the debates about the benefits of omega-3s continue, you have some choices. You can get them from omega-3 "designer" eggs, but those omega-3 fatty acids will be accompanied by a heavy dose of cholesterol. Fish are as good or better a source of omega-3s, and they have less cholesterol than eggs (a 3-ounce salmon portion, for example, has 60 milligrams). And if you do not like fish, or are worried about the methylmercury or PCBs that fish might contain, you can eat flaxseeds themselves, or take fish oil supplements.

THE NATURAL EGG SOLUTION

As a summer camper on a farm in Vermont, I was given the job of feeding about a dozen Rhode Island Red hens, collecting their eggs, and making sure the henhouse and yard were well protected from the local foxes. That was a far cry from the factory-style henhouses that are the source of most supermarket eggs today.

Industrial production protects hens very well indeed. It confines tens of thousands of chickens in cages piled one on top of another in batteries infamous for accumulated feces, feathers, and the overpowering smell of ammonia from the hens' wastes. These conditions have attracted the attention of animal rights groups, some with "chicken liberationist" members who engage in guerrilla tactics to free chickens from their cages.

Even without going that far, almost anything seems preferable to eating eggs produced in this fashion, and "cage free" and "sunlit barns and porches" sound particularly reassuring. In 2000, I was speaking at a conference in New Mexico and joined some of the other participants on a tour of an organic egg farm. This was an education in the deeper meaning of the "cage free" claim on egg cartons. The reality of egg production is that hens have to be confined so they don't wander off, become wet or freeze to death, or get eaten by predators. Sure enough, the hens were not in cages, but many thousands of them were packed together in a crowded indoor space, flapping their clipped wings, fluttering on top of one another, and clucking away. This did not exactly match my bucolic childhood experience, but the place was airy and did not smell bad, and the hens were efficiently laying eggs in the nesting boxes stacked around the edges.

Surely the most bizarre aspect of the marketing of chicken welfare is that egg producers have developed three separate certifying systems to convince you that hens are well treated:

- USDA Certified Organic
- Certified Humane: Raised and Handled
- United Egg Producers Certified (formerly Animal Care Certified)

Certified Organic is the most familiar and the best regulated. If you see the Certified Organic seal on an egg carton, it means the eggs come from hens that eat organic feed, are allowed access to the outdoors and sunlight, and are inspected to make sure the rules are followed. A press kit from Pete and Gerry's Organic Eggs ("produced in the fresh air of the White Mountains of New Hampshire"), for example, explains that their hens "live in spacious barns, with access to organic grain, water and pasture outside." How they manage this on a farm of 100,000 laying hens is difficult to imagine, but a farm that size is small by commercial standards.

Pete and Gerry's eggs are not only Certified Organic but also carry a Certified Humane: Raised and Handled seal. If this seems superfluous, recall that the prices charged for eggs with added value are at least double the price you pay for conventional eggs. Humane certification requires some of the same things as organic certification, but is less restrictive about what the animals are fed. Hens have to be fed a "nutritious diet without antibiotics or hormones" and be "raised with shelter, resting areas, sufficient space, and the ability to engage in natural behaviors" (one can only guess what these might be). The nutritious diet is unspecified, but it does not have to be organic. The points about antibiotics and hormones are superfluous, because laying hens of any kind are only fed antibiotics or hormones when they are sick. But these are good selling points. This seal is sponsored by national and state humane societies and the American Society for the Prevention of Cruelty to Animals. It attests to how the hens are treated, but is less concerned with what they are fed.

> I f you see the Certified Organic seal on an egg carton, it means the eggs come from hens that eat organic feed, are allowed access to the outdoors and sunlight, and are inspected to make sure the rules are followed.

If your egg carton says "United Egg Producers Certified," however, you are in marketing cloud cuckoo-land. The new seal says "United Egg Producers Certified: Produced in Compliance with United Egg Producers' Animal Husbandry Guidelines," and gives the Web site, www.uepcertified.com. This certification system used to be called "Animal Care Certified." It ran advertisements in *Progressive Grocer* explaining that "Animal Care Certified farmers have gone to great lengths to ensure proper care of their hens." Maybe, but these properly cared-for hens are properly cared for in *cages*. The purpose of this program is to make you think commercial egg production is kind to hens. According to the

Web site, those "great lengths" were developed by a scientific committee, although one of unstated membership:

> The committee concluded that depending on the size of the laying hen and the size and style of the cage, hens needed space of 67 to 86 [square] inches per bird. To have moved to this spacing immediately would have created severe egg shortages, market disruptions, and likely major price increases. In due respect for their customers, the egg industry established a phase-in program to implement the space requirements over a 5-year period. Birds housed in cages have ready access to feed troughs directly in front of the cage and water is accessed easily from each cage. Housed in cages, birds seldom require medicine and are never fed hormones or steroids. Antibiotics are only used when birds are ill.

Implementation is to phase in gradually through 2008 and everything mentioned here is standard practice for commercial egg production. Animal Care and United Egg Producers Certifications require some skepticism. You should not be surprised that 80 percent of industrial egg producers are certified this way. This certification merely attests that a company gives food and water to its caged hens.

Egg producers did not want to change the name of the certification system; they were forced to. In 2003, an animal welfare group, Compassion Over Killing, filed a false advertising complaint with the Federal Trade Commission (FTC). "Animal Care Certified," it said, implies that the hens are treated with especially humane care, when they are not. Although the FTC, which regulates advertising, did not formally rule on the complaint, it reportedly encouraged egg producers to make the change voluntarily. A spokesman for the United Egg Producers, Mitch Head, told *The New York Times* that his group had willingly made the change because the FTC review had become "a purgatory" for the industry and was hurting business. He told *The Washington Post*: "We support cage-free eggs as a choice for consumers. We say, let consumers make their own choice. They are making their choice right now, and 98 percent of them are choosing conventional eggs."

Until now, I have not said anything about the most obvious choices you have to make about eggs—color and size. Color is easy; there are only two choices, white and brown. The color of an eggshell is determined by genetics. Some kinds of chickens lay white eggs, others lay brown eggs. Color is the only difference; their nutritional contents are the same. Even so, some stores in my neighborhood get away with charging up to 40 cents more per dozen for brown eggs, because you are supposed to think they are more natural or healthier—even though you throw out the shells anyway. Stores in other areas of the country charge more for white eggs. Take your pick. It makes no difference.

As for size, only two things matter: what you like, and price. The sizes are organized by weight. For a dozen eggs, the small ones are supposed to weigh 18 ounces, jumbos 30 ounces, and the others something in between at 3-ounce intervals. The nutrient content increases with size, so larger eggs have more protein but also more cholesterol than smaller eggs. Larger eggs almost always cost more, but you will need a calculator to figure out the best price by weight. Most recipes call for large eggs, so you have to compensate if you buy other sizes: six medium eggs are equivalent to five large eggs, four extra-large, and three jumbo. The grades—AA, A, or B—refer to cosmetic differences; their nutritional values are the same. Eggs deteriorate with time, especially if they are not kept well refrigerated, and it is best to buy what you need and use them fairly soon. If you do not need many, you can buy eggs by the half-dozen but you are likely to pay more for this convenience.

22

Eggs and the *Salmonella* Problem

The need to use eggs fairly soon after purchase brings us to the second public relations problem confronting the sellers of eggs: *Salmonella*. Not all that long ago, when my kids were small, we would bake cookies together, and they loved helping me clean up afterward by licking the raw dough out of the bowl (it really was delicious). Let your kids do that now and you could be making a big mistake. Times have changed and eggs are nowhere near as safe as they used to be. Egg companies put enticing statements about sunlight and omega-3s on top of the cartons where you cannot miss them, but you need magnifying glasses to read the Safe Handling Instructions printed on the side: "To prevent illness from bacteria: keep eggs refrigerated, cook eggs until yolks are firm, and cook foods containing eggs thoroughly." That warning is usually so unobtrusive that you have to search hard to find it, perhaps because egg companies would just as soon not remind you about safety problems. That the warning is there at all is because the FDA requires it. The FDA insists that producers alert you that eating eggs can make you sick—sometimes very sick—if the eggs happen to be contaminated with a particularly toxic variant of common *Salmonella* bacteria. This species of *Salmonella* turns out to be especially well adapted to chickens. Its formal name is "*Salmonella enterica* serotype Enteritidis," but it is called *Salmonella* Enteritidis for short, and is almost always referred to by its abbreviation, SE. In the United States, SE is responsible for hundreds of thousands of illnesses and a couple of hundred deaths every year.

If SE only landed on the shells of eggs, it would not be much of a problem. You could just scrub the eggs and be done with it. But SE—unlike most other bacteria—sometimes gets into the yolks. If you keep a contaminated egg at room temperature, the bacteria can use the nutrients in the egg to grow and multiply. You kill them when you cook the egg. But if you put a raw egg contaminated with SE into a Caesar salad, a cheesecake, hollandaise sauce, or, alas, cookie dough, you could be in trouble. These bacteria are capable of inducing diarrhea, fever, and cramps within the day or so after you eat them. You may recover and feel better after a few more days, but if you are very young or very old, or have a weak immune system, the infection might spread to your blood and other vital organs and kill you if you do not get medical treatment right away.

The SE problem with eggs is quite recent, and quite unexpected. I used to think of eggs as more or less sterile, and they were. Fresh eggs resist invasion by bacteria. When eggs are newly laid, their shells are covered by a "cuticle" that seals the pores. The cuticle gets scrubbed off during cleaning, however, and bacteria have no trouble getting through the open pores in a washed shell. Even so, once they penetrate the shell they encounter further barriers. To get to the yolk, they have to make their way through two interior membranes, several layers of thick and gluey egg white, and another membrane that surrounds the yolk. This does not happen easily or often and, in fact, is not how SE usually gets into eggs. Instead, SE gets into eggs through the "transovarian" route: infection of the hen's ovaries and of the egg itself as it is being formed in the oviduct. Hens with ovaries infected with SE do not themselves get sick, but once in a while—not necessarily often or always—they shed the bacteria into the egg white that surrounds the yolk. When the hen secretes the shell around the egg white, she seals the bacteria within the egg. You, however, have no way of knowing this unless the egg has first been tested.

Until the 1970s, eggs usually were safe to eat. SE used to be found only in rats and other rodents, but by the late 1960s it had jumped species and started to infect some populations of chickens. Even so, the number of SE-related cases of human sickness was so small that epidemiologists did not worry much about transovarian contamination. From 1976 to 1996, the number of cases of human illness caused by toxic *Salmonella* increased sixfold, and more than 75 percent were linked to foods containing raw or undercooked eggs. That increase has been attributed to changes in egg production linked to industrial farming: the increasing size of chicken operations, the centralization of production that pools the contents of eggs from different farms for commercial distribution (so one SE-infected egg can contaminate the entire lot), and crowded conditions that promote the ability of SE to adapt to new chicken populations. An outbreak of SE in 1994 illustrates how those changes created conditions for widespread illness.

> From 1976 to 1996, the number of cases of human illness caused by toxic *Salmonella* increased sixfold, and more than 75 percent were linked to foods containing raw or undercooked eggs.

That year, more than 200,000 people became ill from eating ice cream made from a contaminated egg mix. The mix turned out to have been trucked in a container that had previously held a "pool" of unpasteurized yolks and egg whites. It would only have taken a few eggs carrying SE to contaminate the entire truckload.

At the time of that 1994 outbreak, the chance of encountering an SE-contaminated egg was 1 in 10,000, but recent safety efforts have halved those odds to 1 in 20,000. As always, whether you think 1 in 20,000 is a remote chance or a clear and present danger depends on your point of view. The industry's Egg Nutrition Center puts its own spin on trying to keep the numbers in perspective: "273,000 people are injured each year from bathroom objects and fixtures; only 125,000 people had problems with egg-related *Salmonella* in 1998." *Only* 125,000? Here is what the American Egg Board says about this risk: "Scientists estimate that . . . only 1 of every 20,000 eggs might contain the bacteria. So, the likelihood that an egg might contain SE is extremely small—0.005% (five one-thousandths of one percent). At this rate, if you're an average consumer, you might encounter a contaminated egg once every 84 years." Maybe, but the USDA counts more than 70 billion eggs in the U.S. food supply each year. Work that out: 0.005 percent of 70 billion means that nearly

4 million eggs could be contaminated with SE. That does not mean that 4 million people will necessarily get sick, but the mere idea should serve as an incentive to cook eggs before eating them.

Indeed, the egg industry, like so many of the industries I've discussed so far, would like you to take responsibility for dealing with SE, rather than preventing *Salmonella* from getting into eggs in the first place. Its publications remind you that proper cooking and handling destroys *Salmonella*. The Egg Nutrition Center publishes handy guides in English and Spanish, which reprint the usual Safe Handling Instructions along with advice that you "Throw out cracked or dirty eggs, avoid foods that contain raw eggs, and wash dishes and countertops thoroughly." You are well advised to follow this advice carefully, but while you are doing so, shouldn't you also ask why the industry isn't taking better care to keep hens free of SE? Preventing *Salmonella* infections is really not all that difficult. Countries in Scandinavia, for example, have fewer problems with SE than we do, largely because they require safety procedures for eggs that start on the farm. These procedures are similar to our HACCP (Hazard Analysis and Critical Control Point) methods; they require egg producers to identify places where *Salmonella* contamination might occur, take steps to prevent that from happening, and monitor to make sure the procedures are followed.

> Indeed, the egg industry, like so many of the industries I've discussed so far, would like you to take responsibility for dealing with SE, rather than preventing *Salmonella* from getting into eggs in the first place.

As they are everywhere, HACCP plans are recent developments in Europe. Late in 1988, a junior health minister in Great Britain, Edwina Currie, infamous for her outspokenness (some would call it indiscretion), announced that most eggs in England were infected with *Salmonella*, a statement that caused egg sales to plummet and enraged poultry farmers who forced her resignation. Indeed, more than half the retail chickens sold in England and Wales at that time carried *Salmonella*, although "only" 15 percent were infected with the Enteritidis strain. The percentage of eggs actually infected with SE, however, undoubtedly was much lower. When it became clear that Currie was pretty much right about high rates of *Salmonella* infection in chickens, the British imposed safety rules and eggs became safer. By 1995, officials were saying that the percentage of infected eggs had dropped to less than 1 percent, and it dropped nearly tenfold to 0.1 percent by 2003.

The U.S. egg industry is dealing with a rate of contamination twenty times lower (0.005 percent), but even this level poses harm that is preventable. Until 2004, keeping eggs safe was left up to the industry to do voluntarily. That year the FDA finally stepped in and required egg producers and processors to use HACCP plans to prevent SE from getting into eggs. Arriving at this point did not come easily, however.

MAKING EGGS SAFE

If you want to understand why government oversight of food safety needs a major overhaul, eggs are a good place to begin. No less than four U.S. agencies are expected to deal with eggs, and in the confusion over who does what, SE sometimes falls between the cracks. The FDA oversees the safety of eggs in their shells ("shell eggs"), but three separate units within the USDA also are involved in the various steps that it takes to move eggs from farm to table: chick breeding (USDA), egg laying on the farm (FDA), cleaning and packaging eggs (FDA for shell eggs, USDA for egg products), transporting them (FDA and USDA for shell eggs, FDA for egg products), wholesale handling and preparation (FDA and USDA), and retail and restaurants (FDA and state health authorities).

> Controlling SE is not rocket science; all it requires is immediate refrigeration of newly laid eggs (to stop bacterial growth), sampling eggs and testing them to see if they are carrying SE, and diverting eggs that test positive out of the supply of shell eggs.

You could have a good laugh about the absurdity of this system if lives were not at stake, but SE can be lethal. And this system is not simply absurd; it does not work. SE could have been stopped in its tracks in the mid-1980s if the food safety system had been even remotely functional. Controlling SE is not rocket science; all it requires is immediate refrigeration of newly laid eggs (to stop bacterial growth), sampling eggs and testing them to see if they are carrying SE, and diverting eggs that test positive out of the supply of shell eggs. In the 1980s, SE was still confined to henhouses in the northeast and it would not have been all that difficult to require companies to do those things and keep *Salmonella* from spreading. With no such actions taken, SE spread throughout the country and more people became ill.

As cases rose in number, government agencies took steps—sometimes grudgingly—to do something about the SE situation. This history involves several government agencies, as shown in the Table on the next page.

Early in the 1990s, the USDA did some experiments to restrict the movement of eggs from flocks that tested positive for SE. In 1995, however, Congress withdrew funding for these efforts and the FDA took over responsibility for tracing and diversion. States moved into the breach. In particular, Pennsylvania, a state that produced about 6 million eggs a year in the 1990s, developed a control program that worked well and showed that SE could be reduced or eliminated.

In 1996, Rose Acre Farms, a commercial egg producer in Indiana, petitioned the USDA and the FDA to create a joint program to reduce SE. The following year, the consumer advocacy group, Center for Science in the Public Interest (CSPI), filed a much stronger petition with two demands: require the cartons of shell eggs to carry a warning label; and require egg producers to use HACCP safety plans to prevent SE infections.

The USDA and FDA did not ignore the petitions; they just did not act on them very quickly. In 1998, the two agencies filed a joint Advanced Notice of Proposed Rulemaking on SE in eggs:

The agencies want to explore all reasonable alternatives and gather data on the public benefits and the public costs of various regulatory approaches before proposing a farm-to-table food safety system for shell eggs.

Any food safety advocate reading this notice in the *Federal Register* would know immediately that nothing was going to happen soon. The regulatory system requires agencies to announce that they plan to propose rules (the "Advance Notice"), collect comments, respond to the comments, actually propose the rules, collect more comments, respond to the comments, write interim rules, collect and respond to further comments, and, eventually, publish final rules. Typically, this process takes years, and the proposed rules for controlling SE were no exception.

A Quarter-Century of Attempts to Control SE in Eggs

YEAR	KEY EVENTS
1980	About 2,000 cases of SE are reported to the Centers for Disease Control (CDC), but safety officials say cases must be multiplied by 20 to 100 to estimate the actual number of illnesses (therefore 40,000 to 200,000).
1986	CDC identifies eggs as the source of SE; reports 6,000 cases (really 120,000 to 600,000).
1987	USDA decides not to require an SE control program.
1988	CDC says SE is epidemic in eggs.
1989	FDA and USDA work on separate control programs; 9,000 cases reported (really 180,000 to 900,000).
1991	USDA starts control program for hens known to have SE; Congress passes law requiring egg refrigeration but USDA does not enforce it.
1992	USDA, Pennsylvania, and the egg industry begin voluntary control programs; these help to reduce SE.
1995	At request of egg industry, Congress cuts funding for pilot programs; 10,000 cases are reported to CDC (really 200,000 to 1,000,000); 17 states report at least a doubling of cases since 1985.
1997	Center for Science in the Public Interest petitions FDA to require Safe Handling label on egg cartons and on-farm HACCP safety rules.
1998	USDA risk assessment estimates more than 660,000 SE cases (range: 126,000 to 1.7 million) and more than 300 deaths.
1999	General Accounting Office criticizes FDA and USDA for inadequate oversight of egg safety; estimates 300,000 illnesses and 200 deaths each year. FDA and USDA require Safe Handling label on egg cartons and refrigeration during storage and transport.
2000	Egg industry lobbies to have government pay to test eggs for SE.
2004	USDA estimates 350,000 cases of SE per year; FDA says 118,000. FDA proposes safety rules for on-farm egg production and handling; says this will cost $82 million annually, but benefits will amount to $580 million.
2005	Under pressure from egg industry, FDA proposes to allow Safe Handling label to be placed on the inside lid of egg cartons as long as "keep refrigerated" appears on the top or side panel; delays implementation of on-farm safety rules.

In 1999, the General Accounting Office, which has long pressed for more effective oversight of food safety, attempted to move the interminable process along by publishing a scathing report on inadequacies in the oversight system for egg safety. The USDA and FDA responded by announcing that they would require Safe Handling labels on eggs (like those demanded in the CSPI petition), and also would require retailers, transporters, and warehouses to keep eggs well refrigerated. By this time, voluntary efforts on the part of egg producers had succeeded in reducing the number of SE-contaminated eggs by half (from 1 in 10,000 to 1 in 20,000), but thousands of illnesses were still being recorded from raw eggs in foods as diverse as tuna salad, bread pudding, lasagna, and chiles rellenos.

In September 2004, seven years after the CSPI petition and nearly six years after the "Advanced Notice," the FDA proposed farm-to-table regulations meant to eliminate SE in shell eggs. Banal as those rules might seem (one example: refrigerate eggs after buying them), they set an astonishing precedent. Marian Burros wrote in *The New York Times*: "For the first time, the federal government has proposed placing responsibility for preventing food-borne illness on farmers rather than consumers." And about time, too.

The new rules apply to producers who have more than 3,000 hens. These producers must raise hens from SE-free chicks, prevent SE from getting into poultry houses, take precautions to prevent SE transmission, control pests and rodents, test for SE, clean and disinfect poultry houses that test positive, divert eggs from SE-positive flocks, refrigerate eggs, and keep records. When a reporter from *Food Chemical News* asked if the FDA would institute some kind of certification seal for eggs that had been tested and found free of SE, an FDA spokesman said: "FDA is here to make sure there is no SE contamination, not to promote a particular product, and a seal is typically a promotion." Egg associations claimed that their members were already taking many of these precautions and assured the reporter that the "chance of encountering an egg contaminated with [SE] remains very small. The possibility of becoming ill from SE can be eliminated with proper storage and cooking." How the rules will play out in practice remains to be seen. In 2005, egg producers convinced the FDA to allow them to remove the Safe Handling warning from the outside of the carton and hide it under the lid.

People like me who care deeply about how foods taste will assure you that a fresh egg from a farm-raised hen is something quite extraordinary, and that no commercial egg comes anywhere close to its taste. If you ever have a chance to buy farm-fresh eggs, do not pass up that opportunity. But most of us buy our eggs in supermarkets where "fresh" is a relative concept. Beyond questions of freshness, it is worth asking whether the more expensive, nutritionally enhanced, more humanely produced eggs taste better. I personally cannot tell the difference but you will have to do some experimenting and decide for yourself.

From a nutritional standpoint, eggs are eggs. Turning eggs into a "designer" food is a great way to get you to pay more for them but there are less expensive and easier ways to get vitamin E, selenium, lutein, and omega-3s from foods. If you do not give a hoot about how the eggs are produced, buy the cheapest ones you can find. The shell color makes no nutritional difference.

If you do care enough about how the hens are treated to pay more for eggs, buy Certified Humane (but *not* United Egg Producers Certified). If you also care about what the hens are fed, or just want to cast your food vote for the organic movement, buy eggs that are Certified Organic. Whatever eggs you decide to buy, don't eat too many of them — or buy the smallest size. Small eggs still have a lot of cholesterol, but less than the extra-large and jumbo sizes.

A final question: What about egg substitutes? These may work for you if you are trying to avoid cholesterol, but they do not really replace the taste or texture of real eggs. If you are satisfied with egg whites, you can buy cartons of them already separated from the yolks; these are handy for making meringues and white omelets. You also can buy any number of other egg substitutes based on pasteurized egg whites. Some have endorsements from the American Heart Association as heart-healthy products. With the yolks separated away, the whites have no fat or

> W hatever eggs you decide to buy, don't eat too many of them—or buy the smallest size. Small eggs still have a lot of cholesterol, but less than the extra-large and jumbo sizes.

cholesterol, so these products come as advertised: fat free, cholesterol free, and, of course, carbohydrate free. Most egg substitutes add stabilizers and thickeners, vitamins to replace those lost from the yolks, carotenes so they are yellow, and, sometimes, spices. If you like the way they taste, they are a reasonable alternative to real eggs. A pound, a bit less than the weight of a dozen small eggs, costs twice as much as real eggs. Overall, if you love eggs but need to keep your blood cholesterol under control, you can eat one egg every day or so, but be sure to get most of the rest of your calories from fruits, vegetables, and grains—all cholesterol free. And until egg producers start following those HACCP regulations to the letter, you might want to play it safe and make sure that eggs are cooked before you eat them.

23

Frozen Foods: Decoding
Ingredient Lists

I f the freezer space in your local supermarket seems to be taking over the store, it probably is. Frozen foods are an industry unto themselves, which like all others is represented by trade and lobbying associations that work hard to promote sales in a consumer environment that values fresh foods. Still, this is a hefty little industry with sales of nearly $30 billion in 2005, an amount that is 20 percent higher than in 1998, and a huge advance over the $1 billion mark first reached in the 1950s. This industry began with Birds Eye frozen vegetables in the 1930s. As refrigerators and freezers moved into mass markets, production of frozen foods expanded to include such things as pastries, meats, fish, sauces, juices, and prepared meals. Today, say the trade associations, "The frozen food industry is limited only by its imagination" and, presumably, by supermarket freezer capacity.

At a P&C Market in Ithaca, small by suburban standards, I measured out the length of the freezer space. In open freezers, I counted sixty feet of prepared meals, thirty of pizzas, twenty of frozen potatoes, but just six of frozen juices (concentrated juice containers are small, after all) and four of frozen vegetables. Ice creams took up another thirty feet of glass-fronted closed cases, each with multiple shelves. This is an impressive amount of supermarket real estate for display cases that must cost a fortune to keep cold, but the space allotment almost exactly parallels sales. Prepared meals and pizzas are the big sellers.

Researchers who work for the frozen food industry have looked into the hearts and minds of supermarket shoppers. Their profound insight: you want hot food on the table no more than five minutes after you begin preparing it, and never more than twenty. Frozen food companies dream up all kinds of prepared meals to grant this wish, and Americans spent close to $7 billion on them in 2004: for example, $1.2 billion for frozen Italian dinners, $508 million for frozen Mexican dinners, and nearly $300 million for frozen pot pies. Ice cream and frozen novelties (popsicles and the like) brought in another $7 billion or so. On a smaller scale, the industry even sold $64 million worth of frozen bagels and $3 million of frozen cookie dough.

That P&C store in Ithaca may have had frozen fruit, but I couldn't find it, probably because I forgot to look for it in the ice-cream freezers. In comparison to frozen meals and frozen desserts, this industry does not sell much frozen fruit (a mere $300 million in 2004) and what it does sell is mostly used as a topping for ice cream. Frozen vegetables, however, bring in $3 billion—about 10 percent of total sales.

I have a soft spot in my nutritionist's heart for frozen fruits and vegetables. They are vastly underrated. At best, they are picked at peak ripeness, flash frozen, and more or less ready to eat whenever you want them. You may have to perform some cooking tricks to compensate for the way freezing changes the texture of a fruit or vegetable. But in the dead of winter I much prefer frozen vegetables to the sad "fresh" ones that limp into Manhattan supermarkets in those cold, dark months, and frozen blueberries always taste better than the ones that pass for fresh in November and are imported from Patagonia.

R esearchers who work for the frozen food industry have looked into the hearts and minds of supermarket shoppers. Their profound insight: you want hot food on the table no more than five minutes after you begin preparing it, and never more than twenty.

What is most reassuring about frozen fruits and vegetables, even as compared with fresh ones, is that you know exactly what you are getting: their ingredients are listed on the packages. By law, the ingredients of packaged foods must be listed in order by weight; the one present in greatest amount is listed first. I admire the ingredient list on frozen corn: "Ingredient: corn." The one for frozen orange juice says, "Ingredient: 100% pure frozen concentrated orange juice." For frozen fruits and vegetables with single ingredients, what you see is what you get.

> For frozen fruits and vegetables with single ingredients, what you see is what you get.

Even better, freezing has practically no effect on the nutritional value of fresh produce. It does not change the number of calories, or the amounts of protein, fat, carbohydrate, fiber, or minerals (calcium and iron, for example). It does reduce the amounts of some vitamins, but not by much. Vitamin C is the most fragile of the nutrients and the one most likely to show losses, but even this one survives pretty well if the freezing is done quickly, the package is not thawed and refrozen before you use it, and you eat the food before its "use-by" date.

FROZEN JUICE

As a general rule, the more that happens to a fruit or vegetable between the time it is harvested and the time you eat it, the more nutrients it is likely to lose. Orange juice is a good example. Do not think for a minute that frozen orange juice is simply squeezed and then frozen. The companies that produce those little cartons extract the juice, pasteurize (flash heat) it, dehydrate it to remove most of the water, and freeze what is left—the concentrate. When you open the carton, you thaw the concentrate, add water, and stir. What happens to the nutritional value of orange juice when you do all that is shown on the facing page.

> Overall, whole fruits are a better nutritional bet than juices, and fresh juices are better than frozen. When you see a juice labeled "pulp free," look for another option.

Orange juice made from concentrate has somewhat less vitamin C than "fresh squeezed" (which, unless squeezed in front of you, usually means treated with pasteurization but not much else), but a standard 8-ounce serving easily takes care of the daily requirement for this vitamin and provides ample amounts of others. The nutritional problem with juice of any kind is that it is extracted from the fruit pulp, which contains most of the fiber and the minerals (calcium, for example) and vitamins (like beta-carotene) that go with it. Overall, whole fruits are a better nutritional bet than juices, and fresh juices are better than frozen. When you see a juice labeled "pulp free," look for another option.

The Nutrients in Fresh Oranges, Fresh Juice, and Juice Made from Concentrate

NUTRIENT	A FRESH ORANGE (1 SMALL)	FRESH ORANGE JUICE (ONE-THIRD CUP)*	ORANGE JUICE FROM CONCENTRATE (ONE-THIRD CUP)
Calories	45	45	45
Vitamin C (milligrams)	51	50	39
Fiber (grams)	2	0.3	0.3
Calcium (milligrams)	40	11	9
Beta-carotene (micrograms)	70	33	17

*One-third cup is just under 3 ounces, but a standard serving size for orange juice is 8 ounces, so the calories and nutrients would be nearly three times higher in a glass that size.

FROZEN PREPARED FOODS

Frozen juices may have excellent nutritional value and a blessedly short ingredient list, but most frozen foods are more complicated. I can understand the appeal of frozen waffles—they are quick to heat up and you do not have a messy bowl and waffle iron to clean afterward. But I am baffled by frozen toast labeled as "ready to eat in 5 minutes." Isn't toast always ready to eat in a minute or two? I also am missing the point of a frozen omelet that "tastes like homemade." Why not just make an omelet yourself then?

Of course an omelet requires a stove, a pan, some butter or oil so it won't stick, and an egg or two (and, perhaps, a dash of pepper, chives, or cheese), and you may not have such things on hand. And yes it is easy to heat up a frozen meal in a microwave. And yes you cannot always get Italian or Mexican food when you want it. But the ingredients in these supposedly homemade-tasting frozen meals stop me cold. Here, for example, is ConAgra's Banquet frozen macaroni-and-cheese meal ("macaroni and rich cheddar cheese sauce"). Take a look at its astonishing but entirely typical contents—just as the package lists them.

INGREDIENTS: COOKED MACARONI (WATER, DURUM SEMOLINA [ENRICHED WITH NIACIN, FERROUS SULFATE, THIAMIN MONONITRATE, RIBOFLAVIN, FOLIC ACID], EGG WHITE SOLIDS), WATER, CHEDDAR CHEESE (PASTEURIZED CULTURED MILK, SALT, ENZYMES, ANNATTO ADDED IF COLORED), DRIED WHEY, CONTAINS LESS THAN 2% OF THE FOLLOWING: DRIED SWEET CREAM (SWEET CREAM, NONFAT MILK, SODIUM CASEINATE), MODIFIED CORN STARCH, WHEAT FLOUR, CHEDDAR CHEESE BLEND (CHEDDAR CHEESE [MILK, CHEESE CULTURE, SALT, ENZYMES, ANNATTO], CREAM, SALT, SODIUM PHOSPHATE, LACTIC ACID, FD&C YELLOW NO. 5 AND NO. 6), BUTTER (SWEET CREAM, SALT), PARTIALLY HYDROGENATED OR LIQUID SOYBEAN OIL, SALT, DISODIUM PHOSPHATE, SOYBEAN OIL, MONODIGLYCERIDES WITH DATEM, CITRIC ACID, BETA CAROTENE (CORN OIL, BETA CAROTENE).
CONTAINS: WHEAT, EGGS, MILK, SOY.

Reading this list is a formidable undertaking, and not just because so many of these ingredients are chemical compounds and not recognizable as food. The brackets inside of parentheses remind me of high-school algebra tests, and the all-capital letters do not make for easy reading. I cannot help but suspect that ConAgra would prefer that you not look at this list or, heaven forbid, think about it. If you do decide to tackle it, you will see that the first three ingredients are macaroni (vitamin-enriched), water, and cheddar cheese. This gives some hope that lurking somewhere in this package is a real food. Maybe, but the remaining ingredients belong on the first floor of a department store. They are cosmetics—dyes to make this product look like real food (FD&C colors, beta-carotene, and annatto); milk additives, soy oils, and thickeners to make it feel like cheese; and emulsifiers and stabilizers to hold the whole thing together (the mysterious "Datem" is an acronym for a particular form of monoglyceride emulsifier). All of this obfuscation is perfectly legal and meets the FDA's labeling requirements to the letter. Manufacturers simply must tell you what is in their products. It is up to you to figure out whether you want to eat products containing such things or whether the ingredients are good for you.

In contrast, the "Contains" list in bold-face type is perfectly clear. By congressional directive, it warns you that this product contains ingredients from foods to which you might be allergic. Since 2004, Congress has insisted that the FDA require food producers to say whether any ingredient in a packaged food comes from any of the eight most common foods that cause allergic reactions: milk, eggs, fish, shellfish, tree nuts, peanuts, wheat, and soybeans. If you are unlucky enough to be allergic to any of those foods, you know how frightening—and life threatening— it can be to be confronted with a product with multiple ingredients and not know what is in it. These lists should help, particularly because Congress required the foods to be listed in plain English. The "Contains" list must specify "milk"—not casein, whey, lactoglobulin, or other euphemisms that turn up in ingredients lists. The list must say "eggs" instead of ovalbumin, mayonnaise, or lysozyme. If you would like food manufacturers to explain more about the chemical ingredients listed on food labels, take up this matter with your congressional representatives. Congress tells the FDA what to do.

Back to the macaroni and cheese: I followed the instructions for microwaving as best I could. This produced a meal that looked exactly like the food on the box top, but tasted nothing like macaroni and cheese as I know it. The macaroni was mushy and the predominant taste was salt.

> If you would like food manufacturers to explain more about the chemical ingredients listed on food labels, take up this matter with your congressional representatives. Congress tells the FDA what to do.

No surprise. If I counted right, sodium or salt (which is sodium chloride) turn up *seven* times on the ingredients list. I checked the Nutrition Facts label. This product contains 1,500 milligrams of sodium, which converts to nearly 4 grams of salt (salt·is 40 percent sodium), meaning that the package provides nearly two-thirds of the maximum I am supposed to have in a day. It also has nearly half the upper limit recommended for saturated fat. Late in 2004, this box did not list *trans* fats from the hydrogenated oil, though it would have to starting in 2006. But: I only paid $1.25 for this meal and it provided 420 calories. Products like these trade cheap calories and convenience for taste and health.

One other box of frozen food caught my eye—a six-pack of Pillsbury Toaster Strudel pastries labeled in bright letters "Made with REAL apples." Really? What else would strudel have? One clue came from a less conspicuous statement: "Real Fruit & Artificial Apple Flavor." If you can stand looking at one more frozen-food ingredient list, try this.

INGREDIENTS: BLEACHED ENRICHED FLOUR (WHEAT FLOUR, MALTED BARLEY FLOUR, NIACIN, FERROUS SULFATE, THIAMIN MONONITRATE, RIBOFLAVIN, FOLIC ACID), WATER, PARTIALLY HYDROGENATED SOYBEAN AND COTTONSEED OIL, HIGH FRUCTOSE CORN SYRUP, CORN SYRUP, CORN STARCH, MODIFIED CORN STARCH, APPLE PUREE (10% OF FILLING), DRY YEAST, SALT, DEXTROSE, WHEY, MILK PROTEIN, EGG YOLK, BAKING POWDER (BAKING SODA, SODIUM ACID PYROPHOSPHATE), CORN SYRUP SOLIDS, YELLOW 5, RED 40 AND OTHER COLOR ADDED, CITRIC ACID, CINNAMON, SODIUM CITRATE, MONO AND DIGLYCERIDES, POTASSIUM SORBATE AND SODIUM BENZOATE (PRESERVATIVES), XANTHAN GUM, NATURAL & ARTIFICIAL FLAVOR, LOCUST BEAN GUM, GUAR GUM, POLYSORBATE 60.
CONTAINS: WHEAT, MILK AND EGG INGREDIENTS.

If you like playing the Where's Waldo game for children, think of this game as Where's the Fruit. The first eight ingredients are flour, water, two kinds of hydrogenated oils (those pesky *trans* fats again), sugars, and starches. Then: eureka! The ninth ingredient is apple puree. This may make up only 10 percent of the filling, but the package label did not tell a lie: apple puree is made from real apples. Everything else is a concoction of starch, sugar, oil, and food additives disguised as apple strudel. If you are an adult, the choice is yours: you can read the label and decide to buy and eat this product, but this "strudel" is clearly meant for children. The box top is illustrated with a cartoon shark from *Shark Tale*, a DreamWorks movie for kids, and with an advertisement for a free *Shark Tale* watch for two box tops and $1.25. Turn the box over, fill out the coupon for the watch, and "Wrap this 'round your fin and you'll be chief of the reef." Unless you examine the ingredient list very closely, you might think you are giving your kids something good for them. But this product has little redeeming nutritional value beyond calories (190 per pastry) and the few nutrients added in fortification. Its main attraction is that it is fast and cheap. Some frozen foods are better than others. If you want healthier frozen foods, look for packages with short ingredient lists.

The bewildering ingredient lists on frozen food packages are only the beginning of what can be learned from decoding their labels. Food packages also have Nutrition Facts labels. These require a separate discussion and a digression into the meaning of calories, the topic to which we now turn.

> **If you want healthier frozen foods, look for packages with short ingredient lists.**

24

A Digression into Calories and Diets

T he FDA requires the labels of frozen foods to list ingredients; these lists provide clues to the nutritional quality of the products. Before tackling the other part of the food label—the Nutrition Facts—a digression into calories seems much in order. Because the calories in foods influence body weight, because being overweight is a problem for so many people, and because dieting is so much a part of modern American life, calories matter. Packaged foods list calories, but fresh foods do not come with Nutrition Facts labels. Restaurant meals also do not disclose calories, although fast-food places (the ones that make everything the same way and in the same size) sometimes have brochures or Internet sites that provide nutrition information.

Calories require special discussion because they are invisible; you cannot see, taste, or smell them. So the only way to get a feel for them is to deal with numbers and to do some counting. To get started on the numbers, let's leave the supermarket for a moment and take a detour into the realm of popular diets, beginning with the low-carbohydrate diets so successfully promoted by the late Dr. Robert Atkins.

In the summer of 2003, when the low-carbohydrate diet craze was nearing its peak (but nobody knew that yet), I attended a meeting in Aspen, Colorado, sponsored by *Fortune* magazine. At dinner one night, I was seated next to a healthy-looking and only slightly overweight business executive whose table behavior reminded me of my kids during the worst of their picky eating phases. Normally, I go "off duty" at dinner parties and just try to enjoy my food, but he made sure I noticed his eating habits. He pushed away anything on his plate that might be "contaminated," not with peas as my kids did but with carbohydrates. He carefully set aside anything that might contain the forbidden starches or sugars, not only the rolls and potatoes but also the especially delicious grilled carrots and beets. Only then did he dig into the buttered filet mignon. Just my luck, I thought, another Atkins dieter. In a minute he will be telling me how much weight he has lost eating this way. Sure enough. Pleased as could be, he said he had just lost eleven pounds in two weeks on the Atkins diet.

Off duty as I was trying to be, I did not point out that his vegetables had only tiny amounts of sugars, too little carbohydrate to make any difference. I also did not point out that there was no way he could have lost that weight as body fat. If the weight loss came from anything but water, it had to be because he was eating fewer calories than usual, and not because he was eating less carbohydrate. If low-carbohydrate diets (or any other kind) work, it is because they help you to reduce the number of calories you eat. When it comes to weight loss, it's the calories that count.

But calories are so hard to understand that I've come to think of them as the "C word." Nobody wants to talk about them. Diet gurus would much rather have you think that what you eat

> If low-carbohydrate diets (or any other kind) work, it is because they help you to reduce the number of calories you eat. When it comes to weight loss, it's the calories that count.

matters more than how much you eat; they never mention calories unless they have to. Calories are too intangible, are much too abstract, and require too many numbers to explain easily, a problem made even more difficult by confusing names and definitions. What follows is what I find most useful for understanding the calories on food labels and in diet plans.

WHAT ARE CALORIES?

Calories are a measure of the energy value of food. In this, they are something like temperature (which measures the energy stored in air, water, or food as heat). Just as you use degrees Fahrenheit or Centigrade/Celsius to tell you whether it is hot or cold outside, you can use calories to tell you how much of a food you should be eating. But unlike temperature, you have no easy way of measuring calories in food. Short of doing elaborate laboratory tricks, the best way to tell if you are getting the right number of calories is by weighing yourself on a scale. If your weight stays about the same over time, you know that you are eating enough calories to balance your body's need for them. The energy you use to go about your daily activities also is measured in calories. It helps to have a good feel for both kinds—the calories you eat and those you expend.

To begin with, all foods—except water and beverages flavored with artificial sweeteners—come with calories. Any food that contains carbohydrates, proteins, and fats has calories because those parts of food store energy. Calories measure the amount of that energy. Carbohydrates and proteins store the least amount of energy: both yield about 4 calories per gram. Food fats have more than twice as much: 9 calories per gram. That is one reason why fat is considered fattening; its calories are more concentrated than those of either protein or carbohydrate.

> The body stores excess calories—no matter where they come from—as body fat.

But carbohydrates and proteins also can be fattening if you eat too much of them. The body stores excess calories—no matter where they come from—as body fat.

This is a good place to note that alcohol also is a source of calories. Alcohol has more calories than either carbohydrate or protein, 7 per gram, but the body deals with them in a somewhat different way than it does with the calories from food. Drink too much alcohol and its calories may be used to make fat in your liver—a beer belly. But let's ignore alcohol for now and just stick with the calories in foods, diets, and bodies.

From what I know about the way calories work, I was almost certain that my Aspen dinner companion had not lost much weight as body fat. I guessed this from knowing two numbers:

- *2,000 to 3,000 calories a day*: the range of calories that maintains body weight in most people (you need more calories if you are bigger or more active, and fewer if you are small or more sedentary)
- *3,500 calories per pound*: the number of calories in one pound of body fat

From this information, I knew that to lose 11 pounds, my dinner companion would have had to eat 11 times 3,500 *fewer* calories than the amount he needs to maintain his usual body weight. On average, distributed over 14 days, this deficit would amount to 2,750 calories per day. This means that he would have had to eat 2,750 fewer calories than he usually eats—every day for two weeks—to achieve that 11-pound weight loss. But if he typically needs 2,750 calories a day (a quite plausible number), the only way he could lose 11 pounds of body fat would be to enter into a total fast—consume absolutely nothing except water—during those two weeks. Yet there he was at this dinner, enjoying his Atkins-allowed, high-fat, high-calorie meat, butter, and, when the dessert came, whipped cream (but not the forbidden fresh, sweet raspberries that came with it). Even if avoiding carbohydrates helped him cut calories below his usual intake, most of the lost 11 pounds had to be nothing more than the water that typically pours off the body on low-carbohydrate diets.

Happily, this early loss of water helps. It made my dinner companion feel that his efforts were succeeding and encouraged him to continue dieting. And he would need plenty of encouragement to stay on that diet during the next few weeks when the excess water is gone and the rate of weight loss slows down. It takes hard work to eat less. In contrast, the science of dieting is easy. Diets are about calories. Eat too many, and weight goes up. To lose weight, you have to eat fewer calories than your body needs ("eat less"), use up more calories than usual by increasing your physical activity ("move more"), or, even better, do both. If a diet plan helps you lose weight, it is because it helps you to eat fewer calories.

THE NAME CONFUSION

I have no polite way of saying this: calories are a mess to explain, beginning with what to call them. The term that everybody uses to describe the energy content of food—calories (spelled with a small "c")—is just plain wrong. Only chemists use calories with a small "c." Nutritionists and other scientists use kilocalories (meaning 1,000 calories) or its equivalent, Calories, spelled with a capital "C." So three words are involved:

- calories (abbreviated cal and spelled with a small "c"): the chemists' term
- Calories (abbreviated Cal and spelled with a capital "C"): the nutritionists' term for 1,000 small "c" calories
- kilocalories (abbreviated kcal, sometimes spelled with either a small "k" or capital "K"): the scientific term for 1,000 small "c" calories

Nutrition Facts labels use Calories and calories interchangeably but both mean kilocalories. A kilocalorie/Calorie is 1,000 calories. But in the United States, everyone except chemists uses Kilocalories, kilocalories, Calories, calories, Kcal, kcal, Cal, and cal to mean exactly the same thing—kilocalories. So the term "calories" is ambiguous; it means two things at once: a measurement of energy, and another measurement that is 1,000 times greater. But in practice, the chemist's small "c" calorie is never used to describe the energy in food (if it did, 200 calories on a Nutrition Facts label would have to say 200,000). The energy in food is always measured in kilocalories, so calling them calories (small "c") is just plain wrong. But everybody else does it and you might as well too.

> The energy in food is always measured in kilocalories, so calling them calories (small "c") is just plain wrong. But everybody else does it and you might as well too.

I hope you get that because there is even more to the name confusion. If you travel to other countries, you will find that many of them label the energy content of food products using an entirely different term: "kilojoules" (pronounced kill-o-djool, abbreviated kJ). One of our interchangeable calories/Calories/kilocalories equals about 4 kilojoules (the precise figure is 4.18). Coping with kilojoules is easy; to get calories, just divide by 4. The result will be close enough. In Barcelona, a can of Atún Claro (tuna in vegetable oil) lists a *valor energético* of 829 kJ/198 kcal (if you divide 829 by 4 you get 207 calories, which is not all that far from 198). In London, a package of Sainsbury's Tomato Pasta Sauce lists 601 kJ/144 kcal (divide 601 by 4 and you get 150 calories, a close estimate of 144). Food labels in New Zealand, however, list only kilojoules. A 15-gram packet of Veggie Crisps ("light puffed crisps made from natural Cassava") provides 227 kJ, meaning about 55 calories (57 actually) in a half-ounce serving. Confronted with kilojoules, I just divide by 4 to get calories and do not worry about the few calories that get lost in translation.

Like the hopelessly inconsistent names, the scientific definition of calories is at once ridiculously precise and thoroughly unhelpful. If you had the chance to see Morgan Spurlock's film *Super Size Me* (my thrilling screen debut, brief as it was), you know that Spurlock's crew could not find anyone to interview who had the slightest idea what a calorie might be. So there I am rolling my eyes and attempting to define a calorie for the camera crew. I said something like this:

> A calorie is a measure of the energy content of food. One calorie—the kind you usually see on food labels—is the amount of energy needed to raise the temperature of a liter of water by one degree Centigrade [Even so, I left out the rest of the definition. It continues: . . . from $14.5°$ to $15.5°$ Centigrade (Celsius), at one unit of atmospheric pressure].

This requires more translation but is well worth the trouble, especially because I received many unsolicited complaints from people who did not hear "the kind used on food labels," and thought I was talking about chemists' small "c" calories. Just as a kilocalorie is 1,000 small "c" calories, a liter is 1,000 milliliters. My critics thought I should have said "a calorie is the energy needed to raise the temperature of a gram (which weighs the same as a milliliter) of water by one degree," an amount 1,000 times smaller.

To translate the definition and get to the part that is fun and useful, you can forget about how hot it is outside (the temperature) and where you are in relation to sea level (the atmospheric pressure); these matter only to researchers. Next, you can make the quite reasonable assumption that a liter of water (metric measure) is about the same as a quart (U.S. measure). This is acceptable because they are quite close: a liter equals 1.06 quarts. With that out of the way, the definition begins to make sense: a calorie (kilocalorie) is the amount of heat needed to raise the temperature of a quart of water by $1°$ C.

One more round of numbers and we get to the reason why it is worth going through all this: water boils at 212° Fahrenheit (F), which, in the metric system, is 100° Celsius (C). Now you can see how this works: 100 calories (kilocalories)—the energy content of a medium apple or two regular Oreo cookies—is enough to bring an entire quart of water to a boil! Why the exclamation point? If, like most people, your typical daily intake is between 2,000 and 3,000 calories, the energy you get from food is enough to boil 20 to 30 quarts of water over the course of a day. To put this more concretely: if you eat a frozen dinner worth 600 calories, you will be getting enough energy to boil 6 quarts of water—the entire volume of blood in the human body.

> If, like most people, your typical daily intake is between 2,000 and 3,000 calories, the energy you get from food is enough to boil 20 to 30 quarts of water over the course of a day.

So how come eating dinner does not make your blood boil? The short answer: digestion and metabolism tap off all that energy in extremely small amounts. Most of the energy gets used to power your body functions (thinking, breathing, heart-pumping, digesting, working, playing), but some gets released as heat. The heat keeps your body warm, but not so warm that you cook.

THE MEASUREMENT CONFUSION

Next question: How do food manufacturers know the number of calories in the foods they produce? Answer: not easily. In your body and in those of the plants and animals you eat, calories are governed by the laws of thermodynamics—the branch of science that deals with heat and the transfer of one form of energy to another (food calories into muscle action, for example). Thermodynamics tells you that the amount of heat released from a food when it is completely burned outside the body is exactly the same as the energy released ("burned") inside the body when that food is digested, absorbed, and metabolized. This means that scientists can completely burn foods or parts of foods and measure the heat they release; this heat will be roughly equivalent to the number of calories the food produces in your body. Experimentally, they do this using a gadget invented in the 1800s—a bomb calorimeter, which is a sealed combustion chamber surrounded by water. They burn the food to ash in the chamber and measure the increase in temperature of the surrounding water as calories.

By 1899, scientists had figured out that only four components of food—carbohydrates, proteins, fats, and alcohol—produce energy in the body. Vitamins and minerals in foods do not have calories, and neither does cholesterol. Important as these substances are for other reasons, they are not metabolized by the body in ways that produce energy.

But scientists working for food companies across the world are not madly burning their products in bomb calorimeters to produce numbers to put on food labels. In a bomb calorimeter, the calorie values would be artificially high. Foods are completely burned to ash in the calorimeter, but in the body they are often incompletely digested, absorbed, or metabolized. Some components of the fiber in food plants do not get digested, are not absorbed into the body, and are not converted to energy; they do not have calories that "count." The nitrogen parts of protein molecules also are not used for energy and are excreted in urine; those parts also do not count. The numbers used on food labels compensate for those losses.

To get a feel for what food calories mean, it helps to know that a gram is a relatively small unit of measure. A teaspoon holds about 5 grams, and a tablespoon holds 3 teaspoons, or 15 grams. To repeat:

- carbohydrate has 4 calories per gram (20 calories per teaspoon)
- protein has 4 calories per gram (20 calories per teaspoon)
- fat has 9 calories per gram (45 calories per teaspoon)

At 9 calories per gram, a teaspoon of olive oil—5 grams—should contain about 45 calories, as compared to 20 calories in the teaspoon of sugar you might put in your coffee (actually, both are a bit less because they contain some water, which has no calories). Fats do not sound so caloric when measured in teaspoons, but nobody eats fat in teaspoons; we use tablespoons, which are three times as large. As food labels tell you, one tablespoon of olive oil or any other vegetable oil has 120 calories. Although fats are always rich in calories, not all fats are equally rich. Butter has fewer calories than olive oil—about 100 calories per tablespoon—because it incorporates more water. Olive oil may be one of the healthier fat choices because it is relatively high in monounsaturated fatty acids, but it is not low in calories.

THE BODY-FAT CONFUSION

So what do all these numbers have to do with body weight? Once more: a pound of body fat has about 3,500 calories, and 1 gram of fat has 9 calories. And one last number: a pound is equal to 454 grams. Multiplying 454 grams by 9 calories per gram gives you more than 4,000 calories (4,086 to be precise)—not 3,500. Why the difference? Body fat is a living tissue that contains blood and other fluids as part of its structure; these dilute its energy value. If you make the quite reasonable assumption that about 85 percent of body fat is actually fat, then a pound of fat contains 3,500 calories or so. This is a handy number. If you are watching your weight, it divides neatly into seven parts: 500 calories for each day of the week. To lose one pound of body fat a week, you have to take in 500 fewer calories per day (or increase your activity levels so your body uses 500 more calories than usual).

> To lose one pound of body fat a week, you have to take in 500 fewer calories per day (or increase your activity levels so your body uses 500 more calories than usual).

Knowing all this, I was pretty sure that my Aspen dinner companion had not lost much real weight—that is, weight as body fat. The foods he was eating had plenty of calories, although perhaps not as many as he typically ate before he went on the diet. Most of the 11-pound loss must have come from the change in water balance that occurs during the early stages of diets that restrict carbohydrates. If you are not eating new carbohydrates, the old ones stored in your liver and muscles break down and the water that is packed in with them is released and excreted in urine. Low-carbohydrate diets also cause the kidneys to excrete salts and other molecules out of the body, and it takes water to do this. That is why anyone eating a low-carbohydrate diet can drop close to a pound a day for at least the first few days.

Even so, the relationship of calories to pounds means that genuine weight loss is inevitably a long and slow process. One pound of real weight (meaning body fat) lost in a week means 500 fewer calories a day, the amount in a small piece of steak, a 16-ounce Starbucks Frappuccino, or 4 tablespoons of olive oil. If you eliminate one of these from your daily diet, it is all too easy to eat 500 calories from something else. This is why anyone who is dieting needs courage and support. I wished my dinner companion the best of success with his diet, while I thoroughly enjoyed eating the vegetables with my dinner and the fruit with my dessert.

THE COUNTING CONFUSION

Without a bomb calorimeter or a laboratory of your own in which to perform analytical chemistry, you can only guess the number of calories lurking in your food. By law, processed foods must give you that information in Nutrition Facts labels, but if you eat fresh foods or prepared foods, you will need to use calorie figures given in tables of food composition. If you eat in a fast-food place, you can ask for nutrition information; most of the time, they have it there or on a Web site. But if you eat in a restaurant, your calories depend on what you order and are at the mercy of the cook.

To know how many calories you are eating from foods that do not have Nutrition Facts labels, you need to know three things:

1. The identity and amount of every food and ingredient that went into your meal

2. The precise amount of each food and ingredient that you ate

3. The calories in a standard weight of every food and ingredient in that meal

With respect to the first two requirements, unless you weigh every food and ingredient that you eat, the best you can do is to make educated guesses. The third requires you to use food composition tables developed by one or another laboratory; these report the calorie content of thousands of foods by weight (in grams or ounces).

Food composition tables are available from many sources, but I like to use the ones issued by the U.S. Department of Agriculture (USDA). I like using them for two reasons: the tables are readily available on the Internet, and I know that the scientists who staff the USDA's Nutrient Data Laboratory are exceptionally thoughtful about the problems they must solve in order to produce reliable information. To develop calorie tables, they have to make endless decisions about which foods to sample (from where? how grown? how prepared?), the number of samples needed, and how the samples must be preserved before and during the testing—all in addition to making sure that the tests are done properly.

USDA food composition tables deal with such issues explicitly. Here, for example, is the way they report the calories for one kind of lamb chop: "Lamb, Australian, imported, fresh, leg, sirloin chops, boneless, separable lean and fat, trimmed to 1 inch fat, cooked, broiled." A 100-gram quantity of this option (a bit more than 3 ounces) has 235 calories. How close is 235 calories to the calories actually present in a lamb chop you might prepare yourself or eat in a restaurant? Without a scale or a recipe, you have to guess based on what you think the chop weighs and how it was prepared.

INTERPRETING CALORIE TABLES

Because your caloric intake depends not only on what you eat but also on how much you eat, it is best not to take the calorie numbers in food composition tables too literally. They can never be precise. That not all the calories in fiber count is enough of a reason why laboratories no longer use bomb calorimeters. Instead, they do calculations. Figuring out the calories in peas or whole wheat crackers, for example, requires USDA scientists to measure the amounts of water, minerals, protein, and fat in these foods. To get carbohydrate ("by difference"), they subtract the measured weights from the total weight of the foods. What's left is carbohydrate. Finally, they multiply the grams of carbohydrate, protein, and fat by their standard conversion values (4, 4, and 9 calories per gram, respectively), and add up the calories to get the total calories.

Any process involving so many steps provides a great many opportunities for error, which is why stating energy to the nearest calorie seems silly to me. The numbers cannot possibly be all that precise. Five or ten calories can hardly make a difference in the body. It makes sense to round off the numbers. I saved a recipe for marzipan–pine nut cookies from the spring 2004 issue of *Eating Well*, one that says each cookie contains 113 calories. It may, but only if you follow the recipe to the letter and weigh every ingredient. The recipe calls for tiny cookies made from a teaspoon of dough rolled in pine nuts. Use a bigger spoon or add more nuts and the calories go up. When baked, the cookies are crunchy and delicious. Could anyone eat just one? Not me. Eat two and you double the calories. Eat five and you have taken in one-fourth of your 2,000 or so calories for the day.

INTERPRETING RESTAURANT CALORIES

Fast-food chain restaurants usually have worked out the nutrition information about the items they serve and will give it to you if you ask for it (or refer you to their Web site). They can do this because they prepare their items the same way in every outlet, every day. McDonald's, for example, publishes a brochure, puts nutrition information on the back of its tray liners, and lists ingredients on its Web site for every food it serves. If you look at the charts, you can see instantly that larger portions have more calories.

But regular restaurants change menus frequently, buy foods from different purveyors, and encourage the chefs to cook by "feel" rather than using precise recipes and amounts. It would be impossible for them to provide accurate nutrition information and I think it is unreasonable to expect them to. This, however, makes restaurant calories a challenge. Restaurant meals are invariably higher in calories than you might expect, in part because they contain more fat from cooking oils, butter, and cheese, but also because of the huge serving sizes. If you are worried about restaurant calories, you need to order carefully, and—the key to controlling calories—watch the portion size.

With that said, we end the detour and return to the supermarket. When it comes to packaged foods in supermarkets, calories should be a no-brainer. By law, they have to be listed on the Nutrition Facts labels. But calories are listed per serving, and that can be a problem. The serving sizes listed on package labels are also regulated, but the regulations leave much room for manipulation. From a marketing standpoint, the object of the game is to keep the label serving sizes—and, therefore, the calories—as small as possible within the letter of the law. That is why a bag of my favorite barbecued potato chips lists calories as 150 for a 1-ounce serving. This opaque bag contains 8.5 servings, however, and 1,275 calories. If you blindly reach into that bag, you can easily eat more than 150 calories. This strategy—which is entirely deliberate—not only makes food products appear to be lower in calories than they are but also minimizes the apparent content of fat, carbohydrate, or any other nutrient perceived as undesirable. In 2004, the FDA proposed to close that loophole and make food companies reveal the number of calories in an entire package. If the FDA succeeds in getting this proposal passed, here is what will happen to the label of a 20-ounce soft drink:

> From a marketing standpoint, the object of the game is to keep the label serving sizes—and, therefore, the calories—as small as possible within the letter of the law.

- before: 110 calories per serving (serving size: 8 fluid ounces, 2.5 servings per container)
- after: 275 calories (serving size: one bottle)

The difference seems surprising even when you know that a standard portion size for a soft drink is just 8 ounces. It is easy to be lulled by the 110 calories per serving into thinking that sodas are relatively low in calories. Soda makers would just as soon keep the labels the way they are.

One last thought: much of the nutrition information on package labels comes from the product manufacturers, not from the government.

Should you trust those numbers? Once in a while the USDA and FDA check to see if food labels are accurate, and most of the time the values come close enough. The large food companies do not think it is worth the risk to lie about package contents. Individually wrapped single-serving muffins and cakes are another matter; these tend to err on the side of generosity and to weigh more than it says on the package. If a food looks like it should have more calories than is stated on the label, it probably does. But for the most part, I think it is reasonable to take the calories on food package labels at face value, and pay much greater attention to portion size and to how many of those small servings you are eating.

> If a food looks like it should have more calories than is stated on the label, it probably does.

25

Frozen Foods:
Reading Nutrition Facts

T he list of ingredients is only one part of the label that has to go on food packages. The rest comes under the heading of Nutrition Facts. If you do not know quite what to make of the Nutrition Facts label, join the crowd. The label is so difficult to interpret that the FDA publishes a guide to using it—one that is ten pages long, elaborately color coded, and full of rules and examples. You have to pay attention when you read this guide because you will be tested on your understanding of sample labels. For example, the guide asks you to compare the labels of nonfat milk and 2 percent milk: "Which has more calories and more saturated fat?" [Answer: 2 percent milk.] "Which one has more calcium?" [They have the same amount.]

Some of my more conspiracy-minded friends think the FDA deliberately designed the Nutrition Facts label to be confusing, so you would not know what you are eating, but I see it more as the result of inevitable compromise. You want to know what is in those foods, but food companies are afraid that you will then classify their products as good or bad and reject the "bad" ones. So the Nutrition Facts label tells you what Congress said it had to, as interpreted by the FDA, under pressure from vested interests. The result: a design that confuses more than it helps.

Until 1990, the food industry fought all attempts to require mandatory labeling of packaged foods. Companies only had to label nutrition information if vitamins or minerals were added or the product label claimed that it contained these nutrients. About one-third of food products fit that category. Food manufacturers labeled another third voluntarily, and did not label the last third at all. In 1989, Dr. David Kessler, who later became Commissioner of the FDA, wrote in the *New England Journal of Medicine* that food labels were "so opaque or confusing that only consumers with the hermeneutic [interpretive] abilities of a Talmudic scholar can peel back the encoded layers of meaning."

Congress was supposed to be fixing this situation when it passed the Nutrition Labeling and Education Act of 1990. This act directed the FDA to do something challenging, if not impossible—design a label that would do a great many things at once. The label was not only to inform you about the calories, nutrients, and ingredients in food products but also to

- discourage you from eating foods high in fat—the nutrient considered most problematic at that time—as well as in saturated fat, cholesterol, and sodium (*trans* fat came later)

- encourage you to eat more foods containing nutrients thought to be lacking in American diets—vitamin A, vitamin C, calcium, iron, and fiber

- allow you to compare the nutrient content of a food product to the amount you should be eating in an entire day (the Daily Value)

- fit all of this information on a label small enough to be printed on food packages

As if all that were not enough, the FDA was also, in FDA-speak, to

require the required information to be conveyed to the public in a manner which enables the public to readily observe and comprehend such information and to understand its relative significance in the context of a total daily diet.

Translation: you are actually supposed to be able to understand the label and to know how each labeled product fits into your total diet for the day. All of this would be a tall order for any agency, and the story of how the overworked and overstressed FDA actually responded to this mandate is long and troubling. For the three years following passage of the 1990 act, in what Marian Burros of *The New York Times* called a "soap opera," the food industry fought the use of the Daily Value as a standard for comparison. Food companies fretted that if you understood that a product contained a large proportion of your Daily Value for salt or saturated fat, for example, you might just say no to buying it.

Because the FDA knew perfectly well that it was going to have a hard time designing this all-purpose label, the agency commissioned studies of many alternative formats. These studies reached a complicated conclusion. People said they preferred the label formats that they actually understood the least (according to comprehension tests). The opposite was also true; the formats best understood were the ones that were least liked. The differences, however, were small and, overall, it looked like hardly anyone could understand any of the designs very well. Eventually food companies pressed for a decision on the design of the food label so they could move forward with product development. Under pressure, the FDA chose the label format that seemed the best of a confusing lot, and that is the one now in use.

U nder pressure, the FDA chose the label format that seemed the best of a confusing lot, and that is the one now in use.

In January 1993, the FDA published the rules for the new labels in a *Federal Register* notice that ran to 875 pages. The size of this document alone is enough to tell you that the label was likely to be far too complicated for even the most diligent of consumers to understand. Even at this length, it was clear that the label format would have problems. The consumer advocacy group, Center for Science in the Public Interest, which had been working for years to get nutrition labels on food packages, soon published a guide to the new Nutrition Facts label; this revealed that the design was full of loopholes that food companies could exploit to their advantage.

Frozen food labels illustrate many of those loopholes—frozen yogurt, for example. I am fond of frozen yogurt as an occasional treat, and I like to know what I am eating. So I read food labels, starting with the ingredient list. Consider Häagen-Dazs vanilla frozen yogurt, the brand most readily available in my local supermarkets (the brand is owned by Nestlé, although you would never guess that from reading the package label). Its ingredient list is short and reassuringly recognizable: "skim milk (lactose reduced), corn syrup, sugar, cream, egg yolks, natural vanilla, active yogurt cultures." But if you want to know what the Nutrition Facts mean, you have some work to do. Take a look at the Nutrition Facts label for that frozen yogurt (see Figure on page 300). I have numbered the sections of this label to make it easier to discuss. Let's take a look at the seven sections, one at a time.

Section 1: Serving size For this frozen yogurt, the stated serving size is half a cup (the FDA's platonic ideal), meaning that this pint-size carton is supposed to have *four* servings per container. I actually know people who scoop half-cup portions out of pint or quart containers, freeze them separately, and eat them one at a time. Good for them, but I, alas, cannot bring myself to do such a thing. I am far more likely to polish off half the container (two servings) and, with considerable reluctance, put the rest back in the freezer for another day.

Section 2: Calories The label says 200 calories for that measly half-cup serving—one-fourth of the 800-calorie pint-size carton. The FDA says 40 calories per serving is low, 100 is moderate, and 400 or more is high. So 200 occurs someplace in between moderate and high—let's call it moderate plus. Next come **Calories From Fat** (the label says 40). If you would like to know the percent of calories from fat, you divide 40 by 200 (times 100). This gives you 20 percent of the calories as coming from fat. By these standards, this frozen yogurt is a relatively low-fat product, but it is not low in calories.

Section 3: The "eat less" nutrients You are supposed to limit your intake of Total Fat, Saturated Fat, Cholesterol, Sodium, and, starting in 2006, *Trans* Fat. For these nutrients, less is better. And here is where things get complicated. You are to compare the amounts of these nutrients to their Daily Values, the upper limits recommended for diets that contain 2,000 calories a day. These limits are given at the bottom of the label in the footnote for diets containing 2,000 or 2,500 calories a day (if you need more calories, you get to eat more of these things). The label gives a percent of the Daily Value. My frozen yogurt contains 2.5 grams of saturated fat per half-cup serving, which comes to 13 percent of my

Häagen-Dazs Vanilla Frozen Yogurt
Nutrition Facts (in 2006)

1   Serving Size ½ cup (106g)
    Servings per container 4

AMOUNT PER SERVING

2   **Calories** 200   Calories From Fat 40

                                                        % Daily Value *

3   **Total Fat** 4.5g   7%
       Saturated Fat 2.5g   13%
    Trans Fat 0g
    Cholesterol 65mg   22%
    Sodium 55mg   2%
4   **Total Carbohydrate** 31g   10%
       Dietary Fiber 0g   0%
       Sugars 21g
5   **Protein** 9g

6   Vitamin A 4%   Vitamin C **

    Calcium 25%   Iron **

** *Contains less than 2 percent of the Daily Value of these nutrients.*

* *Percent Daily Values are based on a 2,000 calorie diet. Your daily values may
be higher or lower depending on your calorie needs:*

		Calories:	2,000	2,500
7	Total Fat	Less than	65g	80g
	Saturated Fat	Less than	20g	25g
	Cholesterol	Less than	300mg	300mg
	Sodium	Less than	2,400mg	2,400mg
	Total Carbohydrate		300g	375g
	Dietary Fiber		25g	30g

Calories per gram: Fat 9 · Carbohydrate 4 · Protein 4

Ingredients:

Skim Milk (Lactose Reduced), Corn Syrup, Sugar, Cream, Egg Yolks,
Natural Vanilla, Active Yogurt Cultures.

Daily Value for this nutrient. Is this a lot or a little? The FDA says 5 percent is low and 20 percent is high, so this percentage is in between. But if I eat two servings, everything doubles. Fun, no? And you get to do this for each of the "eat less" nutrients.

Section 4: Carbohydrates The FDA makes no recommendation about carbohydrates other than to set the Daily Value for total carbohydrate at 300 grams (two-thirds of a pound) for diets containing 2,000 calories. This section is one place where you can drive a truck through the loopholes. It is good to eat more of some carbohydrates but less of others. The FDA, however, chose to lump five kinds of carbohydrates together in one 300-gram category.

> It is good to eat more of some carbohydrates but less of others. The FDA, however, chose to lump five kinds of carbohydrates together in one 300-gram category.

- whole grains (good for you)
- refined grains (not so good unless mixed with more nutritious foods)
- natural sugars (not so bad because they come in foods that contain many other nutrients)
- added sugars (not so good because they add calories but no other nutrients)
- fiber (very good for you)

For reasons of politics masquerading as science, the FDA tucked added sugars in with sugars naturally present in food, rather than calling for them to be listed separately, "because no recommendations have been made for the total amount to eat in a day." A close look at the frozen yogurt label explains why the "added sugars" category does not appear on food labels. My half-cup contains 31 grams of total carbohydrate—about 10 percent of my 2,000-calorie Daily Value, which suggests that I can enjoy my serving of yogurt along with plenty of other high-carbohydrate foods: bread, pasta, rice, and a pastry or two. Those 31 grams include 21 grams of sugars, leaving 10 grams to be accounted for. What could they be? Yogurt is a dairy food and dairy foods do not contain the fiber-rich carbohydrates found in whole grains, fruits, and vegetables. So these 10 grams fall into the loophole. They are carbohydrates from the corn syrup too big to get counted as sugars, but small enough to be immediately converted to sugars in the body. This means that a single serving of frozen yogurt has the equivalent of a full ounce of added sugars. Corn syrup is just another name for sugars; it is the second-most abundant ingredient on the list, and "real" sugar comes next.

This yogurt contains zero grams of Dietary Fiber, and zero percent of fiber's 25-gram Daily Value for 2,000-calorie diets. This is no surprise. Fiber only comes from food plants—fruits, vegetables, and grains— never from meat or dairy foods. Fiber, however, is an "eat more" nutrient that you might expect to see listed with the other "eat more" nutrients soon discussed below under Section 6. The FDA chose to list it with carbohydrates because it is a carbohydrate, although of a kind your intestinal enzymes cannot digest.

Section 5: Protein The FDA lists protein on the label, but makes no recommendation for intake and provides no Daily Value. It lists protein for general interest. Protein is so plentiful in American diets that it raises no nutritional issues that need to be dealt with on food labels. The 9 grams of protein in a half-cup of yogurt amount to about one-sixth of my Daily Value for protein, but it is almost impossible to avoid getting more than enough protein if your calories are adequate—even if you are a vegetarian (vegetables have protein, too).

Section 6: The "eat more" nutrients For these vitamins and minerals (and fiber), eating more is better. The frozen yogurt Nutrition Facts say that a one-half cup serving provides 25 percent of my Daily Value for calcium, 4 percent for vitamin A, and less than 2 percent for iron and vitamin C. This is a hefty amount of calcium, but not a good reason to meet your entire calcium requirement for the day by eating the whole pint container along with its 800 calories.

Section 7: The footnotes If you have lasted this long, you get to the part that gives the limits of the "eat less" nutrients you are allowed for diets containing 2,000 or 2,500 calories, and the daily goals for total carbohydrate and fiber. A further footnote reminds you that fat has more calories per unit weight than protein or carbohydrate: 9 calories per gram for fat and 4 for the other two.

So, got all that?

If you read the FDA guide, you will see more about that agency's criteria for deciding whether a food is high or low in nutritional value, or, if you prefer, "good" or "bad." The FDA uses 5 percent and 20 percent of the Daily Value as cut points. If a food contains a nutrient that is 5 percent of the Daily Value or less, the FDA considers that food to be low in that nutrient. If a nutrient is 20 percent or more of the Daily Value, the food is high in that nutrient. The actual percentages can be good or bad, however, depending on whether you are supposed to eat more of a particular nutrient or less of it.

By these criteria, my half-cup of yogurt is low in sodium (good) but also low in vitamin A, vitamin C, iron, and fiber (bad). It is high in cholesterol (bad), but also high in calcium (good). Everything else falls somewhere in between. The label makes no judgment about sugars. Should you consider an ounce of sugars in half a cup good or bad? The Nutrition Facts label leaves this up to you to decide. I say, in the greater hierarchy of good and bad foods, frozen yogurt is no health food, but it is not meant to be; it is a dessert, after all. This is a once-in-a-while food, best savored in small amounts.

> If a food contains a nutrient that is 5 percent of the Daily Value or less, the FDA considers that food to be low in that nutrient. If a nutrient is 20 percent or more of the Daily Value, the food is high in that nutrient.

But therein lies the problem: serving size. The FDA standards for serving sizes are unrealistically small. Food companies like it that way, because small serving sizes on the label make the calories, fats, cholesterol, and sugars look minimal. When it comes to frozen yogurt, I can easily polish off two servings at a clip. This may double the calcium, but it also doubles the calories to 400 (one-fifth of all the calories I need for a day), doubles the saturated fat to one-quarter of my allotted 20 grams, and doubles the cholesterol to 44 percent of my allotted 300 milligrams. A quite reasonable guideline for added sugars is to keep them below 10 percent of total calories for the day. If so, two servings of frozen yogurt take me beyond that limit.

I have no easy solution to the difficulties of reading product labels. Face it, you need to know a lot about nutrition to understand them, and a lot about your own diet (its calorie limit, for example) to interpret them. But they really can be useful if you keep things simple. I begin my label reading with the ingredient list. If the ingredient list on a package of frozen food is long and incomprehensible, I leave the package in the freezer case and move on. Next, I check serving size and the number of servings per package. If the calories seem low, I know to look carefully at the number of servings in the package (they really expect you to eat only one-fourth of that carton?). Then, I move on to the per serving calories, saturated fat, *trans* fat, and sodium—the "eat less" items. If these are big fractions of the Daily Values, I leave the packages where they are, or I do not buy them very often. And I watch the sugars. To keep my intake of sugars below 10 percent of my daily 2,000 calories, I can only eat the equivalent of four tablespoons (about 60 grams) a day. If a serving has close to one tablespoon of sugars (15 grams), you can consider it a dessert and treat it as such.

> To keep my intake of sugars below 10 percent of my daily 2,000 calories, I can only eat the equivalent of four tablespoons (about 60 grams) a day.

So put the package labels to good use. Once you get the hang of reading them, the Nutrition Facts labels give you plenty of information to help you decide what is and is not worth buying.

Processed Foods:
Wheat Flour and the
Glycemic Index

I f you do not immediately head for the peripheral aisles of the super-market and, instead, begin your journey by venturing into its interior, you will find yourself in serious processed-food territory. You may also find yourself in serious shopping trouble. Unless you put blinders on and stick firmly to a list, your shopping cart will soon be filled with food products laden with sugars, hydrogenated fats, salt, and excess calories, those heavily advertised packages that are so profitable for all concerned—except you. Manufacturers and retailers say that processed foods give you what you want and need: easy-to-eat foods that require no preparation and taste better than anything you could make yourself. Processed foods do have some of these advantages, but you had best think of the center aisles as a clever combination of spiderweb and maze. Supermarket aisles are designed to trap you into looking at breathtaking numbers of products in full confidence that if you see, you will buy.

The Tops Market in Ithaca's Pyramid Mall is medium-size by suburban standards, but the interior sections of the store are arranged in fifteen double-sided aisles, each eighty feet long. Once you enter an aisle, you have only two choices; if you do not immediately turn around and escape, you must go all the way to the end. Count this as good exercise; if you go up and down every aisle in the store, you will rack up one-third of a mile. But you will more than compensate for the caloric expenditure by exposure to tens of thousands of products. Every aisle is flanked on both sides with eighty feet of shelves, each stacked six high; these add up to nearly five hundred linear feet on each side, and nearly a thousand feet in total.

We tend to take what is on those shelves for granted, but the quantity and variety of the products they hold inspire awe in visitors to our country. In this store, five of the fifteen aisles contain household goods, cosmetics, over-the-counter medicines, cleaning supplies, and baby-care items. An entire sixth aisle, both sides, contains supplies for pets. The remaining nine aisles are devoted to foods in boxes, cans, and bottles. Along with smaller sections containing such things as sauces, condiments, juices, cooking oils, baking supplies, health foods, canned fish, fruit, and vegetables, entire aisles are devoted to sodas, to snack foods, to cookies and candy, and to breakfast cereals (mostly sugared).

Foods in the center aisles are highly profitable. And why not? They are made with the cheapest ingredients, advertised with the biggest budgets, and manufactured by some of the largest food corporations in the world. These companies pay slotting fees for that center-aisle space, but make up for that expense in sales. You contribute to their income and that of the store every time you move a product from shelf to shopping cart and pay for it at the cash register.

In the context of the center aisles, "processed" is a code word for foods of low or minimal nutritional value—"junk foods" according to those of us who are less polite.

In the context of the center aisles, "processed" is a code word for foods of low or minimal nutritional value—"junk foods" according to those of us who are less polite. Sodas are the prototypes; their calories come from added sugars and they have no other nutrients to speak of. Food companies, food technologists, and, sad to say, many nutritionists will disagree with this meaning of "processed." They will assure you that practically everything you eat is processed in some way and that unprocessed foods are rare exceptions—fruits direct from the tree or vine, vegetables right from the ground, nuts from wherever they come from, meat and fish eaten raw as steak tartare or sushi, raw eggs, or raw milk. Everything else has been processed in some way that changes its form or nutritional value.

I think it makes more sense to lump lightly processed foods together with unprocessed foods. Aging, drying, freezing, canning, and cooking do change foods, but they cause little loss of nutritional value, if any, and they often make the nutrients in foods more available to the body. More extreme processing methods, however, add or subtract components of the food and cause significant changes in nutrient content. Frozen foods can be lightly or significantly processed. Frozen fruits and vegetables, for example, look much like their fresh counterparts and are more or less nutritionally intact, but others, such as frozen meals and frozen pastries, are highly processed and much changed nutritionally.

As I see it, heavy processing does three things to foods: diminishes the nutritional value of the basic ingredients; adds calories from fats and sugars; and disguises the loss of taste and texture with salt, artificial colors and flavors, and other additives. Canned foods also can be lightly or heavily processed; their principal additives are salt (soups, for example) and sugars (fruits).

MINIMAL PROCESSING

I am happy to engage in philosophical discussions about what constitutes a significant change in nutrient content, but I consider pasteurization, cooking, freezing, drying, and canning to be relatively benign processes. Some nutrients are lost, but most are preserved. The cooking and canning of carrots is a good example, as shown in the Table on the next page.

The following Table includes only a few of the eighty or so nutritional components that the USDA measures in carrots, but it illustrates

The Nutrient Composition of Raw, Cooked, and Canned Carrots
(100 Grams)*

NUTRIENT	RAW	COOKED (BOILED)	CANNED (DRAINED)
Calories	40	35	25
Fiber (grams)	3	3	2
Calcium (milligrams)	35	35	25
Vitamin C (milligrams)	6	4	3
Beta-carotene (micrograms)	5,800	8,000	5,300
Sodium (milligrams)	70	60	240

* 3.5 ounces or about two average carrots

some basic points about food processing. The nutrient composition of a food depends on several factors:

- *How much water it contains.* The more water in a food, the more dilute its nutrients. Boiling adds water to foods. The calories are not destroyed by cooking or canning; they are just diluted. So are fiber and minerals (like calcium). But heat destroys vitamin C, and the longer and hotter a food is cooked, the less vitamin C remains (this is also true of some other vitamins).

- *The solubility of nutrients in water.* Vitamin C is water soluble, meaning that it dissolves in cooking water, as do some other vitamins, minerals, and some parts of fiber. Throw out the cooking water, and you throw these out too. The fat-soluble nutrients, like beta-carotene, stay in the food and are not affected by usual cooking methods. I cannot explain why the cooked carrots in the Table appear to have so much more beta-carotene than the raw or canned carrots, but perhaps those particular carrots had more beta-carotene to begin with or the particular cooking method made the beta-carotene more available for testing.

- *The extent of processing.* The more that is done to a food between harvest and eating, the lower its nutritional content will be. Some nutrients, especially water-soluble vitamins, are more sensitive than others to the effects of heat, light, air, and storage. These losses occur in addition to dilution effects.

- *What gets added.* The higher amount of sodium in the canned carrots comes from salt added to compensate for changes in taste (salt is sodium chloride). Many processed foods also contain added sugars and fats.

Raw carrots may have more nutrients than canned carrots, but canned carrots are still worth eating if you cannot get anything better. The nutritional changes caused by minimal processing are relative, and how much these changes matter is debatable. Once processing becomes more extreme, however, its effects are less ambiguous. The center aisles are filled with miracles of food technology that bear little or no resemblance in nutritional content or taste to their starting ingredients. The classic example is what happens when whole wheat is milled to make white flour—the starting ingredient of hundreds of feet of snack foods on supermarket shelves.

HEAVY PROCESSING: MILLING OF FLOUR

Flour producers have some choices. They can take wheat seeds and grind them to a fine powder to make whole wheat flour. Alternatively, they can convert—"refine"—the wheat grains to one or another version of what we call "white" flour. To do this, millers grind the wheat grains but then remove varying amounts of the chaff—the outer, protective, nutrient-rich bran layers of the seed along with the wheat germ (the part that would sprout if planted). Usually 70 to 80 percent of the original wheat grain is left; this mainly includes the inner part of the seed, the "endosperm," which is full of the proteins and starch that are in seeds to nourish the germinating plant until it can make its own leaves and start photosynthesizing. Because removing the chaff also removes nutrients, about one-third of the countries in the world require millers to enrich white flour by adding back one or more vitamins or minerals. In the United States, millers have to add specified amounts of four vitamins (niacin, riboflavin, thiamin, and folic acid) and one mineral (iron). They buy the vitamins from pharmaceutical companies and mix premeasured amounts into the freshly ground flour. The Table shows what happens to the nutritional value of wheat flour as it gets refined into unenriched and enriched white flour.

The Effects of Milling and Enrichment on Wheat Flour
(100 Grams, 3.5 Ounces)*

NUTRIENT	WHOLE WHEAT FLOUR	WHITE FLOUR, NOT ENRICHED	WHITE FLOUR, ENRICHED
Calories	340	360	360
Protein (grams)	14	10	10
Fiber (grams)	12	3	3
Calcium (milligrams)	35	15	15
Vitamin B_6 (micrograms)	340	45	45
Iron (milligrams)	4	1	5**
Niacin (milligrams)	6	1	6**
Folic acid (micrograms)	45	25	180**

*This amount is a bit less than one cup.
**These are added through enrichment.

The milling of whole grains makes the calories go up and everything else go down. White flour has more calories than whole wheat flour because it is more concentrated; it has lost the fibrous bran, which does not weigh much and has hardly any calories (although it has plenty of nutrients). When the bran is taken away, the vitamins and minerals go away with it (and make great animal feed). The result: unenriched white flour has just 55 percent of the folic acid, 43 percent of the calcium, 25 percent of the iron, 17 percent of the niacin, and 13 percent of the vitamin B_6 in whole wheat flour.

Why do we eat white flour rather than wheat flour? The answer: we like it better. White flour bakes more easily, has a longer shelf life (because it has fewer nutrients), has a bland taste that goes better with peanut butter or bologna, and a softer texture that makes white bread and pastries easier to eat. White bread has long been preferred by bakers and their customers, rich and poor alike. Only recently, as I discuss in the bread chapter, have whole wheat breads come back into favor.

The preference for white bread has nutritional consequences: the nutrient losses are significant by anyone's standards. Foods made from wheat flour account for about 20 percent of the calories in the American diet; bread alone accounts for about 9 percent of calories, cakes and pastries for 6 percent, pasta for 3 percent, and pies, crackers, pretzels, and such things for the remaining 2 percent. Most of these are made from refined white flour. As the Table shows, enrichment replaces the lost iron, niacin, and folic acid (as well as riboflavin and thiamin, which are not shown), but no other nutrients. Enrichment standards in the United States assume that all of the other nutrients are so widely available in everyday diets that they do not need to be replaced.

This assumption is more reasonable than it may sound. Relatively unprocessed foods have lots of nutrients and it is easy to get what you need from them—if you eat them. But the lure of the center aisles means that you might choose processed over unprocessed foods, and that is just what the makers of processed foods want you to do. They know that you are more likely to buy processed foods if you think they are good for you, so they go way beyond enrichment and put all kinds of additional vitamins and minerals into everything they can—and then boast of the nutritional value of those additives on the packaging.

> Foods made from wheat flour account for about 20 percent of the calories in the American diet; bread alone accounts for about 9 percent of calories, cakes and pastries for 6 percent, pasta for 3 percent, and pies, crackers, pretzels, and such things for the remaining 2 percent. Most of these are made from refined white flour.

If you are picky about definitions, "enrichment" means adding nutrients to their original levels and "fortification" means adding more, but both terms are commonly used to refer to any addition of vitamins and minerals to processed foods. Whichever term you use, white flour has a lot more folic acid than is found in whole wheat. As I explained in *Food*

Politics, this happened as the result of a fiercely fought compromise over how best to get enough folic acid to pregnant women to prevent the occasional development of neural tube defects in their newly conceived fetuses. These severe defects in spinal closure occur soon after conception and well before a woman even realizes she is pregnant. Women who are eating plenty of folic acid before they become pregnant have a much better chance of delivering an infant without neural tube problems.

The points most debated were the best way to get folic acid to women "at risk" of pregnancy—the choices were dietary advice, supplements, or fortification—and how much folic acid would be needed to prevent the fetal defects. Also at issue was how to track the effectiveness of the folic acid intervention. For no obvious reason, the number of infants born with neural tube defects had been declining steadily for years and was already at a very low level. Eventually, the FDA selected heavier-than-normal fortification as the strategy.

Follow-up studies show that the strategy worked. The average blood level of folic acid among Americans has more than doubled since 1998, when the FDA-mandated fortification started. Also as expected, the number of babies born with neural tube defects has continued to decline. For this and other reasons, food companies will tell you that processing is precisely what you need to have a bountiful, reliable, safe, and nutritious food supply.

I am not one to argue against the choices that the center aisles provide, particularly when so many of those choices are foods I like. Processing comes at a price, however, and not just in nutrient losses. If the milling of wheat was only a matter of losing vitamins, you could take a supplement and not worry about it. But removing the fiber from wheat changes one other property; it makes the carbohydrates in wheat starch easier and faster for the body to absorb, and this has additional health consequences. Let's take a look at what these are.

If you like browsing around the health sections of bookstores, as I do, you cannot help running across books promoting the Glycemic Index (GI) as a way to help you decide whether a food is good or bad for you. On a trip to Australia in 2004, I was amazed to see food packages labeled with "Glycemic Index Tested" symbols and scores, and even more amazed at the examples: Cadbury Schweppes marmalade (GI 55), Top Taste cake (GI 51), Norco macadamia ice cream (GI 37), Ferrero Nutella spread (GI 33), Thorpedo energy water (GI 19), and the like. When it comes to the Glycemic Index, lower is better; these products have scores considered low to moderate, and on that basis are promoting themselves as good for you.

To understand what this is about, you need to know that the carbohydrates in food come in two forms: starch and sugars. Both kinds of carbohydrate are made up of units of sugar; they differ only in the size and number of sugar molecules and, of course, their function. Sugars are "simple" carbohydrates; they are composed of a single sugar, glucose (blood sugar) or fructose (fruit sugar), for example, or two single sugars linked together. Examples of two-sugar sugars are sucrose (common table sugar), made of glucose linked to fructose, and lactose (milk sugar), made of glucose linked to galactose.

Starch, however, is a huge, "complex" carbohydrate made of glucose molecules linked together in long, branching chains. Starch is the carbohydrate you get when you eat potatoes, rice, pasta, bread, crackers, cookies, and cakes. It may help to think of starch as made of multiple chains of glucose molecules meshed together in a great jumble—a gel. When you eat starch, digestive enzymes in your small intestine attack the gel by breaking the glucose links in many places, and then breaking the longer chains into smaller and smaller chains. Eventually digestive enzymes break the whole thing apart into single molecules of glucose itself. Your intestinal wall cannot easily absorb even short chains of two or three glucose molecules linked together, but you can easily absorb single glucose units. Glucose is the primary fuel for your brain and muscles, and your body does everything it can to make sure you have enough glucose available at all times. Once glucose is absorbed from the intestine into the bloodstream, blood glucose levels go up, and your pancreas starts secreting insulin to help get that sugar out of the blood and into your brain and muscles, where it is needed.

When too much glucose comes in at any one time, however, it swamps the ability of the body's metabolism to handle it. If you habitually eat large quantities of foods with rapidly absorbable carbohydrates—refined starches and sugars—the pancreas makes too much insulin. As a result blood sugar drops too far (making you feel hungry). Also, muscle cells start resisting taking in more glucose, and this means that more of this sugar is stored as fat. The result is that you put yourself at risk for weight gain, diabetes (the adult type 2 variety), cardiovascular disease, and other such problems. Fiber slows down the absorption of glucose from the small intestine, which is why a diet high in fiber-containing fruits, vegetables, and grains helps keep such health problems at bay. As with anything having to do with diet and body weight, the key point here is quantity; too much absorbed glucose can promote weight gain, and so can too many calories from any source—protein and fat, as well as carbohydrate.

It is possible to rank foods that contain carbohydrates according to how quickly glucose is absorbed from them. The Glycemic Index is the ranking system. It compares the rise in blood glucose caused by 50 grams of carbohydrate (almost 2 ounces) in the foods you eat to what happens when you eat 50 grams of pure glucose (or some other standard). Researchers define glucose as having a GI of 100. In comparison, some researchers find white breads to have numbers in the 70s to 90s, and whole wheat breads to have numbers in the 50s. This is a numerical way of saying that white bread offers more rapidly absorbed carbohydrates than whole wheat bread—and that eating a lot of white bread is more likely to make you prone to obesity, heart disease, and the like than eating foods lower on the Glycemic Index scale.

In general, the Glycemic Index of processed foods is much higher than that of unprocessed foods, but there are many exceptions. Carrots, for example, have a high Glycemic Index. Carrots have sugars—mostly sucrose but some glucose and fructose—and these are rapidly absorbed. But the total amount of sugars in carrots is so small—less than 5 grams (a teaspoon) in one large carrot—that their rapid absorption hardly matters. You would need to eat at least ten carrots to take in the equivalent of 50 grams of glucose and raise your blood sugar appreciably. In nutrition-speak, the Glycemic Index of carrots may be high, but—enter a new term—their "Glycemic Load" is low.

The Glycemic Load considers the total amount of rapidly absorbable carbohydrate—starch or sugars—in the foods you eat, as well as the Glycemic Index of that food. Because it takes the quantity of food into consideration (and, therefore, calories), the Glycemic Load is the factor that counts. Even potatoes and rice, which have a Glycemic Index in the 90s, have a low Glycemic Load unless you eat a lot of them, because the amounts of starch or sugars they contain are relatively low. To avoid fruits and vegetables because they might have a high Glycemic Index makes no sense; their Glycemic Load is low, and that's what really matters.

Bookstore health sections are full of books that give lengthy lists of Glycemic Index and Load values, but I generally ignore them, because the values they report are so inconsistent from one author to another. The numbers vary depending on who is doing the measuring and how it is done, and they change drastically when you eat more than one food at a time (which, of course, is the typical situation). They also change with preparation and cooking methods.

Take potatoes, for example. The Glycemic Index of potatoes varies with their type, with how they are cooked, and even with whether they are eaten hot or cold. The Table shows the differences.

The Glycemic Index of Potatoes*

POTATO TYPE	COOKING METHOD	GLYCEMIC INDEX
Red	Boiled, cold	56
Unspecified	French fried	64
White (California)	Roasted	72
White (Canadian)	Baked	73
Russet	Baked	77
Unspecified	Instant mashed	88
Red	Boiled, hot	89

*These values are compared to glucose, which has a Glycemic Index of 100. Scale: 55 to 69 is moderate; anything above 70 is high.

You find the difference between cold and hot potatoes and everything else about this idea absurdly complicated? Well, so do I, especially because if you toss some butter or cheese on those potatoes the Glycemic Index will drop (because fat is not a carbohydrate), but the calories and saturated fat will go up. Overall, what matters more than the Glycemic Index of a food is how much of that food you eat.

Even though I do not use the Glycemic Index, there are some things about the concept that I like very much. The Glycemic Index alerts you to the good things that happen when you eat foods with a low Glycemic Load—fruits, vegetables, and whole grains; lean meats and fish; and low-fat dairy products—exactly the foods recommended for good health. The Glycemic Index also alerts you to the undesirable effects of eating lots of starchy processed foods—crackers, pretzels, cookies, and the like—and foods high in added sugars, such as sodas, candies, and desserts. Sugary breakfast cereals raise particular concerns because they have both rapidly absorbable refined starch and added sugars. In anything but small amounts, these foods add calories that you are unlikely to need (because they come with few or no other nutrients and practically no fiber), and they put your metabolism into overdrive to deal with the influx of glucose from the rapid breakdown of starch and sugars. Such problems are best avoided by saving highly processed starchy and sugary foods for special occasions.

> The Glycemic Index also alerts you to the undesirable effects of eating lots of starchy processed foods—crackers, pretzels, cookies, and the like—and foods high in added sugars, such as sodas, candies, and desserts.

27

Sugar(s)

A couple of weeks after my book *Food Politics* came out in 2002, I received an unexpected letter from a Washington, D.C., law firm representing the Sugar Association, a group "committed to integrity and sound scientific principles in educating consumers and professionals about the benefits of pure natural sugar." The letter said that in talking about my book on a radio program, I had made "numerous false, misleading, disparaging, and defamatory statements about sugar," first among them that I "continuously repeat the false and inaccurate statement that soft drinks contain sugar." The letter went on:

> As commonly known by experts in the field of nutrition, soft drinks have contained virtually no sugar (sucrose) in more than 20 years. The misuse of the word "sugar" to indicate other caloric sweeteners is not only inaccurate, but is a grave disservice to the thousands of family farmers who grow sugar cane and sugar beets . . . [If you do not] cease making misleading or false statements regarding sugar or the sugar industry . . . the only recourse available to us will be to legally defend our industry and its members against any and all fallacious and harmful allegations.

Oh my. I am not a litigious person and this letter was most disturbing, not least because the Sugar Association seemed to interpret the word "sugar" in a most unusual way. The ingredient list of a can of Coca-Cola Classic, for example, says that it contains high fructose corn syrup and/or sucrose. The "and/or" means one or the other, because both do the trick. Chemically, they both are sugars and sweet as can be. But in the self-interested logic of the Sugar Association, sugar means sucrose and sucrose alone.

WHAT IS SUGAR, ANYWAY?

To understand how nutritionally silly this is (and why the Sugar Association did not follow up on its threat), you need to know that at least three different sugars are involved in the hairsplitting over "sugar" versus other sweeteners that have calories. The first is sucrose—common "refined" table sugar—the product extracted from sugarcane and sugar beets. When you say "sugar," the Sugar Association—which represents the growers of sugarcane and sugar beets—wants you to think sucrose. But that would be misleading. Any nutrition or biochemistry book will tell you that "sugar" refers to many kinds of "caloric sweeteners"—caloric, because they have calories. Sucrose itself is a double sugar (disaccharide) composed of two single sugars (monosaccharides), one of them glucose (blood sugar) and the other fructose (fruit sugar). In sucrose, the glucose and fructose sugars are stuck together. In high fructose corn syrup (HFCS) and other sweeteners made from corn, the glucose and fructose are separate. Be-

> Any nutrition or biochemistry book will tell you that "sugar" refers to many kinds of "caloric sweeteners"— caloric, because they have calories.

cause enzymes in the digestive tract quickly split sucrose into its constituent sugars, your body can hardly tell the difference. The Table on the next page gives the percentages.

Composition of Sucrose Versus HFCS*

SWEETENER	FRUCTOSE	GLUCOSE
Sucrose	50%	50%
42-HFCS	42%	53%
55-HFCS	55%	42%

*Source: Corn Refiners Association, www.corn.org.

Sucrose, fructose, and glucose are sugars. One or another of these sugars, singly or together, also show up in foods as dextrose (another name for the glucose derived from corn), fruit juice concentrates, honey, molasses, and, of course, high fructose corn syrup and other corn sweeteners. All are sugar(s). The parenthetical(s) is the one result of the Sugar Association's letter. Although this group did not follow up on its threat, I now use the plural form when discussing caloric sweeteners. As Richard Keeler, then the head of the Sugar Association, assured me when we met a few months later, his group is glad that I am now speaking more precisely. I'll bet.

THE UBIQUITOUS CORN SWEETENERS

Let me take up the matter of corn sweeteners—corn syrup with varying proportions of glucose and fructose—because there are so many misunderstandings about them. I view corn sweeteners as an especially inexpensive and ever present form of sugar(s), but nothing more sinister. Corn syrup starts out as cornstarch. Starch, as I explained in the previous chapter, is a complicated gel-like carbohydrate molecule made of enormous numbers of glucose sugars linked together in chains, some straight and some branched. But starch is not sweet. So chemists treat cornstarch with enzymes to break the gel into smaller and smaller pieces. This process ends up as corn syrup, a mixture of glucose and small starches (chains of just a few glucose molecules).

Corn syrup is sweet, but not as sweet as sucrose, and not nearly as sweet as fructose. To make it sweeter, chemists treat corn syrup with other enzymes to convert some of its glucose to fructose—about 42 percent. With further treatment, they can produce syrup that is 55 percent fructose. The sugar percentages in 42-HFCS and 55-HFCS do not add up to 100 percent because some small starches—chains of glucose—still remain.

You metabolize fructose somewhat differently than glucose, leading some scientists to believe that fructose and, therefore, high fructose corn syrup, is the culprit in rising rates of obesity. Perhaps, but nothing so complicated is needed to explain the effects of corn syrup on weight gain. Sucrose and corn sweeteners both end up as glucose and fructose in the body, and both are rapidly absorbed forms of carbohydrate. Also, both are common constituents of junk foods, and add nonnutritious calories to the diet. Whether or not the biochemical differences between corn syrup and sucrose matter, one thing is clear: we eat a lot of corn sweeteners. Corn sweeteners have calories and so do the foods that contain them.

If corn sweeteners have anything to do with obesity, it is surely because processed foods are loaded with them, and lots of people are eating lots more of such foods. As the Sugar Association made clear in its letter to me, the labels on soft drinks may say "high fructose corn syrup and/or sucrose," but soft drinks have not contained sucrose for years; they contain high fructose corn syrup. In 1980, when rates of obesity were just starting to rise, the U.S. food supply provided an average of 30 gallons of sugary soft drinks per capita, but the amount rose to 35 gallons in 2003. The food supply now provides an average of 200 calories per person per day from the high fructose corn syrup in soft drinks alone.

Corn sweeteners come from corn, obviously, and U.S. farmers grow a lot of this crop. In 2004, they produced 11.8 billion bushels of corn (a bushel is about 35 quarts). Most of this is used to feed animals; only about 6 percent of the corn produced in the United States is used to make corn sweeteners. This small percentage, however, has made a big difference in the food supply. The differences over time are summarized in the Table on the next page.

The food supply now provides an average of 200 calories per person per day from the high fructose corn syrup in soft drinks alone.

Caloric Sweeteners in the U.S. Food Supply (Pounds Per Capita),
1980 to 2004

SWEETENER	1980	2004
Total caloric sweeteners	120	142
Refined sugar (sucrose)	84	61
High fructose corn syrup	35	78
Others (honey, maple syrup, etc.)	1	1.4

Source: USDA, at www.ers.usda.gov/briefing/sugar/Data/Table50.xls.

In the twenty-four years from 1980 to 2004, caloric sweeteners in the U.S. food supply increased from 120 pounds to 142 pounds. These 142 pounds include sugars from all sources—cane, beet, corn, honey, and maple trees—and is the amount available in the food supply for every man, woman, and child in the country. As the Table shows, the availability of refined (cane and beet) sugar dropped by 23 pounds, but the supply of high fructose corn syrup more than doubled. High fructose corn syrup not only accounts for all of the 22-pound increase in caloric sweeteners in the food supply but has also displaced considerable amounts of sucrose. You can see why the Sugar Association is so worried about protecting the interests of sugarcane and sugar beet producers. You also can see why nutritionists like me are so concerned about sugars in general and corn sweeteners in particular—they have calories.

> The 142 pounds of sugars available to every American (even babies) means that your adult share is close to half a pound per day.

And you do not have to look much further than calories from sugar(s) to explain why Americans are gaining weight. The 142 pounds of sugars available to every American (even babies) means that your adult share is close to half a pound per day. This means that average availability is about 700 calories a day from sugars alone, and 200 of them go into soft drinks. But before you become too alarmed, remember that these are supply figures (production plus imports, less exports) and do not necessarily reflect what any one person eats. The USDA estimates that average daily intake of sugars per person is 31 teaspoons—17 from corn syrups and 14 from sucrose. This works out to about 5 ounces in total and a "mere" 500 calories per day—but still one-quarter of the average daily caloric needs. Whatever the exact figure for consumption of sugars, their calories are high enough to suggest guilt by association. All those calories from sugars—whatever their food source—must surely have something to do with weight gain. How could they not?

Sucrose and corn sweeteners may both be sugars, but the Sugar Association cares deeply about the difference. For one thing, sucrose and corn syrups are represented by different lobbying groups. Sucrose is more expensive than corn sweeteners and it is safe to assume that its producers like it that way. As a result of decades of highly effective lobbying, the price of both kinds of sweeteners is supported by the government, but in quite different ways. The government has long protected American growers of sugarcane and sugar beets in two ways: a quota system that restricts the import of cheaper sugar from foreign producers, and a loan program that supports the price of domestic sugar. These methods make the cost of table sugar three times higher than it would be on the free market and means that products made with sucrose are more expensive to produce. You pay a share of those increased costs when you buy foods sweetened with sucrose at the supermarket.

> All those calories from sugars—whatever their food source—must surely have something to do with weight gain. How could they not?

In contrast, corn producers receive subsidies that encourage them to grow even more of this crop than can be sold. This tends to drive down the price. The effect on the wholesale price of this sweetener is remarkable. Early in 2005, a pound of beet sugar (sucrose) cost 24 cents, but a pound of high fructose corn syrup was only about half that amount—13 cents per pound. The low wholesale cost explains why food companies love to put corn sweeteners in their products. The more corn sweeteners in a product, the cheaper the product is to make. If a food product does not cost much, you are more likely to buy it—and to buy it in larger sizes and more often. That is why low prices, wonderful as they are for your food budget, are not so wonderful for your calorie budget: they encourage you to eat more than you should. If corn sweeteners have any special role in weight gain, it is most likely because they are added to so many food products, and products containing corn sweeteners do not cost much.

I like sweet foods and I am especially fond of raw cane sugar sprinkled on cereal or unsweetened yogurt, but I try to be careful about how much sugar I use. Sugars of any kind provide 4 calories per gram (120 per ounce), but have no other nutritional value. And it is all too easy to eat sweeteners in prodigious amounts, thereby driving healthier foods out of your diet, adding unneeded calories, and forcing your metabolism to go into glycemic overload. Sugars are not poisons, but they are best taken in small doses.

That is why I am astonished by the vast quantities of sugary foods sold in supermarkets. The next time you are at a grocery store, try pacing off the linear feet devoted to sweet foods. Here, for example, is what the Tops Market at the Pyramid Mall in Ithaca looked like just before the Christmas holidays in 2004. Holidays or not, this store shelves candy in sections twenty to thirty feet long in three different aisles, as well as in special displays at the ends of aisles, at the store entrance, and at every checkout counter. In this one medium-size market, an inventory of shelf space devoted to sugary foods—just in the center aisles—produces the list summarized in the Table on the next page.

Measured by shelf space, a quarter of all food products in the center aisles of this store are high in sugar. And this count of linear feet did not include the store's bakery section, with its cakes, pies, cookies, and doughnuts, or the refrigerators packed with sweetened milk drinks and sodas, or the freezer cases full of ice cream and frozen treats.

But the high percentage alone does not do justice to the way this store pushes sugary foods. In that pre-Christmas season, the store greeted you at the entrance with red-and-green packages of soft drinks stacked like a Christmas tree (twenty feet of shelf space), not far from a special holiday display of candies in red, green, and gold foil wrap (six feet long, five shelves: thirty feet). You collected your shopping cart next to a wall of soft drink packs (fifty feet). At the outside end of one aisle—prime real estate for impulse buys—the store displayed boxes of sugars for holiday

Space Allotted to Sugary Foods in One Supermarket's Center Aisles

PRODUCT	LINEAR FEET OF SHELF SPACE
Non-diet sodas	400
Cookies	360
Candy	350
Cereals, sweetened	200
Juice drinks	125
Cake and cookie mixes	120
Snapple and sports drinks	110
Packaged baked goods	70
Jams and jellies	70
Cocoa, lemonade, Kool-Aid mixes	70
Sugar, syrups	65
Toaster pastries	30
Chocolate chips	20
Frosting mixes	15
Total feet of sugary foods	2,005
Total feet of food products	8,000 (rounded off)
Percent sugary foods	25

baking (sixteen feet), and another end section displayed cake, frosting, and candy mixes (twenty-eight feet). At the end of a third aisle you had to navigate around nine bushel baskets full of hard candy, also wrapped in holiday colors.

In case you missed all those chances to add sugary foods to your cart, more awaited you at the cash registers. Five of the store's checkout counters displayed candy and chewing gum on shelves four feet long, nine per section: thirty-six feet each, or another 180 feet of sweets. Although that was the holiday season, only the colors differ; the stores find reasons for similar candy displays all year long. If you find yourself buying more sugary foods than you realized or intended, it is because you cannot avoid them. Consider all of these products as expensive ways to buy sugar.

Sweet is sweet, and candy is candy, and sweet foods have a place in healthy diets. But I cannot help saying what the Sugar Association chooses to call "disparaging and defamatory" things about sugars—but that I view as facts backed up by plenty of research—when the makers of such foods pretend they are good for you, invoke "science" to argue they are harmless, and lobby as heavy-handedly as anyone in Washington has ever seen to make sure no nutritionist or government agency suggests otherwise.

MAKING SUGAR(S) LOOK HEALTHY

One summer afternoon, I was called by my university's development officer (the chief fund-raiser) to ask if I would meet with an alumnus who owned a candy company and wanted some nutrition advice. Of course I would. His company makes candies for kids—the inexpensive, brightly colored ones that come in packages you can play with. I loved things like that when I was a kid and, awful as I now think they are, I cannot bring myself to get upset about them as an occasional treat. They are candy and this company is not pretending that its products are anything else. But his question for me was this: Should his company be adding vitamins to its candies? His competitors were doing this, and were promoting their candy as healthier than his. He was worried about market share but also about the ethics of putting vitamins into candy. He *should* be worried about the ethics of that idea; I am too.

I had just done a house-sit for some friends in California and, I must confess, could not help but browse through their kitchen cabinets (with this book in mind, of course). There, I found health-food store gummy bears with added vitamins, herbs, and even dried vegetables (in microscopic amounts). I also found a product I had not seen before: Shark's Fruit Snacks "Made with real fruit juice." I went right to the label. The gummy sharks did indeed start out with fruit juice from concentrate, but the rest of the ingredients were corn syrup, sugar, partially hydrogenated vegetable oil (*trans* fats again), and the usual artificial colors and flavors. I did the math: 52 percent of the calories in this "snack" come from sugars. They may have vitamins, but these are candy, not health foods.

The makers of such products know that you will buy them because they look like they are better for your kids than regular candy. This strategy also works for things you might buy for yourself. Take a look, for example, at the ingredient list for Kellogg's Nutri-Grain Honey Oat & Raisin Granola Bars. I've marked the added sugars in bold.

> Granola (Rolled Whole Oats, Crisp Rice [Rice, **Sugar**, Salt, **High Fructose Corn Syrup**, Malt Flavoring], **High Fructose Corn Syrup**, **Brown Sugar**, Partially Hydrogenated Soybean Oil, Rolled Whole Wheat), Raisins, **Corn Syrup**, Partially Hydrogenated Vegetable Oil (Soybean, Cottonseed and Palm Kernel Oil), **Sugar**, **Fructose**, **Corn Syrup Solids**, Glycerin, **High Fructose Corn Syrup**, **Honey**, **Dextrose**, Natural and Artificial Flavor, Salt, Fractionated Coconut Oil, Soy Lecithin, Nonfat Dry Milk . . . [the remaining ingredients are seven vitamins and iron].

I did not highlight the raisins on this list, although they are naturally high in sugars. Overall, I would characterize this product as a low-fat cookie with added vitamins. You are supposed to think that adding vitamins makes such products healthier, but are they? This question gets us into the realm of philosophy: Is a vitamin-supplemented junk food better than a regular junk food? Take Kool-Aid, for example—it is nothing but sugar water with added vitamin C.

Like any philosophical question, this one can be argued from multiple points of view. Mine is that food categories should be clearly distinguished from one another, and that adding vitamins confuses them. Cookies, candy, and other sweets are sweet snacks or desserts. So are sweet drinks (which, according to the Center for Science in the Public Interest, are equivalent to candy in liquid form). Adding a few vitamins to desserts could lull you into thinking that it is fine to eat sweets instead of more nutritious foods that naturally contain a much wider range of vitamins and other good things. Adding vitamins to sugary foods blurs the distinctions among food categories, and moves desserts into the nutritional mainstream—everyday foods instead of those best eaten occasionally. This, of course, is just where the makers of vitamin-supplemented, high-sugar products want them positioned. Adding vitamins is an "eat more" strategy; it is not really about your health. If you need more vitamins (and most people do not), you are better off getting them from healthier foods or a multivitamin supplement than from candy or Kool-Aid.

This is why I was not pleased when New York City cut a $166 million deal with Cadbury Schweppes to make Snapple the exclusive drink sold in the city's 1,200 public schools. This deal, made directly with the mayor's office, was announced soon after food advocacy groups won what had seemed like a major victory: they had gotten the Board of Education to forbid sugary soft drinks to be sold in New York City schools. Cadbury Schweppes moved right in to pour Snapple into that gap. Shortly after I expressed my dismay about this development to a reporter who quoted my remarks in *The New York Observer*, I received a call from the Board of Education's legal counsel asking me why I could possibly have any objections to Snapple drinks. Snapple, he said, was juice—not a soft drink. Really? I asked to see the labels.

A few days later, I received a letter from Steven Jarmon, Snapple's vice president for communications, assuring me that "Snapple 100% Juiced! Beverages meet New York City's nutritional guidelines—some of the strictest and most progressive in the country," and that the products were "Made with 100% juice . . ." He was kind enough to send me the product labels. The Snapple Fruit Punch made for the New York City schools, for example, indeed was juice at one time, but no more. Its label says it is made from six kinds of fruit concentrates, plus flavor additives, vitamins, and calcium—and no added sugars. You do not need to add sugars to fruit concentrates. To make "juiced" products, food chemists process fruit juice until it is basically fruit-flavored sugar, and then reconstitute it. "Fruit concentrate," according to the U.S. *Dietary Guidelines*, is a euphemism for sugars.

This Snapple drink has 170 calories in 11.5 ounces, and more sugars than in a 12-ounce Coke. Like other soft drinks, each Snapple contains 40 grams of sugars—well more than an ounce. The amounts matter. Soft drinks account for 40 percent of the sugar(s) intake of children and adolescents, and fruit drinks account for another 12 percent. The percentages are slightly different for adults, but soft drinks and fruit drinks together account for

As soon as you start thinking of soft drinks as desserts, you may find it hard to tolerate their presence in school vending machines or to let children drink them all day long.

more than 40 percent of sugar intake for everyone. Whether you consider Snapple a soda or a fruit drink, children only have to drink one can to reach the upper limit of their recommended sugar allowance for the entire day.

Nutritionally speaking, Snapple, added sugars or not, vitamin-supplemented or not, is a dessert. As soon as you start thinking of soft drinks as desserts, you may find it hard to tolerate their presence in school vending machines or to let children drink them all day long. But the sugar, soft drink, and juice drink industries are determined to do everything they can to make sure that you do not think of soft drinks this way. They do not want you to think bad thoughts about sugar, ever.

CONFUSING THE SCIENCE

If health authorities actually advised you to "eat less sugar," you might be inclined to follow their advice. The sugar industry's job is to convince you and government agencies that there is no reason for anyone to eat less sugar(s), and it is relentless in doing so. The industry argues through its trade associations and lobbyists that science does not find sugar to be harmful, and it uses a scientific review done by the USDA in 2001 to support that view. This review concluded that sugars alone—meaning sugars considered independent of their calories or of the foods that contain them—do not raise the risk of diabetes, heart disease, or obesity. But this is like considering the effects of fire independent of the effects of heat. The effects of sugars cannot be understood in isolation from calories or from the other caloric ingredients in sugary foods.

Attributing a disease to any one food or food component is always problematic because diets contain many foods, and foods contain a great many components that singly and collectively can affect health. Even so, plenty of other research, circumstantial evidence, and direct observations about sugars and health should be enough to convince anyone other than an industry defender that sugary foods add unneeded calories to the diet, cause metabolic problems, and promote weight gain. Common sense tells you that eating ounces of sugars at any one time—without the modulating effects of fiber and other food components—will raise blood sugar beyond where it needs to be, add unnecessary calories, and encourage weight gain.

If it makes good sense to cut down on sugars and their principal sources—soft drinks, juice drinks, cookies, cakes, candy, and ice cream—shouldn't the government say so? Until recently it did say so, but the price of good advice and common sense proved too high in the face of industry pressures. In *Food Politics*, I recounted an episode from the Starr Report to illustrate the extraordinary access of the sugar industry to officials at the highest levels of government. On a federal holiday, said the report, a Florida sugar producer (whose companies just happened to have contributed more than $1 million to the election campaigns of both Democrat and Republican parties) had no trouble getting a telephone call through to President Bill Clinton while he was otherwise occupied with the White House intern Monica Lewinsky. Sugar industry contributions to political parties and election campaign funds help to explain why federal dietary advice about sugar intake is such a sensitive topic.

You probably have never heard of the *Dietary Guidelines for Americans,* or have only the vaguest idea of what they are. This is because they are meant as a policy statement about diet and health for government agencies, food companies, and nutritionists, rather than as a tool for public education. In contrast, the USDA invented the Pyramid food guide to translate the policy into a dietary action plan for the public. The first edition of the *Dietary Guidelines* appeared in 1980 as a joint project of two federal departments: the USDA and the Department of Health and Human Services. Subsequent editions appeared in 1985 and 1990. In 1990, Congress required the two agencies to revise the guidelines at five-year intervals. If you enjoy language games, you may be amused by what has happened to the sugar guideline over the years, as displayed by the Table on page 330.

In 1980 and 1985, the guideline contained just four words—"Avoid too much sugar"—a clear "eat less" message and still excellent advice. But look at what happens as the guidelines are revised. The number of words increases and the message becomes less direct and more confusing. By 2005, sugar has disappeared as a separate guideline and is now a "key recommendation" in a chapter on carbohydrates. Could politics have anything to do with this? Because most lobbying goes on behind the scenes, it ordinarily takes deep investigation to attribute such changes to industry interference, but the sugar industry does not bother to hide what it does.

Evolution of the U.S. Dietary Guideline for Sugar, 1980 to 2005

YEAR	SUGAR GUIDELINE	NUMBER OF WORDS
1980	Avoid too much sugar	4
1985	Avoid too much sugar	4
1990	Use sugars only in moderation	5
1995	Choose a diet moderate in sugars	6
2000	Choose beverages and foods to moderate your intake of sugars	10
2005	Choose and prepare foods and beverages with little added sugars or caloric sweeteners, such as amounts suggested by the USDA Food Guide and the DASH [Dietary Approaches to Stop Hypertension] Eating Plan	27

For the year 2000 version, the scientific committee developing the guidelines suggested these words: "limit your intake of sugars." When sugar lobbyists argued that science did not support "limit," the agencies changed the word to "moderate." A USDA official told me that it just wasn't worth taking on the sugar industry to fight about one word. The difference between "limit" and "moderate" may be semantic and not matter much, but this example—and the legal challenge sent to me— illustrate the absurd lengths to which this industry will go to protect sales of cane, beet, and corn sugars.

In many ways, the 2005 sugar guideline is an even better example. The scientific advisory committee developing the basis for the guidelines said these things about sugars (all are direct quotes from the September 2004 committee report):

- The healthiest way to reduce calorie intake is to reduce one's intake of added sugars . . . they all provide calories, but they do not provide essential nutrients.

- Although more research is needed . . . studies suggest a positive association between the consumption of sugar-sweetened beverages and weight gain.

- Most . . . studies have found that an increased intake of added sugars is associated with increased total energy intakes.

- The preponderance of . . . data available suggest that added sugars (particularly in beverages) are associated with an increase in energy intake. As a result, decreasing the intake of added sugars (particularly in beverages) may help prevent weight gain and may aid in weight loss.

Despite the scientific jargon ("preponderance of data," "positive association," and the like), the committee's message is clear: the more sugars you eat, the more calories you will take in, and the more weight you will gain. You might think that a reasonable guideline based on such statements would say "eat less sugar," and suggest doing so by cutting down on soft drinks, juice drinks, and other sweet foods. But if the *Dietary Guidelines* said something this direct, the responsible government agencies would be under siege by lobbyists for sugars and every other product whose sales might be jeopardized by that advice. It cannot be a coincidence that in the 2005 guidelines, the agencies chose to sandwich advice about sugars between uncontroversial recommendations to choose fiber-rich foods and practice good oral hygiene. To their credit, the agencies edited the *Dietary Guidelines* to distinguish natural from added sugars, to show in a Table that soft drinks are the biggest source of sugars in American diets (33 percent of added sugars), and to list the euphemisms under which sugars are hidden on food labels (corn syrup, fruit juice concentrates, invert sugar). But they left it up to you to figure out how to use the USDA Food Guide and DASH Eating Plan,

> To their credit, the agencies edited the *Dietary Guidelines* to distinguish natural from added sugars, to show in a Table that soft drinks are the biggest source of sugars in American diets (33 percent of added sugars), and to list the euphemisms under which sugars are hidden on food labels (corn syrup, fruit juice concentrates, invert sugar).

assuming that you even know what they are. Such are the realities of dietary advice.

I cannot resist pointing out that the concern about too much sugar in the American diet is not new. In 1942, a committee of the American Medical Association saw fit to comment on what it viewed as an alarming eleven-fold increase in sugars in American diets since 1821—to 108 pounds per capita per year (just 60 percent of present levels). The committee was especially concerned about the rapid increase in the per capita supply of soft drinks to three 6-ounce bottles—remember those?—per week. It said:

> Indiscriminate and uncontrolled supply of poor food for between-meal eating cannot be condoned with impunity anywhere . . . Restrictions in the use of sugar will help improve the nutritive quality of American diets. From the health point of view it is desirable especially to have restriction of . . . consumption of sweetened carbonated beverages and forms of candy which are of low nutritional value. The Council believes it would be in the interest of the public health for all practical means to be taken to limit consumption of sugar in any form in which it fails to be combined with significant proportions of other foods of high nutritive quality.

Ah for the good old days. This advice made sense in 1942, and it still does.

SELLING SUGAR(S)

If you cannot help liking sweet foods, it is for a good reason. Humans are born with a predilection for sweetness to stimulate sucking reflexes. Breast milk is sweet because it contains lactose, a double sugar of glucose and galactose. So it is normal to like sweet foods.

But marketers encourage supermarket displays of sugary foods with advertising expenditures large enough (or so it seems) to end world poverty. In 2004, for example, PepsiCo spent $212 million on media advertising for soft drinks; it spent an additional $142 million for Gatorade (which is basically sugar water with a little salt). Coca-Cola spent $246 million to promote Coke products and $45 million for Sprite. Mars spent $73 million to advertise Snickers bars, and Altria's Kraft Foods allotted $50 million for Jell-O, $21 million for Kool-Aid, and $11 million for Crème Savers Candy. These figures are only for measurable media advertising. The USDA estimates that for every dollar the companies spend that way, they spend another two dollars on marketing strategies like coupons, slotting fees, trade shows, and direct mail; if so, you have to multiply all those numbers by three to get the big picture.

> Humans are born with a predilection for sweetness to stimulate sucking reflexes. Breast milk is sweet because it contains lactose, a double sugar of glucose and galactose. So it is normal to like sweet foods.

Late in 2004, Coca-Cola said it would "return to world-class marketing" and spend an additional $400 million a year to boost flagging sales of its products, but market analysts thought that amount would not be nearly enough and that $600 million would be needed to accomplish that task. I have trouble getting a feel for amounts of money that large. If you take just the $11 million Kraft/Altria spent advertising Crème Savers—one candy product among thousands on supermarket shelves—it still amounts to more than five times the largest amount of money ever spent by the U.S. government on the Five-a-Day for Better Health campaign to encourage people to eat more fruits and vegetables. Does spending that kind of money in marketing get people to buy the advertised products? It most definitely does. And you hardly have a chance against the onslaught of marketing methods that companies can buy with that kind of money.

That is because enticements to buy sweet foods in supermarkets do not end with advertising, product placements, and coupon campaigns. They also include the ways foods are priced. Foods containing corn sweeteners are cheap, and soft drinks—the principal source of caloric sweeteners in American diets—are especially cheap to make. And why not? Water is practically free, corn syrup costs only pennies per bottle, and flavor additives are used in tiny amounts. The main costs to manufacturers are in packaging and labor and, of course, in advertising and marketing. That is why bigger sizes are almost always a bargain; the cost of the actual ingredients in the product is trivial compared to the costs of bringing the product to market.

Coping with this situation calls for firm determination. To make it easier on yourself, you can decide never to set foot in the aisles devoted to soft drinks and candy. If you must have sweet drinks, stick with juices (preferably the ones with pulp). But nutritious as they are, fruit juices still have sugar calories—about 100 in 8 ounces—and those calories add up. To avoid sugars in other foods, you will have to read ingredient labels. If an ingredient ends with "syrup" or "–ose," it's a sugar; if it is honey or fruit concentrate, it is still sugar(s). If you want package labels to be easier to understand, you will want to join the campaign of the Center for Science in the Public Interest. In 1999, this group petitioned the FDA to establish a Daily Value of 40 grams for added sugars. This, of course, is precisely the amount in just *one* 12-ounce soda—the equivalent of two of those 1942 bottles. It is disappointing—but not surprising—that the FDA has not acted on this petition.

> That is why bigger sizes are almost always a bargain; the cost of the actual ingredients in the product is trivial compared to the costs of bringing the product to market.

28

Cereals: Sweet and Supposedly Healthy

I f you want to keep up with the latest developments in food market-ing, the processed cereal aisle is the best place to begin. Early in 2005, I came across a box of Post Frosted Shredded Wheat with a big heart on its front panel. But instead of the usual "Helps lower choles-terol or the risk of heart disease," which appears on practically all boxes of cereals aimed at adults, this one said: "Lose 10 lbs. The Heart Healthy Way (see back for details)." I immediately turned the box over: "That's right! Research by a leading cardiologist shows that people who ate 2 bowls of Post Healthy Classics cereals each day, as part of a reduced calorie diet, LOST 10 LBS* and reduced their risk factors for heart disease . . ." You can do this at home, the box tells you, in just three easy steps:

- Replace 2 meals a day with a serving of any Post Healthy Classics cereal, ½ cup fat-free milk and fruit.
- Focus on portion control at mealtimes.
- Add more physical activities into your day.

Good advice. Replacing a meal with a cereal serving (presumably just one) will surely reduce your caloric intake. Eating less and moving more is always an effective way to lose weight, and quickly. But I badly wanted to know what the research showed. I followed the asterisk to this: "*Weight loss achieved over a 12 week period. 50% of subjects lost 10 or more lbs . . . Consult your physician before starting any diet or exercise program . . ." This was followed by the Web address, and I went right to it. The Post company is owned by Kraft Foods (which, in turn, is owned by Altria) so I was not surprised to find myself at the Kraft site, and it took only a few clicks to identify the leading cardiologist as Dr. James Rippe of Tufts University and the Rippe Lifestyle Institute. Rippe's institute conducts clinical studies for many corporate clients, Post among them.

Anyone would lose weight under this study's conditions, cereal or no cereal. Rippe's research subjects were eating just 1,400 or 1,500 calories a day, well below the usual 2,000 to 2,500 calories a day needed by most adults. So Kraft/Post/Altria is not misleading you; its marketers just want you to think that there is something special about Post cereals that will help you lose weight. You can eat nothing but candy bars and lose weight if you do not eat too many of them during the day.

> Y ou can eat nothing but candy bars and lose weight if you do not eat too many of them during the day.

The advertising of ready-to-eat cereals as weight-loss products must be understood as an especially creative attempt to increase sales in a dismal business market. Four companies control 83 percent of commercial cereal sales: General Mills (32 percent), Kellogg (31 percent), Post/Kraft/Altria (14 percent), and Quaker/PepsiCo (6 percent). Big Four Cereal explains why all those boxes look alike and are priced alike. This may appear as peaceful coexistence, but these companies are endlessly jockeying for a greater share of what everyone considers a "soggy" market for breakfast cereals. The peak year for cereal buying was 1994. Sales of Big Four Cereals fell by 5 percent between 1997 and 2002 and by another 2 percent just from 2004 to 2005 (a year in which sales of store brands increased by 2 percent). Marketers would like to reverse these downward trends.

You might think that dropping cereal into a bowl, pouring milk onto it, and sitting down and eating it is so easy and quick that even a child can do it, but apparently this is not easy or quick enough for today's busy people. Bagels, toaster pastries, and anything else that can be eaten on the run give breakfast cereals stiff competition. Corporate cereal marketers have to work hard to make their products catch your eye—and the attention of your children—among competitors' boxes mixed in with the less expensive store brands, and all crowded together on hundreds of feet of shelf space. Thanks to slotting fees, the hard-to-reach top shelves often hold the less profitable high-fiber, reduced-sugar products aimed at health-conscious consumers. The Big Four Cereal companies pay for prime, eye-level real estate for heavily advertised cereals targeted to a mass audience. Nearly all decorate their boxes with large hearts and banners proclaiming health benefits. The bottom shelves hold the larger packages, but sometimes are reserved for the cereals marketed to small children. You can see this convenient placement in action any time toddlers are let loose in the cereal section. They recognize their "own" cereals by the cartoons on the front panel and the banners advertising how much like "candy" these cereals can be: "sweetened," "fun-colored," or "fun-filled" with marshmallows or chocolate. These are cereals gone processed and a far cry from what whole grains do for health.

THE VALUE OF BREAKFAST CEREALS

Let me confess right away that I am not much of a breakfast eater in the typical sense. I do not wake up feeling hungry and usually do not feel like eating until later in the morning than most people do. I am well aware that everyone says breakfast is the most important meal of the day, but I am not convinced. What you eat—and how much—matters more to your health than when you eat. But you are an adult; children are another matter. Many studies show that children who eat breakfast have better overall diets, are healthier, and learn better than children who do not. The research on the importance of breakfast for adults, however, is less conclusive, not least because so many such studies are sponsored by cereal companies. Cereal companies not only have a vested interest in getting you and your children to eat breakfast; they also want you to think that breakfast means *cereal*.

W hat you eat—and how much— matters more to your health than when you eat.

Cereals do indeed contribute to nutritious breakfasts (but so can other foods). Cereals—wheat, corn, and rice—are the starchy agricultural basis of civilization; their calories and nutrients feed the world. Add soy or other beans and you have a protein as good as any that comes from an animal. Add a fruit or milk to your cereal and you have the entire range of required nutrients. Adults who habitually eat whole grains have lower rates of heart disease than those who do not. But the full nutrient value only comes when the grains are whole or unprocessed, and are "good carbs." Once the outer layer of the grain has been removed, the starch calories come with fewer nutrients and have been converted to rapidly absorbable "bad carbs." Even though refined wheat flour is enriched with five nutrients, and white rice is parboiled to drive the nutrients from its bran into the starch, most of the fiber and some of the nutritional value has been lost. Processing cereal grains into flakes, circles, and puffs often makes the starches even less nutritious. Whole grains help protect against disease and the metabolic problems sometimes caused by rapid absorption of carbohydrates. Highly processed grains do not.

Wheat production is subsidized by the government and grains are abundant and cheap. But processing makes grain foods last longer without spoiling so manufacturers prefer them that way. When manufacturers add sugar and vitamins and put cereals into attractive boxes, they "add value" and can charge more for them. And much is at stake. Here are some examples of annual sales of popular ready-to-eat breakfast cereals.

Sales of the Top Five Ready-to-Eat Breakfast Cereals in the United States, 2003[*]

BRAND	UNITS SOLD	SALES
	Millions of units	Millions of dollars
Cheerios (General Mills)	101	$290
Frosted Flakes (Kellogg)	89	$237
Honey Nut Cheerios (General Mills)	75	$235
Honey Bunches of Oats (Post)	79	$212
Cinnamon Toast Crunch (General Mills)	53	$165

*Numbers are rounded off.

The amount of shelf space devoted to such products and the size of their advertising budgets also tell you how much is at stake for their manufacturers. In 2003, advertising spending for the top five cereals ranged from more than $7 million for Kellogg Frosted Flakes to $42 million for General Mills Honey Nut Cheerios. Overall, advertising spending for breakfast cereals defies belief. In 2004, Kellogg spent about $255 million, General Mills $250 million, Post (Kraft/Altria) $120 million, and Quaker (PepsiCo) $75 million—just for media advertising. If these numbers really do have to be multiplied by three to account for the costs of slotting fees, coupons, trade shows, and direct mail, the Big Four Cereal companies are paying well over $2 billion a year to get you to buy breakfast cereals. The absurdity of this expense—which, given the sales figures, is obviously worth it to the companies—explains much of the absurdity of health claims on cereal boxes.

Breakfast cereals are supposed to be good for you, and the relatively unprocessed ones still are, but most are now so thoroughly processed and sugared and filled with additives that they might as well be cookies. You can hardly find a cereal without added vitamins, so let's call them vitamin-enriched, lowfat cookies. Some *are* cookies. Post's Oreo O's, for example: "Extreme creme taste cereal with marshmallow bits made with the genuine taste of Nabisco Oreo." You will be relieved to learn that this cereal is "Cholesterol free, excellent source of six B vitamins, and iron & zinc for growth." Of course it is cholesterol free; cereals are plants and cholesterol comes only from animal foods. The first three ingredients are corn, oat, and wheat flour, but these are followed immediately by sugar and marshmallow bits; sugars in one form or another turn up six times in the list of ingredients.

Breakfast cereals are supposed to be good for you, and the relatively unprocessed ones still are, but most are now so thoroughly processed and sugared and filled with additives that they might as well be cookies.

Nutrients are a major selling point for ready-to-eat cereals, so I had best say something about the whole question of added vitamins and minerals. Virtually all breakfast cereals add some. Without question, nutrient-fortified cereals contribute to the nutrient intake of Americans. They provide a significant fraction—5 to 20 percent—of the four vitamins and iron that companies are required to add to white flour, as well as others like vitamin B_6 and zinc that companies add voluntarily. One cereal serving usually takes care of 10 to 25 percent of the amounts you need of those particular nutrients for an entire day, and "Total" types give you 100 percent of the Daily Values. You still have to get the rest of the nutrients you need from other foods or from supplements. Are cereals the best way to get these few vitamins and minerals into your diet? I prefer mine from less-processed foods—you get all the ones you need that way along with the other good things, like fiber and phytochemicals, that you can never get from processed breakfast cereals.

Oreo O's, for example, have virtually no fiber (less than a gram per serving) and that amount is typical. Besides calories, the main virtue of cereals is fiber, which comes from the outside bran layers of seeds—the parts that are discarded when flour is refined. Fiber does good things for your digestive system and slows down carbohydrate absorption, but through 2004, the flour in most breakfast cereals was refined and the fiber scarce. Late that year, General Mills announced that its cereals, among them sweetened ones like Lucky Charms and Honey Nut Cheerios, soon would be made with whole grains. "Whole grains," said *Advertising Age*, "are the food industry's next holy grail"—the key to boosting sales in a declining market.

Whole grains? In January 2005, I found the first of the new line of General Mills cereals in a local store: Basic 4, "A **delicious** blend of sweet and tangy **fruits**, crunchy **nuts** and a wholesome variety of **grains**." Basic 4, say little tokens in the "Goodness Corner" General Mills places in the upper right corner on the front of its cereal boxes, is a "good source" of whole grain and fiber. And the ingredients do sound promising, with cornmeal, wheat bran, and whole grain barley and oats among those first on the list. But together they provide just 3 grams of fiber in a 200-calorie serving (240 with skim milk). That does not seem like much, considering that plenty of other cereals have more, among them General Mills Total Raisin Bran with 5 grams of fiber in 170 calories. Basic 4 may be "a low fat part of your heart healthy diet," but that does not make it a health food. The fruit and nuts do appear in the top half of the list of 44 ingredients, but the rest are preservatives, artificial colors and flavors, the added vitamins and minerals—and sugars, of course. Basic 4 lists 14 grams of sugars per serving (1 tablespoon) and sugars appear nine times in its list of ingredients (twelve if you count the natural sugars in raisins, cranberries, and dried apples).

The sugars in Basic 4 are added, but Nutrition Facts labels do not distinguish between natural and added sugars; the 1 tablespoon of sugars per serving in this cereal is typical of most presweetened types. Total Raisin Bran has 20 grams of sugars per serving but that is in part because raisins are naturally sweet; raisins have 100 calories per ounce, and 80 of those calories come from naturally occurring sugars. From the industry standpoint, cereals are a great way to add value to sugars; if you like your cereals sweetened, it is much less expensive to add your own.

It is not easy to figure out what the deal is on sugars in breakfast cereals these days. Public concerns about the role sugars play in obesity have made cereal companies take notice of the amounts added, and most have reduced the sweetness to the minimum they think you will tolerate. The sugars in Basic 4 work out to less than 30 percent of the calories in the cereal; in the ultra-sweet world of Big Four Cereals, this percentage is low. Oreo O's have 12 grams of sugars per 110-calorie serving, less than a tablespoon; this may not seem like much but the sugars comprise 44 percent of the calories. It helps to have a calculator with you in the cereal aisle.

Cereal companies surely must manipulate serving sizes to their own advantage, but I cannot figure out the logic to their system unless it is to minimize the apparent sugar content. Some cereals are puffier than others and take up more space in the bowl, but that cannot be the entire reason why the serving sizes are so inconsistent: ½ cup (Post Great Grains), ⅔ cup (Kellogg's Low-Fat Granola), ¾ cup (Quaker Life), 1 cup (Post Alpha-Bits), 1¼ cups (Kellogg's Rice Krispies),

> From the industry standpoint, cereals are a great way to add value to sugars; if you like your cereals sweetened, it is much less expensive to add your own.

1⅓ cups (General Mills Total Corn Flakes), or 24 biscuits (Kellogg's Frosted Mini-Wheats). The weights of these servings vary from 1 to 2 ounces, and the sugar content from 3 to 20 grams. Go figure. I can't.

I like crunchy breakfast cereals and am happy to see that high-fiber ones are readily available—usually on the top shelves and out of reach of small children. I look for three things in ready-to-eat cereals: a short ingredient list (besides the vitamins that manufacturers are required to add), lots of fiber, and little or no added sugars. The fiber is easiest; every big company makes cereals that have at least 20 percent of the day's fiber goal—their names almost always include the words "fiber" or "bran." "Whole grain," as I will soon explain, does not necessarily mean "high fiber." Sugars are a problem: I would much prefer to add my own sugar to cereals, but it is difficult to find unsweetened cereals except in a store's health food section. But if you see an ingredient list on a Big Four Cereal with zero sugars, watch out: the cereal may contain artificial sweeteners like aspartame or Splenda (I deal with these in a later chapter). Overall, most Big Four Cereals are vitamin-enriched desserts, but cleverly marketed with claims for health benefits that may have some scientific justification, though only in the context of everything else you eat or do.

HEALTH CLAIMS: WHOLE GRAINS VERSUS FIBER

Claims about nutrient contents help to sell breakfast cereals, which is the real reason why companies add more vitamins and minerals than they are required to. But claims that food products can help prevent disease are even more effective sales techniques. It is no accident that practically every Big Four Cereal aimed at adults displays a heart on the front of almost every box. Post Raisin Bran, for example, displays a big spoonful of cereal in front of a large red heart with a banner: "May help REDUCE the risk of HEART DISEASE because it is rich in fiber." You have to look carefully to find the small and indistinct qualifying statement required by the FDA: "Diets rich in fiber-containing grain products, fruits and vegetables and low in saturated fat and cholesterol may reduce your risk of heart disease, a disease associated with many factors." Translation: this cereal helps prevent heart disease if you eat a good diet anyway.

The real reason for health claims is well established: health claims

> The real reason for health claims is well established: health claims sell food products.

sell food products. In my book *Food Politics,* I told the story of how Kellogg got around FDA restrictions on health claims in 1984 by working directly with the National Cancer Institute to allow these words on packages of All-Bran cereal:

> The National Cancer Institute believes eating the right foods may reduce your risk of cancer. Here are their recommendations: Eat high fiber foods. A growing body of evidence says high fiber foods are important to good health. That's why a healthy diet includes high fiber foods like bran cereals.

The result? A 47 percent increase in the market share of All-Bran within the first six months of using the claim. This message was not lost on Big Four Cereal companies.

Cereal boxes did not always display hearts and health claims, and the Kellogg claim broke a long-standing barrier. Prior to 1990, the FDA did not allow claims about disease prevention on food packages. The Nutrition Labeling and Education Act of 1990, the law that gave us Nutrition Facts labels, forced the FDA to authorize health claims on food package labels. Before that act, the FDA viewed claims for the health benefits of foods as equivalent to claims for the health benefits of pharmaceutical drugs. If a food label said that the product could reduce the risk of heart disease or cancer, the FDA expected the company to prove it with scientific studies, just as it expected pharmaceutical companies to do with drugs said to reduce cholesterol levels. Food companies knew that this would be impossible. There is no way they could possibly prove that eating a particular breakfast cereal prevents heart disease or cancer. How could it? A cereal is only one food consumed by people who eat many different foods and who also differ in many other genetic and behavioral ways that can affect the risk of these diseases.

Instead, companies lobbied for the right to "inform the public" about the health benefits of their products. When Congress was about to enact the labeling law, food companies pressed hard for permission to make health claims. Congress agreed, and said the FDA would have to authorize health claims that were backed by "significant scientific agreement." Congress directed the FDA to consider approving ten specific claims about nutrients and health that were most requested by food companies.

The FDA reviewed the science and approved some of the claims, but denied others. Food companies that were affected by the denials complained and continued lobbying. Eventually, two subsequent acts of Congress and numerous court decisions further weakened the FDA's restrictions on health claims. In 1994, the Dietary Supplement Health and Education Act authorized structure/function claims—claims on the labels of herbal and other supplements that the products might improve some structure or function of the body. In response, food companies successfully sued the FDA for the right to make "structure/function" claims for foods. In 1997, the FDA Modernization Act required the FDA to allow health claims that could be "substantiated" by statements made by federal agencies or the National Academy of Sciences (now called the National Academies). This may sound impressive, but it is a less restrictive standard than "significant scientific agreement."

After 1997, practically any time the FDA said no to a petition for a health claim, the company took the FDA to court, and the courts usually ruled in favor of the companies—on First Amendment grounds of freedom of speech. Any sensible person might think that the Founding Fathers devised the First Amendment to protect political dissent rather than the right of food marketers to use overblown health claims on cereal boxes. But that is how the courts interpret this constitutional amendment, and the FDA chose not to press alternative legal arguments.

> It is one thing to say, as federal agencies do, that eating whole-grain foods is associated with protection against heart disease and cancer, but quite another to demonstrate that eating a specific breakfast cereal will protect you against those diseases.

The results began to appear on supermarket shelves in 1999. That year, General Mills said it intended to claim that some of its cereals protected against heart disease and certain cancers because they contain whole grains. Whole grains, as I explained in the chapter on food processing, are just that: they are whole or ground seeds of wheat, corn, rice, or other crop plants and contain all of the nutrients and fiber in those seeds. It is one thing to say, as federal agencies do, that eating whole-grain foods is associated with protection against heart disease and cancer, but quite another to demonstrate that eating a specific breakfast cereal will protect you against those diseases.

The ingredient list of the General Mills Basic 4 cereal, for example, starts out like this: cornmeal, wheat bran with other parts of wheat, whole grain barley, whole grain oats; these are followed by forty other ingredients. This cereal does indeed contain whole grains, but it is not especially high in fiber. Under the terms of the Modernization Act, however, the FDA had little choice but to acquiesce. General Mills celebrated with a full-page advertisement in *The New York Times*:

> A whole new way to defend yourself. The FDA agrees that eating whole grain foods like Cheerios, Wheaties and Total as part of a low fat diet may reduce your risk of heart disease and some cancers. So help defend yourself with a good whole grain breakfast from General Mills.

With the FDA in passive "agreement" and no longer requiring rigorous scientific justification for health claims, the amount of whole grain necessary for a cereal to qualify for the claim is difficult to deduce. In 2005, General Mills announced that all of its cereals would be made with whole grains and reprinted all of its boxes with banners saying so. This meant that Cocoa Puffs and Count Chocula cereals now had 1 gram of fiber per serving, instead of zero. These cereals do have whole grains, but not much fiber. Late in 2005, the FDA said no to a petition from General Mills asking for permission to label its cereals as "good" or "excellent" sources of whole grain. The agency said it wanted to think first about what companies would have to put in cereals and snack foods in order to call them "whole grain."

Does putting "whole grains" on a cereal box help to sell it? Yes, it does. In the two months following the release of the 2005 *Dietary Guidelines for Americans*, sales of whole grain cereals increased by 16 percent. As companies began marketing more and more cereals with health claims, mostly for prevention of heart disease, they also introduced structure/function claims previously allowed only for dietary supplements. In spring 2004, I found boxes of General Mills Raisin Bran Total with this banner on the front panel: "HELP MAINTAIN A HEALTHY IMMUNE SYSTEM with 100% of vitamin E and Zinc." This cereal may have more vitamin E and zinc than other Raisin Bran types, but will it really fix your immunodeficiency condition if you happen to have one? Of course not, but do not bother looking for a disclaimer. In passing the Dietary Supplement Act of 1994, Congress specified that structure/function claims do not have to be accompanied by statements that put the supposed benefits in the context of the total diet. So the box does not have to say that the rest of your life has to be healthful to gain immune system benefits from this particular cereal.

The General Mills marketing department especially likes health claims; the one for Corn Flakes Total in spring 2004 said "LOSE MORE WEIGHT with 100% Daily Value of Calcium." This statement did come with a disclaimer, but I had to put glasses on to read it: "as part of a reduced calorie diet." Not to be outdone, Post (Kraft/Altria) sponsored the study showing how you too can lose ten pounds by eating a Post sweetened cereal—when you eat less and move more, of course.

WHAT ABOUT ORGANIC CEREALS?

I bought a box of Cascadian Farm organic Wheat Crunch: "Crispy *organic* whole wheat and rice flakes touched with brown sugar." The front panel comes with three symbols of healthfulness: a red "heart healthy" design, an FDA-approved health claim ("In a low fat diet, whole grain foods like Wheat Crunch may reduce the risk of heart disease"); and a USDA Certified Organic seal. The seal means that the ingredients were grown without pesticides, herbicides, or chemical fertilizers, and were not genetically modified or irradiated. It also means that the farm was inspected, in this case by someone from the Washington State agriculture department, to make sure its production methods were consistent with USDA organic standards.

The first ingredient in this cereal is organic whole wheat, followed by organic rice, and, if I counted right, eleven added vitamins and minerals. Four of seven other ingredients are added sugars: organic naturally milled sugar (cane sugar and brown sugar), organic cane syrup, organic honey, and organic molasses, but these add up to just 6 grams per serving, low by the standards of most processed cereals. Like most processed cereals this one does not have much fiber—just 2 grams per serving.

The box lists the distributor of Cascadian Farm as a company called

Small Planet Foods in Washington State. Small Planet sounds great—local and environmentally friendly—and I wanted to know more about it. Oops. The company was sold to General Mills in 1999. This sale, as I learned from the Cascadian Farm Web site (www.cascadianfarm.com), "afford[ed] us the opportunity to bring our products to even more people around the country." No doubt.

The General Mills purchase made me wonder if organic cereals differed in other ways from cereals made from conventionally grown crops. In July 2005, I bought boxes of the company's Cascadian Farm Honey Nut O's and Honey Nut Cheerios at the Wegmans market in Ithaca, and did a quick comparison.

> O rganic ingredients do not convert processed cereals to health foods, but if you care about how foods are grown, organic cereals are worth looking for.

Conventional Versus Organic "O" Cereals Made by General Mills

PER 1 CUP SERVING (1 OUNCE)	HONEY NUT CHEERIOS CONVENTIONAL ($2.69 for 14 ounces)	HONEY NUT O'S ORGANIC ($3.99 for 12 ounces)
Calories	120	120
Fiber (grams)	2	2
Sugars (grams)	11	8
Price per ounce	19¢	33¢

This tells you that there are only two differences between the two cereals: the organic ingredients and the price you pay for them. Nutritionally speaking, both are processed cereals, and indistinguishable for all practical purposes (the difference in sugars is only half a teaspoon and not worth fussing about). The nearly twofold difference in price explains why Big Four Cereal is so interested in acquiring organic line extensions. Organic ingredients do not convert processed cereals to health foods, but if you care about how foods are grown, organic cereals are worth looking for. I look for cereals higher in fiber than the one in the Table. General Mills makes some (Cascadian Farms Hearty Morning, for example), as does Kellogg, which owns the Kashi line of organics.

Supermarkets like Wegmans separate the organic and high-fiber cereals from other Big Four Cereal (and small cereal) products and stock them in special health food sections. Research shows that the "healthier" options sell better that way. There you might find Uncle Sam Toasted Whole-Grain Wheat Flakes with flaxseed providing a hefty 2,000 milligrams of omega-3 fatty acids per 2-ounce serving. This cereal has a total of just seven ingredients (whole wheat kernels, whole flaxseed, barley malt, salt, and three vitamins) with a lot of fiber per serving—10 grams—and less than 1 gram of sugars. The box sports something I had not seen before in the United States: a "Low Glycemic" seal. This comes from Glycemic Solutions, a research group in Washington, D.C., that tests foods (and pet foods) containing sugars and starches to see how much of a rise in blood sugar—glycemic response—you get when you eat them. After tasting the cereal, I had no trouble believing that it does not produce much of a glycemic response. I thought it was good, but could use some sugar.

You may also have to go to the health food section to find the granolas and mueslis. These start out with oats, wheat, other grains, or soy, and sometimes add seeds, nuts, dried fruits, or all three. Some are organic, some not. These cereals are crunchy and delicious, as well you might expect for something toasted in oil and sweetened with the more "natural" forms of sugars—juice concentrates, fructose, raw sugar, cane sugar, honey, or maple syrup, and, sometimes, all of the above. The big issue with granolas and mueslis is calories. Depending on the ingredients, the calories can run to 150 or so for a tiny one-quarter cup serving. If you care about calories, these products are best used sprinkled on fruit or yogurt and not piled into a bowl the way you might with a puffier cereal.

ON DEALING WITH CEREALS

By this time, you can appreciate why I so enjoy the cereal aisle. I like reading the health claims on the processed cereals and wondering what marketers will dream up next. The packages are, in their weird way, fun to look at. They represent the best thinking of marketers about how to get you to eat processed cereals, to believe that they are good for you, and to insist that nothing else will do for breakfast.

Fortunately, the slotting-fee system makes it easier to find the healthier options. All you have to do is look for the worst real estate and reach high or off to the sides for the ones with short ingredient lists, lots of fiber, and not much sugar. Check the health food section to see if the store offers organic options, and choose them to encourage more environmentally friendly food production. If you like your cereal sweeter, you can always add your own sugar and still come out ahead. High-fiber, whole-grain cereals, with milk and fruit added, make a fine breakfast and one that is a lot more nutritious than a bagel or roll made with processed flour, or a pastry loaded with fat and sugars.

Let me close with one last comment about the "Goodness Corners" on boxes of General Mills cereals. The three little round tokens on the front of the boxes display health messages like "good source of whole grains," "low fat," "excellent source of iron," "12 vitamins and minerals," and so forth. The tokens are clever. The FDA has rules about such statements and General Mills follows them, but the same claims could be made for any food of comparable nutritional value, unprocessed as well as processed. You have to credit the company's marketers for adding vitamins and finding other ways to make even their most sugary cereals look like health foods.

But that is not all that cereal companies do to make their products look healthier. They also get medical and health organizations to endorse—or appear to endorse—the health benefits of their products. How that system works comes next.

> High-fiber, whole-grain cereals, with milk and fruit added, make a fine breakfast and one that is a lot more nutritious than a bagel or roll made with processed flour, or a pastry loaded with fat and sugars.

29

Packaged Foods:
Health Endorsements

Because health claims increase product sales, food companies also use alliances with medical authorities to appeal to health-conscious adults in the same way that they use alliances with sports celebrities to appeal to kids. But cereal, snack food, and drink companies get plenty of active assistance in marketing their products from health professionals. Let's take one more look at cereal boxes, beginning with General Mills Cookie Crisp. General Mills does not bother to pretend that Cookie Crisp is anything other than a cookie, and one that offers "a mouthful of chips in every bite" at that. Even so, a side panel on the container displays a red heart with a white check mark, and these words:

> **American Heart Association.** Meets American Heart Association food criteria for saturated fat and cholesterol for healthy people over age 2. While many factors affect heart disease, diets low in saturated fat and cholesterol may reduce the risk of this disease.

This and other such statements on the boxes of processed foods can be there for only one purpose: to convince you that these foods are good for you and your children. What is the American Heart Association logo doing on a box of sugary cereals aimed at children? Let's take a look.

The American Heart Association authorizes its "food criteria" statement on many General Mills cereals, among them such sugary treats as Lucky Charms, Count Chocula, and Cocoa Puffs. The statement also appears on cereals like Kellogg Frosted Mini Wheats and Quaker (PepsiCo) Frosted Shredded Wheat. Like all breakfast cereals, which are based on plant seeds, these are low in saturated fat and cholesterol. Plant oils are low in saturated fat and never have cholesterol. But these cereals are not low in calories or sugars. Sugars have calories. Calories contribute to weight gain. Obesity is a risk factor for heart disease.

But these are not the only surprising products that carry American Heart Association endorsements. In February 2004, I received a form letter from PepsiCo addressed to "Dear Influencer," announcing the first entry in its partnership with the American Heart Association for new product development: Rold Gold Heartzels. Packages of these heart-shaped pretzels, released just in time for Valentine's Day, carried the association's endorsement right over the heart design on the front of the pretzel package. These are a salty snack, even if less salty than other kinds of pretzels. Salt, as I will explain in the next chapter, causes blood pressure to rise in some people; high blood pressure increases the risk for heart disease and stroke.

So why, you might ask, is the American Heart Association involved in food endorsements? This is, after all, a venerable (since 1915) organization of medical and health professionals who volunteer their time and expertise to help the public reduce the risk of heart disease and stroke and the disabilities and deaths caused by these diseases. American Heart Association volunteers work hard to promote better access to disease treatment, to generate resources for research, and to support policies that encourage disease prevention. Its endorsement of food products as heart healthy would be expected to inspire confidence in consumers—and to stimulate sales of the endorsed products.

Setting up criteria for distinguishing "good" from "bad" foods is not nearly as simple a task as it might seem. Personally, I would not know how to begin to do something like this. I would have no trouble characterizing pure sugar and soft drinks as "bad" because they contribute calories but no other nutrients, but just about every other food contains at least some useful nutrients along with its calories. Foods vary greatly in their nutrient composition; some foods have more of one nutrient, while others have more of another. Establishing distinct cutoff points does not always make sense, especially when considering foods that are highly processed. And what about added nutrients? Does adding a few vitamins to a product made with refined flour make it as nutritious as something made with whole grain? Obviously not, but such problems did not seem to discourage the American Heart Association. It accepted the challenge and established its own criteria. To qualify for the association's endorsement, cereals and snack foods must

- be low in fat (less than or equal to 3 grams)
- be low in saturated fat (less than or equal to 1 gram)
- be low in cholesterol (less than or equal to 20 milligrams)
- have a sodium value of less than or equal to 480 milligrams for individual foods (20 percent of the Daily Value for a 2,000 calorie diet)
- contain at least 10 percent of the Daily Value of one or more of these nutrients: protein, vitamin A, vitamin C, calcium, iron, or dietary fiber

On the basis of these criteria, sugary cereals qualify because they are low in fat, saturated fat, cholesterol, and sodium; nearly all add one or another of the specified vitamins and minerals to levels of 10 percent to 25 percent of the Daily Values. Although fiber helps products like Rold Gold Heartzels to qualify, cereals do not have to have 10 percent of the Daily Value for fiber; they qualify on the other criteria. The criteria say nothing at all about sugars or refined carbohydrates. Requiring products to meet limits for sugars and refined carbohydrates would exclude the sugary cereals and some of the snack foods and drinks that the American Heart Association currently endorses—as well as the income derived from them.

The income is the sticking point. In *Food Politics*, I traced the history of controversy over the American Heart Association's food certification program, largely centered on the fees companies pay for participation. At the time I was researching that book, the association listed the fee schedule on its Web site. In 2000, it asked companies to contribute $7,500 per product for the first year of certification, and $4,500 for annual renewals, and companies got discounts if they paid the fees for more than ten products in one year. According to *The Wall Street Journal*, the association charged the same fees in mid-2004.

The American Heart Association, however, no longer provides that information on its Web site, and confirming the current fee schedule was not easy. For weeks I made telephone calls, left voice messages, and sent e-mails to national and local offices. Eventually a spokeswoman got back to me to say that the same fee schedule is still in place. The American Heart Association is doing important work to promote heart health, and I find it depressing that arrangements with food companies are not more transparent. This is particularly so because the food certification program is likely to provide only a small fraction of the association's annual income, reported as $653 million in 2004, one-third from donations.

But whatever the big cereal and snack food companies do have to pay for the endorsement, the cost is trivial in comparison to other advertising expenses. Companies can deduct the fees from their taxes as business expenses or, perhaps, as charitable donations. However the companies manage the fees, there can be little doubt that they consider the money well spent. On Mother's Day in 2004, PepsiCo displayed the American Heart Association Heartzels endorsement in a full-page color advertisement in *The New York Times*: "We [Heartzel] you Mom! . . . o grams *trans* fat, 10% of the Daily Value fiber and iron, 100% great taste." A marketing official from Frito-Lay/PepsiCo told a reporter from *Advertising Age* why the company displays the American Heart Association endorsement so prominently on the front of the Heartzels package. He said: "Health professionals are very trusted by consumers, and we want to help them help consumers place [Frito-Lay] products in their lives." Surely the American Heart Association has better things to do than to encourage people to eat Frito-Lay products, even if the organization uses the food certification funds for the worthiest of purposes.

I said earlier that the American Heart Association endorsement appears on sugary cereals from General Mills, Kellogg, and Quaker/PepsiCo. Noticeably absent from this collection are sugary cereals from the fourth major producer of ready-to-eat breakfast cereals—Post. There is a reason for this omission. In addition to setting nutritional criteria that products must meet in order to qualify for endorsement, the American Heart Association also sets criteria for social responsibility. Because cigarette smoking is a major risk factor for heart disease, the American Heart Association refuses to certify food products made by tobacco companies. This criterion firmly excludes breakfast cereals made by Post. Post, as I keep reminding you, is owned by Kraft Foods, and Kraft Foods is owned by Altria. Altria, you need to remember, owns Philip Morris cigarettes.

> Because cigarette smoking is a major risk factor for heart disease, the American Heart Association refuses to certify food products made by tobacco companies. This criterion firmly excludes breakfast cereals made by Post.

But that does not mean that Post cereals lack apparent "endorsements" from health organizations. Take a look at Post cereals like Honey Nut Shredded Wheat and Frosted Shredded Wheat. Both cereals have banners on the front saying "Helps reduce the risk of heart disease because it is rich in whole grains." Now look at the side panel. There, in bold letters, is **American Diabetes Association.** Can this be an endorsement of these presweetened cereals? Not at all. You have to look at the small print. Post, it seems, is:

A proud sponsor of
American Diabetes Association
Cure * Care * Commitment
www.kraftdiabeticchoices.com

The Web address takes you to Kraft "Life Can Still Taste Great!" products that meet the dietary requirements of people with diabetes. These are mostly sugar-free products, but they also include Post whole grain cereals, which happen to be presweetened. A visit to the Web site of the American Diabetes Association (www.diabetes.org) explains its relationship to Post. The association runs a corporate recognition program to thank the 150 or so companies that contribute to its operating funds each year. These are listed according to the size of the annual donation, with categories ranging from $15,000 to more than $750,000. Drug companies dominate the list, especially at the highest tiers, but plenty of food companies also participate. Kraft Foods appears in the second tier, called the "Banting Circle" after Dr. Frederick Banting, the Canadian pioneer in diabetes research. Companies at that level contributed at least $500,000 in 2004.

After hearing me speak about this sponsorship arrangement with Post cereals, Jane Brody, who has long reported for *The New York Times* Science section, wrote in September 2004 that the American Diabetes Association seemed like "a surprising bedfellow for a sweetened cereal, even one made from whole grain." The association, she said, told her it had changed its policy and would "no longer automatically permit such statements from companies that contribute to it." Perhaps, but more than a year later I was still finding the acknowledgment of Post's sponsorship of the American Diabetes Association on new boxes of Honey Nut and Frosted Shredded Wheat cereals.

I can well understand why Kraft might think it worthwhile to have something that looks like an endorsement (even if it is not) from the American Diabetes Association on its cereal boxes. But what criteria does the American Diabetes Association (ADA) use for permitting its name to be used in this way? It is instructive, if dismaying, to find the answer to this question in an interview given in May 2005 by Richard Kahn, the association's chief scientific and medical officer, to an unidentified writer from *Corporate Crime Reporter* (CCR). Two brief excerpts from their lengthy discussion will give you the idea.

> CCR: Do you allow the companies to put the ADA label on their product?
>
> KAHN: For some companies, we will allow them to indicate that they are a proud sponsor of the American Diabetes Association . . . If it is

a food company, it would be only on a product that meets our food guidelines, which are that the product has to be low in saturated fat and reduced in calories . . .

CCR: Why not just say that you are not going to take money from companies that are causing these problems [diabetes]?

KAHN: If we want to prevent diabetes, reduce the prevalence of obesity, help find the cure to diabetes, we have to get funds from someplace.

Progress report: During spring 2006, the American Diabetes Association reconsidered its sponsorship policies and removed its logo from Post (Kraft/Altria) cereal boxes, but American Heart Association endorsements remained on cereals and snack foods produced by companies that were not involved in marketing cigarettes.

30

Snack Foods: Sweet, Salty, and Caloric

T he huge SG Superstore in San Gabriel, California, caters to a largely Chinese-speaking immigrant community. The store prints all of its signs in Chinese characters as well as in English, and the one over aisle 14B says: SPEAR ASPARAGUS, MUSHROOMS, COOKIES, CANNED FISH, and—get this—JUNK FOOD. Chinese-speaking colleagues tell me that a more accurate translation of the characters for the last two words is "snack food," but the shelves hold exactly what you would expect: crackers, chips, pretzels, cookies, and the like.

"Junk" may seem unfairly pejorative when applied to foods you like to eat, but it works for conveying the idea that you would be better off eating something else. In nutrition-speak, junk foods are those of low nutritional value relative to their calories. They have lots of sugars (calories but no nutrients), starches (calories but not many nutrients), or fats (lots of calories), and are so heavily processed that they bear little resemblance to the starchy cereal grains or potatoes listed as their starting ingredients.

Processing "adds value." The growers of grains get only a few cents out of every dollar you spend on food, so government subsidies make the difference for many of them between earning a living and not. But subsidies also act as an incentive to grow more food; this increases supply and lowers the cost of the raw ingredients. Starchy root vegetables also are inexpensive as raw ingredients. But if you grind, refine, freeze, can, or cook these foods, and put them in a package with a well-advertised brand name on the label, people will pay a lot more for them. Take potatoes, for example. Raw, whole potatoes do not cost much and hardly seem profitable to anyone, but look what happens when manufacturers process them to "add value."

The Shelf Price of Potatoes, Raw and Processed, Key Foods Market, New York City, December 2004

POTATO TYPE	PRICE PER POUND
Idaho, raw	$0.79
Del Monte, canned new	$1.42
Ore-Ida frozen wedges	$2.49
Pillsbury (General Mills) mashed, box	$3.01
Ore-Ida frozen twice-baked	$4.30
Lays (PepsiCo) chips	$4.77
Lays Kettle cooked chips, extra crunchy	$5.14
Lays Ruffles chips, baked	$6.37
Lays Olean light chips (with the artificial fat, olestra)	$7.65
Terra (Hain Celestial) Yukon Gold chips	$10.21

The more than tenfold range in the price of potatoes from the raw ones you cook yourself to those that are peeled, canned, cooked, sliced, mashed, or fried into chips encourages food companies to make even more processed foods. Each year, American manufacturers introduce about 20,000 new products into supermarkets. In a typical year, these products might include 3,000 new candies; 3,000 snack foods; 2,000 soft drinks, juice drinks, and dairy drinks; 1,000 bakery products; and more than 100 new versions of breakfast cereals. Many such products are "line extensions"—variations in packaging or flavors (barbecued or cheese-flavored potato chips, for example). Most new products fail within a short time, but some succeed and repay the investment of their manufacturers. New products, as I explained earlier, are a "buy more" (and, therefore, an "eat more") strategy.

All too often, snack foods come at a nutritional price. The junk food aisles are filled with processed foods rich in "bad" carbohydrates (I put "bad" in quotation marks because these foods are not devoid of nutritional value; they just have fewer nutrients or more sugars, salt, and calories than the unprocessed versions). Counterintuitive as it may seem, whole potatoes are nutritious. They are not particularly high in calories; an ounce has just 30, because potatoes contain so much water. But take off their skins and there go the nutrients. Fry them in high-calorie cooking oil as chips or french fries, and the calories can run to 150 per ounce. With the fibrous skins gone, potato starch is quickly converted to glucose

> Counterintuitive as it may seem, whole potatoes are nutritious.

in the mouth and intestinal tract, and rapidly absorbed into your body. Eat too many skinless potatoes at one time and they can raise your blood sugar faster than your metabolism can handle it. Just like sugars, processed potatoes and other starchy foods are best eaten in modest amounts.

Because the basic ingredients are cheap, junk foods are highly profitable and companies want to sell more of them. Companies pay supermarkets to devote entire aisles to such products, which is why you see so many stores with hundreds of linear feet of potato chips, cookies, and crackers. And they spend a fortune promoting these products. Consider, for example, the annual sales and advertising figures for some of the best-selling snack foods in America, as indicated in the Table on the next page.

Sales like these make it easy to understand how a company like Campbell can spend $16 million a year to promote Pepperidge Farm Goldfish, or how Kellogg can spend $24 million just to promote Cheez-Its. Companies do get their money's worth. Spending $9 million to promote Oreo Cookies seems like a bargain next to sales of more than half a billion dollars a year. Kraft Foods makes many of the best-selling cookies and crackers, and in 2004 this company spent more than a billion dollars on marketing—but sold $32 billion worth of products worldwide. (Its parent company, Altria, spent $135 million promoting Philip Morris cigarettes, and these brought in $57 billion in sales that year.) On a smaller scale, Frito-Lay snacks brought in $9 billion for PepsiCo in 2003, just in North America. Do these expenditures influence preferences for such foods? If you do not respond to food marketing, you would be highly unusual; most people do.

Snack Food Sales and Media Advertising Expenditures, 2003[*]

PRODUCT (COMPANY)	SALES	MEDIA ADVERTISING
	Millions of units	Millions of dollars
Oreo Cookies (Kraft/Altria)	524	$9
Chips Ahoy Cookies (Kraft/Altria)	356	$3
Ritz Crackers (Kraft/Altria)	329	$17
Cheez-Its (Sunshine/Kellogg)	320	$24
Wheat Thins (Kraft/Altria)	277	$18
Goldfish (Pepperidge Farm/ Campbell Soup)	258	$16
Nature Valley Bars (General Mills)	147	$8
Chewy Granola Bars (Quaker/PepsiCo)	138	$13
Nutri-Grain Bars (Kellogg)	109	$25

Numbers are rounded off.

In part as one consequence of food marketing, snacking—eating between meals and after dinner—has become an increasingly common practice. Nutritionists already worried about this trend in the early 1980s before the obesity epidemic took off. At that time, about 70 percent of Americans reported eating at least one snack during the day, and snacks accounted for 20 percent of daily calorie intake. These foods accounted for smaller percentages of intakes of most nutrients, however, meaning that many of their calories were nutrient poor or "empty." The most popular snacks among teenagers in the early 1980s included baked goods, dairy desserts, and salty snacks, but also included more nutritious foods like milk, fruit, fruit juices, and bread.

M ore snacking is good news for the makers of snacks, but not such good news for waistlines. Snacks provide extra calories that most people do not need.

Since then, snacking has become even more common, and the snacks more junky. Now, more than 80 percent of Americans snack at least once a day, the average number of snacks is up by 14 percent, snack calories account for 23 percent of total calorie intake, soft drinks and juice drinks lead the pack—and the proportion of daily calories from salty snacks has doubled. More snacking is good news for the makers of snacks, but not such good news for waistlines. Snacks provide extra calories that most people do not need.

SELF-ENDORSEMENTS: PEPSICO'S "SMART SPOTS"

Health organization endorsements are such an effective marketing strategy that PepsiCo invented its own. The company spent $10 million in 2004 to develop "Smart Spot" labels—green circles with white check marks saying "Smart choices made easy." The spots now identify 200 or more PepsiCo products as "smart choices." The company explains to dietitians that these green symbols make it

> easier for your clients to spot food and beverage choices that contribute to healthier lifestyles . . . more than half of PepsiCo's new product revenues are coming from Smart Spot products . . . PepsiCo is committed to have at least half of its new U.S. products carry the Smart Spot symbol.

You might readily agree that Tropicana orange juice and Quaker Oats cereal qualify for Smart Spots, but you might wonder about some of the others: Tropicana Smoothies (48 grams of sugars and another 14 grams of carbohydrates per 11-ounce serving), Quaker Chewy Granola Bars (1 gram of fiber accompanied by cottonseed oil and nine kinds of sugars), Gatorade Energy Drink (salted sugar water), and Aunt Jemima Butter Lite Syrup (25 grams of sugars per quarter cup). The Rold Gold Heartzels pretzels that I discussed in the previous chapter qualify for the spots, and so do the baked (as opposed to fried) versions of Cheetos, Doritos, and Potato Crisps. All of these products meet the company's nutrition criteria, which are based on "authoritative statements from the FDA and the National Academy of Sciences."

In practice, PepsiCo's criteria pretty much adhere to FDA guidelines for calling products "low" or "reduced." To qualify, a product must have no more than zero grams of *trans* fat, 1 gram of saturated fat, 60 milligrams of cholesterol, or 270 milligrams of sodium per serving, and must have no more than 35 percent of its calories from fat. Alternatively, the product may have any of those nutrients at a level 25 percent below the level in the original version. I wonder if independent evaluators would consider PepsiCo products "smart" choices from a nutritional point of view—or just agree that this is "smart" marketing.

To be fair, PepsiCo does not explicitly claim that its Smart Spot–labeled sodas, sports drinks, juice drinks, cereals, or snacks are good for you. I learned this on a cross-country flight to Los Angeles, when I found myself sitting next to a man reading a stack of documents prominently displaying the PepsiCo logo. He told me he worked for PepsiCo analyzing trends that might affect new product development. When I told him that I thought the Smart Spots might mislead consumers into thinking junk foods were health foods, he accused me of being cynical and said I misunderstood the situation. PepsiCo, he said, does not claim that Smart Spots identify foods as healthy; the spots just mark the better choices. The spot, he said, means that PepsiCo considers Gatorade to be a better choice because it has about half the calories and sugars of a regular Pepsi. Fortunately for him the plane landed before he had to endure hearing more about my skepticism that small nutritional improvements in junk foods really do make them better choices.

PepsiCo explains the rationale behind its Smart Spots strategy this way: "If the rudder on a ship is slightly moved it will change the course and destination of the ship . . . Likewise the principle of *small changes making big differences in outcome* is true in health." The company gives an example on the Smart Spot Web site (www.smartspot.com): if you substitute Baked Lays Potato Crisps for Lays Regular Potato Chips, you will save 40 calories per ounce. Make this substitution once a day, and you save 40 calories, which over the course of a year adds up to a 4-pound weight loss. Although the Web site cites references to scientific studies, none of them demonstrates that substituting Baked Lays for regular potato chips helps people lose weight, no doubt because a difference of 40 calories a day is too small to make a dent in the 3,500 calories you need to reduce to lose a pound of body fat. Small dietary changes— like substituting one slightly "better" junk food for another—may indeed make a difference to your health, but only if you make many such changes throughout your entire diet.

Whether the average consumer cares about the subtle distinction between the "healthy" or "better" meaning of the Smart Spot, PepsiCo thinks its healthier products will sell well. As a PepsiCo executive told *Nutrition Business Journal* in 2004:

> S mall dietary changes—like substituting one slightly "better" junk food for another—may indeed make a difference to your health, but only if you make many such changes throughout your entire diet.

Our eyes have been opened to new opportunities that we have . . . Since *Tostitos* are usually eaten with salsa . . . you have lycopene [a phytonutrient from tomatoes] and other types of health products. What we're looking at is what is the right way to communicate that to consumers. You will definitely . . . see us becoming more aggressive in the area . . . Fundamentally, we sell a lot of whole grain products, products with healthy oils and vegetables, so there is a story there.

The Smart Spot Web site lists an impressive group of physicians on its "Blue Ribbon Advisory Board," among them its chair, Dean Ornish (Preventive Medicine Research Institute), and Kenneth Cooper (Cooper Aerobics Center); another member is Thomas Foley (former ambassador to Japan). They and others must believe that the Smart Spots do more than just sell PepsiCo products; they will also promote wiser food choices among consumers. Perhaps, but I am unaware of evidence that such campaigns succeed in that purpose.

One apparent benefit of "healthy" label campaigns is to encourage food companies to reformulate their products in order to qualify. The National Heart Foundations in Australia and in New Zealand, for example, run a Pick the Tick program much like the food certification program of the American Heart Association (see previous chapter). Rather than having one set of criteria that apply to all food products, however, the Australia and New Zealand programs have separate sets of guidelines that apply to different categories of foods, among them cereals, cereal bars, crackers, and cookies. For example, the program only awards Ticks (Australian for check mark) to breakfast cereals with less than 2 grams of sugars and 130 milligrams of sodium per ounce. Cookies and crackers can have no more than 5 grams of sugars per ounce and 120 milligrams of sodium per ounce. Few American processed cereals, cookies, or crackers would meet these standards.

Researchers from these foundations report that manufacturers developed new products precisely formulated to qualify for the Heart-Tick logo. As a result, hundreds of tons of salt have been removed from the food supply. You might expect that doing this would make it easier for people to eat less salt, but the effects of the program on the salt intake of individuals, or on their health, are not yet known. People might compensate by eating other high-salt foods. Or, if they think a snack food is healthier, they might eat more of it, thereby canceling the gain in nutritional benefits.

In 2003, PepsiCo announced "Great News! America's favorite snacks have 0 grams Trans fats . . . That's right, America's favorite fun snacks have all of the great taste and crunch you've come to know and love with none of the Trans fats . . . zero, nada." The ad illustrated bags of Frito-Lay potato chips, Doritos, Tostitos, Fritos, Ruffles, and Cheetos, each with one of these words underneath: "zero, zip, zilch, nada, nil, none." *Trans* fats, you may recall from the margarine chapters, are the bad ones formed when vegetable oils are hydrogenated. Because *trans* fats raise the risk of heart disease, the FDA required Nutrition Facts labels to disclose the amount of these fats in food products, starting in January 2006. At that point, listing *trans* fats on food labels might discourage sales. So PepsiCo jumped the gun and got a head start on what other snack makers were sure to do by 2006.

Eating less *trans* fat from Cheetos and Doritos or less salt from chips makes good nutritional sense, but taking them out of food products as soon as possible makes even better marketing sense. I thought it might be easy to misinterpret those zeros, zips, and nadas in the PepsiCo ad as implying that you can now eat all the Lays snacks you want because the *trans* fats are gone. It is great that they are (and they should have been gone a long time ago), but removing the *trans* fats can make you forget that these snacks still have plenty of calories—and lots of salt. And salt is involved in its own set of health issues.

The American Heart Association's allowance for sodium in its endorsement program is generous; products may contain up to 480 milligrams per serving, an amount that is 20 percent of the Daily Value. The new Heartzels pretzels have half that amount, but a 1-ounce serving still contains 10 percent of the daily sodium allowance. An ounce of pretzels or potato chips is not much—just a handful. If you eat snack foods at all, it will not take long for you to eat more salt than is healthy, and often much more than is good for you.

Salt is 40 percent sodium and 60 percent chloride, and both of these nutrients are essential in the human diet. But salt is even more essential for the processed food industry. Adding salt to processed foods constitutes an "eat more" strategy all on its own; it makes foods taste better because it heightens flavors, reduces bitterness, and enhances sweetness. Salt is perfect for processed foods. It is cheap. It keeps foods from becoming discolored, and it extends shelf life. Even better, it binds water and makes foods weigh more, so you pay more for heavier packages.

> If you eat snack foods at all, it will not take long for you to eat more salt than is healthy, and often much more than is good for you.

But according to the overwhelming majority of scientific committees that have examined the question, eating too much salt raises the risk of high blood pressure and, therefore, heart disease and stroke—at least in some people, some of the time. In 2005, the *Dietary Guidelines* advised Americans to "Consume less than 2,300 mg of sodium per day" (the equivalent of about 1 tsp of salt), and "Choose and prepare foods with little salt." The guidelines explained:

> Reducing salt is one of several ways that people may lower their blood pressure. The relationship between salt intake and blood pressure is direct and progressive without an apparent threshold. On average, the higher a person's salt intake, the higher the blood pressure. Reducing blood pressure, ideally to the normal range, reduces the risk of stroke, heart disease, heart failure, and kidney disease.

A guideline this restrictive is bad news for the makers of snack foods. Although most companies provide lower-salt alternatives in their lines of processed foods, these do not sell well. Executives of Kraft Foods, Campbell Soup, and PepsiCo all tell me the same thing. Their consumer research shows that unless food products are salty enough—and reach what the snack food industry calls the "bliss point"—people do not like the way the foods taste. Experts on taste perception say that this is because most people are accustomed to high salt levels in processed and prepared foods. Unprocessed foods are relatively low in salt, and only about 10 percent of the salt in the American diet comes from salt added at the table; the other 90 percent is already added in processed foods where it cannot be avoided. Flavor experts say you can get used to the taste of foods with less salt, but it takes several weeks to do so; they also say that it is much easier to get used to increasingly salty foods than it is to get used to those with less salt. So food companies keep the salt content of their products tuned way up. The makers of sweet foods have a similar problem, which is why manufacturers add artificial sweeteners when they reduce the sugars in processed foods.

The Salt Institute, an industry lobbying group, promotes consumption of salty foods in the usual way such groups operate: it lobbies against guidelines to restrict salt, sends articles extolling the benefits of salt to health professionals, sponsors research studies that invariably give favorable results, and files lawsuits against government agencies that advise salt restriction. Its chief strategy is to spin the science. Salt, it says, raises blood pressure in only a few people and poses a health problem only if you do not get enough of it. The Salt Institute says that the science is so conflicted that there is no need to bother with restrictions. This approach is typical for a trade association with vested interests and, as always, the science is subject to interpretation. But in this case, virtually all national and international health agencies—among them the USDA, the U.S. Department of Health and Human Services, the Institute of Medicine, and the World Health Organization—tell you to eat less salt and ask food companies to make it easier for you to do so by reducing the amount of salt in their products.

In 2005, the Center for Science in the Public Interest published a comprehensive report on the science and politics of salt, along with a call for federal action. We are eating more salt than ever, the report says, and the salt content of processed foods continues to rise. If Americans reduced salt consumption by half, we could "save an estimated 150,000 lives per year. That in turn would reduce medical care and other costs by roughly $1.5 trillion over 20 years." The barriers? "We like salt . . . and the Salt Institute wants to keep it that way." Snack foods are an expensive way to buy salt, but that works just fine for the companies that make them.

COOKIES

As already noted, one way food companies attempt to increase sales is by developing "line extensions," tempting variations on favorite items. Oreo cookies from Kraft/Altria are a good example. I like them, and you no doubt do too. They sell brilliantly. But publicly traded companies are required to demonstrate growth every quarter, so it is not enough for Kraft Foods to sell half a billion dollars worth of Oreos every year; it has to find ways to sell more of them all the time. Line extensions help. In 1990, you could only find six varieties of Oreo cookies in supermarkets; by 2003 there were twenty-seven. Oreos come with chocolate filling, fudge filling, vanilla filling, and colored fillings for holidays; they come flavored with mint and peanut butter, in mini sizes and double sizes, in cup and cone shapes. You can also buy Oreos in breakfast cereals, ice cream, yogurt, and candy bars.

And then there are the Oreos that Kraft promotes as good for you. In 2004, Kraft, like PepsiCo, announced that it would remove the *trans* fats from its snack foods and late that year I bought a package of *trans* fat–free, reduced-fat Oreos. These had 1.5 grams of fat per cookie, half the amount in the regular cookies, and one-half gram less of saturated fat. The package said "reduced fat, no *trans* fat," which made them sound like diet cookies, but I checked the calories. Regular Oreos have 53 calories each; these have 50 calories, a difference that can hardly be measured. The "reduced versions" may have a bit less fat, but they still are cookies; they have sugars and calories, but do not taste nearly as good as the regular versions, at least to my palate.

Kraft marketers are also creative in finding other ways to make cookies look like health foods. Early in 2005, I found a small box of NEW! OREO Carb Well Chocolate Sandwich Cookies, labeled as 6 grams

"Net Carbs" and 100 calories per serving. To accomplish this feat, Kraft replaced the sugars with maltitol, an indigestible (except to intestinal bacteria) sugar alcohol, and two artificial sweeteners, acesulfame potassium and sucralose (Splenda). Ignore "Net Carbs" for the moment; I deal with them in connection with health foods (Chapter 37). For now, pay attention to the calories. Regular Oreo cookies have 160 calories per serving; a serving is three cookies. Kraft may have replaced sugars with artificial sweeteners, but cookies still have calories. What feat of food technology did Kraft perform to reduce the calories to 100 per serving? None, as it happens. They simply changed the serving size to two cookies, instead of three. Eat these cookies instead of the classic Oreos and you save 3 calories each. Taste them, read the ingredient list, and decide for yourself if you think 3 calories are worth boasting about.

DEALING WITH JUNK FOODS

I eat my share of junk foods and have my favorites. But junk foods are what they are and I wish companies would stop mucking around with them to make them look healthier. When I said this one time to a PepsiCo marketing official, he accused me of being against food marketing altogether. I am not, but I do object to the selling of junk foods in the guise of "better for you" health foods. Companies may boast in ads and on packages that they are making better-for-you changes to help you eat more healthfully, but the changes are unlikely to produce much of a health benefit unless you make a great many of them in your overall diet. Junk foods are once-in-a-while foods and the effects of taking out the *trans* fat, for example, depend a lot on what companies replace it with, and what else you eat.

At what point do product tinkerings convert a junk food to one that is not? Once you get beyond soft drinks, which are sugary waters with no other nutritional value, categorizing foods as junky or not brings up problems that require much splitting of nutritional hairs. Some crackers, chips, and cookies are better than others, but deciding among them puts you on a nutritional slippery slope. Baked Lays chips have less fat and, therefore, fewer calories than the regular kind, and if you are someone who eats bags of chips at a time, they might make a nutritional difference (but watch out for the salt). I like potato chips and have a particular fondness for the ones at the higher end of the price range (especially the thick ones fried in olive oil and seasoned with rosemary), and baked chips just do not do it for me. If I am going to eat potato chips at all, I would rather eat ones I like—just not too many at once. If I am in the mood for Oreo cookies (this happens, especially if they are right in front of me), I would rather eat a couple of the old kind than any of the doctored new ones. The regular ones taste better to me and do not leave me feeling deprived.

Supermarkets, however, do not make it easy to eat just a couple. In July 2005, the P&C market in Ithaca sold a package of regular Oreos—forty-five cookies—for $3.39; that came to 7.5 cents per cookie. Eating only three cookies, however, requires you to defy the Law of Portion Size: the more cookies in front of you, the more you will eat. For $5.23, the store also sold a box of twelve "single-serving" packages. These were more expensive at 11 cents per cookie, but the individual packets contained six cookies. Faced with a package of six, you are likely to eat them all along with their 320 calories.

I suppose I could try to substitute Mini Oreos for the larger ones, but mostly I try to stay out of the junk food aisles. If you do find yourself corralled in them, you will have to read the package labels carefully if you hope to make "better" choices. I look for items with short ingredient lists, whole grains, and as little sugar or salt as possible. Such products do exist. I like the crunchy taste of Finn Crisp crackers (from a Finnish company) made from precisely three ingredients: whole grain rye flour, yeast, and salt. I also like the chips you sometimes find in health food sections of supermarkets, for example, Green Mountain Tortilla Chips; its three ingredients are masa harina corn flour, non-hydrogenated canola oil, and salt, this last giving you just 5 percent of the Daily Value for sodium per ounce of chips. Compare these to Wheat Thins (Kraft/Altria): enriched flour, soybean oil (now free of *trans* fat), four kinds of sugars (sugar, high fructose corn syrup, corn syrup, malt syrup), salt (11 percent of the Daily Value for sodium), several color and other additives, and vitamins, of course. If you love junk food, by all means eat and enjoy it—just not too much at a time, not too often, and without kidding yourself that it is good for you.

> Eating only one serving, however, requires you to defy the Law of Portion Size: the more food in front of you, the more you will eat.

31

Foods Just for Kids

You would never know it by going to a supermarket, but children are supposed to eat the same foods their parents eat. Dietary recommendations, such as the *Dietary Guidelines* and pyramid food guide, apply to everyone over the age of two. Once children are past infancy and can chew and swallow foods without choking (which usually happens by age two), they should be eating the same healthy foods that everyone else in the family is eating—just less of them and with a few minor modifications: leave out the salt, sugars, and peppery spices; mash the foods or cut them into small pieces; and make sure the foods are well moistened so children will not choke on them.

Children do not need added salt or sugars. They do not need soft drinks, juice drinks, desserts, candy, sweetened cereals, or fast food. And yes, they will eat "adult" foods, the healthier kinds that grown-ups eat, if given the opportunity to eat such foods early and often. If you offer healthy foods, your children will have the chance to eat them. If you offer junk foods to your children, they will eat junk foods.

If you offer healthy foods, your children will have the chance to eat them. If you offer junk foods to your children, they will eat junk foods.

Surveys of what American children are eating these days reveal dismaying trends. In contrast to the diets of children in the 1950s, for example, the diets of up to 80 percent of today's young children are considered "poor" or "in need of improvement," and their diets get worse as they get older. Many American children do not eat enough fruits, and nearly 80 percent do not eat enough vegetables. A great many—if not most—are taking in more calories than they use up in physical activity. The reasons for this trend are well established: fewer organized meals at home, more meals eaten outside the home, more fast food, more soft drinks, larger portion sizes, and more snacking—all of which promote higher calorie intake from less nutritious foods.

Trends in snacking are particularly striking. Since the late 1970s, the proportion of young children eating snacks increased from 76 to 91 percent, and snacks account for more and more of children's daily calories. Three-quarters of American children say that they—not their parents— decide what they will eat for breakfast, and more than 60 percent say they do not eat three meals a day. How did this happen? These trends have been driven in part by economic and other changes in society that took women out of homes and into the workforce and that cause everyone to work longer hours, thereby making "convenience" in meals a necessity. They also are in part a consequence of corporate pressures to sell more food in an overabundant—and highly competitive—marketplace. One result of such pressures is to market foods directly to children.

MARKETING TO KIDS

Right at the entrance to the Morton Williams Associated Supermarket near where I live its managers have placed the cutest little red shopping carts with flags saying "Customer in Training." In training? Any child old enough to push one of those carts does not need training. Children already know what to ask for from the thousands of televised food commercials most have been exposed to since infancy, as well as from food tie-ins on toys, books, clothes, and games. Even the most health-conscious parents I know—those who say they never let their kids watch TV, never take them to McDonald's, and never bring kids' cereals into the house—are astonished when their children ask for brand-name food products. They cannot imagine how their children learned to recognize the cartoon characters on cereal boxes or pictures of Ronald McDonald.

Marketing to children is so much a part of our culture that most of us do not even notice it. We are not supposed to notice it, and if the marketing is truly effective, we will not notice it. As a result, if you are like most parents I know, you hate taking your kids to supermarkets. Such outings are bound to cause conflict, tantrums, and public humiliation — unless, of course, you give in and let your kids have whatever they want.

Marketing to children is an old story, but two aspects are new: the methods have increased in sophistication and intensity, and it is now *your* children who are the targets of food marketers. In 1957, Vance Packard's then shocking exposé, *The Hidden Persuaders*, described what happens "when mother and child come out of their [store-induced] trances and together reach the check-out counter." As a store manager explained to him:

> There is usually a wrangle when the mother sees all the things the child has in his basket and she tries to make him take the stuff back. The child will take back items he doesn't particularly care about such as coffee but will usually bawl and kick before surrendering cookies, candy, ice cream, or soft drinks, so they usually stay for the family.

Today even more, Customers in Training know exactly what they are supposed to want, starting with breakfast cereals. Consider, for example, three boxes from three Big Cereal makers:

- Froot Loops "Marshmallow Alien Berry with Funtastic Marshmallows and Fun Colored Bits" (Kellogg)
- Count Chocula "chocolaty cereal with spooky-fun marshmallows" (General Mills)
- Oreo O's "Extreme creme taste cereal with marshmallow bits" (Post/Kraft/Altria)

These three cereals have much in common. Their boxes are covered with beautifully designed cartoon characters (Toucan Sam, Count Chocula, Creme Team), all shown with arms raised above their heads throwing cereal right at you. All three cereals use candy for enticement;

all use "fun" marshmallows to attract attention. All three boxes have games on the back panels—also "fun."

Millions of dollars of advertising go to promote such cereals, but the companies also use more sophisticated forms of marketing. Count Chocula, for example, comes with directions about how to use the box tops to earn money for schools. And unless you closely monitor your children's Internet habits, you might not realize that the Oreo O's box sends kids to its Web site (www.postopia.com), where they can spend hours playing dozens of cereal-enriched games linked to cartoon and movie features. The site does offer full disclosure in fine print: "This page contains commercial advertising of Post products we sell."

THE MARKETING-TO-KIDS INDUSTRY

As I explained in *Food Politics*, marketing to children is big business and comes with its very own research enterprise, rationale, budget, and code of ethics. Research on how to market foods to children is simply breathtaking in its comprehensiveness, level of detail, and undisguised cynicism. This research, which involves interviews, focus groups, and direct observations of children's food preferences and behavior (some of it done by having kids wear cameras), invariably concludes that marketing enormously influences kids' choices of brands and food categories, particularly of the heavily advertised breakfast cereals, soft drinks, candy, snacks, and fast foods. Entire books summarize this research and explain how to apply its findings to campaigns that most appeal to boys and girls of different ages.

> Research on how to market foods to children is simply breathtaking in its comprehensiveness, level of detail, and undisguised cynicism.

Marketers justify direct appeals to children as an education in "street smarts," as an expression of freedom of speech, and as good for the American economy. Advertising expenditures for foods marketed directly to children can only be estimated, but two researchers, Susan Linn, the author of *Consuming Kids*, and Juliet B. Schor, author of *Born to Buy*, guess that marketers spend about $15 billion a year to promote all products aimed at children, with about half that much spent to promote food products. They describe how companies that specialize in marketing to children come together at an annual Kid Power Exchange conference to figure out how to protect themselves against opposition to their efforts and to give each other prizes for the most effective campaigns. The conference Web site (www.kidpowerx.com) explains that its organizers "take pride in creating a total experience that encompasses all areas of marketing, promotions, market research, e-commerce, and branding . . . that just might mean the difference between your marketing success and failure." This industry is not just about marketing; it is about marketing to children.

As for ethics, food companies participate in the Children's Advertising Review Unit (CARU) of the Council of Better Business Bureaus, which sets voluntary guidelines for self-regulation. CARU guidelines say, among long lists of other such things, that advertisements to children should be truthful and not misleading, should not create unattainable expectations, and should not be designed to get children to pressure their parents to buy products. For foods in particular, the guidelines say that commercials should encourage good nutritional practices, depict the product within the framework of a balanced diet, and show snacks as snacks, not as meals. These sound just fine, but nobody outside of the industry believes that they are either followed or enforced, which is not surprising given that CARU is funded by the companies it supposedly regulates. Analyses of food marketing practices cite many examples of advertisements by the makers of breakfast cereals and other foods targeted to children that violate one or another of the CARU guidelines.

Advertisements are supposed to sell food products, and companies have three goals in mind for marketing strategies: creating brand loyalty, getting kids to pester their parents to buy the products, and giving kids the idea that they are supposed to eat packaged foods rather than unprocessed, home-cooked foods. Let's examine how these work.

BRAND LOYALTY

Even the ahead-of-his-time Vance Packard could not have imagined the extent of the research that goes into selling sweetened cereals, "fruit" snacks, salty snacks, candies, cookies, and sodas to children these days. Food marketers dearly want kids to want their products, and brand loyalty is a good place to start. They hope that if kids grow to recognize and desire a brand when they are young, they will go on wanting it for life. The success of this strategy is best illustrated by kids' breakfast cereals. I saw brand loyalty in action in 2003 when I was invited by the founders of Google, Sergey Brin and Larry Page, to advise them about the nutritional quality of the food they provided as a perk to the thousand or so employees in their Mountain View headquarters. I thought what they were offering was just fine (think: upscale college cafeteria), but I was amazed by what they made available in the twenty-four-hour snack bar: every snack food, soft drink, and kids' breakfast cereal you could imagine—all free for the taking and much appreciated by the late-night programmers (most of them still young enough to postpone the caloric effects of this inadvertent "eat more" strategy).

A year later, David Roth and Rick Bacher launched their new fast-food concept, Cereality, at Arizona State University to satisfy the inner child of college students who want cereal away from home. Since then, Cereality has expanded beyond college campuses. The chain encourages customers to choose their favorite brands and let "pajama-clad Cereologists" fill their orders; customers get to add their own milk. The Web site (www.cereality.com) says: "95% of Americans like cereal. 57% like sex. We've got cereal." They also know what their brand-loyal customers want.

The odd thing about brand-named processed foods is that loyalty to these products has little to do with how they taste. In *Food Politics*, I explained how brand loyalty and taste are so profoundly disconnected that even children can prove it, as neatly shown by a couple of thirteen-year-olds in a prizewinning science fair project. More recently, government-funded university scientists did the same thing in a much fancier version (involving brain scans, no less). Both groups of scientists asked their "study subjects" to say which brand of sodas they preferred; then they asked the subjects to taste sodas in a blind test (in which the subjects did not know which soda they were drinking). Neither study found much of a match. So if you think foods meant for kids taste awful, it doesn't matter. Taste is not the point (and neither is nutrition); the brand is the point.

THE "PESTER FACTOR"

Folks in the marketing-to-kids trade cheerfully refer to the second strategy as the "pester factor." Kids may not have much money of their own, but they can and do influence family buying decisions. Food companies want kids to be asking their parents for products—by sight and by name. The books by Susan Linn and Juliet Schor review the extensive body of research on how to get kids to pester their parents. Researchers divide the practice into two types: "persistence nagging" in which kids repeatedly ask for products, and "importance nagging" in which kids give reasons for wanting them. Persistence nagging increases as children get older. You can see pestering in action in any grocery store. Even toddlers can point to the products they want. Let them loose, and they run right to the cartoon-decorated products they recognize from television, videos, toys, and games. And what happens if you say no? Then, too, they know exactly what to do. This is brilliant marketing in action.

KIDS' CUISINE

Even so, I find the third strategy for marketing to children to be the most insidious. Food companies want kids to think they are supposed to be eating foods made especially for them, not those boring old things eaten by adults and the rest of the family. They want kids to expect foods to be sweet and salty, and to come in "fun" colors, shapes, and packages. ConAgra, for example, wants them eating Kid Cuisine—a TV-type dinner on a tray filled with fun-colored and fun-shaped food objects. This kid-food strategy says everything you might want to know about the reasoning behind Lunchables, those prepackaged "lunch combinations and fun snacks" from Kraft/Altria that can be tossed into lunch boxes and traded in schools. Never mind that they are loaded with saturated fat, salt, and sugars. They are not about nutrition; they are about sales and profits, as made clear by Kraft's nearly $26 million advertising expenditure on Lunchables in 2004—and the $500 million in revenues that it generated.

This "kids are only supposed to eat kids' food" strategy also explains the invention of blue-colored french fries from Ore-Ida/Heinz and, not coincidentally, purple and green ketchups (also from Heinz) to put on them. In the same genre, Kraft/Altria makes macaroni with blue cheese sauce; its box displays the popular cartoon character SpongeBob SquarePants, licensed by Nickelodeon, the commercial television channel aimed at children. Such products are sold as harmless amusements—and that may well be their manufacturers' intention—but their overall effect is to teach kids not to like or to refuse to try the "adult" foods their families are eating. When you hear parents say, "My kid only eats this [particular product] and won't eat anything else," you are witnessing targeted food marketing at its most effective.

If kids eat junk foods and gain weight, the makers and sellers of those products say it is the parents' fault, not theirs. They are not forcing you to buy these foods for your children. If you don't think your kids should have them, it's up to you. Just say no. Really? Try saying that to a parent struggling through a supermarket with a child in tow. Saying no in this situation—important as it might be—can seem more trouble than it is worth. When my children were little, I did not want to fight with them about food, and I do not know anyone who does. If, as I was, you are working full time and are away from your kids most of the day, the last thing you want to do is argue with them about cereals and sodas. In the greater scheme of raising children, buying a box of cereal or a snack food seems harmless enough. So you give in. I certainly did. Marketers know this, and exploit the time-pressured realities of modern life to the hilt.

MARKETING BY STEALTH

Marketing to kids would be less of a concern if American children weren't gaining weight at alarming rates and developing early signs of diabetes, high blood pressure, and heart disease. And marketing would be less troubling if you only had to deal with advertising. But advertising, as I have heard Susan Linn say, "is just so twentieth century—totally passé." Food marketers, as she, Juliet Schor, and others demonstrate, now infiltrate the very essence of childhood. Kids are exposed to food company logos from earliest infancy on diapers, nursing bottles, toys, games, and books. I own a small and treasured collection of food toys: an Oreo Cookie lunch box and Barbie doll, a Coca-Cola Barbie and toy car, M&M dispensers and stuffed toys, and a shelf of "educational" counting books based on products like Oreos, Fruit Loops, or Hershey's Chocolate (this last distributed by Scholastic, the children's book publisher, directly to schools).

These are forms of food advertising visible to anyone paying attention, but twenty-first century methods of stealth marketing are designed deliberately to slip under the radar of parental oversight. The next time you take a child to a cartoon movie, notice what the cartoon characters are eating and drinking. You can bet that the film studio has a deal with food company sponsors (hence: SpongeBob SquarePants on Kraft macaroni and other such products). Food companies arrange for product placements in popular songs and organize word-of-mouth campaigns, contests, cell phone ads, personalized e-mail messages, and endless tie-ins to anything a child might do, none of it accidental.

Part of the stealth is to persuade you that the products targeted at kids are actually good for them. Take the three cereals I mentioned earlier. Count Chocula displays Goodness Corner tokens ("9 vitamins & minerals, excellent source of iron, low fat") and an endorsement from the American Heart Association, but you have to do the math to figure out that sugars comprise 47 percent of its calories. The Oreo O's box says it's "cholesterol free, excellent source of six B vitamins, iron and zinc for growth" (44 percent sugar calories). The particular version of Froot Loops noted here has a similar set of vitamins and minerals but does not make a big deal of them, perhaps because it has no fruit at all and sugars make up more than half—52 percent—of its calories. These cereals are cookies—not only vitamin enriched, but also marshmallow candy enriched.

If kids' breakfast cereals are fortified with added vitamins, can snack foods be far behind? Indeed not. I have on hand a full-page advertisement for Munchies Kids Mix (from Frito-Lay/PepsiCo): a mixed bag of Cheetos, Cap'n Crunch cereal, Doritos, and Rold Gold pretzels.

Mom and Dad, you'll feel great about offering it to your kids because Munchies Kids Mix snack mix is a good source of 8 essential vitamins and minerals, has o grams *trans* fat, and meets nutritional guidelines established by Dr. Kenneth Cooper for sugar, fat, and sodium.

Why Dr. Cooper, the physician who heads the Cooper Aerobic Institute, is doing this is beyond me, but "fortified with fun" or not, such products are best left in the store or reserved for special occasions.

I have not said anything yet about candy marketed to kids. Candy is candy and everyone knows that it is a once-in-a-while treat. It's the candy pretending to be healthy that bothers me; it is still candy. Look at "fruit" snacks, for example, packed neatly in pouches the perfect size for lunch boxes. The word "fruit" goes in quotation marks because there isn't any to speak of. Consider the contents of Trix Fruit Snacks (from Betty Crocker/General Mills) illustrated with the cartoon Trix cereal rabbit. The packages say the snacks are made with real fruit juice, but the ingredients include processed juice made from concentrate (translation: sugars), and the rest of the ingredients also are sugars (corn syrup, sugar, dextrose) and color and flavor additives to make the snacks look and taste something like fruit. There seem to be dozens of such "fruit snack" products, virtually indistinguishable from one another except for the cartoon character on the front. All are candy disguised as fruit; up to 75 percent of the calories can be from added sugars. Such products also come with the addresses for elaborate and engaging Web sites, as does Kool-Aid (100 percent sugar calories, vitamins added, and candy in drinkable form).

> Candy is candy and everyone knows that it is a once-in-a-while treat. It's the candy pretending to be healthy that bothers me; it is still candy.

Rates of childhood obesity have risen rapidly in the United States since the early 1980s and are now considered to have reached epidemic proportions. Children cannot be expected to apply personal responsibility at the grocery store, so intervention has to come from adults. The threat of anti-obesity lawsuits has placed food companies on notice that they need to reexamine their product lines and their marketing practices aimed at children.

As it happens, I am not the only one who says these things. In 2002 and 2003, three large international investment companies—UBS Warburg, JP Morgan, and Morgan Stanley—issued research reports to investors on the effects of anti-obesity lawsuits on food companies. Even if nothing comes of the lawsuits, they said, food companies are vulnerable and need to change their practices. UBS Warburg, for example, said: "We think the winners will be those who successfully capture the change in attitudes in order to halt the spread of this epidemic. The task will be hardest for those whose brands are associated with exactly the foods we should be consuming less of . . . Coca-Cola, PepsiCo, Cadbury Schweppes, Tate & Lyle [the maker of the artificial sweetener, Splenda, and other such ingredients], McDonalds and Diageo (Burger King) . . ." In a later report, its researchers noted:

> Many commentators . . . like to dismiss concerns about obesity as being solely an issue of personal choice . . . [but] the issue for food and drink companies is whether they can adapt . . . or will they be left behind promoting anachronistic processed foods and sugary drinks while their target customer has moved on.

Based on my wanderings through the food business world, I can assure you that food companies have gotten this message loud and clear. But companies cannot address the substance of the problem and make foods that really are healthier, because such foods would be more expensive to make, would cost more to the consumer, and might not sell as well. Instead, companies try to make their products *look* healthier. Expect to see even more vitamins added to foods, and in larger and larger amounts ("Contains 100 percent of the Daily Value!"). As I've already noted, General Mills is making all of its cereals from whole grains— even Count Chocula, Lucky Charms, and Cocoa Puffs—but the fiber content is only 1 gram per serving. PepsiCo has removed the *trans* fat from its snack foods, but the calories and salt are the same. Kellogg has reduced the sugars in its cereals by one-third—from 3 teaspoons per serving to 2. These may be, as the companies argue, better choices, but on balance your kids are still better off eating foods that are less processed.

One indication that profit—not health—is at stake is how rarely big food companies apply sophisticated marketing savvy to promote healthier foods. In fall 2004, as one example, McDonald's took milk out of those dowdy square cartons and put it into curvy 8-ounce plastic bottles printed with a cartoon Ronald McDonald. Sales zoomed. When Wendy's did something similar, its milk sales rose fifteen-fold, an event considered the "most dramatic sales increase for a non-discounted item in fast food history." But much of the increase came from sales of the sweeter chocolate-flavored version. Market analysts considered the experiment a great success: the companies could get children to drink more milk if it came in plastic, single-serve containers "just for kids," and made the milk conform to kids' expectations of sweetness. But we have to ask: Where did those children's expectations of sweetness in drinks come from in the first place?

Food companies are schizophrenic about marketing to kids. While they are scrambling to "health up" their products, they also are hedging their bets by making package sizes larger, adding more candy, and making drinks creamier. While they are promising to stop targeting young children, they continue to promote consumption of soft drinks and snack foods in schools through vending contracts that reward higher sales volumes and consumption of larger-size portions. Whether the "healthier" foods designed for children will get equal marketing attention remains to be seen. In 2005, Nickelodeon licensed the SpongeBob character for use on packages of spinach produced by Boskovich Farms in California. Will doing this make kids want to eat spinach? Candies are still the food products most heavily marketed to children. With those marginally healthier products, however, companies can safely argue that they are offering options, and the choice is up to you.

In mid-2005, I received a press kit from Sunkist (www.sunkist.com) introducing its "grab-and-go" packages of, I could hardly believe it, "fun fruit—

> Candies are still the food products most heavily marketed to children.

100% natural, single serve, fresh-cut fruit and vegetables in fun easy-to-open packages." You could do this at home by cutting up oranges or apples or putting some grapes in a bag, but let's give the company credit for figuring out how to "add value" in convenience to something that might actually be good for kids. Whether the fruit—which "smiles, grins, and giggles," as the packages are labeled—will sell well enough to survive market forces remains to be seen.

Marketing to children, healthy foods and not, crosses an ethical boundary, and companies know it. It is one thing to argue that adults should be exerting personal responsibility, but quite another to demand that of children. An executive of Kraft Foods once called to ask me what I thought the ethical cutoff point was for marketing to children. Was it acceptable to target eighteen-year-olds? Fifteen-year-olds? And so forth down the line. The question suggested that he knew he had an ethical problem. Children younger than eight or ten years have trouble distinguishing advertising from news content, and that confusion continues in some children well into their teens. At the *Time* magazine summit meeting on obesity in spring 2004, the late ABC News anchor Peter Jennings asked that same Kraft executive to answer his own question: Below what age is it unethical to market foods to children? The audience gasped at the response: six.

> It is one thing to argue that adults should be exerting personal responsibility, but quite another to demand that of children.

Half a year later, Kraft announced its new ethical stance: it would no longer market its junkier foods directly to children under the age of twelve. It would start its own "Sensible Solution" labeling program for the healthier options in its food portfolio. Most telling, Kraft would stop advertising its less nutritious foods directly to children ages six to eleven. To the relief of the advertising industry, however, Kraft said it would not reduce its $80 million annual expenditure on that demographic; it would simply market its supposedly healthier choices to them that way instead. When I asked a Kraft executive whether the new ethical marketing standards applied to the Internet, he said not yet, but they were working on that. If I keep saying that Kraft is mostly owned by Altria, which also owns Philip Morris, you will understand why. Regardless of the best intentions of Kraft executives, the parent company has a long history of marketing unhealthy products to children and of strong protection of its bottom line above any consideration of health.

The easiest way to deal with kids' marketing in supermarkets is to follow some simple rules, except, of course, on special, and infrequent, occasions:

- don't take tots grocery shopping or let them near one of those training carts
- if you must take them, set spending limits in advance (one parent I know sets that limit at $1)
- don't buy food products with cartoons and games on them
- don't buy any packaged cereal or snack labeled as "fun"
- don't buy foods just because they are vitamin enriched
- count the sugars (a tablespoon is 15 grams)

And, if you are really serious about what your kids eat, stick to the periphery and

- don't set foot in the center aisles

Bear in mind that food companies would rather you did not notice how they market their products to your kids. If you did, you might see, as researchers tell us, that much of food marketing seems designed deliberately to undermine your authority and to encourage your children to view you as ineffective or stupid. As the Center for Science in the Public Interest explains in its 2003 report, "Pestering Parents: How Food Companies Market Obesity to Children":

> Conflicts arise because the foods that are most heavily marketed to children are low-nutrition foods of which parents would like their children to eat less. Marketers count on children wearing their parents down and on parents giving in and purchasing low-nutrition food for their children . . . [F]ood marketing aimed at children makes a parent's job harder and undermines parental authority. It forces parents to choose between being the

bad guy who says "no" in order to protect their children's health or giving in to junk-food demands to keep the peace.

Analyses of food commercials aimed at children demonstrate that such advertising often promotes "antisocial" and "antiadult" behavior designed to make kids think they know more about what they are supposed to eat than their parents do. As a parent, your job is to set limits but you are up against an entire industry devoted to undermining your authority to do so. Marketing to children does more than make them want certain products; it is meant to change society. It aims to put kids in charge of decisions that you should be making. For this reason alone, marketing to children is worth opposing.

> Marketing to children does more than make them want certain products; it is meant to change society. It aims to put kids in charge of decisions that you should be making. For this reason alone, marketing to children is worth opposing.

With that said, I must point out that it is perfectly possible to teach kids to like adult foods. I've seen it done. It just takes some persistent action by adults who care about kids' health and want to make a difference. The best way I can think of for you to get kids interested in real food—the fruit, vegetables, meat, and dairy foods that you buy along the peripheral aisles of supermarkets—is to teach them how to cook such foods. Even better, teach them how to grow vegetables; radishes growing in a pot on a windowsill can change a child's relationship with food forever, and much for the better.

Short of that, you have to figure out your own sets of rules and compromises. One nutritionist I know compromises by letting her children sprinkle small amounts of their favorite presweetened cereals on top of the unsweetened varieties. But however you decide to cope with the marketing of foods to kids, be sure to talk to your children about what food marketing is for and how it really works.

32

Oils: Fat and More Fat

Toward the height of the low-carbohydrate craze late in 2003, the Tops Market in Ithaca must have thought it was doing a favor for its customers. It installed "low-carb" signs in front of foods without the sugars or starches forbidden on the Atkins or other such diets. I saw these signs helpfully posted in front of bottled waters, diet sodas, and (oops) teas and other drinks sweetened with high fructose corn syrup—sugars! But my favorite was the low-carb sign on the salad and cooking oils. Oils never have carbs. They are 100 percent fat. Happily, the low-carb frenzy did not last long, and may it rest in peace. It's the calories that count, and salad oils have lots of them—a whopping 120 per tablespoon.

By January 2005, when I began taking a serious look at salad oils, the low-carb signs had disappeared and so had most of the low-carb products. That month, I was on a business trip to San Diego. I have no idea what other people do in their spare time on business trips, but I visit supermarkets, and the nearest one to my meeting site was a Vons at Point Loma that I hoped would have a good collection of oils. Indeed, its collection was typical for a medium-size store. I found the oils displayed in a ten-foot-long section with six shelves—sixty linear feet of corn, olive, peanut, safflower, and canola (Canadian rapeseed) oils, a few exotics like walnut and sesame, and a large selection of containers simply labeled "vegetable oil." These last were all soybean oils, but labels are coy about saying so. So here is Food Oil Rule #1: all salad and cooking oils are from vegetable sources, but otherwise unidentified "vegetable" oils are from soybeans. The soy folks must think that nobody wants to cook with soybean oil, and that "100% pure vegetable oil" works better. As long as it has not been hydrogenated—

So here is Food Oil Rule #1: all salad and cooking oils are from vegetable sources, but otherwise unidentified "vegetable" oils are from soybeans.

and if it has, the ingredient list will always say so—soy oil is a good choice for cooking, but I can understand why its makers might worry about image; they produce about 8 billion pounds of soy oil annually, and soy oils constitute about 80 percent of the cooking oil market; they do not want misapprehensions about beany flavors to keep you from buying their product.

Although not a gourmet store by any means, the Point Loma Vons sold thirty-four kinds of olive oils: domestic, imported, virgin, extra virgin, light, extra light, and flavored with garlic, pepper, herbs, orange, or lemon. These ranged in price from 25 cents per ounce for a domestic light olive oil in a large container to 86 cents per ounce for the small bottles of flavored oils. You can pay a fortune for the best quality olive oils, and they are sometimes—but not always—worth it. Olives are a fruit, botanically speaking. The really good oils are freshly squeezed at cool temperatures (cold pressed) from the best ripe olives, poured into dark bottles to protect the oil from light, and never exposed to heat. They contain many of the fruit's natural vitamins and antioxidants. These oils are called "extra virgin" (translation: top quality) or "virgin" (good but not great). When poured, both kinds look green or golden, smell pungent, and taste fruity or peppery. This store carried a pricey Greek olive oil in a dark bottle, labeled "extra-virgin, first cold pressed, acidity 0–0.5%." I did not buy it (I was traveling, after all) but would expect it to taste really good on bread or a salad.

Low acidity is another sign of a good olive oil, but most commercially sold bottles do not mention it. Acidity is a sign of deterioration, as I will soon explain. In the meantime, let me introduce Armando Manni, an Italian film director who owns a company that makes an extra-virgin, low-acid oil from olives grown in Tuscany. He says that a good olive oil is "alive." Expose it to light, heat, or air and you kill its natural antioxidants and destroy the flavor as well as the health benefits. He puts his oil in thin black bottles that hold just 100 milliliters (3 ounces). You are supposed to use up the oil quickly while it is still living. This is why some olive oils are labeled "store in a cool, dark place" and why oils stored in dark bottles or cans taste better and keep longer. Like all oils, olive oils become rancid (deteriorate and smell and taste bad) when exposed to light, heat, and air.

Salad and cooking oils from any source—olives, seeds, or corn—are useful in human nutrition. They are the principal source of one of the fatty acids required in human diets (linoleic acid), and they are low in "bad" saturated fatty acids and high in "good" unsaturated ones. They are the biggest single food source of vitamin E in the American diet. And they make salads and vegetables taste better so you will eat more of these foods. They are, however, a confusing, horrible mess to deal with because they pose all kinds of health issues: calories, health messages, saturation, rancidity, ratio of omega-6s to omega-3s, and health claims. Some oils taste better than others, and cost is also a consideration. Let's take the issues one by one, starting with calories.

THE CALORIE PROBLEM

Dead or alive, olive oils labeled "light" mean they are light in color, not calories. Extra-light olive oil has the same number of calories as every other salad and cooking oil: 120 per tablespoon. Oils are fats and fats have calories, lots of them—9 calories per gram as opposed to just 4 for proteins and carbohydrates. So fat is fattening because it has more than twice the calories of carbohydrate or protein. Calories constitute Food Oil Rule #2: it makes no difference whether an oil comes from soybeans, safflower seeds, rapeseeds, corn, peanuts, walnuts, or olives, or whether an olive oil is "light" or "virgin"; all have the same number of calories—120 per tablespoon.

Calories constitute Food Oil Rule #2: it makes no difference whether an oil comes from soybeans, safflower seeds, rapeseeds, corn, peanuts, walnuts, or olives, or whether an olive oil is "light" or "virgin"; all have the same number of calories—120 per tablespoon.

Even the oils in spray cans have 120 calories per tablespoon. The Point Loma Vons carried fifteen kinds, distinguished from one another by the type of oil and brand, but not much else. I had never looked closely at those products and was astonished by their labels: "no calories, no fat." How could this be? If they were made from soy or any other oil, yet had no fat or calories, they must be some kind of miracle. Oil is just liquid fat and fats have calories, even when the next two ingredients are water (no fat, no calories) and whatever propellant is used to spray the oil out of the cans (no fat, no calories, and—in California at least—no environmentally unfriendly chlorofluorocarbons).

Alas, this miracle turns out to be nothing but a trick of serving size. In the spray-oil world, a serving size is not how much you eat; it is how long you spray—in this case, one-quarter of a second. A quarter-second spray gives you a quarter-gram of fat, but in the FDA's curious way of doing things, nothing below half a gram has to be listed on the Nutrition Facts label. Hence: zero fat. Push the squirt button for a full second, and you spray a full gram of fat into your pan, along with its full 9 calories. The Vons canola spray (a "cholesterol free food") holds 557 quarter-second servings. The Crisco olive oil version, "no stick for fat-free cooking," has less propellant, meaning that you can push the button for half a second for the same quarter-gram of fat. You may well end up using less fat in cooking if you spray the oil rather than pour it, but whatever the amount you use, it will most definitely be fat and will most definitely have calories.

THE HEALTH MESSAGE PROBLEM

The calories are the same in all oils because oils are 100 percent fat. Fat has a bad reputation because of calories and heart disease risk, but because of the requirement for linoleic acid, you must eat the equivalent of a tablespoon of oil or two a day to stay healthy. Fats, even more than carbohydrates, come in categories—they can be good, bad, or neutral for health. Telling the difference takes you into the arcane realm of fat biology, where the terms are so technical that nobody other than a nutritionist or biochemist should be expected to keep them straight. But these terms show up so often on Nutrition Facts labels and on the front labels of salad and cooking oils that it is a good idea to know what they mean. I will explain them as they arise in this discussion. Because there are so many of them, I also summarize them in Appendix 2 for reference.

The word "fat" has two meanings in foods. It is the generic term for any food fat (what scientists call "lipids"). But it also is the specific term for fats that are solid at room temperature and that mostly come from meat and dairy animals. In contrast, oils, which are also fats, are mostly liquid at room temperature and come from plants. All food fats—solid and liquid—are "triglycerides," and triglycerides are used in the body for energy (which is why they have calories).

The building blocks of fats and oils are called "fatty acids." Triglycerides are composed of three fatty acids attached to a backbone of a small sugar alcohol (glycerol), arranged much like the letter E, only with longer arms. The additives that you see so often on food ingredient lists—mono- and diglycerides—are just triglyceride fats with one (diglycerides) or two (monoglycerides) arms missing. Beyond the E arrangement, fats differ in characteristics that affect health, and the manufacturers of oils proclaim these features in messages on food labels. The Table on the next page lists and explains some of the messages that show up most frequently.

The makers of oils want you to forget about the calories and instead think about the healthy features of fat. Fortunately for them (and us), there are at least three good features to think about: essential fatty acids, no cholesterol, and low saturated fat. Everybody needs to eat two particular fatty acids that come only from plants: linoleic acid and alpha-linolenic acid. Most vegetable oils supply plenty of linoleic acid, and some supply the other one as well. Cholesterol is made only by animals so vegetable oils never have any. Eating meat and dairy foods with cholesterol makes your blood cholesterol rise and can increase your risk for heart disease. For some reason (which researchers have not yet been able to explain), saturated fatty acids are worse than cholesterol in raising blood cholesterol. Saturated fatty acids are highly prevalent in meat and dairy fats; all vegetable oils have some, but usually much less.

Health Messages on the Labels of Salad and Cooking Oils

SALAD OR COOKING OIL	HEALTH MESSAGE	WHAT THE MESSAGE MEANS	HEALTH RATIONALE
Any vegetable oil (but usually soy)	"100% pure vegetable oil"	The oil comes from a plant, not from meat or dairy sources	Vegetable fats are better for you than animal fats
Any vegetable oil	"Unsaturated"	The oil contains unsaturated fatty acids as opposed to saturated fatty acids (but all oils are mostly unsaturated)	Unsaturated fatty acids are better for you than saturated fatty acids
Canola oil (Canadian rapeseed)	"Contains omega-3s"	Some fatty acids are of the omega-3 type	Omega-3 fatty acids are good for you
Any vegetable oil	"0 grams *trans* fat"	The oil has not been hydrogenated to stabilize it	*Trans*-fatty acids are bad for you
Any vegetable oil	"No cholesterol"	Of course: vegetable oil never has cholesterol	Cholesterol has no calories, but it is unhealthy for other reasons
Any vegetable oil	"Low carb"	Of course: oils are fats, not carbohydrates	Fat is fat; it still has calories
Olive oil	"Helps prevent heart disease"	Maybe, if you substitute olive oil for other fats and limit daily intake to 2 tablespoons	Monounsaturated fatty acids are good for you (in small amounts)
Spray oils	"No fat, no calories"	A labeling trick	All oils have calories: 120 per tablespoon

Consider that fatty acids come in three kinds of saturation: saturated, unsaturated, and polyunsaturated. Saturation refers to the amount of hydrogen attached to a fatty acid. When all possible sites for attachment are filled, the fatty acid is fully saturated. Saturated fatty acids seem to be more difficult for the body to handle than the unsaturated ones (which are missing some hydrogen); they—or the foods from animals that contain them—may increase the risk for certain cancers as well as heart disease. In contrast, unsaturated and polyunsaturated fatty acids reduce blood cholesterol levels and, therefore, heart disease risk.

Without knowing a thing about its chemistry, you can guess how saturated a food fat might be by whether it is solid or liquid at room temperature and, if it is solid, what you have to do to get the fat to melt. I like to think about saturated fatty acids as stiff and packed solid like flat boards stacked tightly on top of one another. Food fats with lots of saturated fatty acids, like the ones in butter and beef, are stacked solid at room temperature. Butter melts in hot weather, but you have to cook steaks and pork chops to melt their fat. The need for heat tells you that both have lots of saturated fatty acids.

In contrast, food fats that are largely made of unsaturated fatty acids are liquid at room temperature and do not need heat to melt. This is because the points at which the hydrogens are missing give the fatty acid some flexibility. Unsaturated fatty acids are too wiggly to be stacked solid; they slip and slide and flow. Monounsaturated fatty acids (like oleic acid in olive oil), have only one place where hydrogen is missing and, therefore, only one point of flexibility. Olive oil is liquid at room temperature, but if you put it in the refrigerator, it congeals. But polyunsaturated fatty acids, those with two or more points of flexibility, stay fluid even when cold. A highly polyunsaturated fat like safflower oil—in which nearly 75 percent of the fatty acids have two places where hydrogen is missing—is liquid even when refrigerated. This tells you that olive oil has more saturated fatty acids than does safflower oil (13 percent as compared to 6 percent, but both are low in comparison to the 50 percent saturation of butter or beef fat).

Ordinarily, the higher saturated fatty acid content of olive oil might make you want to avoid it, but this oil has other good things going for it that compensate. More than 70 percent of the fatty acids in olive oil are monounsaturated—oleic acid. Oleic acid, for reasons that researchers also have yet to explain, does not increase the amount of cholesterol in blood and may even raise the level of the "good" form of cholesterol (high density, or HDL). This makes the priority order for choosing fatty acids on the basis of their saturation level (1) monounsaturated, (2) polyunsaturated, and (3) saturated.

> **F**ood Oil Rule #3: all fats—no exceptions—are mixtures of saturated, monounsaturated, and polyunsaturated fatty acids. It is just the proportions of their fatty acids that differ.

But fats are not that simple, ever. Fats and oils do not have just one type of fatty acid. Food Oil Rule #3: all fats—no exceptions—are mixtures of saturated, monounsaturated, and polyunsaturated fatty acids. It is just the proportions of their fatty acids that differ. Here are some examples of how the mix works in a sample of salad oils from the Point Loma Vons.

Fatty Acids in Salad and Cooking Oils (Grams per Tablespoon)*

OIL SOURCE	SATURATED	MONO-UNSATURATED	POLY-UNSATURATED
Olive	2	10	2
Canola	1	8	4
Peanut	2	7	5
Sesame	2	6	6
Corn	2	4	8
Soy (vegetable)	2	3	9
Safflower	1	2	11

On salad oil labels, a tablespoon is defined as 14 grams (except for canola, which has 13, for some unstated reason).

Olive and canola oils have the most monounsaturated fatty acids, which makes them good choices, but the others are fine to use too. All of these oils are liquid at room temperature and relatively unsaturated as compared to the fats in meat or dairy foods. They have 1 or 2 grams of saturated fat per tablespoon serving. I have seen oils advertised as having "half the

> I have seen oils advertised as having "half the saturated fat." When you see that on a food label, it means that oil has 1 gram of saturated fat instead of 2.

saturated fat." When you see that on a food label, it means that oil has 1 gram of saturated fat instead of 2. For all practical purposes, the proportion of saturated fatty acids is about the same in any liquid oil, and the difference between 1 or 2 grams per serving does not make much nutritional difference unless you eat oils in large amounts.

THE RANCIDITY PROBLEM

If you keep a bottle of salad oil around too long, it smells bad and tastes nasty; it has gone rancid. Exposure to light, heat, and air destroys the quality and taste of an oil. This happens as a direct result of unsaturation. The more unsaturated and polyunsaturated fatty acids there are in an oil, the more quickly it goes rancid. The more quickly it goes rancid, the shorter its shelf life. So manufacturers do tricks to prevent oils from becoming rancid. They sometimes add extra vitamin E as an antioxidant, but this does not work nearly as well as partial hydrogenation. You may recall that partial hydrogenation is what turns soy oil into margarine, and that partial hydrogenation does two bad things: it turns unsaturated fatty acids into saturated fatty acids, and it creates *trans*-fatty acids—both of which raise the risk of heart disease. That is why a Mazola vegetable/soy oil at the Point Loma Vons carried a reassuring label saying "0 grams *trans* fat."

Rancidity is the reason why you should care about the acidity of olive oils. Low acidity is a sign of an oil that is "fresh," and not rancid. If you are wondering where the acid comes from, here is the answer. Remember that oils are triglycerides made from three fatty acids attached to glycerol (a sugar alcohol)—sort of like a letter E? Well, with light, oxygen, and time, one or another fatty acid can get loose from the glycerol and float freely in the oil. These "free fatty acids" are what get measured as acidity in olive oils. A "low acid" oil has less than 1 percent of its fatty acids unattached and "free." The expensive Greek olive oil that I saw at the Point Loma Vons, for example, had an acidity of 0 to 0.5 percent, meaning that its fatty acids were firmly attached, just as they are supposed to be, at the time it was bottled. A run-of-the-mill olive oil will have no more than 3.3 percent acidity. Anything above that does not taste good. Armando Manni's oils are alive, in his view, because their fatty acids are attached, are protected from getting loose, and are used up before any loosening occurs. Those mono- and diglyceride emulsifiers that you see on ingredient lists are made by forcing fatty acids off the E. Monoglycerides have only one fatty acid still stuck on; diglycerides have two.

Rancidity is also why you do not see high omega-3 oils on supermarket shelves. These oils are so polyunsaturated that they have no shelf life at all. Only one of the canola oils in this Vons Market mentioned omega-3s on its label, even though nearly 10 percent of the fatty acids in canola are omega-3s. Flaxseed oil is richest in omega-3s; more than half its fatty acids are the essential omega-3 fatty acid, alpha-linolenic acid. But flaxseed oil is so highly polyunsaturated and so easily oxidized that it has to be stored in black bottles in a refrigerator. If you find it at all in markets or health food stores, you have to assume that it has been treated in some way to prevent it from going rancid.

Preventing rancidity is why solid shortenings seem to last forever. The Point Loma Vons had a small collection of oxymoronic "solid" vegetable oils. Crisco is a good example; it is labeled "all vegetable," which it is: its ingredients are partially hydrogenated soybean and cottonseed oils and mono- and diglycerides. The partial hydrogenation makes it more saturated—25 percent of its fatty acids are saturated compared to the much lower percentage in untreated oils—and it also introduces *trans*-fatty acids.

Because of concerns about the role of *trans*-fatty acids in raising heart disease risk, shortening manufacturers want to get rid of them. And some have done so. The Vons had a Smart Balance "*trans* fat free" shortening. This was solid but not because it was hydrogenated. Instead, it contained a blend of oils: "soy, palm, fraction of palm and canola." Aha! Palm oils. Nearly 50 percent of the fatty acids in palm fruit oil are saturated, as are more than 80 percent of the fatty acids in palm kernel oil. At this level of saturation, these vegetable "oils" are solid at room temperature. If you see a solid vegetable oil, it has to have a lot of saturated fatty acids. Otherwise it wouldn't be solid.

THE OMEGA-3 VERSUS OMEGA-6 PROBLEM

One more fat complication deserves a look. If you have not heard about the omega-3 versus omega-6 problem, you soon will. Entire books are devoted to warning you about how an imbalance between these two kinds of fatty acids is responsible for practically anything that could possibly be wrong with you: cancer, heart disease, diabetes, arthritis, skin disorders, and more. The ideal proportion of omega-6 to omega-3 fatty acids is not really known but some investigators believe that a ratio of 6 to 1 is best for heart health. But American diets contain at least ten times more omega-6 than omega-3 fatty acids, and up to thirty times more in people who eat a lot of foods fried in oils.

In the fish chapters, I explained that one omega-3 fatty acid, alpha-linolenic acid, is required in the diet because your body cannot make it. The other required fatty acid, linoleic acid, is in a different "family" of fatty acids, the omega-6s. Oleic acid, the principal fatty acid in olive oil, belongs to yet a third "family," the omega-9s, but these are not required in the diet because your body can make them from scratch. All three kinds of fatty acids—omega-3s, omega-6s, and omega-9s—help protect you against heart disease, so it is useful to eat foods that contain all three.

You must eat some linoleic acid (omega-6) and alpha-linolenic acid (omega-3) because these two are starting points—precursors—for making other fatty substances you need. Although these two essential fatty acids differ, the enzymes that work on them are exactly the same. This means that when you eat a lot of linoleic acid (which many people do), it can compete with alpha-linolenic acid for the enzymes that turn alpha-linolenic acid into EPA and DHA, the two longer omega-3 fatty acids that seem especially good for health (and for which fish is the biggest source).

> All three kinds of fatty acids—omega-3s, omega-6s, and omega-9s—help protect you against heart disease, so it is useful to eat foods that contain all three of them.

To prevent this competition, a better balance of omega-6s to omega-3s is needed, perhaps a ratio of 6 to 1. But vegetable oils differ in this balance. The Table gives the proportions of omega-3, omega-6, and omega-9 fatty acids in some oils typically found in supermarkets.

Percentage of Omega-3, Omega-6, and Omega-9 Fatty Acids in Some Salad and Cooking Oils*

OIL	OMEGA-3 ALPHA-LINOLENIC ACID	OMEGA-6 LINOLENIC ACID	PROPORTION OF OMEGA-6 TO OMEGA-3	OMEGA-9 OLEIC ACID
Flaxseed	53%	13%	1 to 4	20%
Canola	9%	20%	2 to 1	56%
Soy	7%	51%	7 to 1	23%
Olive	1%	9%	9 to 1	72%
Corn	1%	54%	54 to 1	27%
Peanut	<1%	32%	At least 32 to 1	45%
Safflower	<1%	75%	At least 75 to 1	14%

Percentages do not add up to 100 because oils also contain saturated fatty acids and other monounsaturated and polyunsaturated fatty acids. Source: USDA Nutrient Data Laboratory at www.nal.usda.gov/fnic/foodcomp/search.

The Table shows that flaxseed oil has four times as many omega-3 fatty acids as omega-6 fatty acids, and would be the best choice for balancing the omega-6s in more commonly used oils, but it goes rancid so quickly that it is not usually available. Canola, with a ratio of two omega-6 fatty acids to one omega-3 fatty acid is an excellent choice, particularly because it is widely available. Soy oil is well balanced in fatty acids but is usually hydrogenated; this destroys linoleic acid and defeats the point. Olive oil has a fairly good balance of omega-6s to omega-3s and also has lots of the heart-healthy omega-9s.

THE HEALTH CLAIM PROBLEM

In 2003, the North American Olive Oil Association petitioned the FDA to allow this health claim for olive oil: "Monounsaturated fats from

13.5 g [grams] per day of olive oil (one tablespoon) may reduce your risk of heart disease when included in a moderate-fat diet low in saturated fat and cholesterol." After reviewing the research, the FDA concluded in 2004 that the evidence for this relationship did not meet its standard of "significant scientific agreement," but that olive oil could use a "qualified" health claim, one that placed the claim in appropriate scientific and dietary context:

> Limited and not conclusive scientific evidence suggests that eating about 2 tablespoons (23 grams) of olive oil daily may reduce the risk of coronary heart disease due to the monounsaturated fat in olive oil. To achieve this possible benefit, olive oil is to replace a similar amount of saturated fat and not increase the total number of calories you eat in a day. One serving of this product contains [x] grams of olive oil.

If you see a statement on olive oils that they are heart healthy, look for that cautious disclaimer, which is sure to be in tiny print.

Back on the East Coast after that San Diego visit, a friend showed me something new and different in the cooking oil aisle—a product called Enova oil. This had an amazing label: "More is burned as energy. Not stored as fat. Diacylglycerol oil." No kidding? I took a fair amount of biochemistry in graduate school, and I was pretty sure that diacylglycerol is just another name for diglyceride, the common food additive—the triglyceride E with one arm missing. If you want to turn soy oil into diglycerides, you just add a lot of glycerol, the small sugar alcohol that forms the backbone of the E. The way I remembered it, diglycerides are digested and absorbed pretty much like triglycerides and are freely interchangeable with them, meaning that they can be converted to triglycerides (meaning fat) in your body. So I could not see why your body would use them preferentially for energy instead of storing them if you ate too much of them. I tried the Web site.

Enova advertisements early in 2005 said "Don't change the way you live . . . just change your oil." Some exploration of the company's Web site (www.enovaoil.com) led to a review of the few research studies, mostly done on animals. These suggest that triglycerides with the middle arm of the E missing go directly to the liver to be burned for energy.

The biochemical details of this rationale and the study results are so complicated that the company's own assessment of the state of the science concludes with the inevitable "More research is needed on the health implications of DAG [diacylglycerol] consumption." Even if the rationale turns out to be correct, and the fatty acids in this oil really are used preferentially for energy, any other calories you eat—from carbohydrates, proteins, or the other fats in your diet—will go straight to fat if you eat too many of them. Enova has exactly the same 120 calories per tablespoon as any other cooking oil. One way or the other, its calories, like all others, count.

Question: Where is the FDA when we need it to help interpret situations like this? Answer: kept under wraps by Congress. If you would like the FDA to keep a sharper eye on health claims on food products, you need to convey that sentiment to your congressional representatives.

SOLVING THE OIL CRISES

In the late 1980s, when health authorities urged everyone to pay attention to fat and eat less of it, they had no way of knowing that this sensible advice would be interpreted as a call to avoid fat entirely and to substitute carbohydrates instead. What we got was what my nutritionist colleagues call the "SnackWell's phenomenon"—fat-free, high-carb, same-calorie cookies consumed with abandon—and the ensuing epidemic of obesity. Next came the low-carb backlash and the return to fat. Both trends focused on *what* you eat—fat versus carbohydrates—and not on what matters more in weight gain: *how much* you eat and, therefore, the calories you consume relative to the ones you use in physical activity.

As with carbohydrates, thinking about fats requires some perspective, even more so than in other areas of nutrition, because fats—and their effects on health—are so complicated. Because of the calories, almost everyone would be better off eating less fat, but avoiding it altogether is not a good idea.

The 2005 *Dietary Guidelines* advise you to choose foods that are "lean, low-fat, or fat-free." Among fatty foods, you are to choose those with unsaturated fats (fish, nuts, vegetable oils) and restrict those with saturated fat, cholesterol, and *trans* fat. The guidelines provide handy tables that show beef and dairy foods as the main sources of saturated fat and cholesterol, and baked goods, snack foods, and margarine as the main sources of *trans* fats. Once again it is worth trying to figure out how to decode a food label. If the label says that the food has more than 20 percent of the Daily Value for saturated fat, leave it on the shelf (if it has less than 5 percent, consider it low fat). If a food has any *trans* fat at all, you will want to eat only a little of it, if any.

> If the label says that the food has more than 20 percent of the Daily Value for saturated fat, leave it on the shelf (if it has less than 5 percent, consider it low fat). If a food has any *trans* fat at all, you will want to eat only a little of it, if any.

Salad and cooking oils are 100 percent fat, but they are low in saturated fat (5 to 10 percent of the Daily Value), do not have *trans* fat unless they have been hydrogenated, and never have any cholesterol. If you do not eat too much of salad and cooking oils, you can decide which ones to buy on the basis of how they taste and how much they cost. All of them are better for you than fats from animal sources. All have about the same nutritional value (linoleic acid, some vitamin E, and antioxidants). Those with stronger flavors like olive oils taste better on salads, but this is a matter of personal preference. Some of the blander ones are better for cooking, and some give off smoke at lower temperatures than others so are not as good for frying. Oils can be reused in cooking but once they get discolored—or any time they smell or taste bad—they are not good for you and you should not eat them. Beyond that, unless you care deeply about minor differences, one salad or cooking oil is much like another and you can choose them on the basis of taste and cost.

> You really only need to consider two things when choosing salad and cooking oils: watch out for those calories (120 per tablespoon), and avoid hydrogenated vegetable oils because of their *trans* fat.

Despite the many different kinds of oils, their complicated structural details and biochemistry, and the range of issues they pose, the choices are simple. You really only need to consider two things when choosing salad and cooking oils: watch out for those calories (120 per tablespoon), and avoid hydrogenated vegetable oils because of their *trans* fat.

Some people also worry a lot about the balance between omega-3 and omega-6 fatty acids, but I am not one of them. That is because I much prefer to get my fats from foods, not processed oils. Omega-6 fatty acids commonly occur in grains and seeds, and you get plenty of them in seeds, nuts, and avocados, which also come with a good balance of omega-9s. The omega-3 fatty acids show up in leafy vegetables in small amounts, but those amounts add up. In American diets, fish is the greatest source, but chicken and eggs are also important sources, even when the chickens are not fed special diets. If I feel like eating flax, I will buy the seeds, not the oil. I like olive oil for bread and salad dressings and cooking (for reasons of taste), and if I want to save money I'll use canola and soy oils as long as they are not hydrogenated. Overall, it always makes sense to look for oils in dark bottles or cans, and to use them up long before they lose life (as Armando Manni might say) as well as taste.

33

Water, Water Everywhere: Bottled and Not

When I see bottled water, I think liquid gold. It is no surprise that supermarkets devote entire aisles of prime shelf space to these products. Their main ingredient costs the producers practically nothing, plastic bottles are cheap (except for what they do to the environment), and you can pay an astonishing amount for them—without even noticing. All told, bottled water has to be the most profitable packaged food item ever invented.

Granted, bottled water does have some advantages over tap water or soft drinks. The bottles are handy and portable, water has no calories, and who knows what is in your local water supply. But in places with good public water systems—and in the United States this means most places—the idea that you need to drink bottled water rather than tap water comes more from smart marketing than from science or public health. And so does the idea that you need to drink water all day long.

You do need to drink water in one form or another to replace the amount you lose when you breathe, sweat, and excrete. This works out to the equivalent of about a liter (a bit more than a quart) of water for every thousand calories you eat. Most people need to drink at least two quarts of water a day. But these quarts do not have to come from water itself; they also can come from food, juice, coffee, tea, soda, and anything else with water in it. Most of the time, you don't have to keep track of how much water you are drinking because water balance takes care of itself. If you need more water, you feel thirsty. You only need to force yourself to drink water in very hot weather, at high altitudes, or when you exercise hard for a long time. And you can easily tell when you need to drink water: your urine will be bright yellow and smelly (if you are well hydrated, urine is pale and practically odorless). Otherwise, the water in food and beverages takes care of fluid needs, which means that hardly anyone needs to drink eight glasses of water a day. But that "hardly anyone" includes not only athletes and mountain climbers, but also children and the elderly, who do not regulate water balance very well. Beyond these exceptions, however, as the Institute of Medicine explains, "the vast majority of healthy people adequately meet their daily hydration needs by letting thirst be their guide."

> Most people need to drink at least two quarts of water a day. But these quarts do not have to come from water itself; they also can come from food, juice, coffee, tea, soda, and anything else with water in it.

Maybe, but the beverage industry finds this relaxed view of your water needs "alarming." Its trade association, the International Bottled Water Association, wants you to drink a minimum of eight 8-ounce glasses of water a day, and it provides a hydration calculator to "prove" that you need to do so. You type in your weight and the number of minutes a day you exercise; the calculator does the rest. The calculator conveniently does not care how hard you exercise, as I learned when I tried it out for myself. What with one errand or another, I think I walk about an hour a day, so I called that sixty minutes of exercise. The calculator's result: I need to drink 100 ounces of water a day—about three quarts or twelve 8-ounce glasses. It tells me that I should be sure to drink water at least six times a day in addition to what I drink with meals and get from food: before breakfast, at mid-morning, before lunch, at mid-afternoon, before dinner, and at mid-evening. Maybe, but if I followed this advice I would not be able to last through an hour of walking, teaching a class, or watching a movie. Hydration calculators are "drink more" strategies, and strategies for the promotion of bottled water at that.

Try as hard as I can, I cannot decide whether bottled water is any healthier than tap water. Tap water is not pure, but neither are most bottled waters. Both start with spring water, and sometimes water from the same spring. At their source, spring waters contain dissolved gases, minerals, and other substances acquired from the soil or air; these are usually harmless. By the time spring water gets to your sink, it has traveled long distances through waterways, reservoirs, and pipes. In this odyssey, it can run into sewage, agricultural runoff, and industrial wastes and take up whatever dangerous microbes and chemicals might be in them.

S ince the early 1900s, local and regional governments have added chlorine to drinking water to kill infectious organisms, and this basic public health measure successfully eliminated threats of cholera, typhoid, dysentery, and the like in all but the poorest and least-developed areas of the world.

Microbes, fortunately, are not much of a worry in industrialized countries. Since the early 1900s, local and regional governments have added chlorine to drinking water to kill infectious organisms, and this basic public health measure successfully eliminated threats of cholera, typhoid, dysentery, and the like in all but the poorest and least-developed areas of the world. But chlorination alone does not destroy cyst-forming protozoa, such as *Cryptosporidium* and *Giardia*, which now contaminate even the most remote back-country streams. Getting rid of them requires stronger chemicals or filtration, and some public water systems do this too (but not New York City; 1.2 billion gallons a day is too much to filter).

In the United States, the Centers for Disease Control and Prevention (CDC) tracks disease outbreaks caused by contaminants in drinking water from any source: public systems, private wells, and bottled products. In 2002, the CDC reported thirty-one outbreaks from nineteen states; these caused more than 1,000 illnesses and seven deaths. Microbes were responsible for most of the outbreaks, but five were due to chemicals that had gotten into the water. Nearly all of the outbreaks were caused by drinking impure water from private wells at camps, trailer parks, or golf courses, but one was the result of drinking bottled water. None—not one—was caused by microbes in a public water supply that year. Despite occasional lapses, the evidence indicates that tap water is free of harmful microbes, and you do not need to filter or boil it before you drink it. As water engineers love to say, "The solution to pollution is dilution." The sheer quantity of water in public (as opposed to private) water systems almost always keeps the level of microbial contamination below anything that might be harmful.

Chemical contaminants, however, are another matter. Ironically, chlorine—the very chemical used to kill microbes in water—is part of the contamination problem and creates its own dilemma. Chlorine itself is benign but it reacts with other chemicals in water to form "disinfection by-products" such as chlorinated trihalomethanes. The more chlorine added to water, the more disinfection by-products get formed, and these are anything but benign. At high concentrations, they cause cancers of the bladder and other organs. They also interfere with reproduction, alter menstrual cycles, reduce the quality of sperm, and cause fetal losses. You would not want your local water authorities to stop chlorinating drinking water because this method is such an effective way to prevent common and uncommon microbial diseases, and water engineers have no easy and equally inexpensive alternatives. Researchers who study the effects of disinfection by-products—and there are many who do this kind of work—actively debate whether the low levels typically found in tap water cause harm and, if so, to what extent. Some say tap water increases the risk of cancer and reproductive problems (although not by much), while others say studies of water and health are so difficult to design and interpret that nobody can really tell.

But there is no debate about whether tap water contains undesirable chemicals. It does. In 2002, the U.S. Geological Survey found antibiotics, hormones, plasticizers, insecticides, and fire retardants in 80 percent of the streams it tested, one-third of them containing ten or more of such chemicals. These streams are not necessarily headed for drinking water reservoirs, but they can and do leak into water systems. The Environmental Protection Agency (EPA) has identified a thousand or so chemicals in tap water, and sets allowable limits for about eighty of the worst of them. You can go to the EPA Web site, click on a map of the United States, and look up reports on the quality of your own city's drinking water. I did this and was relieved to see that the tap water in New York City—which only adds a little chlorine and fluoride to its unfiltered water—is virtually free of microbial contaminants. But it has low but detectable levels of most disinfection by-products (only one type exceeded standards, in the Croton Reservoir), as well as detectable amounts of lead, nitrates, strontium, and any number of other such things. I have no idea whether these pose a health risk and, if so, how serious that risk might be. Neither, apparently, does anyone else. As the U.S. Geological Survey unhelpfully explains, "Little is known about the potential health effects to humans or aquatic organisms exposed to the low levels of most of these chemicals . . ."

What is most disturbing about this level of ignorance is how quickly and how recently the quality of drinking water has been allowed to deteriorate. The EPA says that the number of chemically polluted streams in America increased more than tenfold just from 1993 to 2003. As recently as 1998, the EPA administrator was still defending the safety of city water supplies: "We want the public to understand that standards set for municipal drinking water supplies are mandatory, and are monitored and tested more often than for bottled water." By 2003, however, EPA publications were saying that "threats to drinking water are increasing . . . we can no longer take our drinking water for granted." Using EPA data as a starting point, *Organic Style* magazine asked: "Is your drinking water really safe?" Its investigators collected state and EPA reports on water quality and were horrified by what they found. Their excellent advice: "get a copy of the report from your utility company or have your tap water tested. If you're concerned about the water's safety . . . install a filter."

What this means is that the government no longer guarantees the safety of drinking water. Instead, *you* are responsible for getting your utility's safety report, paying for having your tap water tested, and installing a filter. It makes good sense to do these things, but here is another place where economists talk about "externalized" costs. The government allows companies to dump chemicals into streams and contaminate drinking water, but instead of requiring them to pay for prevention or cleanup, it shifts the burden to you. Your water utility bill does not cover anywhere near the true costs of providing clean water, so you pay for water in three additional ways: in taxes to pay for cleaning up polluted water, in taxes that pay for subsidizing companies that do the polluting in the first place, and in the price you pay for bottled water at the grocery store.

BOTTLED WATER

The bottled water industry uses your legitimate concerns about the quality of city water to convince you that its products are worth what you have to pay for them. Hundreds of national and international companies sell bottled water in the United States, some from as far away as Fiji or Australia. Despite the economic and environmental costs of the transportation, plastics, or glass, annual sales are in the billions of dollars, and bottled water is the fastest-growing segment of the beverage business. The brands vary by source, process, and price, from gallon jugs of store-brand spring water to small bottles of Perrier and Evian. All are just water—but with profit margins of 20 to 60 percent. Companies support their brands with staggering advertising budgets. In 2004, PepsiCo put $22 million into domestic media advertising for Aquafina, and Coca-Cola spent $18 million to advertise Dasani. These amazing sums are spent to promote *water*.

Bottled waters appear to present many choices—bubbles, flavors, and the colors and sizes of packages—but up to 40 percent of them start out as tap water. To create Dasani, for example, Coca-Cola takes water from local city supplies, cleans it up a bit, and tosses in a few minerals. PepsiCo does the same to make Aquafina. Many other brands also are tap waters run through distillation, deionization, reverse osmosis, or some other cleaning system. By law, mineral waters must have at least 250 parts per million dissolved solids. Spring waters—sparkling, still, or mineral—must come from an underground source identified on the label (these are often the same local springs that go into tap water). Sparkling waters contain natural or added carbon dioxide to make bubbles. Seltzer is filtered carbonated tap water, and club soda is the same, but with added minerals. Most bottled waters have been treated to remove chlorine, and

> B ottled waters appear to present many choices—bubbles, flavors, and the colors and sizes of packages—but up to 40 percent of them start out as tap water.

they do not have fluoride unless the labels say it has been added. These differences do not make much nutritional difference. Water is water; it is not an important source of nutrients (except added fluoride). The waters may taste different in subtle ways, and you may prefer one over another, but basically they are all just water.

If there is any meaningful difference at all between one bottle of water and another, it is surely in price. In my Manhattan neighborhood, grocery stores rarely bother with anything so helpful as shelf labels or price stickers. Making a rational choice is hopeless, even with a calculator in hand. I gave up and went to the more consumer-friendly supermarkets upstate in Ithaca. Even there, comparisons are difficult. Some stores label unit prices in quarts, while others do so in pints, liters, milliliters, or gallons. It is so difficult to make sense of the units, fractional bottle sizes, packaging methods, and mineral additives that I cannot help but suspect that the confusion is deliberate. The Table on the next page gives a small sample from one bout of comparison shopping, starting with what Ithaca residents paid for tap water in 2004: $3.46 per 1,000 gallons, or a bit more than three-tenths of a cent per gallon.

Tap water is cheap, so the bizarre range of prices for bottled water must depend on the distance traveled, the package, the company's marketing costs, and—most important—a calculated guess as to what you are willing to pay for it. At the extremes that day, you could buy a gallon container of filtered tap water for 69 cents, or pay nearly $4.00 for less than a quart of water (and, therefore, close to $16 per gallon) imported from Norway in a bottle so elegantly designed that it belongs in a museum. At prices like these, water costs a lot more than gasoline.

Even so, these prices pale in comparison to those I witnessed on a trip to the United Arab Emirates in spring 2005. At a brunch at the Burj Al Arab Hotel in Dubai (the hotel you see on travel posters that looks like a spinnaker sail), we asked for water with our meal and the waiter handed us a handsome parchment folder—the water menu. Just as you might see on a wine list, the menu provided lively descriptions of each of twenty-four bottled waters, mostly from European countries. The prices started at what seemed like a modest 15 dirhams (about $4.00 at the exchange rate that day) for a bottle of Niksar, a Turkish spring water

Water Price Comparison, December 2004

BRAND	CLAIM ON LABEL	CONTAINER SIZE	OUNCES	PRICE PER GALLON
City of Ithaca	Tap water			$0.003
Store brand	Spring water	Gallon	128	$0.69
Store brand	Spring water with fluoride	Gallon	128	$0.89
Store brand	Spring water (6-pack)	Pint	16	$2.52
Dasani (Coca-Cola)	Purified water enhanced with minerals	Liter	32	$5.28
Fiji	Natural artesian	500 milliliters	17	$6.80
S. Pellegrino	Sparkling natural mineral water, Italy	750 milliliters	25	$7.56
Saratoga	Sparkling spring water, New York	12 ounces	12	$10.56
Voss	Artesian water, Norway	800 milliliters	27	$15.56

whose "therapeutic qualities have been known for over 1400 years," but the bottle contained only 300 milliliters and worked out to $13 per liter or $51 per gallon. The most expensive option was a liter bottle of mineral water from Chateldon, "the oldest source in France exclusive to King Louis XIV . . . also a curative water for nerve and skin problems," conditions no doubt brought on by its 95 dirham cost—$27 per liter and $103 per gallon. For a mere 30 dirhams ($31 per gallon), you could get a liter of Scottish Highland Spring water from "a protected underground source beneath the Ochil Hills, where no farming has been permitted for the last 20 years and is now certified organic." Certified organic *water*? The menu, alas, did not disclose the certifying criteria.

You might not mind paying ridiculous prices if bottled water is better than tap water, but nobody outside the beverage industry who has looked closely at the comparison thinks that it is. Dubai is on a desert along the

Persian Gulf (or, as they call it, the Arabian Gulf), and its tap water comes from desalinated seawater. It tasted fine to me and I would expect it to, given that country's high level of technological development.

Back home, I went to the Bolton Point Municipal Water Plant on Lake Cayuga in central New York to see for myself how one facility purifies water, treats it to remove sediments, filters it, and tests it for contaminants before it travels to public water supplies in the surrounding communities. Bolton Point water tastes clean, wet, and refreshing. When you drink water like that, you cannot imagine why anyone would pay a price hundreds or thousands of times higher to drink anything else.

For this and other reasons, Ian Williams, the United Nations correspondent for *The Nation*, views bottled water as "ostentatiously useless," "environmentally deleterious," and a "complete insult to our intelligence." He points out that you can buy bottled water from Greenland

> alleged to be melted glacier water. Think about it. Why should water that has been lying around since the last Ice Age, or maybe even the one before, collecting dioxins, lead, radioactive fallout, polar bear poop, and for all anyone knows, the occasional dead Inuit or Viking, set any acceptable standard for purity?

Without going that far, the quality of bottled water does bring up some uncomfortable issues. The FDA—not the EPA—is responsible for overseeing the safety of bottled waters, but these products are not high on this agency's regulatory agenda. FDA standards are weaker than those of the EPA, which may be why the FDA so confidently says bottled waters are

U nder current federal regulations, bottled waters do not have to be tested as rigorously as tap waters or disinfected to the same extent.

safe. Surveys by state, university, and advocacy groups, however, suggest otherwise; while they agree that most bottled waters meet tests for safety and quality, they find many exceptions. In 1999, for example, the National Resources Defense Council (NRDC) tested more than 1,000 bottles of 100 brands of bottled water, and found *one-third* to exceed allowable limits for one or more regulated chemical or biological contaminants. Under current federal regulations, bottled waters do not have to be tested as rigorously as tap waters or disinfected to the same extent. Waters packaged and sold within the same state are left to the states to regulate; some do this rigorously, and some don't. The bottled water industry is largely self-policed and it is a wonder—and a tribute to the safety of the tap water that is the basis of most bottled products—that problems do not occur more often.

Some of my friends who live in upstate New York depend on wells for their running water, and their tap water reeks of sulfur. Bathing in it makes you feel like you are in a European spa, but it is not something you would want to drink. They drink bottled water. Friends and relatives who live near Chicago, where Lake Michigan is the source of the tap water, disagree about how it tastes, in part because their communities are served by different water treatment systems. Some from Evanston say the taste has deteriorated since the invasion of the Great Lakes by zebra mussels; it does not taste of shellfish exactly, but they describe its taste as steely or metallic. They too drink bottled water. But cousins of mine who live in Hyde Park, which is served by the Chicago water system, think their tap water tastes better than bottled water. Zebra mussels or not, untreated sewage is a much greater hazard in the Great Lakes, but Chicago officials report that not a single biological or chemical contaminant in the city water supply exceeds federal limits.

Natural waters are naturally impure and the impurities make them taste better.

In taste tests, municipal water supplies routinely win over bottled waters—once the tap water has been aerated with a whisk or poured into a pitcher and allowed to stand overnight to get rid of the chlorine and its smell (you can do this at home). Like any taste sensation, the taste of water is highly subjective, but most people find distilled (purified) water to taste flat. Natural waters are naturally impure and the impurities make them taste better. In the best-tasting spring waters, the impurities stimulate—but just barely—a sweet or other pleasant sensation in the mouth. Soft waters are low in minerals and taste better than hard waters, which have iron, calcium, magnesium, and other dissolved salts. Adding tiny amounts of these minerals to distilled water (as many companies do) improves the taste but makes little nutritional difference; the Nutrition Facts labels usually display a complete set of zeros. When minerals do show up on the label, you can expect the water to taste slightly salty or bitter. If the label shows calories, it means that sugars have been added and the water has been converted to a soft drink.

So how to choose? Drinking water unquestionably poses a dilemma, and one that I cannot easily resolve. Sometimes I drink tap water, sometimes bottled. I like the taste and bubbles of some bottled waters, but I am not convinced that drinking bottled water is healthier than drinking tap water. Neither bottled water nor tap water is regulated to the extent it should be. This dilemma is not one you can fix with a choice at the grocery store; this one needs politics, big time. As Ian Williams might say, think about it: this is America. You are supposed to have clean, safe drinking water. If you do not (and the only way to find out is to ask or do your own research), it is because companies are allowed to contaminate waterways and nobody is stopping them. Complain. Join advocacy groups. Contact your mayor's office. Write your congressional representatives. But do not expect any help from the bottled water industry in getting companies to stop dumping wastes into public water supplies. The International Bottled Water Association wants you to leave the industrial polluters to their own devices:

> Comprehensive groundwater resource management is critical to maintaining this renewable natural resource . . . No industry should be identified as a threat to the water resource without the benefit of sound scientific evidence of the impact on the groundwater quality and quantity which therefore diminishes the resource for other users.

In other words, they say, you should not be worrying about polluters; trust us and buy bottled waters.

MARKETING WATER: HEALTH BENEFITS

The Europeans are way ahead of us in marketing bottled waters for their health qualities. The labels of some bottles of Dolomiti "acqua minerale naturale oligominerale" from Italy, for example, display a Gerber baby–like infant to indicate that these contain "microbiologicamente pura" mineral water for babies. This is water with tiny amounts of a few minerals and should be just as effective as tap water for keeping babies hydrated, although at a higher cost. For adults, Sanfaustino water (also from Italy) offers bottles containing half a gram of calcium per liter. Drink eight glasses a day, as the company hopes you will do, and you will take in 80 percent of your Daily Value for calcium—"without adding the calories, fat, carbs, cholesterol, lactose, or sugars found in other food and beverage sources" (and, of course, all the other nutrients that come with food).

I am indebted to the Global Public Affairs department of Nestlé (no relation) for letting me know about its new "osteoporosis initiative," Contrex water. If you drink 1.5 liters of Contrex every day, you will get 729 milligrams of calcium and be well on your way toward meeting your daily calcium needs. Nestlé's marketing manager in North America, Mike Hoynes, sent a package containing a liter of this water to one of my dietitian colleagues. The enclosed flier said:

> HELLO my name is Contrex . . . Je suis francaise [sic]. I am sourced from the Vosges Mountains in Contrexéville, France . . . As an all-natural mineral water, the minerals found in me are naturally occurring. Nothing fortified here!

The package contained a personal letter to my colleague asking her to complete a feedback card which would be entered into a drawing to win $250, an incentive to taste the water and recommend it to her clients. The letter said the water is "best enjoyed when chilled." I tasted it. It is a hard mineral water and does taste better cold. Natural or not, this is an expensive way to take a calcium supplement.

Unsweetened water—from tap or bottle—has no calories, and if you drink water rather than soft drinks, you can save the calories for eating foods. But this does not make water a weight-loss product. I am fascinated by a brochure from the company that makes Brita water filters. It says, "You're trying hard to reach your weight loss goals. What works? Water works . . . Brita water works to help curb hunger and improve metabolism to help you achieve your weight loss goals and maintain them over time." Water might indeed do this if—and only if—you also reduce your calories. As the work of Barbara Rolls has shown, it's the water in *food* that fill... ...ger, and makes you feel full, and fruits ...est in water—another good reason for

...ther to laugh or cry when I received ...tritionist spokesperson for a new bot-...y Water—a "natural form of weight

...further. It actually aides [*sic*] the ...g the appetite, increasing meta-...rmation ... [It] combines with ...t, Hydroxycitric Acid ("Super ...es and is completely ephedra-...Skinny Water 30–60 minutes ...diet, combined with the nor-

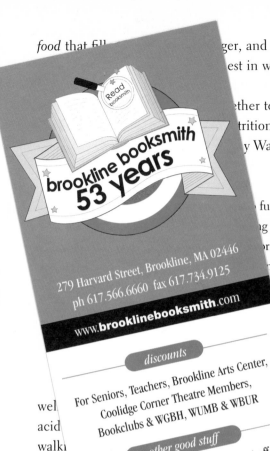

wel... ...ne who believes its claims), acid... ...confirm that hydroxycitric walki... ...g calorie-free water and ever a... ...healthy weight, I do not ...ed the invitation.

...TER: ECO-BENEFITS

In Augus... ...stores in the United States wo... ...water, "Ethos: Help-ing childr... ...tarbucks customers to the inte... ...f safe drinking wa-ter for 20 p... ...inated water is re-sponsible fo... ...eople, and these cause the dea... ...ay. Starbucks ex-pects to dona... ...ars to help countries de-velop clean wa... ...ne head of a nonprofit "cause marketing" firm explained what this is really about to *USA Today*: "More and more marketers are looking for ways to appeal to consumers on an emotional level by indicating that they support the sorts of causes that consumers support." Starbucks will sell 700-milliliter bottles of Ethos for $1.80 and donate 5 cents of that amount for this purpose. This means that you pay nearly $10 per gallon for Ethos water, of which about 20 cents goes to the worthy cause. If you care about this issue, consider drinking tap water and donating the cost of bottled water directly to international agencies devoted to providing clean water to everyone.

BUT WHAT ABOUT THE BOTTLES?

You may have heard that plasticizers, the chemicals used to make plastic bottles soft, are "endocrine disrupters." They interfere with sex hormones and could be responsible for health problems such as early sexual development, reduced sperm counts, and cancers of the breast and testes—all of which seem to be increasing in human populations. In 1996, the EPA considered concerns about plasticizers to be so serious—but so unstudied—that it ranked endocrine disruption as one of its top research priorities. Since then, researchers have confirmed that some of the chemicals used in making plastic bottles are indeed "estrogen active," and that they can leach into bottled waters.

But wait! Before adding plasticizers to your list of water worries, consider this: the amounts that get into water from plastic bottles are measured in nanograms—billionths of a gram. Besides, investigators in Germany have discovered that these chemicals are ubiquitous in foods as well as in water, but that the amounts present are not at all related to the type of packaging. These investigators suggest that the endocrine disrupters are more likely to come from pesticides (note: another reason to choose organics), disinfectants, and cleaning agents than from plastic bottles. Bottled water, say other researchers, accounts for less than 10 percent of the total amount of endocrine disrupters in the food supply. As Rolf Halden, an environmental scientist at Johns Hopkins, concludes: "people should be more concerned about the quality of the water they are drinking rather than the container it is coming from."

Whether nanogram amounts of endocrine disrupters really are responsible for health problems seems unlikely, but is a question that cannot be easily investigated. Plasticizers occur in so many foods that everyone consumes them, which makes it difficult to compare their levels in people who do and do not drink bottled water. Halden notes that endocrine-disrupting chemicals leach out more easily when plastic is heated. Most people drink bottled water cold or at room temperature, temperatures at which chemicals do not diffuse out as easily. Avoiding bottled water is not going to make much difference in your body burden of endocrine disrupters because they are so common in foods—whether or not the foods come in plastic containers. Here too the only recourse is political action. Tell the EPA to institute more effective controls to prevent industries from dumping these chemicals in places where they can drift into either food or water.

So if you need the convenience of bottled water, enjoy its taste, appreciate the shape or color of the bottle, revel in the status it conveys, and do not care about its cost, by all means buy it. Bottled water is just water. If you are trying to quench your thirst, and still do not care about cost, the choice is a toss-up between tap water and the bottled kind—unless, of course, you live in a community where the tap water tastes bad or does not meet safety standards. That is something you need to find out for yourself. Alternatively, you can play it safe and install a water filter, as *Organic Style* advised. If you still prefer to drink bottled water, you might as well buy the cheapest kinds, as they are no worse. But be sure to pick the ones with added fluoride to protect your children's teeth.

34

"Healthy" Drinks: Sugared and Artificially Sweetened

O ne day in fall 2004, I could not help but admire a truck double-parked outside my neighborhood convenience store. Painted on its sides were six-foot-tall bottles of Glacéau Vitamin Waters in an array of jewel-like colors, each more beautiful than the next. This was marketing at a breathtaking level of sophistication. Bottled water is expensive enough, but beverage companies can sell it at a higher price by adding minerals, and they can sell it at an even higher price by adding vitamins and herbal supplements—and then by promoting the health benefits of these additions. Energy Brands, the company responsible for that gorgeous truck advertisement, positions Glacéau SmartWater as an "electrolyte-enhanced" health food, even though any vegetable would be a better source of its few added minerals. The label of Buzz Water from Canada, "The World's First Caffeinated Spring Water," hints that its caffeine jolt will be healthy because it comes with bits of magnesium, potassium, sodium, and seventy other minerals. These are smart waters, even more smartly marketed.

You do need vitamins and minerals in your diet, about thirty of them altogether. These are best obtained from foods that also supply the dozens of other nutrients you need or are good for you—sources of energy (carbohydrate, fat, and protein), essential fatty acids (components of fat), essential amino acids (components of protein), fiber, and a host of phytochemicals. If you eat enough of a variety of foods and are otherwise healthy, the chance that you will be deficient in any vitamin or mineral is small. Deficiencies of vitamins and minerals rarely occur among people with adequate calorie intakes (iron may be one exception because it is lost in menstrual blood). Difficult as it may be to believe, eating more vitamins or minerals than are needed does not make healthy people healthier. But it is human nature to think that if eating some vitamins and minerals is good, eating more of them has to be better, especially since it is not possible to know the nutrient content of the food you eat with any degree of precision. Marketers know this about human nature, and they take full advantage of any doubts you might have about the nutritional quality of your diet.

If drinking minerals seems like a good idea, drinking vitamins might seem even more so. But there is one problem: vitamins taste awful. You can test this for yourself at home. Dissolve a vitamin pill in a glass of water and try drinking the concoction: it cries out for sugar. Once manufacturers add sugars to water, they are creating a soft drink. Surely Kool-Aid (a product of Kraft/Altria) is the historic prototype; it is sugar water supplemented with vitamin C. Unless vitamin waters are artificially sweetened, the first two ingredients are invariably water and sugars—sucrose, fructose, crystalline fructose, high fructose corn syrup, or fructose-glucose syrup.

> Difficult as it may be to believe, eating more vitamins or minerals than are needed does not make healthy people healthier.

If manufacturers add artificial sweeteners instead, they are creating a diet soft drink. PepsiCo's Propel Fitness Water adds several vitamins and calcium along with a bit of sugar and some artificial sweeteners to make it drinkable; it is a vitamin-enriched diet soft drink and a highly profitable one; PepsiCo spent nearly $38 million to advertise this one product in 2004 and Wall Street analysts gave it much credit for a PepsiCo growth spurt in 2005.

But let's go back to that truck. Without nearly that level of expense, look at how Energy Brands markets Glacéau Vitamin Waters. The waters are virtually identical except for their additives, but each comes with its own color-coded health theme: "Endurance" (peach-mango), "Rescue" (green tea), "Revive" (fruit punch), "Focus" (kiwi-strawberry), and so forth. All are water and fructose sugar along with various vitamins, minerals, and herbs; this makes them vitamin-enriched or herbal-enriched sugar waters with about half the calories of a regular soft drink—but in exceptionally pretty bottles. From 2002 to 2005, sales of Glacéau waters tripled, perhaps because, as one commentator put it, "the beverage aisle is basically tired."

Once companies start adding vitamins to sugar water, it is only a small step to putting vitamins into carbonated soft drinks. In August 2004, I received a mailing from public relations officials of Cadbury Schweppes alerting me to their latest product, 7UP PLUS:

> The idea for this product came directly from consumers, at least 6000 of them . . . [T]hese consumers . . . told us their ideal carbonated beverage would contain juice and added nutrients while being lower in calories. Although 7UP PLUS is not intended to be a replacement for healthy beverage choices such as milk, juice or water, we feel it provides a more balanced choice for those consumers still seeking fun and refreshment with flavor.

They said that 7UP PLUS is a "low calorie carbonated beverage with fruit juice, vitamins and minerals . . . sweetened with Splenda . . . with a mixed berry flavor and a fun pink color." Fruit juice? You have to look hard. There is just enough juice in 7UP PLUS to squeak by the FDA's famous "jelly bean rule," which says that food companies cannot put vitamins into candy, sodas, or other such products in order to market them as healthy. So there is juice in 7UP PLUS—all of 5 percent. Credit Cadbury Schweppes for ingenuity; the company was the first to figure out how to enrich soft drinks with nutrients but evade the jelly bean rule. More such products are sure to follow.

It is not impossible to make a healthier soda but it is more expensive. Instead of adding a little juice to sugary soda water, manufacturers could add a little soda water to juice. A small company, Fizzy Lizzy, does this quite nicely. Its owner, Liz Marlin, makes "Sparkling Juices" by diluting fruit juices about one-third with soda water (two parts juice, one part soda). The company's grapefruit juice drink, for example, is 70 percent juice and is made with only four ingredients: water, ruby red grapefruit juice, white grapefruit juice, and natural flavors. But watch those calories; a 12-ounce bottle still holds nearly an ounce of sugars.

JUICE AND NON-JUICE

When I was a kid, I was given about 6 ounces of orange juice every day to take care of my daily requirement for vitamin C. Today, children still are the biggest consumers of fruit juices, and 6 ounces is still a reasonable amount. Six ounces, however, is about what the average toddler drinks, and some drink much more. When it comes to juice, more is not better. Indeed, the American Academy of Pediatrics is so worried about the sugars and calories in fruit juices that it issued a juice advisory in 2001. Parents, pediatricians say, should give only 6 ounces of juice a day to children up to age six and no more than 12 ounces to children ages seven to eighteen, and should never give children vitamin-enriched sugar waters as a replacement for juice.

In moderation juices are good for you, but a walk through supermarket juice aisles can be quite confusing. Supermarkets usually stock juices in three places: frozen concentrate in freezer cases (discussed in the chapter on frozen foods), "fresh" juices in refrigerated cases (so they do not spoil), and juice drinks in bottles or cans in the beverage aisles. You can take your pick on the continuum from "fresh" 100 percent juice to juice-flavored sugar water that contains no juice at all.

Real juice is just that—100 percent—with nothing else added. Although you can find fresh-squeezed fruit and vegetable juices in specialty stores (and nothing compares with their tart flavor and freshness), supermarket juices are "fresh" in quotation marks. This is because an almost fresh product like Tropicana/PepsiCo "100% Pure Florida Squeezed Orange Juice" has been pasteurized before putting it into a carton. Pasteurized juices lose some of the taste of truly fresh juices, but they retain nearly all of the vitamins, minerals, and phytochemicals in

The more pulp a juice retains, the better its nutritional value.

the fruit or vegetable from which they were extracted—except for the nutrients that stick to the fiber in the pulp. The more pulp a juice retains, the better its nutritional value. Some "fresh" juices undergo a further processing step: they are reconstituted from frozen concentrate. These are almost as nutritious as the non-reconstituted but have lost even more of the flavor. They are cheaper, of course. On the basis of taste and, to a lesser extent, nutritional value, the priority order for juices is (1) fresh-squeezed, (2) squeezed and pasteurized, and (3) reconstituted from concentrate. Price goes the same way; you pay more for taste and freshness.

Fresh and near fresh juices of any kind naturally contain a wide range of nutrients—vitamins, minerals, and phytochemicals. Healthful as they are, they contain sugars. Sales dropped when people went on low-carbohydrate diets. To restore sales, juice companies have work to do and adding a few extra nutrients to juices is a terrific marketing strategy. PepsiCo is particularly adept at using this strategy. This company produces special Tropicana orange juices designed to "meet your unique health needs." These products contain added vitamins A, C, and E and calcium ("Healthy Kids"); B vitamins and potassium ("Healthy Heart"); and vitamins C, E, and echinacea ("Immunity Defense"). Do you need the extra vitamins? Only if you are deficient in them. Deficiencies of these vitamins are rare among Americans who, if anything, tend to eat more food than is required to meet nutritional needs. In the juice aisles, extra vitamins are calorie distracters—they make you forget that juice has calories and is best consumed in limited amounts.

On the basis of taste and, to a lesser extent, nutritional value, the priority order for juices is (1) fresh-squeezed, (2) squeezed and pasteurized, and (3) reconstituted from concentrate. Price goes the same way; you pay more for taste and freshness.

Once you leave the refrigerated cases, you are in more heavily processed juice territory. The beverage aisles are stocked with cans and bottles of liquids that started out as real juice but have since been pasteurized, concentrated, frozen, reconstituted, diluted with water, and loaded with additives. These products range from 100 percent juice (from concentrate) to much lower percentages. Fortunately, the labels make it easy for you to tell the difference. If the label on the front of the package says "100% juice," the product is made from juice (concentrate, usually), and you will see that printed in big letters so you cannot miss it.

If you do not see "100% juice" on the front label, the product does not have much (or any) juice in it and you are dealing with a juice drink. But to find that out, you have to turn the container around and look at its Nutrition Facts label; the percent of juice is printed right at the top. Coca-Cola's Minute Maid orange drink, for example, is just 3 percent juice from concentrate. PepsiCo's Tropicana Twister, "Naturally and artificially flavored juice beverage from concentrate," is 10 percent juice. Libby's Kerns All Nectar Guava, "Good source of calcium," is 13 percent juice from concentrate. The rest of the ingredients in such products are sugars and sweeteners, colors and flavors, and an occasional added nutrient.

In beverage aisles stocked with canned and bottled juices, you have to be especially wary of labels that say "100%" but are not followed by the words "juice" or "fruit juice." A "100% Joe's Road Stand Original Lemonade" is actually less than 3 percent juice from concentrate, and some "juice drinks" have no juice at all. The front label of Tang (Kraft/Altria), which comes in fruit-colored packages, says "100% vitamin C, good source of calcium." That sounds like juice but Tang is a mix of colored sugars with added vitamins and calcium—but no juice.

Fruit-flavored sports drinks are much the same. The label of PepsiCo's fruit-colored and fruit-flavored Gatorade drinks asks:

What exactly does Gatorade do for an athlete? Good question. It's scientifically formulated to replace more of what you lose when you sweat. By providing fluids and electrolytes to promote complete rehydration and carbs to refuel working muscles, Gatorade helps keep you going longer and stronger. Nothing rehydrates, replenishes, and refuels athletes better.

Maybe, but try water for rehydration; it works better than anything to replace lost fluids. For replenishment of "fuel" (which presumably means calories from "carbs" or any other source), try food. Electrolytes are another matter. These are minerals in your blood—like sodium, potassium, and chloride—that keep its acidity balanced. You lose them when you sweat (sweat tastes salty, right?). All but the most vigorously exercising and sweating people would not even notice those losses because everyone has plenty of electrolytes to begin with. Gatorade Orange Sports Drink contains these electrolytes (which I put in italics):

Water, sucrose syrup, glucose-fructose syrup, citric acid, natural orange flavor with other natural flavors, *salt, sodium citrate, monopotassium phosphate*, yellow 6, ester gum, brominated vegetable oil.

If you are an athlete working out for an hour or more, Gatorade might replenish your sodium, potassium, and chloride more quickly than food can do, but not by much; an 8-ounce Gatorade provides just 1 percent of the Daily Value for potassium (30 milligrams) and 5 percent of the Daily Value for sodium (110 milligrams). Electrolytes are plentiful in food. A carrot, for example, provides 230 milligrams of potassium and 50 milligrams of sodium. If you are not doing vigorous athletics, any vegetable should do the trick. This particular version of Gatorade may be orange in color, but it is not orange juice. Gatorade is a salt-supplemented sugar drink, but with fewer sugars and calories than a regular soft drink. On that basis, PepsiCo markets it as a better choice than, presumably, a non-diet Pepsi, and backs up that contention with a hefty advertising budget—$142 million in 2004.

DIET DRINKS: CHEMICALLY SWEET AND "LITE"

Beverage marketers view "diet" as the "D word." "Diet" does not make most people—especially men—want to buy beverages. So they dream up euphemisms, starting with "lite." The best diet drink is water; it has no sugars or calories and is as light as can be.

> The best diet drink is water; it has no sugars or calories and is as "light" as can be.

To make juice or soft drinks "lighter," manufacturers add water to them (you can do this too, and at home). This is precisely how PepsiCo makes Tropicana Light 'n Healthy orange juice, which has one-third less sugar than regular Tropicana juice. The company takes two parts regular juice, adds one part water, and puts the diluted juice into a new container. Obviously, "light" juices have less juice, and water is a cheap ingredient so production costs are lower; PepsiCo sold $25 million worth of these products in 2004. Premium Light Minute Maid (Coca-Cola) is made the same way. Both "light" products end up as 42 percent juice but supermarkets sell them right next to the 100 percent juices, and at the same price. This practice greatly upsets the Florida citrus trade associations that represent producers of 100 percent orange and grapefruit juices. These groups want diluted juices to disclose that fact prominently on front labels.

Adding water also is the strategy behind "mid-calorie colas" like Coca-Cola C2 or Pepsi Edge, introduced in 2004 but considered "dead" by 2005 because they pleased neither dieters nor non-dieters. These are Coke and Pepsi line extensions with the corn sweeteners and calories diluted with water, and with artificial sweeteners added to make up for the taste of the missing sugars. Coca-Cola C2, for example, came sweetened with half the high fructose corn syrup of a regular Coke, but also with all three of the leading artificial sweeteners: sucralose (Splenda), aspartame (NutraSweet, Equal), and acesulfame-K (K is the chemical abbreviation for potassium).

Artificial sweeteners convert beverages to diet drinks (because they reduce the calories from sugars). The label of Fruit$_2$O (Kraft/Altria) may say that it is a "Naturally fruit flavored spring water beverage," but it is sweetened with things not found in nature—sucralose and other "nonnutritive" (no calorie) chemicals. That brings us back to the dreaded "D word." Companies avoid using it even though diet drinks have become the focus of soft drink company marketing efforts. In 2005, Coca-Cola introduced a new diet cola that it hoped would appeal to men—Coca-Cola Zero ("zero calories, zero carbs, zero sugar, zero color, and zero caffeine"), and PepsiCo introduced Sierra Mist Free. Both were sweetened with aspartame and acesulfame-K. Neither did well.

The FDA says all nonnutritive sweeteners are safe at current levels of use, and they may well be, not least because they are used in extremely small amounts. But testing is invariably done by the makers of the products, rather than by the government or independent testing agencies, and their studies leave much room for interpretation. Without question, safety studies of anything consumed in tiny amounts are difficult to do. Consider what scientists would have to do to determine the effect of artificial sweeteners on human health. They could compare the health of people who did and did not consume artificial sweeteners in the past, but the differences, if any, would probably be too small to reach statistical significance. Or they could recruit people willing to consume artificially sweetened foods and drinks over a period of many years, and then compare the health of that group to the health of an equally large and otherwise comparable group of people who never consume such chemicals. Alternatively, they could give pills containing artificial sweeteners to one group but not to another and make sure the groups do not eat anything else with artificial sweeteners that might complicate the study design. Forget it. These kinds of studies are too complicated, too expensive, and too difficult to interpret to even attempt.

Instead, scientists speed up the process by giving large amounts of artificial sweeteners to experimental animals. Such studies are always subject to the criticisms that people are not rats and that nobody ever consumes as much sweetener as the animals do. But even when animal studies suggest that smaller amounts of artificial sweeteners are harmful, which they sometimes do, many people do not care: they still want to be able to consume these chemicals.

Why people like artificial sweeteners so much is worth its own research study. These substances are not natural. They do not really taste like sugars and have undertones and aftertastes that I and plenty of other people find unpleasant. And what good do they do? They do not seem to help control weight. If anything, they are associated with gaining weight. I am not saying that artificial sweeteners cause weight gain; I just mean that their use has risen in parallel with rising rates of obesity. Artificial sweeteners may give you the illusion of doing something useful to avoid sugars and control your calorie intake. But it does not take much food to make up for the calories you save, and the sweeteners do not help with what really matters in weight control: eating less and being more active. Whether or not they do any good, they are very much with us. So let's take a look at them, starting with a bit of history.

The use of artificial sweeteners in soft drinks began in the 1960s with cyclamates, but the FDA banned these chemicals in 1970 because studies suggested that they caused cancer in rats and mice. Saccharin came next. Coca-Cola used saccharin to create Tab in 1963. You can still find saccharin in Tab and in the pink packets of Sweet'N Low on restaurant tables, but this sweetener has been otherwise superseded by newer and more stable chemicals—aspartame (NutraSweet, Equal), acesulfame-K, and sucralose (Splenda).

In thinking about any of these sweeteners, it helps to remember that it took an act of Congress to keep saccharin on your table. In 1977, the FDA learned the hard way about Americans' love for artificial sweeteners when it proposed to ban saccharin because studies had just suggested that it—like cyclamates—caused bladder cancers in rats and mice. As a result of an earlier congressional decision, in 1958, the FDA had no choice but to take immediate action to ban saccharin. In 1958, Congress passed the Delaney amendment to the food and drug laws, which required the FDA to ban any substance shown to cause cancer—in people or in animals—from the food supply. But in 1977, saccharin was the only artificial sweetener allowed on the market, and millions of people were adding it to coffee and tea or drinking it in soft drinks like Tab.

The response to the FDA's proposed ban was immediate and forceful. More than 100,000 saccharin users wrote letters to Congress complaining about the proposed infringement on their freedom of choice. These letters were generated by an exceptionally vigorous media campaign led by the Calorie Control Council, the trade association for the diet drink industry. This campaign, which reportedly cost $890,000 for public relations and $1.14 million for congressional lobbying in its first three months, mocked the science. According to the council's two-page advertisement in the March 13, 1977, edition of *The New York Times*, the rats were fed

more than the amount a human would receive from drinking 1,250 twelve-ounce diet beverages a day over a lifetime! That's 117 gallons of liq-

uid, or over 4,000 packets of saccharin a day for a lifetime! . . . Nevertheless, the FDA still proposes to ban saccharin. If you find this action ridiculous, you're not alone. It's just another example of the arbitrary nature of
BIG GOVERNMENT.

At that point, Congress introduced more than fifty bills to stop the FDA
from taking action against saccharin, and it passed the Saccharin Study
and Labeling Act of 1977. This kept saccharin on the market but required a
warning label: "Use of this product may be hazardous to your health. The
product contains saccharin which has been determined to cause cancer in
laboratory animals." In December 2004, I asked Donald Kennedy, the editor of *Science* magazine, about those events because he had been commissioner of the FDA at the time. His e-mailed response said,

> Those were the good old days, no? . . . The Calorie Control Council was
> a pioneer for euphemistic titles . . . You may not know this but Diet Coke
> [he means Tab] and regular each cost 25 cents at the time, but the saccha-
> rin needed to sweeten the former cost 1.5 cents less than the sugar in the
> regular version. Six percent margins in the grocery business are huge —
> that's why they worked so hard even though diet drinks were only 17% of
> their market by volume.

That 1.5-cent difference amounted to 6 percent of the 25-cent cost.
Since then, substitution of high fructose corn syrup for sucrose has
reduced the ingredient cost of regular soft drinks, and more stable artificial sweeteners have replaced saccharin
in diet drinks. Coca-Cola still uses saccharin in Tab, but switched to aspartame
when it introduced Diet Coke in 1982. In
2005, the company introduced Diet Coke
Splenda, sweetened with a mixture of sucralose and acesulfame-K. Various kinds
of diet Pepsis also use aspartame, sometimes along with acesulfame-K.
No matter who makes them, diet soft drinks contain either aspartame,
acesulfame-K, or sucralose, sometimes singly but more often in combinations of two sweeteners.

> **N**o matter who makes them, diet
> soft drinks contain either
> aspartame, acesulfame-K, or sucralose,
> sometimes singly but more often in
> combinations of two sweeteners.

Nevertheless, the Calorie Control Council is still hard at work protecting sales of saccharin. I speak from personal experience. In 1997, Cumberland Packing, the owner of Sweet'N Low saccharin, gave a $5,000 scholarship to the New York University (NYU) department I then chaired, designated specifically for a minority student studying nutrition. One of my responsibilities as chair was to raise money for such purposes. Although I was concerned about potential conflicts of interest in accepting funds from food companies, I thought that a reasonable policy might be to accept money from any source as long as the funds were used exclusively for student scholarships and I had no role in deciding who was to receive them. That hands-off policy, however, proved insufficiently protective when Cumberland Packing issued a press release on its new partnership with NYU.

Michael Jacobson, the head of the Center for Science in the Public Interest (CSPI), saw the press release and called to remind me that cancer is rife in minority communities. A group of independent experts had just reviewed the research and agreed with the views of previous groups that saccharin did indeed increase the risk of cancer in experimental animals. How, he asked, could I expect to provide an impartial evaluation of the safety of saccharin if my department accepted funds from the company that sold it? How, indeed.

I declined further scholarship money as politely as I could, but Cumberland was not pleased. Its chief official wrote directly to the NYU president: "We are very disappointed that as a result of this desperate attack by the CSPI, worthy students will not be offered this valuable opportunity to subsidize their studies in the area of chronic diseases affecting the African American population." The Calorie Control Council wrote me that it was "astounded to learn that New York University has refused to accept a scholarship to have been awarded by Sweet'N Low to a minority student . . . The scientific research on saccharin soundly supports its safety."

Well, yes and no. Saccharin is a weak promoter of cancer in laboratory animals. It is consumed daily by millions of people who freely choose it above sugars or other kinds of artificial sweeteners. It is made by an industry skilled at using scientific uncertainties to reassure you that saccharin is perfectly safe. But everyone in or out of the "calorie control" sweetener industry agrees that high doses of saccharin promote cancer in rats and mice. The disagreements center on what that means for people who habitually drink Tab or use Sweet'N Low. Because studies of saccharin and human health cannot give unambiguous answers to that question—it is never possible to prove that a substance is perfectly safe—regulatory agencies have two choices. They can apply the "precautionary principle" and ban saccharin until it is proven acceptably safe (the approach of the 1958 Delaney amendment). Or, in the absence of clear evidence of harm, they can allow you to keep consuming saccharin and hope that it does not turn out to be harmful to human health (the approach of Congress when it exempted saccharin from the Delaney amendment).

Regulatory agencies, which are increasingly expected to consider the needs of industry as well as public health in their decisions, generally favor the latter approach, and industries encourage them to do so. In 1996, the Calorie Control Council asked for elimination of the warning labels for saccharin and the FDA agreed, "consistent with the Administration's 'Reinventing Government' initiative which seeks to ease burdens on regulated industry and consumers." In 1998, the Calorie Control Council petitioned the National Toxicology Program to remove saccharin from its carcinogen listings and, in the absence of evidence for overt harm to people, the program did so in 2000.

The saccharin saga is worth recounting because it explains much about current views of the three artificial sweeteners most commonly used in diet drinks: aspartame (NutraSweet, Equal), acesulfame-K, and sucralose (Splenda). All are organic (carbon-containing) chemicals that happen to fit nicely into receptors in the mouth that respond to sweet tastes; all stimulate sensations of sweetness. The receptors perceive these chemicals as 200 to 600 times sweeter than sugars and as tasting enough like sugars so all but the most finicky eaters (of which I, alas, am one) do not mind the difference. All three have passionate devotees, and equally passionate critics. All come from companies engaged in bitter fighting over patent issues, advertising claims, and market share. The Calorie Control Council says the sweeteners taste sweet and clean (or taste like sugar), help control calorie intake, do not promote tooth decay, are useful for people with diabetes, and are FDA-approved and, therefore, safe.

The chemicals do not, in fact, promote tooth decay, and they are FDA-approved. Beyond that, not everyone agrees with the council's position, as I will now explain, one sweetener at a time.

ASPARTAME

Of the three common sweeteners, the most controversial is aspartame. It is sold commercially as NutraSweet and as a table sweetener in the pale blue packets of Equal. Aspartame was discovered accidentally in 1965, as many sweeteners are, by a scientist at Searle who licked his finger in the laboratory. Monsanto bought Searle and its products in 1985. By the time the patent ended in 1992, aspartame was used in more than 5,000 products and generated $1 billion in annual sales. Monsanto sold Equal to Merisant in 2000.

Aspartame has three components: two amino acids—aspartic acid and phenylalanine—and an attached methyl group. The amino acids are identical to those in any food or body protein, and methyl groups are also common components of foods and human bodies. When you eat aspartame, digestive enzymes split it into its three components. The two amino acids are either broken down for energy or assembled into body proteins. The methyl part is converted to methanol and then to formic acid, a substance that can be quite toxic in high concentrations. But large numbers of studies in the 1970s and 1980s showed that none of the three parts did harm, even among people who habitually drank diet sodas. Although most of these studies were funded by industry, many went through rigorous peer-review processes before publication. More recent studies in rats purporting to link aspartame to several forms of cancer are preliminary and difficult to interpret. Overall, it is still highly debatable whether any of the separate components of aspartame might cause harm—except to people with phenylketonuria, the genetic inability to metabolize phenylalanine. Such people know they have this problem, so aspartame products come with a warning: "Phenylketonurics: Contains Phenylalanine."

I have a hard time thinking of any other reason why aspartame might cause problems in the amounts typically consumed, but lots of people say it makes them feel dizzy, gives them headaches, or causes other unpleasant symptoms. Between 1980 and 1995, the FDA received more than 7,000 such complaints, but I am not aware of any scientific studies that confirm them. Dr Pepper diet soda is one of the few soft drinks that uses aspartame exclusively (usually aspartame is paired with acesulfame-K or sucralose). If you feel bad after you drink a diet Dr Pepper or eat or drink something with aspartame, the remedy is easy; read labels carefully and avoid such foods.

Whether or not aspartame causes demonstrable harm, I do not like its bitter aftertaste and I tend to be uncomfortable with artificial anything when it comes to food. But this particular substance has been so weirdly maligned that I almost feel sorry for it. In the mid-1990s, a letter signed by "Nancy Markle" began circulating on the Internet and dozens of copies have been sent to me over the years. This letter provides a long list of diseases purportedly caused by the methanol released by aspartame (it does release methanol, but in tiny amounts, and so do lots of other foods). The logic of the accusation is simple: "People who use aspartame have problems. They quit using it, and their problems usually go away." This letter and that kind of thinking apparently convinced many readers that aspartame is poison. In October 2004, scientists in Scotland criticized the letter in an editorial in the *British Medical Journal*. Within hours, the journal's instant-response Web pages were flooded with testimonials from people who reported bad personal experiences with aspartame and cited the Markle letter. For them the remedy is simple; do not buy drinks sweetened with aspartame.

At the risk of eliciting a similar flood, I have to agree that drinking a few diet sodas made with aspartame does not seem harmful. But despite the lack of confirmed scientific evidence for harm, I also do not knowingly eat foods containing it or other artificial sweeteners. Safe or not, they are phony. They are examples of dietary dishonesty and I can well understand why they make so little difference to body weight. If you eat foods containing them, you may think you have saved lots of calories, and not even realize that you are making up for them by eating more calories from food.

ACESULFAME-K

The CSPI says that acesulfame-K belongs in the category of additives it deems "unsafe in amounts consumed or . . . very poorly tested and *not worth any risk.*" The FDA approved it for use in foods in 1988. In 1996, CSPI asked for more safety testing on the grounds that the original studies that led to its approval dated from the 1970s and were of "mediocre quality." Acesulfame-K is absorbed from the digestive tract, not metabolized, and excreted intact in urine, raising questions about what it might be doing in between. In 1998, the FDA said "none of the objections raised issues of fact that justified granting a hearing or otherwise provided a basis for revoking the regulation," and approved its use in beverages. The FDA considers it safe. On ingredient lists, you almost always find acesulfame-K paired with aspartame (as in Coca-Cola Zero) or with sucralose (Diet Coke Splenda).

SUCRALOSE

The FDA approved sucralose in 1998 and allowed it to be marketed in drinks and in table form (the yellow packets) as Splenda, which has done splendidly ever since. The "–ose" ending makes sucralose sound like sugar and Splenda is advertised as "Made from sugar, so it tastes like sugar." It may start with sugar, but that is not how it ends up. Sucralose is chlorinated, which makes the "sugar" unavailable to digestive enzymes and difficult to absorb or metabolize (hence: no calories); it is mostly excreted intact.

You can buy bags of Splenda in the same way you buy bags of sugar. The product contains a small amount of the chemical mixed with a fluffy non-digestible filler. Unlike other artificial sweeteners, the filler lets you bake with Splenda but only if you do not care how things taste. If it helps you lose weight, it may be because you will not want to eat foods baked with it. Admirers of Splenda are legion, however. The product's advertising budget in 2004 was more than $30 million and the marketing is so effective that supplies cannot keep up with demand. Splenda outsells other sweeteners by a wide margin; it earned $160 million in 2003, compared to $66 million for Equal/aspartame and $53 million for Sweet'N Low/saccharin.

Late in 2004, Merisant, the company that owns Equal, sued Splenda for misleading consumers with false advertising. Splenda, the suit argued, does not contain sugar, does not get its sweetness from sugar, and uses phosgene, a poison gas, in its chlorination process. The Sugar Association, which represents producers of cane and beet sugar (sucrose), not only filed a similar suit, but also set up a Web site (www.truthabout-splenda.com) questioning the product's safety. Whole Foods Markets refuses to carry Splenda products because sucralose is not metabolized and, therefore, could be potentially unsafe, is more than minimally processed, and is ideologically incompatible with the company's philosophy of selling "the highest quality natural and organic products available." Mine too.

SUGAR ALCOHOLS AND STEVIA

Although not used in commercial diet drinks, a couple of other artificial sweeteners are worth mentioning. Low-carbohydrate diet fads encouraged companies to put sugar alcohols, long used in chewing gums (because they do not cause tooth decay), in foods. Maltitol, sorbitol, xylitol, and other carbohydrates ending in –ol rather than –ose are sugar alcohols and have no calories because you cannot easily digest them. The bacteria in your digestive tract can, however, so expect a laxative effect if you eat too much of them. Is this worth the calories they save? Other than in chewing gum, I don't think so.

I get asked all the time about stevia, an herbal sweetener said to have been used in Paraguayan rituals since the fifteenth century, and now available in health food stores in liquid concentrates and powders that you can add to your own foods and drinks. Its admirers are furious that the FDA has turned down at least three requests to approve it, each time because of lack of safety information. Canada and the European Union also deny approval. Its marketers get around FDA restrictions by selling stevia as a dietary supplement, which means that its contents, safety, and label claims go virtually unregulated. In a health food store, I picked up a Wisdom Herbs booklet that says stevia is "one of the most beneficial plants on earth" because it strengthens the immune system, enhances the body's natural production of vitamins, promotes regularity, supports liver health, and helps control formation of free radicals, among other benefits—all this and sweetness too. CSPI thinks that small amounts are "probably" safe (that word again), but does not endorse its use. Neither do I.

When it comes to messing about with drinking water, I grow wary. I am far from convinced that added nutrients convert sugar water to a health food, and I also think the cost of such products borders on the absurd. If you think you need vitamins, take a daily multivitamin supplement and save the money. It is easy to deal with juices; choose the freshest 100 percent juices you can afford, don't drink too much of them (12 ounces a day is more than enough for an adult), and leave everything else — juice drinks, sports drinks, buzz drinks — where you found them. Do not let your children drink more than 6 ounces of juice a day, and do not let them drink "juice" drinks at all except, perhaps, as an occasional treat — just like any other candy or dessert. I also am reluctant to give anything with artificial sweeteners to children. These chemicals have never been tested on children, nor can they be, and their effects on growing children are unknown. If they do turn out to be harmful, children will be most vulnerable to their effects. Why take a chance?

As should be evident by now, I am not a fan of artificial sweeteners. I don't like the way they taste, can't believe anything that tastes so "chemical" can be good for you, and prefer what I eat to be metabolized — broken down and rendered harmless before it is excreted. Yes, sugars (and their calories) are a problem in the American diet. And yes, the FDA has approved artificial sweeteners because there is no compelling evidence that they cause harm at current levels of intake, at least in adults. And yes, many people with diabetes, whose diets are restricted in sugars, no doubt think that artificial sweeteners are a gift from heaven. But I do not like the dietary deceptiveness. If a food tastes sweet, it ought to be sweet because it contains sugars. Foods with artificial sweeteners fool you into thinking they contain sugars when they do not. They may encourage you — and your children — to think that if foods are not sweet, they are

> **D**o not let your children drink more than 6 ounces of juice a day, and do not let them drink "juice" drinks at all except, perhaps, as an occasional treat — just like any other candy or dessert.

not edible. And children especially may learn to think that if a drink is not sweet, it is not drinkable.

Eventually researchers may find that fooling the body about sugar induces harmful physiological changes. Alternatively they may not, and will discover that artificial sweeteners are perfectly safe. Time will tell, but for now these chemicals are just not my thing. When I want to eat something sweet, I'll take sugar(s) any time. At least I know sugars are metabolized in the body. The single virtue of artificial sweeteners is their absence of calories, but I can think of better ways to avoid calories. Drink water, for example.

35

Teas and Coffees:
Caffeine to Eco-Labels

T he Key Food store on Avenue A in Manhattan's East Village is small by national supermarket standards, but devotes 20 feet of one 80-foot aisle to coffees (with 7 shelves) and teas (with 8 shelves), totaling up to 148 linear feet of shelf space. This store must know its customers. Coffees and teas are a good excuse for taking a drug, in this case a rather mild one—caffeine. These products are not just drugs, of course. Teas and coffees are the basis of elaborate social rituals, some of them having to do with health. These rituals are so important that they apply equally well to the decaffeinated varieties.

But teas and coffees have meanings that extend even beyond caffeine and rituals. Coffee has become a symbol of some of the least attractive aspects of our globalized world. To enter the coffee section of a supermarket is to be confronted with the products of an especially raw form of globalization in action. Coffee is the prototype of a commodity produced by farmers in the poorest of developing countries for the benefit—economic as well as social—of people living in much wealthier nations. At the moment, this particular manifestation of globalization works just the way it is supposed to: you can buy coffee at relatively low cost, but at the expense of the poor farmers who produce it. These days, so many farmers in developing countries are producing coffee that supply greatly exceeds demand. The oversupply has forced prices below the cost of production, and places the livelihoods of farmers at risk. Everyone, even the largest corporate coffee producers, considers the current situation a crisis.

If worrying about the plight of coffee farmers in Peru or Rwanda seems like more than you want to take on just to buy a pound or two of coffee, you can ignore where your coffee comes from. You can simply decide among beans or ground, caffeinated or decaffeinated, or flavored with vanilla or hazelnuts. Only if your local supermarket happens to carry such products, will you have to deal with certification labels that alert you to one or another aspect of the crisis: Certified Organic, Fair Trade, Rainforest Alliance, Shade Grown. Certified products cost more, but might be worth the price if you care about such issues. Or, if you want your coffee stronger and fresher, you might want to skip the supermarket and buy it from specialty stores. Whatever you decide, the product you savor or bring home comes with an astonishing amount of baggage, not the least of which is a long cultural history based on how coffee delivers caffeine.

COFFEE AND CAFFEINE

The late, great food writer Alan Davidson sums up the cultural history of coffee in one phrase: "A rich mythology, full of dancing goats and sleepy monks." The myth is too good not to repeat. It begins with Kaldi, a herder of goats in the highlands of Ethiopia. Soon after his goats ate berries from a certain tree, they got frisky and did not sleep. He took seeds from the tree to the dozing abbot of a nearby monastery, who brewed them up and drank the concoction. The rest is history.

Myth or not, the tree was *Coffea arabica*, which grows in temperate climates. Its beans are about 1.5 percent caffeine by weight. The alternative kind is *Coffea robusta* from the tropics, which is higher in caffeine—about 2.5 percent. The taste and aroma of coffee depend on the type (arabica tastes better), where it is grown, how ripe the beans are when they are harvested, and how they are processed. The fruit of either type, called cherries because they are red, contains two seeds—the coffee beans. The cherries must be picked by hand and processed immediately to dry them and remove the outer hulls. The remaining "green" coffee beans must be roasted to bring out their flavor. After that, you or your coffee seller take the beans and grind them to fine pieces. To make coffee, you add boiling water to the grounds, thereby performing a hot-water extraction of the caffeine and the many other chemicals that make freshly brewed coffee smell so good. Some of the rituals have to do with details of the roasting, grinding, heating of the water, brewing method, and brewing time, all of which incite passionate debates among coffee aficionados. Pharmacologically speaking, however, these rituals are really about how best to deliver caffeine.

Caffeine is a mild "upper." It perks up your central nervous system, and makes you feel more alert, energetic, and cheery. Caffeine is common in plants but coffee, chocolate, and tea have the most. The amounts you can extract from coffee or tea vary widely and depend on the type, how much you use, and how long you brew. The range is at least ten-fold, from 30 milligrams for a small cup of weak tea to more than 300 milligrams for some of the larger and stronger Starbucks drinks. Caffeine also is added to soft drinks; in these, you know exactly how much you are getting. Energy drinks made for adults, like Red Bull, put about 80 milligrams in an 8-ounce can. Coca-Cola, Pepsi-Cola, and other soft drinks marketed to children have less—30 to 40 milligrams in 12 ounces.

In the middle of that range, caffeine stimulates but does not bother most people. Take in more than your personal limit, however, and you may feel nervous, shaky, and sleepless. People react to caffeine in different ways and by this stage in your life, you undoubtedly know how much of it you can handle and at what time of day. The more caffeine you drink, the more you become accustomed to it, and the harder it is to give up. Caffeine crosses the placenta and fetuses cannot metabolize it, which is why doctors advise pregnant women not to drink coffee (when I was pregnant, I couldn't stand the smell of it

> The more caffeine you drink, the more you become accustomed to it, and the harder it is to give up.

anyway). It has stronger effects in some children, although researchers consider the overall effects of caffeine in children to be "modest and typically innocuous." The low amounts of caffeine in tea make this brew tolerable for practically everyone.

There is something about coffee—perhaps just the caffeine—that makes researchers try hard to find something wrong with it. My files are full of papers claiming that coffee raises the risk for heart disease, heartburn, cancer, infertility, fetal growth retardation, spontaneous abortion, breast lumps, osteoporosis, ulcers, and any number of other health problems, but the observed effects are so small and so inconsistent that the studies are not very convincing. Instead, well-designed studies tend to show no harmful effects—on blood pressure, for example. Caffeine given as a drug is a weak diuretic (urine inducer), though the amounts in all but the strongest coffees are too low to do that. Most likely, the water in coffee is what increases urine volume. The same logic applies to caffeine as an appetite suppressant; doses at drug levels work, but the caffeine in coffee is too dilute to have much of an effect. One peculiar finding is that decaffeinated coffee produces many of the same pharmacological effects as regular coffee, which means that chemicals other than caffeine must be responsible. One non-caffeine chemical in coffee appears to stimulate the receptors in the brain that respond to opioid drugs. This could explain why coffee is so popular; it makes you feel good when you drink it.

Complicating an overall assessment of the health effects of coffee are studies showing the benefits of drinking it—for people with asthma, for example. Coffee, as a plant extract, contains polyphenolic antioxidants that could be beneficial. As with so many studies of foods and health, research on coffee and health is hard to do. Coffee is not a consistent product of food technology; its contents are "alive" in the sense that they vary with plant biology and brewing conditions. Also, the physiological effects of coffee depend on everything else you do. Researchers insist that if you are someone who regularly drinks coffee, you are also likely to smoke cigarettes, drink too much alcohol, eat too much saturated fat and cholesterol, and be inactive. If you find yourself bristling at this generalization, so do I. I drink coffee (admittedly weaker than most of the kinds at Starbucks) but do not fit any of those other categories. You too can enjoy coffee and have a healthy lifestyle.

About 30 million Americans are considered daily "gourmet" coffee drinkers, many of them dropping into Starbucks, for example. I prefer milder coffee. Still, I cannot help but notice how Starbucks has convinced practically everyone else in the world that strongly roasted coffee is better. The business side of Starbucks is truly impressive. In 2004, the company operated more than 8,500 stores in 34 countries, bought nearly 300 million pounds of coffee beans, and sold more than $5 billion worth of coffee, tea, and accompaniments. Starbucks is so ubiquitous that at least six units are located within a half mile of where I live, two of them famously across the street from each other at Astor Place. In the United Arab Emirates in May 2005, every shopping mall I visited in Dubai had a Starbucks café, all packed with caffeinating customers.

Other aspects of Starbucks are less impressive. The company's business success is based in part on selling "added value" milk and sugar as well as coffee. Black coffee has practically no calories to speak of but it picks up calories fast as soon as you add sugar, milk, or cream. Starbucks provides a nutrition chart if you ask for it and it also puts Nutrition Facts on its Web site (www.starbucks.com). These should be required reading. A cappuccino espresso made with steamed and foamed whole milk has a quite reasonable 150 calories (plus 20 calories for every teaspoon of sugar you add). But a "tall" (12-ounce) caffè latte breve has 420 calories, three-quarters of them from fat, and its 23 grams of saturated fat exceed a full day's allowance. A "venti" (20-ounce) breve vanilla crème is one serious dessert; it has 790 calories (one-third of the daily need) and 38 grams of saturated fat (nearly two days' allowance), and this is without the whipped cream, which adds another 100 calories and another teaspoon of saturated fat. These drinks are caffeinated milk and sugar, and best shared among several friends.

DECAFFEINATED COFFEE

If caffeine bothers you, decaf is an option. I am not particularly sensitive to caffeine in amounts under 150 milligrams or so, and I think I must metabolize it fairly quickly, but I know plenty of people who say they get jittery in response to the smallest amounts. Coffee can never be entirely decaffeinated, but it can come close.

Coffee roasters decaffeinate beans using any one of several different processes. These processes come in two categories: direct and indirect. Both begin with beans that have been steamed to soften them and open up their "pores." Direct decaffeination methods soak the beans in something that extracts the caffeine—water, solvents like methyl chloride or ethyl acetate (the coffee industry no longer uses benzene or other solvents linked to cancer), high-pressure carbon dioxide, or triglycerides (fats). Indirect methods extract the caffeine from the beans with water, treat the water with something that removes the caffeine, and add the water back.

Decaffeination methods of any kind extract the flavor components along with the caffeine, so the flavors have to be replaced in some way. Here is what coffee roasters have to do to decaffeinate coffee beans and add back flavor by an indirect "water process":

- soak green coffee beans in very hot water for several hours to leach out the caffeine (along with other flavor components)
- drain off the water
- treat the water with a solvent, or run the water through a bed of activated charcoal ("Swiss water process"), to remove the caffeine
- heat the water to steam off the solvent and caffeine, or treat with charcoal to get rid of both
- add the solvent-free and caffeine-free water back to the beans and soak them until they reabsorb the flavor chemicals
- dry and roast the beans in the usual manner

All of these processes work well for removing most—never all—of the caffeine. Usually less than 1 percent is left, and this should not be enough caffeine to bother anyone. Decaffeinated coffee is a trade-off between caffeine and flavor. The more caffeine that disappears, the more the flavor disappears too. Adding back the extracted water is supposed to replace all the desirable flavor components, but even the most casual consideration of the steps in the process should tell you that decaf can never taste like the original coffee. Many people think that decaf tastes just fine. I do not. I much prefer the real thing. So do other people, apparently. On average, American adults drink more than three cups of coffee a day, but hardly any of that is decaf.

> **D**ecaffeinated coffee is a trade-off between caffeine and flavor. The more caffeine that disappears, the more the flavor disappears too.

You may think, as I once did, that tea means tea bags or packages of loose tea. I had no idea that to the tea industry, tea means "ready to drink" (RTD)—the kind in bottles, cans, or cartons, invariably sweetened, and competing with soft drinks. These account for 62 percent of all tea sales in the United States. The rest comes largely from those little boxes on supermarket shelves: regular, instant, specialty (including chai), and herbal, sometimes decaffeinated, and occasionally Certified Organic or Fair Trade. In most supermarket coffee and tea aisles, tea means tea bags. If you want loose teas, you have to look hard for them or go to larger supermarkets or specialty stores.

Tea comes with both myth and mystique. In 2737 B.C., so the story goes, Shen Nung, the Chinese emperor, happened to be sitting underneath a tree (guess what kind) while a servant was boiling water for him to drink. When a leaf of the *Camellia sinensis* fell into his cup of hot water, he drank it anyway. So much for mythology.

The health mystique is more interesting. On September 30, 2002, for example, the front section of *The New York Times* carried a full-page ad from the Tea Council of the USA. The ad said:

> Are you drinking enough tea? You've probably known all along that tea is good for you. But you may be surprised to learn that there is a growing body of scientific evidence to support your feelings . . . Recent studies suggest a beneficial link between tea consumption and cardiovascular health, reduced risk of certain types of cancer, and increasing bone density . . . Shouldn't tea be a major source of fluids in your diet?

The council is the public relations arm of the Tea Association, a trade group that, among other things, works to "represent the tea industry against harmful allegations . . . and proactively address the general public on tea related issues." The council's purpose is to promote tea drinking through "the furtherance of tea science and the establishment of tea as a healthy beverage."

The ad referred to research presented at a symposium on tea and human health held in 2002, sponsored by several government and professional organizations but paid for—no surprise—by a grant from the Tea Council. The papers from that symposium and one that followed a year later appeared in supplements to a leading nutrition journal. They review evidence that antioxidants extracted from tea might reduce the risk for cancer and heart disease, and "may also play a beneficial role in other conditions, including dental caries, osteoporosis, cognitive function, and weight maintenance"—an impressive accomplishment for hot water poured over a spoonful of dried leaves.

The papers focus on the effects of flavonoids, antioxidants similar to the ones in soybeans that are present in most tea leaves. Like the studies of flavonoid antioxidants in soybeans (and other food plants—chocolate, for example), some of the studies of tea flavonoids show health benefits while others do not. This line of research is still in its infancy, but it is consistent with the burgeoning interest of researchers in the health benefits of phytochemicals in food plants. As a group of cancer researchers explained in a paper published in the British medical journal *Lancet* in 2004, "We believe that anticancer agents designed by nature and used for several thousands of years with little toxicity may prove useful in treating and preventing cancer." That kind of statement is all it takes to encourage tea sellers to seek FDA approval for a health claim—in this case, for green tea as a protective agent against cancer.

GREEN TEA: THE HEALTH CLAIM

Teas come in three types—black, oolong, or green—but they all come from the same leaves. The only difference is in the way the leaves are processed. To make black teas, growers pick the leaves, bruise and roll them, let them sit for hours to oxidize or "ferment" (in quotes because no bacteria or yeast are involved), and dry them. To make oolong teas, growers allow the leaves to be only partially oxidized. Green teas, however, are not allowed to oxidize at all. The growers steam the freshly picked leaves to stop oxidation and dry them immediately. I once visited a tea plantation in southern China known for producing a green tea of exceptional quality. Tea workers rifled through the bushes to pick only the freshest new leaves of perfect size. Within minutes, the leaves were steamed, dried on a hot wok, and put in packages. You put a few green tea leaves in the bottom of a cup, pour in simmering water, and watch the leaves unfurl, float to the top, and slowly settle. Delicious.

Because green teas are "fresh," they have higher levels of certain phytochemicals than other forms of tea. In 2004, Dr. Sin Hang Lee, who owns a company that markets green teas for their health benefits, petitioned the FDA to allow a "qualified" health claim that drinking 40 ounces of green tea a day will help reduce your risk of cancer. Qualified health claims are those for which "significant scientific agreement" does not exist; they require a qualifying disclaimer to put them in context. Green tea, said Dr. Lee, contains a naturally occurring antioxidant, EGCG (epigallocatechin gallate), that "may reduce the risk of certain forms of cancer." He asked the FDA to approve this qualifying statement: "There is scientific evidence supporting the health claim although the evidence is not conclusive."

As is customary in such cases, the FDA conducted a lengthy review of the research linking green tea to cancer prevention. Late in June 2005, the FDA said that no credible evidence supported a health claim for green tea and most cancers, but that "very limited" evidence supported the claim for cancers of the breast and prostate. The FDA allowed what the American Herbal Products Association referred to as a "highly qualified" claim. In this case, "highly qualified" is an understatement. If the label on a package of green tea says the product can help reduce the risk of breast cancer, the FDA requires it to add:

> Two studies do not show that drinking green tea reduces the risk of breast cancer in women, but one weaker, more limited study suggests that drinking green tea may reduce the risk. Based on these studies, FDA concludes that it is highly unlikely that green tea reduces the risk of cancer.

If the label makes a claim for green tea and prostate cancer, the qualifying statement is:

> One weak and limited study does not show that drinking green tea reduces the risk of prostate cancer, but another weak and limited study suggests that drinking green tea may reduce this risk. Based on these studies,

FDA concludes that it is highly unlikely that green tea reduces the risk of prostate cancer.

What is going on here? Politics again. The FDA's grudging "approval" of this claim must be understood as a response to congressional insistence that the agency allow claims for which some—but not necessarily compelling—research exists. Experience shows that when the FDA denies such claims, the petitioning companies take it to court— and usually win on the grounds of freedom of speech. In granting the claim in this manner, the FDA was surely trying to head off a court case. Never mind that qualified health claims are completely baffling. As long as nobody takes them too seriously and they help sell food products, companies love to use them.

It would be wonderful if tea could perform health miracles, but even without them this brew is lovely to drink. The flavonoid or EGCG content of any tea is a mystery, however, as the amounts are neither tested nor labeled. You might as well choose a tea by how it tastes. If you want a green tea that is "fresher" and likely to contain lots of antioxidants, you have to go to specialty shops (or online) and be willing to pay more for it and, sometimes, much more. At the time of the FDA decision, Dr. Lee's Web site (www.teaforhealth.com) was selling 125 grams (about one-quarter pound) of "high antioxidant" green tea for $54—about $200 a pound. No wonder he thought a health claim would be useful.

CHAI

Chai (pronounced ch' eye) is the new best seller among teas, a black tea of Indian origin sweetened with honey, vanilla, and spices, and mixed with milk or cream. Chai has become so much a part of the tea vocabulary that the seller of one line of products is lobbying hard to get the word into American dictionaries (the one other odd word on the tea shelves is already in dictionaries—bergamot, a citrus peel extract used to flavor Earl Grey tea). Chai, say its makers, is perfect for American tastes, by which they

> Chai, say its makers, is perfect for American tastes, by which they surely must mean that it is sweet—very sweet—and high in calories.

surely must mean that it is sweet—very sweet—and high in calories. Chai usually is both, and Starbucks chai drinks are perfect examples.

Starbucks Tazo Chai Drinks, "Tall" (12-Ounce Size), July 2005[*]

TAZO CHAI DRINK	MILK	CALORIES	SUGAR (GRAMS)
Green Iced Tea	None	60	15
Chai Latte	Nonfat	170	34
Chai Latte	Whole	210	34
Chai Latte Breve	Cream	320	26
Chai Crème Frappuccino	No whipped cream	280	45
Chai Crème Frappuccino	Whipped cream	370	47

[*]*Figures are from information posted at www.starbucks.com. One tablespoon of sugar is about 15 grams, and an ounce is about 30 grams.*

Putting a tablespoon of sugar in 12 ounces of tea gives you just 60 calories, but it does not take much more sugar, milk, or cream to get you into calorie levels more appropriate to meals than to drinks. The 12-ounce "tall" is Starbucks' smallest size, of course, and you have to scale up for the 16-ounce "grande" and 24-ounce "venti" (this chai drink is 24 ounces, not the usual 20). If you choose the Venti Chai Crème Frappuccino with whipped cream, you do not get twice what is in the 12-ounce drink, but you do get 640 calories and about 3 ounces of sugar—86 grams. This is (or was) tea, but I doubt it will help you prevent cancer.

HERBAL TEAS

If the tea is anything other than black, oolong, or green, it is not really a tea: it is a tea-like herbal drink extracted from leaves, stems, or any other part of aromatic plants. The plant parts are simply dried, which makes them "natural." Herbal teas do not have caffeine and are supposed to make you healthy or feel good. Drinking herbal (or any other) tea is calming; the water is hot and you have to wait for it to cool or sip it slowly. Whether herbal teas have any special health benefits beyond patience is debatable, however. The chemical content of herbal teas is not well defined, and some components may be good for you, while others may not, as I explain in the chapter on dietary supplements. My guess is that whatever effects herbal teas might have, good or bad, they are likely to be too small to merit even the most highly qualified health claim. Choose a tea because you like the way it tastes, and save your food worries for another category.

CAFFEINE POLITICS: ECO-LABELS

At the 2004 Fancy Food trade show in Manhattan, I picked up a brochure from Zhena's Gypsy Tea. All of her teas, from Gypsy Love to Passionate Peach are Certified Organic and Fair Trade: "At Zhena's Gypsy Tea we want to make a difference in the world . . . When you sip a cup of Zhena's Gypsy Tea . . . you will be loved. You will belong. You will hear children laughing, and you will join hands with the world . . ." I also visited the Peace Coffee booth, which specializes in Organic, Fair Trade, Shade Grown products from cooperatives that engage in "an alternative approach to coffee based on the belief that coffee should reward your taste buds while respecting coffee farmers and the environment."

Sorting out the new eco-labels takes some effort. There are lots of them and they have to do with one or another pesticide, labor, or wildlife protection issue, but rarely with all of the issues at once. Here is a brief summary of the most common ones on packages of coffee and tea.

Some Eco-Labels on Coffees and Teas

ECO-LABEL CERTIFICATION	FOLLOWS ORGANIC RULES?	AVOIDS CHEMICAL PESTICIDES?	TREATS WORKERS RESPONSIBLY?	PAYS FAIR PRICES?	PROTECTS BIRD HABITATS?
Certified Organic	Yes	Yes	Optional	Optional	Optional
Bird Friendly	Yes	Yes	Optional	Optional	Yes
Shade Grown	Optional	Optional	Optional	Optional	Yes
Fair Trade	Optional	Optional	Optional	Yes	Optional
Rainforest Alliance	Optional	Optional	Yes	Optional	Yes

Certified Organic you know about from previous chapters. There are good reasons to buy organic coffees and teas, even if they cost more. Most teas and coffees are imported from countries where pesticide use is not always well regulated—meaning that the beans and leaves are often loaded with undesirable chemicals. Certified Organic tells you that the farmers' growing practices followed standards for use of fertilizers, pesticides, and land, and that the farm has been inspected to make sure those rules were followed. The Smithsonian Migratory Bird Center in Washington, D.C., gives Bird Friendly certification to Certified Organic coffee growers who also protect trees inhabited by local and migrating birds (typically, growers cut down shade trees on coffee plantations to be able to produce greater yields; this destroys bird habitats). Shade Grown addresses the same issue, but the plantations do not have to be organic.

Fair Trade certification is about making a decent living; the coffee growers must be paid above-market prices for their crops. Most—but not all—Fair Trade coffees and teas are also Certified Organic and Shade Grown, but they do not have to be. This brings us to Rainforest Alliance certification, which deals with labor as well as environmental concerns. Growers must pay workers above-market rates, pay men and women equally, and allow workers to organize; they also must adhere to the country's child labor laws. Although their growing methods must protect the environment and help conserve wildlife, they do not necessarily have to meet organic standards. All of these labels are backed up by inspection systems, and all are recommended highly by Consumer's Union (the publisher of *Consumer Reports* and rater of eco-labels at www.eco-label.org), but none of them covers everything, so you have to pick your issue.

> Fair Trade certification is about making a decent living; the coffee growers must be paid above-market prices for their crops.

It is too bad there are so many labels, because if they got together they might receive greater attention from the coffee industry. In the summer of 2004, I received a letter from Niels Christiansen, then the vice president of public affairs for Nestlé: "As you may be aware . . . coffee prices have reached an historic low, which leaves many coffee farmers and their families facing an extremely difficult situation. This is a matter of concern for Nestlé." This opening made me think I was being asked for a donation, which seemed surprising from a company that had earned $33.5 billion just in the first half of 2004. But no, Christiansen was writing to tell me about Nestlé's initiatives to help coffee farmers. Nestlé was hard at work to increase the worldwide demand for coffee, buy beans directly from farmers, support crop diversification, and invest in coffee-producing countries. Nestlé, he said, helps the countries from which it buys coffee; it generates employment, creates demands for goods and services, and promotes safety and quality standards. He enclosed a copy of the company's report on these issues, *Faces of Coffee*.

It is hard not to be skeptical about Nestlé's good deeds in developing countries, given its history of pushing infant formulas on poor women who would be better off breast-feeding (a long-standing problem I discussed in *Food Politics*). Let's just agree that the situation with coffee prices should alarm everyone who cares about such things. From 1962 to 1989, an International Coffee Agreement regulated coffee production. This pact suffered its share of graft and corruption, but did help to keep prices stable. When the Cold War ended, the United States stopped worrying about Soviet influences in developing countries and withdrew from the agreement, which promptly collapsed and let the free market reign. Production immediately increased beyond demand, and prices fell. As Nestlé explains, "The contrast between the flourishing profits of coffee companies and the rising poverty among farmers has made headlines around the world."

The problem, according to Nestlé, is trade barriers, some of which close off markets for crops grown in developing countries: "The brunt of famine and poverty will fall most heavily on those who depend most on growing low-grade crops unless, and until, a more liberalized system of world trade allows them a viable alternative." Maybe, but Nestlé firmly opposes Fair Trade prices: "if on a broad basis coffee farmers were paid fair trade prices exceeding the market price, the result would be to encourage farmers to increase coffee production, thus further depressing prices."

You do not have to be trained in economics to find something troubling about this logic, which is one of the reasons why Fair Trade coffees and teas seem so attractive. At a cost to you of pennies a cup, these products promise a living wage to coffee farmers. How effective they are in doing so, however, is a different question. *The Wall Street Journal* did an analysis of the cost of one pound of Fair Trade coffee in mid-2004. The reporter paid $8.49 for the coffee at the grocery store. Of this amount, $3.49 went to the store itself. The remaining $5.00 went to the wholesaler, whose expenses came to $4.80; this yielded a profit of 20 cents. The $4.80 in expenses included the amount paid to the coffee producer—$1.44. Although this payment is only 17 percent of the retail cost, it is almost certainly higher than the coffee producer might get from Nestlé or anyone else. Is the premium price you pay at the grocery store for Fair Trade coffee worth it? Yes, if you feel deeply about such matters.

DEALING WITH THE TEAS AND COFFEES

Eco-labels are about how food is produced. If Certified Organic constitutes an agricultural critique of conventional food production, eco-labels extend the critique beyond pesticides to issues having to do with labor and wildlife. If you want pesticides out of your food, if you care about having birds in the air, if you would like farmers in developing countries to be paid decently, and if you feel you can afford them, you will choose eco-labeled coffees and teas. You will cheerfully join what food marketers are now calling LOHAS, customers who choose foods on the basis of Lifestyles of Health and Sustainability. If you see yourself in that category, you have plenty of company. According to the marketers that run the LOHAS Web site (www.lohas.com), you are among the 30 percent of American adults who make "conscientious purchasing and investing decisions based on social and cultural values," and who collectively spend nearly $300 billion annually on products perceived as fitting those values. LOHAS helps to explain why organics are the fastest-growing segment of the food industry, and sales of Fair Trade products are doing well, thank you. Eco-labeled products may account for less than 5 percent of coffee sales, but the percent-

> If you want pesticides out of your food, if you care about having birds in the air, if you would like farmers in developing countries to be paid decently, and if you feel you can afford them, you will choose eco-labeled coffees and teas.

age is rising and puts the conventional food industry on notice. This is good news for anyone who cares about how food is produced as well as how it tastes.

I have discussed the eco-labels at some length because you will be seeing them on more and more food packages and because teas and coffees elicit concerns about environmental and labor issues much more than they do about health. I cannot think of a compelling health reason for drinking or not drinking tea, or for choosing one over another (but watch out for the calories in the chai drinks). And unless you drink large amounts of strong, heavily caffeinated coffee, it too raises no particular health alarms—except when it gets turned into a high-calorie dessert.

36

Infant Formula and Baby Food

I f your children are grown, as mine are, you are not going to care much about infant formulas and baby foods (at least until grandchildren come along). But the feeding of babies is a fascinating subject in its own right, and so is the marketing of infant formulas and baby foods. The infant formulas sold in American supermarkets are the visible manifestation of decades of controversy over the ways formula companies market their products, especially to women in low-income countries. Their sales techniques were (and still are) so aggressive and manipulative, and the possible consequences so potentially harmful, that United Nations agencies had to step in and negotiate an international code of ethics for marketing infant formulas. Similarly, the simple, bland ingredients now found in those little jars of baby food are the visible result of years of complaints about the unhealthy additives these foods used to contain, now almost entirely gone. If you use baby foods at all, you really have only one question to answer: organic or not (and how much you are willing to pay for organic options). Beyond that, everything else about infant formulas and baby foods is about marketing and, therefore, politics, interpretation, and point of view—all generating endless controversy.

Underlying the controversy is the unpleasant reality for the companies that make infant formulas and baby foods: the market for these products is severely limited. For these products, the usual methods for corporate growth do not work. The companies that make infant formulas and baby foods cannot easily attract new customers or persuade old customers to buy more and eat more. For formulas, the size of the market depends entirely on the number of babies born each year and the proportion that are not breast-fed. But formula companies have no control over how many babies are born, so the only way they can increase sales is to discourage breast-feeding (hence the need for an international code of ethics). Sales of baby foods also depend on the number of babies born. But older infants and toddlers eat those foods just for a year or two, so the only way baby food companies can increase sales is by promoting use of their products for longer time periods. With these kinds of constraints, the companies that make formulas and baby foods compete fiercely to hold or increase their share of an extremely restricted market.

INFANT FORMULA

Infant formulas are flashpoints for contention for three important reasons: they are largely unnecessary (most mothers can breast-feed their infants); are less perfect than breast milk for feeding babies; and are more expensive than breast-feeding. Breast milk is nutritionally superior to formula, but from a marketing standpoint it has one serious disadvantage: it is free. Beyond one-time purchases of breast pumps, storage bottles, or special clothing, nobody makes money from it.

For mothers who cannot, should not, or do not want to breast-feed, formula is a socially and nutritionally acceptable substitute. But formula companies do not restrict the promotion of formulas only to mothers who need to use these products. In subtle and not-so-subtle ways, they promote the use of formulas to all pregnant women and new mothers. This is not hard to do. Breast-feeding takes some getting used to, breast milk takes a few days to come in after birth, and the milk does not come with Nutrition Facts labels. All of this can be worrying, as can be the many kinds of social pressures against breast-feeding in Western societies (for example, that breast-feeding is "dirty" or inappropriate in public). Even the slightest suggestion that infant formulas are nutritionally better for babies or more convenient for families is enough to undermine confidence and instill anxiety in a new mother who might otherwise breast-feed. Formula giveaways in doctors' offices and hospitals are well known to discourage mothers from nursing their infants, which is why breast-feeding advocates so strongly oppose such practices.

Formulas do serve a useful purpose, however, and they do support infant growth. Cow's milk, however, does not. Untreated milk from cows (or goats or sheep) contains too much protein, fat, salt, and other minerals for an infant's digestive tract to handle. The animal's milk must be diluted; it also must be heated to "denature" the proteins (loosen up their structure) and keep them from forming indigestible clumps with the fat. Before the 1800s, when formula makers figured out how to dilute, denature, and mix cow's milk effectively, an infant who could not be breast-fed by its mother or a surrogate wet nurse had practically no chance of surviving. As soon as the makers of cow's milk formulas were able to demonstrate that formula-fed infants grew just as well as breast-fed infants, they knew they had a terrific marketing opportunity. They formed alliances with doctors to promote the use of formulas to all mothers, not only to those who were unable to breast-feed. Formula feeding soon became a common practice and, among many groups, the norm.

To use formula properly, you need enough money to buy it, enough education to know how to mix or dilute it, a supply of clean water for the mixing or dilution, and a refrigerator to keep the prepared formula cold so microbes will not grow in it. Without these items, formulas can be too dilute, too concentrated, or too contaminated to maintain infant health; they can kill the very infants they were meant to save. That is why formulas are a poor substitute for breast milk in low-income areas, why marketing them to low-income women borders on the unethical, and why the United Nations developed the International Code of Marketing of Breast-Milk Substitutes in 1981. Eventually, U.N. member countries agreed to abide by the code (the United States was the last holdout and did not sign on until 1994 out of fear that international standards might set a precedent that might adversely affect U.S. corporations). Despite the code, formula companies persist in finding ways to get around it, and international breast-feeding advocates continue to document and publicize code violations. As I explained in *Food Politics*, whole shelves of books describe the past and present history of the actions of formula makers—particularly the largest of such companies, Nestlé—to sell their products in low-income countries to mothers who do not need them and would be better off breast-feeding their infants.

Convenience, however, is often a sufficient reason for mothers to choose to use infant formulas, and the products do reproduce the nutrient content of human milk fairly well, except for certain irreplaceable factors that help protect infants against infection. Modern formulas are stable mixtures of emulsified vegetable fat, milk or soy protein, sugars, and vitamins and minerals. They come as powders or concentrates that require mixing or dilution, or as ready to feed. Because formulas (if used in place of breast milk) are the only source of nutrition for infants, they have to contain everything babies need to grow. If they lack even one essential nutrient, as happens on occasion, babies can become ill and die. To make sure that formulas are complete, the FDA closely regulates and monitors their contents. The result is that all brands of infant formulas must have a virtually identical nutritional composition. The nutritional similarity of infant formulas poses another marketing problem for their makers. If the products are all the same, it makes no difference which brand you buy.

> The nutritional similarity of infant formulas poses another marketing problem for their makers. If the products are all the same, it makes no difference which brand you buy.

SOY FORMULA

The same is true of soy formulas. These were developed as an alternative for infants who cannot digest or are allergic to the proteins in cow's milk formulas. Some—but not all—infants who are allergic or sensitive to cow's milk formulas thrive better when fed soy formula. Soy formulas replace the proteins in cow's milk with proteins from soybeans; they replace the sugar in cow's milk—lactose—with corn syrup or cane or beet sugar. The added vitamins and minerals are the same as those in cow's milk formulas. Like milk-based formulas, one soy formula is much like another. They are also more like milk-based formulas than you might guess. Denatured soy proteins are not all that different from denatured milk proteins and both can cause allergic reactions in sensitive infants. The American Academy of Pediatrics says that soy formulas are just as good as milk formulas, but have no particular advantage for preventing allergies or any other problems. Except for allergy problems (which may require special formulas), either milk-based or soy-based formulas work about as well for feeding infants who are not breast-fed or who are only partially breast-fed.

Despite their fundamental similarity, the choice of soy- or milk-based formulas generates strong opinions. Some people believe that soy formulas are superior because they are vegetable based and uncontaminated by animal hormones. Others argue in favor of milk-based formulas out of concern that the estrogen-like chemicals in soybeans may not be good for infants. As in many areas of nutrition, questions about the effects of soy formulas are difficult to resolve. Soybeans are plants. Plants contain phytochemicals, and some of the ones in soybeans are flavonoids that behave like estrogens in the body. Could the estrogen-like flavonoids in soybeans be harmful to infants? The quick answer is that soy formulas have been fed to infants for decades with no apparent evidence of harm.

With that said, I am aware of only one research study that has looked at this question directly. This study, which was funded in part by the Infant Formula Council (a trade association of formula makers), examined more than thirty measures of the health and reproductive ability of young adults aged twenty to thirty-four who had been fed either soy- or milk-based formulas as infants. The investigators did not find any statistically significant differences between the two groups. These findings, they said, should be "reassuring about the safety of infant soy formula." Even though this result would be more reassuring if independent investigators had come to the same conclusion, it seems clear that if soy formulas cause problems at all, the problems are too subtle to measure easily. The same is true of possible benefits; if there are any special benefits of soy formulas, they too are not obvious.

Could the estrogen-like flavonoids in soybeans be harmful to infants? The quick answer is that soy formulas have been fed to infants for decades with no apparent evidence of harm.

Because most mothers in the world still breast-feed their infants, the infant-formula market is not large; worldwide sales are estimated to amount to under $8 billion annually, of which half is generated in the United States. Besides its large proportionate share, the U.S. infant-formula market is unusual in other ways. For one thing, the U.S. government buys half of all formulas sold in this country in order to provide them at no cost to low-income mothers enrolled in the USDA's Special Supplemental Nutrition Program for Women, Infants, and Children (familiarly known as WIC). The WIC program serves about half of the 4 million or so infants born in the United States each year.

These halves (half the formulas and half the infants), however, do not mean that your taxes pay for half of $4 billion in annual sales. Formula companies give the government steep discounts—sometimes up to 95 percent of the cost. The companies bid for state WIC contracts, and the one that offers formulas at the highest discount wins the bid for that state. All WIC participants in that state will be given the winning brand.

Why would companies agree to such enormous discounts? Two reasons: they establish brand loyalty and do not lose much money on the deal. WIC, as it happens, does not provide all of the formula that a child needs. Participants have to buy their own formula to make up the difference, and they invariably choose the brand given to them by WIC. One unanticipated result of these arrangements is that supermarkets in areas with large numbers of WIC participants tend to charge more for the brand of infant formula covered by the state contract. Another is that infant formula becomes a fungible commodity, one that can be exchanged on the open market for cash, and these products rank high on the list of those most frequently stolen from supermarkets. Some stores keep infant formulas under lock and key and you have to ask for them if you want to buy them.

Formula companies also agree to the kickback arrangement because they can afford to; the industry is highly concentrated and, therefore, highly profitable. Given the similarity of products, the relatively fixed number of infants who need them, and the short time infants use infant formulas, it is not surprising that only a few companies are in this business. In the United States, just three companies account for an extraordinary 99 percent of annual sales: Mead Johnson/Bristol-Myers Squibb (Enfamil) with 52 percent of the market, Ross Products/Abbott Laboratories (Similac, Isomil) with 35 percent, and Carnation/Nestlé with a 12 percent share. A fourth company, Wyeth, supplies house brands for Wal-Mart, Kmart, and other national chain stores. Concentration in any industry invariably increases profits (because of size efficiency, if nothing else) and the three Big Formula companies do not want any other companies nibbling at their market shares. In 2001, for example, the courts scolded Mead Johnson for placing fliers in doctors' offices implying that generic infant formulas were deficient in nutrients (they cannot be; all formulas are the same).

SPECIAL FATTY ACIDS (ARA AND DHA)

Competition for market share explains why formula companies want to put distinctive nutrients in their formulas—especially nutrients considered "conditional." A conditional nutrient is one that might have some benefits under some circumstances. Even if the health benefits are minimal or questionable, they can be used in advertising. That is the principal reason why so many formulas now have fatty acids added, in this case ARA (the omega-6 arachidonic acid) and DHA (the omega-3 docosahexaenoic acid—the same one that is in fish oil). These two fatty acids are normally present in breast milk, and there is some evidence, weak and questionable as it is, that they specially promote infant brain development and vision. Formula makers got the FDA to agree that ARA and DHA are normal components of food (which they are) and, therefore, are generally recognized as safe (GRAS). This means that companies could add ARA and DHA to infant formulas without having to prove that these fatty acids really do anything beyond the ordinary.

Apparently the FDA agreed to the GRAS petition with some reluctance, as indicated by its Web site's answer to the question, "What is the evidence that addition of DHA and ARA to infant formulas is beneficial?"

The scientific evidence is mixed. Some studies in infants suggest that including these fatty acids in infant formulas may have positive effects on visual function and neural development over the short term. Other studies in infants do not confirm these benefits. There are no currently available published reports from clinical studies that address whether any long-term beneficial effects exist.

Most of the research focuses on the omega-3 fatty acid DHA. A highly authoritative scientific review by independent investigators in 2005 concluded that the existing studies "supply some evidence that is *not inconsistent* with a causal connection between DHA availability and cognitive function, but they do not show causality" (my emphasis). "Not inconsistent" appears to be the important descriptor. The authors use it again in evaluating studies of the infants of breast-feeding mothers who received DHA supplements. "Results of human breastfeeding studies, though seriously confounded, are *not inconsistent* with a need for supplementation, but the studies do not provide direct or clear evidence" (my emphasis again). The best they could say was that "small differences in brain concentrations of DHA . . . may result in subtle effects that currently are difficult to detect but could be significant."

The ambiguous science is no deterrent to formula makers, however. International formula makers advertise their DHA-fortified products as "the smart formula for smart babies" or "makes your baby healthy and smarter," illustrated with photographs of babies working at computers, reading business newspapers, or wearing mortarboards. In the United States, the company that produces these additives tells dietitians that DHA and ARA are "touching the lives of more than 5 million babies worldwide. Currently, most major U.S. formula brands contain these important nutrients . . ."

Much of the evidence for the benefits of added fatty acids for human infants comes from studies sponsored by formula companies. One such study admits to finding no difference in mental or motor development among three-year-old children who had been fed formulas with and without ARA and DHA. Perhaps because the study was funded by Ross Products (Abbott Laboratories), the researchers framed this conclusion as a positive result: "ARA and DHA support visual and cognitive development through thirty-nine months." In other words, having them is as good as not having them. But adding fatty acids increases sales and allows companies to up the price. With so few companies in this game, it is not surprising that the cost of infant formulas is as consistent from one brand to the next as their contents (except in WIC areas). Early in 2005, I got out my calculator and worked out the cost per ounce of formulas sold in my local grocery stores. The prices mostly varied with convenience. The cheapest formulas were powdered and required mixing—15 cents per ounce. The most expensive—50 cents per ounce—were ready-to-feed formulas with added ARA and DHA.

The Average Retail Cost of Infant Formulas, Per Ounce, 2005

FORMULA TYPE	COST PER OUNCE
Powdered (requires mixing in water)	15¢
Concentrate (requires dilution in water)	20¢
Ready-to-feed (milk- or soy-based)	30¢
Ready-to-feed (milk-based, lactose-free, with added ARA, DHA, and iron)	50¢

SOME CAVEATS

Beyond the difference in cost, does it matter which level of convenience you choose in an infant formula? It might. Powdered formulas are not sterile. In this they differ from concentrate and ready-to-feed formulas, which have been heated to sterilize them. In 2002, the FDA warned pediatricians that powdered-milk formulas could be contaminated with *Enterobacter sakazakii*, a type of bacteria that causes rare but terrible and sometimes fatal infections in infants, especially those who are premature, weak, or in hospitals. The FDA says it is not aware of any *E. sakazakii* infections in healthy full-term infants in home settings. Reports from other countries, however, suggest that even healthy babies may sometimes acquire such infections. Powdered formulas do not carry warnings although their labels do tell you to throw out any formula that is not used during the first hour in which it was prepared. This is good advice.

Infants, of course, should never be given cow's milk or anything other than breast milk or commercial infant formulas that meet FDA specifications. The FDA particularly warns against use of products like Better Than Formula Ultra Infant Immune Booster 117. Although this product is sold as a dietary supplement, the FDA thinks the "better than formula" claim makes it sound like a formula substitute. It is not. The FDA also warns against using infant formulas made in China; it found some to contain less protein, fat, calcium, and magnesium than the amounts stated on the label and needed by babies.

BABY FOOD

Baby foods are about the easiest products in the supermarket to deal with. Most stores in the United States carry only one or two brands, usually Gerber and either Beech-Nut or Heinz. Their ingredients are the same and their #1 (2.5-ounce), #2 (4-ounce), and #3 (6-ounce) sizes are identical. Other than price, the only real decision you have to make is whether to choose organic. This unusually uncomplicated situation is the result of the unique role of baby foods. They are strictly for convenience. Surprising as it may seem to anyone who thinks a baby cannot survive without commercial baby foods, at least half the infants in the world are weaned to foods prepared at home. They do just fine. Home-prepared baby foods work well as long as they are suitably cooked, pureed, moistened, and not allowed to sit around for too long. Take bananas, for example: there is not much point in buying pureed bananas in a jar when you can so easily mash a banana with a fork. The "Graduates" diced foods in jars, and the freeze-dried "mini" fruit and vegetable snacks sold for toddlers, also are not about need. Toddlers can and should be eating table foods and do not require commercial foods made "just for them" at that age, or later. With that said, I can think of many situations when it would be handy to have jars of baby foods available and many reasons why harried parents would want to use them.

Whether you use commercial baby foods or make your own, you no doubt have questions about when to start using them. Pediatricians say that you should not even try to give "solid" food (meaning anything other than breast milk or formula) to babies until they are old enough to recognize a spoon, swallow thicker or pureed foods, and turn their heads away when they are not hungry. Most babies can do these things by the time they are four to six months old. But practically everyone other than the most committed of breast-feeding mothers tries to sneak solid food into babies much earlier. At least three reasons account for the startling disconnect between advice and practice: social pressure to get as many calories into babies as quickly as possible (this might have made sense when babies were more at risk of infections and weight loss, but it makes little sense now), the hope that solid food will induce babies to sleep through the night (it won't), and, not least, manipulative marketing by the makers of baby foods.

If you are a new mother, the goal of baby-food marketers is to encourage you to believe that commercial products are easier for you to use (which they may well be) and are scientifically designed to be better for your baby (perhaps, but not necessarily). On the "better" claim, I am impressed by how much the baby-food market has changed since my children were small. Then, baby foods were packed with sugar, salt, starchy fillers, and other food additives. Over the years, consumer complaints and lawsuits induced baby-food makers to get rid of unhealthy ingredients. The desserts still have sugars and starches, but most other baby foods are now remarkably simple. Many just have one or two ingredients—carrots and water, for example. For the most part, what you see in baby foods is what you get, and babies eating them will be exposed to the flavors of real foods (at least those in jars). So if the convenience is worth the price, they pose no nutritional problems.

The similarity in contents and sizes across brands makes it hard for baby-food companies to "add value" or do much else to increase sales. In supermarkets, the different brands all cost about the same. Price-fixing is illegal, so let's call this either a remarkable coincidence or an example of carefully arranged noncompetition in the corporate interest. How much the products cost depends on where you live. I have seen jars of baby foods in Manhattan priced twice as high as the same jars sold elsewhere in the country.

The uniformity of sizes, contents, and prices across brands explains why business analysts consider the baby-food market to be "boring." For one thing, even with a relatively stable birth rate of about 4 million per year, baby-food sales are declining in the United States, perhaps because with nothing special about the products, parents have caught on that table foods work just as well. For another, Gerber completely dominates the market with a 65 percent share (bringing in more than $1 billion in sales in 2004). Gerber benefits from a level of brand recognition and loyalty greater than for any other U.S. product, even Coca-Cola. Among the runners-up, Heinz has just 17 percent of the U.S. market (but is the largest producer of baby food worldwide), and Beech-Nut just 15 percent. Finite as the market is, the three major players are businesses; businesses must grow; and Heinz and Beech-Nut would dearly love to have a larger market share.

In 2000, Heinz and Beech-Nut attempted to merge their baby-food businesses to compete with Gerber. The Federal Trade Commission (FTC), whose job it is to make sure that business competition is conducted fairly (as in honest advertising, for example), asked the courts for an injunction to stop the merger. The FTC said that unless the companies could show that the merger would not reduce competition in the baby-food industry, it would violate antitrust laws. Because an obvious purpose of the proposed merger was to eliminate competition between Heinz and Beech-Nut, the court said the merger would not be in the public interest, and blocked it. The court decision in this case makes interesting reading. It reveals, for example, how concentration in an industry leads to cooperation around certain matters that protect profits and why, as a result, baby foods look alike and are priced alike. As the judge explained:

> When Heinz attempted to market a premium all-organic product known as "Earth's Best," Gerber's immediately launched its "Tender Harvest" line and offered special incentives to retailers if they agreed to discontinue the Heinz product. The launch . . . failed, and Heinz sold the product line at a $10 million loss. When Beech-Nut ran advertisements illustrating differences between its products and Gerber's in terms of their nutritional

value, Gerber retaliated by lowering prices . . . driving Beech-Nut's volume down dramatically. Beech-Nut officials testified that this experience taught them to adopt a less competitive posture . . .

With birth rates relatively stable, baby-food makers are desperate for growth opportunities. Heinz sees the half of the world's infants who are still eating homemade food as a "significant upside opportunity." The company's best shot at realizing that opportunity is to convince mothers that its baby foods are "more nutritious and safe than anything they can do themselves." Heinz is not alone in such efforts. Gerber spends a fortune to convince health professionals as well as families that good infant nutrition requires babies to eat commercial baby foods, preferably Gerber's. My files are packed with symposium reports, surveys, and articles from leading professional journals describing inadequacies in infant diets, problems of childhood obesity, and the complications of feeding guidelines—all sponsored by Gerber and all hinting that many nutritional problems can be solved if babies were just fed Gerber baby foods.

> Heinz sees the half of the world's infants who are still eating homemade food as a "significant upside opportunity."

THE ORGANIC ALTERNATIVES

To date, the most effective method for baby-food makers to add value and charge more is to make the foods organic, which is why you can find organic options available in many stores (although by no means all). In February 2005, the largest supermarket near where I live sold a jar of Beech-Nut carrots in the #2 (4-ounce) size for 75 cents, but charged $1.09 for the same size jar of organic carrots from Earth's Best (now owned by Hain Celestial)—a premium of 34 cents or 45 percent. Prices in a Washington, D.C., Safeway were lower, but the percent differential was about the same. At the Tops Market in Ithaca, organic options cost just pennies more, but even a few pennies add up. Are the organic varieties worth the extra cost? By this time, you can guess that I will say they are, but in this case especially I think the choice is easy. If you do not want your children eating pesticides, you will choose organic baby foods. So, apparently, will other parents. Sales of organic baby foods increased by 57 percent from 2001 to 2005.

In this view, I also have plenty of other company, starting with the Environmental Protection Agency (EPA). The EPA is particularly concerned about pesticides in children's diets. Children eat more fruits and vegetables for their size than adults. They are exposed to proportionately greater amounts of chemicals that act as neurotoxins, endocrine disrupters, and carcinogens. However harmful these chemicals might be, they will almost certainly cause more severe problems in children than in adults. That is why the EPA monitors the exposure of children to pesticides and sets standards to ensure that current levels of pesticide use will not harm them. Advocacy groups also test baby foods and publish reports about their pesticide contents. The Environmental Working Group notes that babies eat hundreds of jars of baby food in their first year of life and provides answers to the question, "Guess how many pesticides they eat in that yummy mush?" It and the National Resources Defense Council have complained for years that the EPA's standards are too lenient and that pesticides in baby foods constitute an "intolerable" risk.

They too get plenty of support for such contentions, and from no less an authority than the prestigious National Academy of Sciences. In 1993, this group produced a study of pesticides in the diets of children that came to unusually forceful conclusions. The EPA, said the National Academy, needed to

> modify its decision-making process for setting tolerances so that it is based more on health considerations than on agricultural practices . . . Children should be able to eat a healthful diet containing legal residues without encroaching on safety margins. This goal should be kept clear.

European pediatric societies also argue that commercial food products designed for infants and young children "shall not contain any substance in such quantity as to endanger the health of infants and young children."

The implication here is obvious: choose organics. But does eating organic food really protect children against pesticides? So it seems. In 2003, researchers compared the levels of pesticide "excretion products" in the urine of preschool children who were fed organic or conventional diets. The urine of those fed conventional foods contained six times as many pesticide residues as were found in the urine of children who ate organics. The investigators said their study "demonstrates that dietary choice can have a significant effect on children's pesticide exposure . . . Consumption of organic produce represents a relatively simple means for parents to reduce their children's exposure to pesticides." In 2004, the attorneys general of four states (New York, California, Connecticut, and Massachusetts) petitioned the EPA to tighten its standards so as to better protect children against food pesticides. Bill Lockyer, the attorney general from California, said, "Government has no greater duty than to safeguard the health and safety of its children. It's time for the federal government to step up, do the right thing, and honor that duty." While waiting for your own state to act and for the EPA to set more stringent standards, you can take matters into your own hands: you can buy organic baby food.

> Whatever you do, it is always a good idea to postpone giving young children soft drinks, sugar waters, juice drinks (and even juice in large amounts), fast food, salty snacks, sugary cereals, and desserts for as long as you possibly can.

Beyond organics, I leave it to your pediatrician to advise you about which formulas to use, which weaning foods to start with, and how to manage the daily ups and downs of infant and child feeding. Whatever you do, it is always a good idea to postpone giving young children soft drinks, sugar waters, juice drinks (and even juice in large amounts), fast food, salty snacks, sugary cereals, and desserts for as long as you possibly can.

37

Supplements and Health Food

One day when I was on my way to the nearest ATM, I noticed a sign in front of my local General Nutrition Center (GNC) store: "Vitamin E is safe and beneficial . . . Overwhelming evidence supports that vitamin E is safe and has proven health benefits." These words might seem to state the obvious—vitamin E is an essential dietary requirement so of course it is safe—but I knew exactly why the GNC had posted that sign. I had just seen a full-page advertisement in *The New York Times*, using almost exactly the same words, and paid for by the Council for Responsible Nutrition, the vigilant trade and lobbying association for the dietary supplement industry.

The ad and the sign were damage control, part of the industry's response to a big review of clinical trials of vitamin E supplements that was about to be published in a well-regarded medical journal. The review's startling conclusion: people who took high doses of vitamin E—more than 400 international units (IU) per day—were *more* likely to die during the course of the trials than people who took less or none. Survival depended on dose. People taking the much smaller amounts recommended for prevention of vitamin E deficiencies (20 IU per day) were *less* likely to die during the course of the trials than people who took higher doses. Above 400 IU per day—precisely the amount in a typical vitamin E capsule—the risk of dying increased with increasing doses of vitamin E.

No wonder this called for damage control. The 400 IU dose of vitamin E is a top supplement seller and considered an industry standard. Worse, this study was only the latest of several to point out the downside of taking fat-soluble vitamins in amounts greater than those available from food (other such studies continue to appear). Unlike water-soluble vitamins, which you readily excrete in urine, the fat-soluble vitamins—vitamins A, D, E, and K—are stored. Ingest too much of them and they can build up to harmful levels. Several clinical trials using beta-carotene, the fat-soluble pigment in plants that gets converted to vitamin A in the body, also reported more deaths among people taking large amounts than among those who took smaller amounts or none. The vitamin E researchers concluded:

> In view of the increased mortality associated with high dosages of beta-carotene and now vitamin E, use of any high-dosage vitamin supplements should be discouraged until evidence of efficacy is documented from appropriately designed clinical trials.

To the makers and sellers of dietary supplements, those were fighting words, and the council's ad began with this usual first line of defense—attacking the science. It quoted experts arguing that this was only one study, a "backward-looking analysis that combined numerous trials with different types of patients, including many who already had chronic ailments" and "selected not to employ a vast number of studies that show no harm from vitamin E and a great deal of benefit." The council recruits experts who interpret the science in its favor, of course, but as is usually the case the arguments do contain small grains of truth.

The science of supplements is never unambiguous, mainly because this research, like so much of the other research I have discussed in this book, is difficult to do. When researchers compare the overall health of people who take supplements to those who do not (in what they call "observational" studies), the ones who take supplements often appear to do better. But when they conduct clinical trials in which they give supplements to one group but placebos to another, and track the two groups for years to see what happens, the results are quite different. Clinical trials rarely show much benefit from taking supplements and, as in the case of beta-carotene and vitamin E, sometimes show harm.

The most likely explanation for the different results is that people who take supplements are healthier to begin with. If you take supplements, studies show, you probably are well educated, physically active, a nonsmoker, a light-to-moderate drinker (if you drink alcohol at all), and reasonably well-off financially—all traits associated with better health. Health habits cluster. If you do one good thing for your health, you probably do others. But relative to the benefits of a good diet, regular exercise, and not smoking, the effect of a vitamin supplement is small.

> Clinical trials rarely show much benefit from taking supplements and, as in the case of beta-carotene and vitamin E, sometimes show harm.

The supplement industry, however, tends to ignore or attack inconvenient research results. It much prefers personal testimonials and favorable observational studies. Supplement trade associations and companies work hard to convince you that your diet is deficient in nutrients, that this deficiency threatens your health, and that supplements are the solution to whatever ails you. Wyeth, for example, the maker of Centrum multivitamins, conducts its own studies to demonstrate how badly you need supplements. One of its studies concluded that $1.6 billion could be saved in annual health care costs if older people took vitamin supplements. As it happens, Wyeth makes Centrum Silver, a supplement marketed to older age groups. In March 2004, the company's public relations people were kind enough to write me a personal letter enclosing a copy of that published study. A few months later, they sent me another letter, this one with a report of a Wyeth-sponsored conference on "Micronutrient Intake in America: An Emerging Public Health Problem." The "problem" this conference addressed was "suboptimal nutrition," a condition said to lead to metabolic abnormalities (rather than overt clinical symptoms)

> Supplement trade associations and companies work hard to convince you that your diet is deficient in nutrients, that this deficiency threatens your health, and that supplements are the solution to whatever ails you.

that can be corrected by—you guessed it—supplements. Whether suboptimal nutrition really leads to metabolic abnormalities that need to be corrected to improve health is debatable, but it is very much in Wyeth's interests to encourage you to think so and to take supplements as a result.

If you are like the majority of adults in the United States—60 percent or more—you already take supplements of one kind or another. You probably take them because you do not eat right all the time, because you are worried that you might not be getting all the nutrients you need from your diet, because you think some nutritional insurance is a good idea, or because you feel that taking supplements does something positive for your health—all quite understandable reasons. But—and here is where the difficulties arise—you almost certainly expect the supplements you take to do you some good, and you no doubt assume they are safe. If you are health conscious and follow the news, you probably also pay attention to media accounts of the latest research. If any of these statements describes you, you are the supplement industry's core customer.

Because industry sales are exquisitely sensitive to media reports, supplement trade associations fret about how research results might affect your expectations and assumptions. Sales of vitamin A supplements, for example, plummeted in the wake of the disappointing results of the beta-carotene trials, which were widely reported in the media. The Council for Responsible Nutrition, whose job it is to protect the industry against public relations disasters, is diligent in finding ways to blunt the impact of reports like the one about increased death rates among people taking high doses of vitamin E.

Its *New York Times* ad defending vitamin E went on to say: "Your safety is also assured because the manufacturing, labeling, health claims, and advertising of vitamin E are regulated by the Food & Drug Administration and the Federal Trade Commission." Coming from this particular lobbying group, a statement like this is shameless. As I related in *Food Politics*, this same Council for Responsible Nutrition (irresponsible would be more like it) lobbied for years to undermine the FDA's ability to regulate dietary supplements—that is, to weaken the very federal oversight that the ad was using as evidence for the safety of its products. Furthermore, this same council wrote the language for—and got

Congress to pass—the 1994 Dietary Supplement Health and Education Act (DSHEA, pronounced d'shay), the law that forced the FDA out of the business of doing much to ensure that supplements have what they say they have, do what they say they do, and are safe.

DSHEA AND ITS CONSEQUENCES

What I am about to say is an exaggeration, but only a slight one. As a result of the council's success in lobbying Congress, you can go into your garden, pick some spinach, dry it, and sell it in a Popeye-illustrated package labeled "All-natural herbal supplement! Promotes muscle strength!" and no federal agency is going to stop you. This is true, even if your product becomes widely distributed throughout the United States and earns you millions of dollars. While visiting a game park in South Africa in 2005, I learned that elephant dung is used locally as a remedy for migraine headaches. All I would have to do to market a supplement made from this substance—Natural remedy! Used by African tribal groups for centuries!—would be to inform the FDA that I am selling this "new dietary ingredient" and explain why it might reasonably be expected to be safe (and I get to choose the evidence to back up my contention). As long as not too many people die from eating this product, no federal agency is going to pay much attention.

You think this scenario is far-fetched? Consider that it took the FDA ten years to get ephedra (ma huang) off the market, despite thirty or so deaths and hundreds of reports of illness among young people who took it as an "upper" or to lose weight. During that decade, the leading manufacturer of ephedra products, Metabolife, spent millions of dollars lobbying to keep it on the market. Only when it seemed that ephedra might have had something to do with the death of Steve Bechler, a twenty-three-year-old pitcher for the Baltimore Orioles, was enough public outrage generated to allow the FDA to finally ban ephedra.

For the supplement industry, this ban meant a loss of $800 million in annual sales, which helps explain why the industry is still fighting the ban in the courts. In 2005, a federal judge in Utah (where Senator Orrin Hatch, the architect of DSHEA, is the principal protector of the interests of that state's supplement companies) ruled that ephedra could be sold there because the FDA had failed to prove that low doses caused harm.

Nevertheless, the national ban was a wake-up call, and some supplement makers now think that a stronger FDA would be a good thing, mainly to counter the "myth" that the FDA has lost control over supplements. Why any industry would want a weak FDA is beyond me, when it is so obvious that strong federal regulation builds consumer confidence. Supplements need that. But this industry, like many others, does not always act in its best long-term interest.

I would not call the FDA's loss of control a myth. Congress passed DSHEA in 1994 on the basis of two quite questionable assumptions: that supplements are basically harmless, and that supplement makers are honest. The law does not require supplement makers to demonstrate the safety or efficacy of their products. Instead, it makes the FDA responsible for proving supplements harmful—in court (on the basis of evidence from clinical trials or reports of harm to many individuals)—before doing anything about them. While DSHEA did

> Congress passed DSHEA in 1994 on the basis of two quite questionable assumptions: that supplements are basically harmless, and that supplement makers are honest.

not allow supplement labels to claim that products prevent, cure, or treat disease, it expressly allowed them to be marketed with "structure/function" claims—claims that the product supports some body structure or function—that appear almost the same as FDA-approved health claims. Although supplement labels are forbidden to say that the product prevents heart disease, they are allowed to say that it "promotes heart health." The labels cannot say that the product prevents colds or AIDS, but they can say that it "supports a healthy immune system." If you find the difference too subtle to distinguish, that is the point. The purpose of DSHEA was to be able to market the benefits of supplements, whether or not backed up by science.

Supplements brought in more than $60 billion in worldwide sales in 2004, of which nearly $21 billion was spent in the United States alone. The U.S. figure represents a doubling since 1994. But the rate of growth— the figure that Wall Street cares about—has declined almost steadily from a peak of 14 percent in 1997 to just under 4 percent in 2002. Since then, growth has recovered a bit, fueled by supplement sales through mail order, private health practitioners, and the Internet, but it has not returned to its previous highs. The industry's need for damage control in response to bad news about vitamin E supplements is understandable for business reasons; retail sales of vitamin E dropped by 7 percent in 2004, and by another 33 percent in the first half of 2005.

But research is not the only threat to this industry. Integrity is too. Supplement makers are supposed to follow Good Manufacturing Practices, meaning formulating their products according to defined chemical criteria and making sure that the products contain what the labels say they do. But because neither the government nor the industry sets standards for the contents of supplement products, what is in those containers is on the honor system.

PRIVATE TESTING OF SUPPLEMENTS

One result of DSHEA is that the FDA no longer routinely checks up on supplement products. A private company, ConsumerLab.com, has taken advantage of the regulatory gap; it tests product samples and discloses its methods and the results of its studies to the public on its Web site. The lab's stated mission is "to identify the best quality health and nutrition products through independent testing," and it tests a variety of nutritional supplements, functional foods, and personal care products. It performs its own comparisons and also conducts commissioned studies for which companies pay a fee. Early in 2005, I paid $24 for a year's subscription to the ConsumerLab.com Web site, which allowed me access to the complete collection of the company's reports on all products, not just to the summaries (which are available to everyone at no cost). I consider this money well spent. The reports make astonishing reading. No matter what kind of supplements the lab chooses to analyze, it finds that some samples—and sometimes most samples—do not actually contain what their labels say they do.

ConsumerLab.com tested multivitamin supplements, for example, and found one-third of the samples to have levels of nutrients below the amounts stated on the labels. Some products contained nutrients that did not dissolve (so the body could not use them), or were contaminated with lead or other toxic metals. The lab reported similar results for herbal products. Some samples of echinacea supplements contained something other than echinacea. Only 25 percent of ginkgo supplements and 40 percent of St. John's Wort samples had what they were supposed to. The lab congratulated the makers of Korean ginseng because *only* 17 percent of their samples were contaminated with pesticides; previous tests had found 60 percent to be contaminated. Among twenty-five samples of oil supplements, six did not have the stated amount of beneficial fatty acids or were rancid. Nearly a third of probiotic ("friendly" bacteria) samples had less than 1 percent of the claimed number of live bacteria. Whether creatine supplements really do "build lean muscle mass" is open to argument, but the science may not matter; only 50 percent of the samples had what was claimed, and one sample did not even have 1 percent of the amount indicated on the label. It is a relief of sorts to learn that all samples of whey protein supplements were labeled properly, but these products—packaged in tough, masculine cans that look like they belong in garages—are not complicated to make, much less to describe on a label; they are just milk protein, sometimes chocolate flavored.

With these kinds of results available for anyone who has $24 and access to the Internet, it is not hard to see why the Council for Responsible Nutrition has asked the Federal Trade Commission to investigate ConsumerLab.com's "deceptive business practices" and supposed lack of transparency in its business dealings. Says the council: "ConsumerLab. com's entire business model is a shake-down, based upon threat and deception." The irony of this complaint is striking. If you want to know who is responsible for the "anything goes" state of supplement regulation, and an absence of federal oversight of this industry that is so profound that private companies like ConsumerLab.com can move into the breach, I put the Council for Responsible Nutrition right at the head of the list. Because of the industry's shortsighted actions, the supplement marketplace is virtually unregulated. The result is that no federal or private agency can assure you that the supplements you buy are as advertised.

Early in 2005, I said something like this on a call-in radio show aired in Mendocino County, California, a place where, the host told me, many listeners take supplements and strongly oppose government interference in their right to take whatever they please. One clearly upset caller, who identified herself as someone who worked in the supplement business, said I was unfair to talk about the industry as if it were one entity, when most supplement makers and sellers are honest, most supplements are safe, and any health food store clerk knows which products are best. I freely concede the possibility that most supplement companies make decent products, but unless you subscribe to the ConsumerLab.com Web site, how are you—or store clerks—supposed to know which ones they are? Some clerks may know their business, but in my experience many do not. Instead, they rely on store copies of *Prescription for Nutritional Healing*, a book that consists of descriptions of supplements said to be useful for treating any condition you can think of, but that makes no pretense of critically reviewing the science or guaranteeing product contents.

Even the most responsible store clerks have their work cut out for them. Knowing the science of supplements is no easy matter, not least because there are thousands of products and few have been studied carefully. The products that are best understood are nutritional (vitamin and mineral) supplements. These work splendidly for correcting evident nutrient deficiencies, but few people in the United States have health problems resulting from deficient intake. Food is plentiful in this country and most Americans eat more than enough of it to meet vitamin and mineral requirements. Iron deficiency in young children and in women of child-bearing age is the one notable exception, and even its prevalence is low. Nevertheless, most health authorities recommend taking a daily multivitamin as a form of nutritional insurance, and most American adults do so, at least occasionally. It is hard to argue against this practice, and I won't. Multivitamins are supplements that combine large proportions—often 100 percent or more—of the daily recommendations for twenty or more vitamins and minerals in a single pill. These—and single nutrients in similar amounts—are safe and, if nothing else, act as powerful placebos. They might do some

B ut, as the science increasingly shows, nutrient supplements are safest and most effective in small amounts. When it comes to supplements, more is not necessarily better.

good, and the confidence they provide could be good for your health all on its own. But, as the science increasingly shows, nutrient supplements are safest and most effective in small amounts. When it comes to supplements, more is not necessarily better.

HERBAL SUPPLEMENTS

Beyond vitamins and minerals, the value of supplements gets much harder to assess. There are thousands of products, each with its own claims for health benefits, folklore, and mystique. Although some have been used for millennia in Asian traditional medicine, they may not work the same way in a Western context. Some years ago, I co-taught a course in complementary and alternative nutrition that dealt with such products, and I quickly became convinced that only an extraordinarily well-trained specialist can understand even a small fraction of them. The best we nonspecialists could do was to teach students how to find whatever information is available about a product of interest and how to assess the reliability of that information.

One conclusion seems inescapable. When it comes to herbal supplements, the more carefully the research is designed, the fewer benefits it shows. Disappointing research results, according to *Nutrition Business Journal*, are a big reason for disappointing sales of many herbal products: "Not only did ephedra disappear from the market, once-popular herbs like St. John's Wort, ginkgo, ginseng and

> One conclusion seems inescapable. When it comes to herbal supplements, the more carefully the research is designed, the fewer benefits it shows.

echinacea slid again, with equivocal news about efficacy and labeling partly to blame." In 2005, a well-designed clinical trial found that supplements of echinacea did nothing to alleviate symptoms of the common cold. This particular disappointing result prompted one critical editorial writer to argue that current research on supplements allows for no "demarcation of the absurd," meaning that there is no point at which proponents of supplements will admit that science does not support their benefits. Supplement research, he said, is characterized by "repeated clinical trials, redundant systematic reviews of implausible methods, and indeterminate conclusions," and it is high time to replace all this with science based on "wisdom and common sense." But well-designed clinical trials are bad news for the supplement industry. Sales of echinacea had fallen by more than $50 million a year since 1999, and the latest study would only be expected to accelerate that trend. And further bad news was surely forthcoming; regulators are said to be taking a closer look at the possibility of banning kava, *Citrus aurantium* (bitter orange), comfrey, and other herbal supplements that had been reported to cause problems.

Research is a worry for the supplement industry as a whole, but herbal products have been hit especially hard; their sales have been relatively flat—increasing or decreasing by a few percentage points—for several years in the United States (in European countries like Germany and France that reimburse patients for the cost of herbal medicines, however, sales are lively). The few industry bright spots are specialty products targeted to an aging population—things like probiotics, fish oils, and glucosamine (said to be helpful in treating joint pain). If ConsumerLab.com's analyses lead to publicity about the unreliability of the contents of such products, these products also could be in trouble.

One intriguing observation about the supplement industry is that its market is still divided among a great many companies—more than 800 of them, hardly any of which bring in more than $20 million a year. There is still a place in this industry for backyard products such as my hypothetical spinach or elephant dung supplements. The industry leader by far is NBTY, owner of Nature's Bounty, Vitamin World, and numerous other brands; these earned $910 million in sales in 2004—still a tiny amount by the standards of large food companies. Companies blame their small size and slow growth on media-induced consumer confusion about supplements, the bad press about ephedra, and concerns about the lack of regulation. Chickens coming home to roost, I would say. Having won DSHEA and the almost complete deregulation of its products, the supplement industry is in the awkward position of having brought its current troubles on itself.

Where that leaves you is another matter. You have to decide for yourself whether you need supplements and which ones to take. If you want to take them, you are better off buying ones made by relatively large pharmaceutical companies that have the most to lose if ConsumerLab. com finds problems with their labeling or contents. Otherwise, you must do your own research or rely on the research of others (I've given some suggestions for where to start in the endnotes to this chapter). I know plenty of people who take supplements and swear by them, but I mostly avoid them. I much prefer to take my nutrients in the form of foods. Occasionally after a spate of badly cooked business dinners I will pop a multivitamin, but that is about all. I can understand taking multivitamins for their broad range of nutrients in recommended amounts, but taking supplements of individual nutrients makes no sense to me (unless your doctor tells you that you are deficient in iron or some other vitamin or mineral). All nutrients are needed to make your body work properly; you need every one of them, and the best place to get them is from relatively unprocessed foods that still have their original vitamins, minerals, fiber, and phytochemicals. As for herbs and all those other non-nutrient supplements, you take your chances on what is in them, but as long as the amounts are small, they are unlikely to be harmful. With supplements of any type, small is especially beautiful.

> As for herbs and all those other non-nutrient supplements, you take your chances on what is in them, but as long as the amounts are small, they are unlikely to be harmful.

HEALTH FOODS

Toward the finale of the low-carb dieting mania early in 2004, I bought a box of Dreamfields "Healthy Low-Carb Living Authentic Pasta" because its label said, "Now you can eat all the pasta you want without all the carbs you don't." This pasta, the box said, had only 5 grams of "digestible carbs" (also called "net carbs" on some packages) per serving. But it also said that a 2-ounce serving had 42 grams of carbohydrate. What could possibly have happened to the other 37 grams? The box promised "With Dreamfields, fewer carbohydrates get absorbed into your system, much like whole grains." You don't absorb carbohydrates from whole grains? Since when?

Pasta is wheat flour. The first ingredient in Dreamfields is enriched semolina—wheat flour. However quickly absorbed, carbohydrates produce 4 calories per gram and this pasta has 42 grams of them per serving. Next on the list of ingredients comes a "fiber blend" of inulin, guar gum, xanthan gum, carrageenan, and pectin, followed by the sugar alcohol, sorbitol—all somewhat indigestible carbohydrates. You may not be able to digest these substances easily, but your intestinal bacteria can. That is why a 2-ounce serving of this pasta has 190 calories, 88 percent of them from carbohydrates. I can only think of two explanations for the label claims on the box. Perhaps Dreamfields' marketers do not understand what happens to food in the body. Or perhaps they do know but are taking advantage of customers who do not know. Slowly absorbed carbohydrates like the ones in this particular pasta may be better for you, but they still have calories. "Low-carb" is a calorie distracter. You are supposed to think the calories don't count, but they do.

> "Low-carb" is a calorie distracter. You are supposed to think the calories don't count, but they do.

Low-carb pasta (surely an oxymoron) is in the category of health foods known in the trade as "lesser evils"—foods with fewer unwanted calories, fat, *trans* fat, sugars, salt, or, as is the case of this pasta, carbohydrates. *Nutrition Business Journal* tracks sales of such products, as well as those in two other health food categories: natural and organic, and functional. Natural and organic, you know about from earlier chapters. The so-called functional foods are those to which manufacturers add ingredients like oils, artificial sweeteners, indigestible starches, cholesterol reducers, soy or milk (whey) proteins, phytochemicals, and other such things to enable them to take advantage of "qualified" health claims permitted by the FDA. Sales of lesser-evil and functional foods have done well in recent years and foods in these two categories combined brought in about $85 billion in sales in 2004. If you routinely buy such foods, you are among that select group of customers the health food business calls LOHAS (Lifestyles of Health and Sustainability).

If you are LOHAS, you buy low-carb products as well as energy and nutrition bars, vitamin- and mineral-fortified foods and beverages, soy foods, and practically anything with a health claim. This makes you part of the health food industry's cherished demographic base. You may be choosing these foods for reasons of health, but this industry views your health concerns as a business opportunity. Nancy Childs, a business school professor writing in *Nutrition Business Journal*, says that functional foods for obesity, for example, promise their makers

> a double reward—eligibility for qualified health claims and possible reimbursement under Medicare as a disease treatment. They also offer . . . balance to food company product portfolios, thereby limiting corporate liability on both legal and stock valuation fronts.

Her concern about corporate liability refers to the potential for claims against companies that their products might cause obesity or poor health. She reassures the makers of functional foods that "Consumer interest in obesity-fighting products will not wane, and consumer patterns of faddish over-response should remain the norm."

Like many people, I had the idea that functional foods, like supplements, were made by small, innovative companies. Maybe, but the top seller of functional foods is none other than PepsiCo. This company holds an impressive 25 percent share of the market for products like Quaker cereals and fortified Tropicana juices that qualify for FDA-approved health claims. Lagging well behind—with market shares ranging from just 7 to 4 percent—are Coca-Cola, General Mills, Kellogg, Kraft, and international companies like Nestlé and Groupe Danone. The control of this market by such companies makes sense if you think about what it is they are selling. The most popular functional foods are soft drinks, sports drinks, breakfast cereals, snacks, energy bars, and juice drinks. About three-quarters of breakfast cereals make heart-health claims for the whole grain or fiber that has been added to make them "functional." Many of these products are basically sugar water or sugary foods that might as well be cookies—but with ingredients added or subtracted to make them appeal to LOHAS customers who would not otherwise choose to buy such products. It is no accident that the advertising budgets for Balance Bars (Kraft/Altria) and PowerBar (Nestlé) exceeded $12 million each in 2003.

ConsumerLab.com has taken a look at these products as well. In 2001, the company found that hardly any of the "vitamin waters" it tested actually contained what the labels said they did, and some had only 20 to 50 percent of the amounts of nutrients listed. Power and energy bars may bring in $2 billion in annual sales, and most of them test out just fine, but the contents of a few of them do not match what is on their labels. Half the fat in most bars is saturated and some is *trans*. Like the Dreamfields pasta, many bars targeted to low-carb dieters have misleading "net carb" calculations. Some do not disclose their content of sugar alcohols, and some have so much of these additives that they are almost certain to produce laxative effects or gas. Some are so highly fortified with vitamin A or D that ConsumerLab.com advises against giving them to young children.

Even if I had not seen these results and warnings, I would have problems with power and energy bars. I do not care for their taste or texture. *Consumer Reports* says that its test panels judge the bars as tasting "gritty, chalky, or . . . chemical." I agree. When I ask friends and colleagues why they buy the bars, they say: "Because I know they are healthy and I don't care how they taste." Well, I do. I consider them vitamin-supplemented, fiber-supplemented cookie bars, and I can't see the point of eating indigestible carbohydrates flavored with artificial sweeteners. If I think I need more vitamins, I prefer to take a multivitamin supplement. If I need a hundred or so calories in a hurry, I much prefer a banana, a handful of nuts, or, for that matter, a delicious candy bar (I am particularly fond of peanut bars, toffee, and chocolate-covered ginger). This is not to diminish the value of some of the lesser evils—low-fat milk and yogurt, for example—but beyond such things, most foods posing as health foods raise the same philosophical question as vitamin-supplemented candy: Does adding vitamins really make a food better for you? Real foods *are* health foods and do not need to be made functional to be good for you. They are functional just the way they are.

> Real foods *are* health foods and do not need to be made functional to be good for you. They are functional just the way they are.

38

Bread: The Bakery

F riends in upstate New York were telling me that the Price Chop-per supermarket in Cortland had an in-store bakery that produced wonderful "artisanal" bread, the kind made slowly, from basic in-gredients, under the careful supervision of experienced and committed bakers. Artisanal bakers take four simple ingredients—flour, water, salt, and yeast—and turn them into loaves so crusty, chewy, elastic, and fra-grant that nothing could possibly taste better. Forget low-carbohydrate di-ets. This is bread, the staff of life, and worth the trip to wherever you have to go to find it.

But artisanal bread at a chain supermarket? The very idea deserved investigation, so I headed up to the Cortland Price Chopper one snowy February day. The store is about thirty miles southwest of Syracuse in a shopping center that also houses Kmart, Wal-Mart, Applebee's, JCPen-ney, and a tractor supply company—not a place where I would expect to find bakers hovering over bread that takes days to make. Once inside the enormous store, I looked for the bakery. The search took me past the specialty shops lined up along a far peripheral aisle. These sold pizza, salads, coffee, rotisserie chicken, deli items, and bagels, which you could eat in a nearby seating area decorated with paintings by local schoolchildren. The pizza place was giving out free samples, so I tasted one. This pizza was baked right there, but it tasted like standard commercial pizza, thick crusted, loaded with cheese, and a bit soggy. This did not bode well for the bakery, which I finally found way at the back of the store.

By itself the bakery was the size of a medium New York City grocery store and a handsome sight. It displayed many kinds of loaves and rolls, fresh out of steel ovens set up in plain view. In front of them, a couple of workers were shaping dough on a table covered with flour. One popped a tray of dough into a machine that instantly formed it into perfect rolls. The bakery manager pointed to a pound block of butter sitting next to baskets of sliced bread on a counter, and invited customers to help themselves. I took him up on the offer.

As with any other food, bread is a matter of personal preference. These breads, as I soon learned, were made from the basic four starting ingredients and ought to have been splendid. But I thought the best of the lot were just competent: good but not great. They were soft-crust breads with a smooth consistency and a comforting yeasty smell—like breads you might make at home using a bread machine. To its credit, this bakery knew its limitations. It only baked soft-crust breads. For the more complicated hard-crust breads, the store bought partially baked ("par-baked") loaves made by La Brea Bakery, a company based in Los Angeles. The breads are frozen solid, trucked cross-country, and delivered to the store to be baked right there.

This operation seemed like a big chunk of store real estate and personnel—a trained baker ran the place—to devote to finishing off the baking of par-baked, frozen breads or baking freshly made varieties that cost only a little more than commercial sliced bread, of which Price Chopper also sold plenty. The purpose of the bakery, the store manager told me, is service to customers, and people drive for miles, as I just had, to buy freshly baked bread from this place. I could only conclude that an in-store bakery has to be one terrific loss leader. Without question, it is marvelous theater. It is great fun to watch the bakers do their thing and even more fun to eat what comes out of the oven at the dramatic climax. The aroma of freshly baked bread is enough to make any customer happy, hungry, and in the mood to head to the far back corner of the store, passing aisles and aisles of products, and filling shopping carts along the way. The quality of the bread is decidedly secondary.

The quality *has* to be secondary. Bread baking is an art. To make great bread, bakers have to know how to handle any number of hard-to-control variations in ingredients, temperature, and humidity. With years of experience and much trial and error, they develop a feel for working with the variations. Supermarkets are well aware that skilled bakers are hard to find, so they compensate, as this one did, by mechanizing, automating, and using preprepared ingredients. Their breads may look and smell better than commercial sliced products, but how bread tastes depends on the skill and training of the baker. Theater, not bread, explains why the Wegmans supermarket in Ithaca has a wood-fired brick oven in its bakery. Customers get to watch employees putting logs in that fire all day long, and to experience what Matthew Reich of New York City's Tom Cat Bakery calls the "romance" of bread. But stoking wood takes less skill than coaxing that oven to produce superior bread, and some of that bread comes frozen from Los Angeles.

In her book for home bakers, *The Bread Bible*, Rose Levy Beranbaum points out that it is "utterly amazing that flour, water, yeast, and salt, judiciously proportioned, transform into the most perfect loaf of bread . . . Bread is like life—you can never control it completely." The late food historian Alan Davidson explains bread making as a process of "deceptive simplicity," dependent as it is on the biology of yeast and the invention of agriculture, wheat domestication, milling machinery, and baking ovens. Skilled bakers are only the last step in this long saga of human progress.

THE ART OF BAKING

The baking of wheat bread depends on a unique property of the wheat grain—its gluten content. Wheat (as I explained in the chapter on processed foods) has three layers: the fibrous bran, the nutrient-rich germ, and the endosperm filled with starch and proteins. The important proteins in wheat are glutens. These are unusually long, coiled, springy molecules that can be worked into gas-entrapping networks. The gases are a by-product of the digestive action of yeast on the wheat starch (the process called "fermentation"). When bakers make fresh bread, they take those four simple ingredients—wheat flour, water, yeast, and a little salt—measure them out in the right proportions, mix and knead them together, allow the yeast to ferment and puff up the dough, punch down the dough, cut it to size, shape it, let it rest, make it up into its final shape, "proof" it by letting it rise again, and then bake, cool, and store it. Every step of this process requires close attention, a feel for how the yeast is working, and inordinate amounts of time. The baking of good bread takes so much time that it is easy to understand why commercial bakeries would want to speed up the process, which they do by mechanizing every step they can and tossing in any number of additives to compensate for rushing something that is best not hurried.

In my experience, artisanal bread bakers are a passionate, obsessive, and testy lot, disdainful of anything resembling a shortcut. They are artists. They have to be; their customers appreciate great art. My food aficionado friends in New York City argue endlessly about the relative merits of bread from Amy's, Tom Cat, Balthazar, or Sullivan Street, and how these compare to the ones produced by Acme in Berkeley; BreadLine in Washington, D.C.; Zingerman's in Ann Arbor; or the frozen ones from La Brea. As for me, if I go to a New York restaurant and am presented with a basket of pane pugliese from Sullivan Street, instantly recognizable by its dark, crisp crust that leaves crumbs all over the table, and its porous, stretchy interior, I know right away that the place must be serious about food.

Curious to know what is involved in producing bread like this day after day, I asked Mark Furstenberg, the master baker who owns Bread-Line, to explain how he does it. He writes:

> Bread is made from the simplest imaginable ingredients: flour, yeast, water, and salt. The difference between good bread and bad bread is the most expensive ingredient—time. What the big bakeries do is to replace time with stabilizers, dough softeners, preservatives, and other chemicals so the bread develops quickly and evenly and stays on a supermarket shelf looking and feeling fresh—even if it isn't. Bakers like me put additions into bread—whole wheat flour and rye, raisins or currants, herbs or olive oil—only for flavor. Only for flavor—not to replace time.

At best, supermarket in-store bakeries can produce breads somewhere in between such exalted heights and the commercial sliced breads typically on their shelves.

SLICED BREAD, BROWN AND WHITE

The starting ingredient for wheat bread is wheat flour. If all three parts of the grain—the bran, germ, and endosperm—remain after grinding, the flour is whole wheat. White flour is "refined." It contains 70 to 80 percent of the components of the original grain and is mostly endosperm (the nutrient-rich bran and germ are mostly removed). White flour bakes into lighter and softer loaves, but these are nutritionally inferior to those made from whole grains. If you look at all the foods made from white flour in the United States, they account for nearly one-fifth of the calories in American diets, so nutrient losses from that proportion of calories could lead to deficiencies. To compensate in part for the losses, the U.S. government requires white flour to be enriched with the five nutrients least likely to be available from other foods in the diet: the vitamins niacin, riboflavin, thiamin, and folic acid, and one mineral—iron. If you eat white bread, rolls, cookies, or cakes (or, for that matter, pretzels), you are eating enriched white flour. As a result of enrichment policies, hardly anyone in the United States is likely to be deficient in those particular nutrients.

> White flour bakes into lighter and softer loaves, but these are nutritionally inferior to those made from whole grains.

A century ago, white bread was considered food for the rich, and was priced accordingly. As milling became more mechanized, the cost dropped and white bread became available to everyone. Wonder Bread introduced sliced white bread into the American market in 1930, and this form of bread soon dominated the market. It also spawned its own vocabulary ("the greatest thing since sliced bread"), gadgets (toasters), and cuisine (grilled cheese sandwiches). Eventually, nearly all of the bread sold in supermarkets was made from refined white flour, bleached and treated with softeners and preservatives.

My well-worn 1964 edition of the *Joy of Cooking*, with the pages in the bread section stained and annotated from my long-ago experiments in bread baking, contains plenty of advice about the value of whole grains. Its authors, well ahead of their time in this and other matters, were early believers in "health foods." They advised readers to "bake with whole grains" and "cut down on refined starch," especially because "whole-grain cereals are no more costly than highly processed ones." By the 1970s, the demand for breads that offered better taste, texture, and nutritional value had grown to the point where an increasing number of commercial bakeries were adding whole wheat varieties to their sliced-bread product lines.

Today, breads are a typical supermarket commodity, by which I mean that stores sell them in a bewildering array: white or brown, plain or premium, natural, organic, low carbohydrate (surely an oxymoron), with or without one or another part of the wheat grain, and with corn, potato, oats, soy, peas, barley, flax, millet, triticale (a cross between wheat and rye), buckwheat, nuts, raisins, zinc, calcium, or just about any other grain or nutrient you can think of. Many supermarket breads include partially hydrogenated soybean oil (with those dreaded *trans* fats), and more and more—and not necessarily the "lite" ones—are adding the artificial sweetener sucralose (Splenda).

B ut if you get out a calculator and convert everything to ounces, you quickly discover that the nutrient contents of supermarket breads are much alike.

All of these variations can make comparative shopping an annoying undertaking. Bread comparisons are especially difficult because some list the serving size as one slice, but others list two, and the weight of the slices can vary by as much as twofold. But if you get out a calculator and convert everything to ounces, you quickly discover that the nutrient contents of supermarket breads are much alike. The calories work out to 70 to 80 calories per ounce, a difference that hardly matters. Some are a little saltier, some are a little sweeter, and some are a lot more cluttered with seeds and things, but otherwise they do not differ significantly. Nearly all contain high fructose corn sweeteners, and many feature molasses or honey. The clutter and sweetness are there for a reason: to disguise the unpleasant chemical taste of dough conditioners and preservatives that keep the breads soft and free of molds for weeks at a time (and we Americans do like our foods sweet). The remaining ingredients are cosmetics to make the bread look attractive.

From a culinary standpoint, bread is about aroma, taste, and texture, and it is possible for commercial sliced breads to achieve these with a minimal number of ingredients. The Cortland Price Chopper's shelves of commercial sliced breads, for example, carried a Heidelberg Organic Flaxseed bread with the shortest possible ingredient list—organic wheat flour, water, organic flaxseeds, sea salt, and yeast—advertised as "Old World taste hand made in America" with not a preservative in sight. You would have to eat this bread fairly soon before it goes stale, but you can expect it to taste like real bread. Bread is supposed to be eaten soon after it is baked, and it is meant to be a fresh commodity, purchased frequently and used right away (or frozen immediately and used later).

Nutritionally speaking, bread is about calories, with a few nutrients included for good measure. All breads give you calories, with 75 percent of them coming from the carbohydrates in that starchy endosperm (the rest come from protein and a bit of fat). Other than calories, the nutritional value of any particular bread depends on whether the flour is refined or whole wheat. White bread has lost most of the fiber and the nutrients that did not get replaced by enrichment, but the differences are not great. Because of the way food labeling rules work, the amount of fiber in one bread or another does not look all that different once you convert everything to ounces. The labels of breads made from white flour say they have 1 gram of fiber per ounce, but this is rounded up from about half a gram. Whole wheat breads, which list 2 grams per ounce, probably have three or four times as much fiber as white breads. Premium breads are designed to look like they are loaded with nutrients and fiber, but you have to read labels carefully to find the ones that really are high in fiber and made from whole wheat flour.

To repeat: other than the kind of wheat, commercial breads are much the same. The bread industry, however, classifies soft sliced breads into distinct categories:

1. Soft white breads made from processed enriched white flour (non-premium)
2. Soft Italian and French breads made from processed enriched white flour
3. Soft premium enriched white sandwich breads
4. Soft enriched white breads made with whole grain (new in 2005)
5. Soft whole-grain sandwich breads

In the Table on the next page, I've given one example of bread from each of the first four categories and, because it is so complicated, three examples from the fifth category. To figure out whether a bread has anything in it worth eating beyond the calories from the carbohydrate and protein in wheat, it helps to look for the first ingredient, the total number of ingredients, and the amount of fiber. Except for the amount of whole grain, the differences are subtle and do not matter much (my comments are in brackets).

Wonder Bread is the historic prototype of the soft white bread category. Its first ingredient is enriched white flour followed by twenty-one others (of which seven are from the enrichment). The + in the Table stands for the indeterminate number of dough conditioners. Try figuring out how many or what they are. The label just says "may contain sodium stearoyl lactylate, calcium dioxide, calcium iodate, diammonium phosphate, dicalcium phosphate, monocalcium phosphate, mono and di-glycerides, ethoxylated mono and diglycerides, calcium carbonate or datem." Never mind. These keep bread "fresh." You would not expect this bread to have much in the way of fiber, but the label lists 1 gram per serving. Here is where bread labels get tricky. The serving size is two slices so I'm guessing that these together provide just enough fiber (a little more than half a gram) to get rounded up to 1. In 2005, the package still had the USDA's old Food Guide Pyramid on the back. It's hard to believe that Wonder Bread is what USDA nutritionists had in mind when they wrote about grain foods, but the package said:

Overall, Wonder Bread offers a versatile, convenient, affordable way to get the 6–11 servings from the Bread, Cereal, Rice, and Pasta Group as rec-

Selected Examples of Commercial Sliced Bread: Ingredients, Fiber, and Health Claims

BREAD Ingredient Listed First	TOTAL # OF INGREDIENTS	GRAMS FIBER PER OUNCE	LABEL CLAIM OR ADVICE [MY COMMENTS]
Wonder Bread Enriched wheat flour	22+*	About ½	"Excellent source of calcium" [it is added]
Wonder Italian Enriched wheat flour	35*	0	"Try 3 slices a day" [grain servings, yes; whole grain servings, no]
Pepperidge Farm White Original Unbrominated unbleached enriched wheat flour	19*	0	"Low fat, cholesterol free" [of course]
Sara Lee Whole Grain White Enriched bleached flour	33*	1.5	"Good source of whole grains," "good source of fiber, vitamin D & folic acid," "excellent source of calcium" [all added]
Baker's Inn Seven Grain Unbleached enriched wheat flour	42*	1	"Good source of 7 minerals and vitamins" [added]
Arnold Stone- ground 100% Whole Wheat Whole wheat flour	14	2	"Great news! In a low fat diet, whole grain foods like this bread may reduce the risk of heart disease" [if the rest of your diet is healthy]
Wegmans 100% Whole Wheat Stoneground whole wheat flour	22	3	"Two slices contain 80 mg of EPA & DHA omega-3 fats" [fish oils? in bread?]

*The starred figures include the seven components of enriched white flour (flour, malted barley flour, and five nutrients: iron, niacin, thiamin, riboflavin, and folic acid).

ommended in the USDA Food Guide Pyramid. Wonder Bread . . . a terrific "foundation food" for a balanced, nutritious diet that will help you and your family build strong bodies.

The Wonder Italian Bread is much the same but specifies four dough conditioners along with thirty-one other ingredients, among them a truly generous collection of emulsifiers, thickeners, and fresheners topped off with sesame seeds.

The Pepperidge Farm white bread is considered premium because it is made with unbrominated unbleached flour. Wheat flour, as it happens, is naturally yellow-brown in color and gradually turns white (which many people prefer) as it ages—but that takes precious time. Aging also makes the dough easier to handle. To speed things up, commercial bread makers add bleaching agents—chlorine compounds, peroxides, and bromates (hence: brominated). You pay more for unbleached flour because it costs more to store flour while it ages and whitens. Whole Foods markets do not sell products made with bleached or brominated flour, but more for reasons of keeping things natural than for anything to do with health. The whitening agents are unlikely to be harmful because they disappear or become inactive when stored or baked, but they are part of the additive mix that sometimes gives breads a "chemical" taste.

Despite the expensive flour, the Pepperidge Farm white bread and others like it include such unnatural things as high fructose corn syrup, partially hydrogenated soybean oil, and an emulsifier and preservative or two. This particular bread includes a "trivial" (according to the label) amount of butter, which seems odd to add to a bread with a "low-fat, low-cholesterol" claim. The claim itself is odd. Bread usually has hardly any fat to speak of and, since wheat is a plant, no cholesterol.

B read usually has hardly any fat to speak of and, since wheat is a plant, no cholesterol.

In 2005, in response to the *Dietary Guidelines* admonition to "consume at least 3 ounce-equivalents of whole grains per day," as well as to technical innovations that allow whole grains to be milled to an exceptional degree of fineness, Wonder Bread introduced a 100 percent whole grain bread for "white bread fans." This really is not white bread but the company is hoping that white-bread lovers will not be able to tell the difference. The bread is loaded with dough conditioners and is very soft.

Not to be outdone, Sara Lee introduced a whole new category of sandwich bread—the apparently oxymoronic "Whole Grain White" with "all the Fiber and many nutrients of 100 percent whole wheat bread with the taste and texture of white bread!" I spoke with a Sara Lee representative who was giving out free samples of the bread at a meeting of nutrition educators in summer 2005. This bread, she explained, is designed to be "transitional," to get customers used to its slightly chewier taste. People who like soft white bread are particularly finicky. In taste tests, the company was able to push the fiber to 3 grams in two slices, but anything above that amount elicited complaints. I thought the bread had a better texture than the standard soft white breads, but I am not one who usually eats the old kind. If transitional breads convince people to eat more whole grains, this could be a tiny step in the right direction.

Commercial bakers add back pieces of the wheat bran or cracked wheat (whole grains broken into smaller pieces) to give white bread the appearance of whole wheat. These "reconstituted" breads look natural and healthy but are little more than white breads in disguise.

From the Sara Lee experience, it seems clear that whole grains pose a problem for companies that sell mass market breads—many people do not like eating whole grains. This is one reason why the "whole grain" sandwich bread category is so complicated to deal with. As interest has grown in the health benefits of whole wheat flour, bakers do tricks to make white breads look like whole wheat breads. Commercial bakers add back pieces of the wheat bran or cracked wheat (whole grains broken into smaller pieces) to give white bread the appearance of whole wheat. These "reconstituted" breads look natural and healthy but are little more than white breads in disguise. The Baker's Inn Seven Grain bread, for example, is packaged in an earthy brown paper bag with a window so you can see its thick seed covering—but its first ingredient is white flour. The label lists 2 grams of fiber per serving, but the serving size is unusually large (44 grams), so it has just over 1 gram per ounce—the usual amount. The fiber in this reconstituted bread comes from additives:

whole wheat flour (ingredient #3), cracked wheat (#4), wheat bran (#10), and a bunch of minor (less than 2 percent) ingredients: sunflower seeds, barley flakes, rye flour, rolled oats, flaxseed, millet, triticale, and buckwheat flour. This is white bread with forty-two ingredients to give it the aura of whole wheat.

In contrast, the "100%" in the Arnold Stone-ground 100% Whole Wheat Bread tells you that it really is made entirely from whole wheat flour, although this one puts in additional cracked wheat, high fructose corn syrup, molasses, and the usual emulsifiers and preservatives. The "100%" also means that it has the full 2 grams of fiber per ounce. This bread qualifies for an FDA-approved health claim, albeit one with careful caveats that I've put in italics:

> Eating whole grains is an important part of a healthy diet. *In a low fat diet,* whole grain foods like this bread *may* reduce the risk of heart disease. Diets rich in whole grain foods *and other plant foods and low in total fat, saturated fat, and cholesterol may* help reduce the risk of heart disease and certain cancers.

Translation: if you include this bread in your otherwise healthy diet, you might be doing yourself some good.

Wegmans, the privately held East Coast chain whose owners are unusually sensitive to the health concerns of its customers, makes a 100 percent whole wheat bread with the same claim about reducing the risk of heart disease and certain cancers, but also with something I had not seen before on a bread ingredient list: "refined fish oil [fish oil, gelatin, tocopherols (vitamin E), natural flavor, citric acid & sodium ascorbate (preservatives)]." According to its label, the bread has 80 milligrams of EPA and DHA in two slices, much less than the 1,800 milligrams you would get in a 3-ounce serving of farmed Atlantic salmon, but close to the 100 milligrams you might get from 3 ounces of canned light tuna in water. Fish oil may seem like a strange thing to put into bread, but there is no accounting for what will sell food products. I tasted a slice. I did not find it fishy, but the bread was soft to the point of stickiness. I prefer fish as a source of omega-3s.

Whole grains used to be an important part of daily diets, but the average daily intake of whole grain breads and cereals has declined by more than half since the early 1900s. In more recent years, bread has been especially hard hit by low-carbohydrate diet trends. Sales of white bread alone fell by nearly 7 percent from 2003 to mid-2005. Eating less bread worries nutritionists almost as much as it worries bread companies. Because practically everyone eats bread, this food accounts for 14 percent of the fiber in American diets, making it the largest single source. High-fiber diets are good for health; they promote healthy bowel function and reduce the risk of heart disease and bowel cancers. If people eat less bread, they will miss out on fiber and the other nutrients that come from whole grains.

In an effort to reverse this trend, the 2005 *Dietary Guidelines for Americans* tell you to

> Consume 3 or more ounce-equivalents of whole-grain products per day, with the rest of the recommended grains coming from enriched or whole-grain products. In general, at least half the grains should come from whole grains.

Ounce equivalents? In USDA-speak, this means one slice of bread, one cup of dry cereal, or one-half cup of cooked rice, pasta, or cereal. On a 2,000-calorie diet, you are supposed to have six ounce-equivalents of grains every day, half of them from whole grains. This means that three 1-ounce slices of 100 percent whole wheat bread should take care of your whole-grain requirement for an entire day. But watch out for those ounces. If you eat a large bagel, which can easily weigh 6 ounces, you will be eating six ounce-equivalents of grains—the full day's allotment. If the bagel is 50 percent whole wheat or more, it takes care of your three whole-grain equivalents for the day.

Whole grains, according to the guidelines, are foods made from "the entire grain seed"—the bran, germ, and endosperm. If the seed "has been cracked, crushed, or flaked, then it must retain nearly the same relative proportions of bran, germ, and endosperm as the original grain to be called whole grain." By this standard, the only breads in the Table that qualify are the 100 percent whole wheat breads from Arnold and Wegmans. The others may add back pieces of the wheat seed, but not necessarily in the same proportions as the original. If you are looking for real whole grain breads, look for 100 percent on the label, whole wheat flour as the first ingredient, 2 grams of fiber per ounce, and the heart disease health claim. Anything else is a reconstituted white bread with varying amounts of whole grains added.

> **If you are looking for real whole grain breads, look for 100 percent on the label, whole wheat flour as the first ingredient, 2 grams of fiber per ounce, and the heart disease health claim.**

COPING WITH THE BREADS

So what's wrong with a reconstituted white bread with whole grains added? Not much, if the bread tastes good. Bread is one place where my nutritional correctness weakens. No question, 100 percent whole wheat bread is the better nutritional choice, always and often. And yes, white bread has too little fiber, too few nutrients for its calories, and too many carbohydrates absorbed more rapidly than one would like. But I cannot think of anything that tastes as good as a painstakingly made, freshly baked white bread with a good texture and a hard, dark crust.

> **No question, 100 percent whole wheat bread is the better nutritional choice, always and often.**

The trick is finding one. That may not be easy unless you are lucky enough to live in a city that has a passionate, obsessive baker or two or, failing that, a commercial bakery devoted to making a high-quality product.

I live near an outlet of Le Pain Quotidien ("daily bread"), the French-Belgian bakery chain, which posts this sign over its baguettes: "Hand made in small batches, several times daily, contains organic wheat flour, sea salt, yeast, and water." This bodes well for the taste and quality. The ingredients add up to only four, and there are no dough conditioners, no preservatives, and no trace of dozens of other additives. This is just bread, and good bread at that.

The largest commercial artisanal bread bakery in New York is Tom Cat. The company makes excellent breads with simple ingredients, no preservatives, and good taste and texture. The scale of operations is impressive. The company stores silos of flour on its premises, and deals in futures markets in flour, butter, and chocolate. It makes more than twenty different kinds of dough, forms it into nearly 400 products, and delivers fresh breads and pastries each morning to more than 600 locations. Tom Cat is huge by the standards of a two-shop artisanal bread bakery like Sullivan Street, but small in comparison to commercial sliced-bread companies. Its owners say they could not maintain the quality of their products if they grew any bigger.

If you do not live in an area with bakeries like these, you can consider buying partially baked, frozen loaves as one alternative. There are good reasons why supermarket bakeries (and some restaurants) use them: frozen breads are cheaper than freshly made breads, smell delicious while they are baking, and give customers the illusion that the breads will be something quite special. As long as they do not force real bakers out of business, I am for them. La Brea makes its par-baked products by mixing the dough and shaping, proofing, and baking the loaves until they are about 80 percent done, but not yet browned. At that point, the breads come out of the oven and are flash frozen. Some (but not all) breads freeze well if the freezing is quick. Supermarkets can and do pop the prefrozen loaves in the ovens to finish the baking throughout the day, and some sell frozen loaves in freezer cases for you to do the same thing in your oven at home.

La Brea boasts of having won taste tests; its breads came out first in blind tastings against fresh breads conducted by the *San Francisco Chronicle* in 1997 and 2001. But bread aficionados complained that the judges used the wrong criteria for assessing quality, and anyone who has ever eaten a baguette from Acme, the bread company in Berkeley, would surely agree that it beats anything previously frozen (or, for that matter, anything made anywhere). Since then, La Brea has been bought out by an international company and competitors say its quality has declined.

Mark Furstenberg says that if he lived in a place where good bread was unavailable, he would order it by mail from Zingerman's, the remarkable specialty store in Ann Arbor, Michigan, that supplies the best of the world's most delicious products, some of them made right there. You can order the breads from the company's Web site (www.zingermans. com). They arrive a day or two later, says the company's mail order spokeswoman, "protected by the very crusty crust, the bread's own natural preservative." You heat the bread in a 350 degree oven for fifteen or twenty minutes to "help steam up the bread and make it taste just like it came out of the ovens at our bakehouse." Or, she says, you can freeze them for later use, put them "in that 350 degree oven for forty minutes or so and enjoy!"

I try to avoid supermarket breads but if these are your only choice, you have to deal with what you find. Nearly all commercial sliced breads will be loaded with cosmetic ingredients. If you care about taste, look for commercial breads with the fewest ingredients and the lowest number of additives. If your first consideration is nutrition, choose breads labeled 100 percent whole wheat. Anything else will be white bread reconstituted to a lesser or greater extent. You can pick the breads you like and forget about small distinctions that make little difference. Just keep in mind that even the best breads have 70 to 80 calories per ounce, that slices taken from whole loaves may weigh more than one ounce, and that larger slices have more calories—and will have even more when you cover the bread with butter, olive oil, or peanut butter.

> If you care about taste, look for commercial breads with the fewest ingredients and the lowest number of additives.

39

Prepared Foods: Salads and More

cannot help thinking that the real purpose of the Whole Foods stores in Manhattan (or of stores like it anywhere else) is to sell prepared foods—"take-out" foods that you collect from hot or cold bins, scoop into containers, and pay for by the pound. One cold day early in 2005, I wandered into the Whole Foods store in Chelsea and took inventory of what that section had to offer: at least twenty prepared salads, dozens of meats and dishes cooked Indian or Asian style, and a salad bar with four kinds of lettuce and nearly fifty vegetable, meat, cheese, and fruit ingredients to add—all sold at $6.99 a pound. If those options did not satisfy, I could take eight kinds of soup from a cart, sushi made right in front of me, and any number of meats, fish, vegetables, and salads from a deli counter. The take-out salads and Indian dishes looked especially delicious. I wanted to taste all of them, but they were posted with prominent "no samples" signs. This required action. I introduced myself to the man changing the salad bins, got passed up the chain of command, and eventually was handed a tray covered with pill cups filled with hot and cold foods. Pig heaven.

The foods were good—really good—and for good reason. They had been made in the store kitchen that morning by employees who get to invent and share recipes, decide what they like, try out new items, and keep track of what customers like. Some are trained chefs, and one was taking classes at a local culinary academy. They were happy to show off their work. I went back to the counters and bought several of the items I liked best, took them home, stuck them in the refrigerator, and reheated them later for another round of tasting. The salads held up pretty well, but the hot foods were not as tasty as I remembered. No getting around it, most food tastes better when it is fresh.

The secret of good take-out food can be expressed in four words: good ingredients eaten soon. This rule applies to any preprepared food, whether from a supermarket, a take-out place—Chinese, Mexican, Italian, or any other ethnicity—or a deli, fast-food outlet, or restaurant selling sandwiches, pizza, or the finest of gourmet cuisine.

> The secret of good take-out food can be expressed in four words: good ingredients eaten soon.

Finding out how the best take-out restaurateurs pull this off required a conversation with my friend Maury Rubin, who owns the City Bakery in Manhattan, a place famous for its pastries but also for its array of unusually interesting prepared foods that you serve yourself and can eat right there or carry out. The essential difference between take-out food and restaurant food, he says, is this: in restaurants, food is cooked (or the cooking gets finished) only when you order it, but take-out food has to be prepared in advance. City Bakery makes all of its prepared foods first thing in the morning, keeps them well refrigerated, and brings them out as needed during the day. So Maury's challenge is to guess how much food customers will buy in any one day. If he makes too little, customers will be disappointed. If he makes too much, he has to throw it out.

If New Yorkers are smug about what the city offers, access to an enormous variety of take-out food is one reason. But you can now buy prepared foods in practically every supermarket in America. As a rule you get exactly what you pay for. Early in 2005, I found prices ranging from $2 per pound (inedible and scary) to $12 per pound (spectacular). At the middle to high end, the food is reasonably well prepared and closely supervised. At the low end, the less said about it the better. Before I would knowingly eat take-out food, I want to know three things about it: Who makes it? Is it safe? What is in it?

If you ask these questions, be prepared for unexpected answers. My nearby Morton Williams Associated may not produce foods that meet the culinary standards of Whole Foods or City Bakery, but you can see the cooks hard at work in a kitchen right next to the deli counter. Stand there and you can smell what's for lunch. The cooks are proud of what they make: "Go ahead, try it!" The foods are a bit high in fat for my taste, but quite fresh and tasty, and the price is a reasonable $5.99 a pound. In sharp contrast, salads in a small supermarket a couple of blocks away cost $1.99 a pound. These arrive twice a week from some unnamed supplier. As the deli clerk explained, "They don't have to come every day. Salads have their life." Yes, and I dearly hope it's a short one. If salads are acidic enough (think cole slaw or sauerkraut), they hold up well, but I would not want to eat a seafood salad that had been sitting there for three or four days, even on ice. As I discovered, that twice-a-week delivery system is all too typical. For example, a deli clerk at a Washington, D.C., Safeway that follows the same plan shrugged and said, "That's how they do it these days."

Supermarket delis are a relatively recent innovation, coming into their own in the 1980s. At first, they just offered meats and cheeses. Even in 1992, less than a quarter of American supermarkets offered take-out meals, although nearly 40 percent had bakeries and 60 percent had delis. Today, more than 80 percent of supermarkets offer what they call home meal replacements, in part to help make up for the decline in food sales that occurred when people began to eat more meals outside the home. The prepared-foods sections of supermarkets add value, and lots of it. Supermarkets can charge a good deal more for carrots if they cook the vegetables and add a little butter and parsley, and they can double the price of a piece of salmon with some heat and a bit of lemon.

Many supermarkets prepare at least some of the foods in their own kitchens. Like the bakery, this gives the impression that fresh cooking is in progress, when it may just be reheating. The smaller of the two Tops Markets in Ithaca, for example, makes pizza, sandwiches, and rotisserie chicken in its deli section, but the hot foods arrive frozen from a nearby central kitchen and are reheated on-site. I have no doubt that it is easier to manage take-out sections that simply reheat food rather than cooking it from scratch, but reheated foods never taste as good as those made fresh. And, like all foods, they will still need to be handled carefully so they stay safe.

HOW SAFE ARE TAKE-OUT FOODS?

The big mystery of take-out foods is not why people might get sick from eating them, but why more do not. Any food with multiple ingredients exposed to air, sneezes, and probing fingers is inviting bacteria to multiply. Yet surprisingly few people report becoming ill from eating prepared foods. The apparent safety can be attributed to two reassuring factors: most microbes are harmless, and most people

> The big mystery of take-out foods is not why people might get sick from eating them, but why more do not.

have healthy immune systems that can handle them. Even so, I am wary of eating take-out foods at most places.

I much admire the prepared foods sold at Marks & Spencer stores in London, and some years ago I took a visiting executive from that company on a tour of several supermarkets in my Manhattan neighborhood. I suspected the comparison would surprise her. New York stores are pressed for space, but that hardly excuses a lack of basic cleanliness. Early one morning, we arrived at a visibly unswept and mouse-infested store and pointed to some tired-looking salads in the deli counter. Are those made every day? Oh yes, the clerk said. Were those made this morning? They are running late today, he said. Could we buy what was there? Indeed, we could. I thought my British guest would faint on the spot.

Happily, that particular store is now out of business, but you can find others like it all over the country. Even in the best situations, take-out foods are open to whatever microbes care to drop in. But hazards can be reduced to practically zero if the place makes the foods fresh, keeps them appropriately cold or hot, tosses the foods out when they have been sitting around too long, and pays an employee who takes special pride in keeping the display clean, and who watches over it like a hawk. Such places exist, and you can tell at a glance if you have landed in one. One method for evaluating the safety of prepared foods is easy: if the foods don't look fresh, don't buy them.

In New York, the kitchens responsible for making take-out food are licensed and inspected by the State Department of Agriculture and Marketing. Restaurant kitchens, however, come under the purview of local health departments. New York employs 115 inspectors to deal with the state's more than 28,000 grocery stores. Inspection visits are not announced:

> O ne method for evaluating the safety of prepared foods is easy: if the foods don't look fresh, don't buy them.

> Food Inspectors are quick to spot insanitary [sic] meat grinders, meat or milk cases which are too warm, unsafe soup or salad handling procedures . . . Evidence of rodent or insect activity at the store will bring enforcement, as will . . . improper facilities to allow employees to practice good personal hygiene.

Given the ratio of inspectors to stores, they don't do too badly. Maury Rubin tells me his off-site pastry-dough kitchen gets inspected two or three times a year.

If state inspectors do find violations in the supermarkets they visit— and surely they must—you will not easily discover what they are. The department does not post outcomes on its Web site. Restaurant violations are another matter. The New York City Health Department fully discloses inspection results, and it is fun to look up your favorite places and see how they fared (or read about them in the occasional surveys of the least-sanitary New York restaurants conducted by the *Daily News*). If the restaurant is still open, you can assume it passed the most recent inspections, although it may have had to correct some of its procedures in response to evaluations saying things like "personal cleanliness inadequate," "in-use food dispensing utensil improperly stored," "cold food held above 41°F," or "evidence of live mice present." In Los Angeles, the Department of Health Services requires restaurants to post letter grades on their front doors that reveal whether the place's level of compliance with safety standards is average (C) to superior (A)—scarlet letters, indeed.

But the overall safety of take-out food remains a mystery unless some reporter starts nosing around. In 1999, Marian Burros of *The New York Times* took samples from salad bars and sent them off to a lab to be tested for total bacteria (an indicator of poor temperature control), *E. coli* (fecal contamination), yeasts and molds (spoilage), *Staphylococcus* (dangerous), and *Listeria* (also dangerous). The results: half the samples had bacteria counts that exceeded guidelines, many tested positive for yeasts and molds, and one tested positive for *Staphylococcus*, but none had *Listeria* or *E. coli*. High bacteria counts may trigger a "yuck" response, but these make the food unsafe only if they are the bad kind. But her reports of the attitudes of store managers did little to inspire confidence. The managers said they were "shocked, shocked" by the findings, and they denied or excused the results, or blamed others.

New York City is not alone in having such problems. A Connecticut survey found 28 percent of salad bars to be reusing foods from previous days in violation of guidelines, and the *Milwaukee Journal Sentinel* found practically all the salad bar samples it had tested in that city to be loaded with bacteria, although only one had *E. coli*. This is either good or bad news, depending on how you view such things.

At this point, I called the New York City Department of Health and spoke with a representative who assured me that only about 10 percent of the places the agency inspects are out of compliance with cleanliness, temperature, insect, or rodent rules. But 10 percent of the restaurants in New York means that several thousand restaurants are out of compliance with safety standards in any given year. These violations may induce nausea, but are not necessarily dangerous. Inspectors do find harmful bacteria occasionally in sprouts ("a problem"), seafood salads, smoked fish, and the end pieces of cold cuts. The department sent me some summaries, and these show a steady decline in outbreaks of food-borne disease in New York State since the early 1980s—162 food-borne disease outbreaks from all sources in 1982, but just 38 in 2003. Among places that cause problems, retail stores account for just a small fraction. From 1980 to 1999, inspectors found only 19 disease outbreaks caused by eating food from retail stores—an average of one a year. Given that there are

28,000 such places, this looks pretty good (unless you were one of the people caught in an episode). It is, however, likely to be an underestimate as so many episodes of food-borne illness go unreported.

Food safety requires eternal vigilance, and it troubles me that nobody beyond an occasional reporter seems to be worried much about the safety of take-out foods. Newspaper accounts and off-the-record comments of inspectors suggest that the potential for transmitting bad bacteria is quite high, but how many episodes of food poisoning occur — or how serious they might be — is not easy to discover. The worst example I know about occurred as the result of deliberate tampering. In 1984, followers of the guru Bhagwan Shree Rajneesh, who had moved into a town in the state of Oregon, attempted to influence the outcome of a local election by sprinkling *Salmonella* over salad bars at ten restaurants. This caused at least 750 people to become ill. None died, but dozens were hospitalized, and all but one of the restaurants soon went out of business. Even so, the results were kept hush-hush for thirteen years because federal officials did not want to give anyone ideas.

Nobody wants to talk openly about such problems, because exposing gaps in food safety puts places out of business. Fortunately, you can make some good guesses about the safety of prepared foods on your own. If take-out foods are made on-site, look fresh and clean, and are watched over by a hovering employee, the risk is likely to be small (although never zero). You will pay more for take-out food in such places, but the food is likely to taste better and you are more likely to survive eating it.

ARE PREPARED FOODS GOOD FOR YOU?

Today, nearly half the food dollar is spent on foods prepared outside the home, and what those foods contain matters a lot. Prepared foods, no matter where they are sold, tend to be higher in calories, fat, saturated fat, salt, and sugars, and lower in fiber and some vitamins and minerals than in meals prepared at home. And if you habitually eat prepared foods, your diet is likely to be worse than that of people who do not — unless you choose carefully.

But choosing carefully is not so easy. In case you have not noticed, supermarket take-out foods do not come with Nutrition Facts labels or

P repared foods, no matter where they are sold, tend to be higher in calories, fat, saturated fat, salt, and sugars, and lower in fiber and some vitamins and minerals than in meals prepared at home.

with complete ingredient lists. They do not have to. If you are unlucky enough to have a serious food allergy to peanuts or anything else, you have to ask how the food is made and hope that nobody makes a mistake. I can understand why labeling would be difficult for employee-generated recipes that change from day to day based on available ingredients, but the real reason why the makers of prepared foods would just as soon not disclose contents is that you might not buy the foods if you knew what was in them. In 1998, the Center for Science in the Public Interest (CSPI) sprang a pop quiz on its *Healthletter* readers: "Which has the most artery-clogging saturated fat? (a) Macaroni & cheese side dish, (b) Parmesan creamed spinach, (c) Meatloaf & brown gravy." Answer: "The Parmesan creamed spinach is one of the worst vegetable side dishes we've ever seen" (two-thirds of a day's saturated fat allotment). CSPI's analyses of the nutrient and calorie contents of restaurant and take-out meals, from chains to mom-and-pop Chinese, Greek, and Italian restaurants, yield the same result: if someone else prepares the food, you have no idea what is in it. Even salads and vegetables from take-out places will almost certainly have more calories, fat, sugar, and salt than you would use at home or, for that matter, believe possible.

I learned this the hard way. Some years ago, that same *New York Times* reporter, Marian Burros, had the clever idea of inviting some nutrition professors and doctoral students to lunch and embarrassing us by proving that even trained nutritionists have no idea what we are eating. We met her at a classy downtown Italian restaurant where she instructed us to order and taste every item on the menu, from club sandwiches to lasagna. Oh yes, and we were to tell her how many calories and grams of fat each dish contained. I knew we were in trouble when she ordered a second set of lunches to send off to a laboratory for testing.

Trouble understates the matter. I would never have come close to guessing that the innocent-looking and entirely delicious risotto would turn out to have 1,280 calories and 110 grams of fat—for *lunch*. Most diners in that restaurant also ordered salads and desserts, not to mention wine and cappuccinos. My chef friends had no sympathy for my disbelief that a quite small rice dish could contain a full 4 ounces of fat. "Marion," one said, "if you knew anything at all about restaurant cooking, you would know how they make risotto; the cooks simmer rice in olive oil, finish it with a handful of butter, and top it off with cheese. That's why it's so good." It was very good, but without knowing such things, mere mortals are likely to underestimate the calories in take-out and restaurant foods, sometimes by staggering amounts.

From the standpoint of calories, take-out foods are a mixed blessing. The variety of items at a prepared-food counter or salad bar encourages you to sample a little of this and a lot of that (an "eat more" strategy), but paying for them by the pound helps curb that tendency. On the other hand, the items that weigh the most are the ones with the most water (and, therefore, the fewest calories). Tomatoes, for example, have lots of water and are not an economical choice at a salad bar—fresh, delicious, and nutritious as they may be.

But if you are concerned about calories, the best way to keep them down is to keep the portion size under control. The more food you put into that take-out container, the more calories you get. Even salads and vegetables have calories, and a great many of them if you choose foods loaded with mayonnaise or salad oil. This may seem absurdly self-evident, but only in theory. In practice, you are likely to eat what is in front of you, even if the foods have far more calories than you want or need.

THE PORTION-SIZE PROBLEM

Earlier, I mentioned the Law of Portion Size: the more food in front of you, the more you will eat. When you take items from a salad bar, you are choosing your own portions—and making a guess about how much food you will want to eat. But this guess is likely to be more accurate than any guess you try to make about the calories in that salad. The connection between portion size and calories is so important, and so poorly understood, that it is worth taking a closer look at what it means. For this discussion it is easiest to use fast foods as an example. Unlike restaurants and take-out bars, fast-food chains make the same items in the same sizes day after day. That is why they are able to give you nutrition information if you ask for it. If you do, you can see what happens to calories as the sizes get larger, which is the reason for the CSPI's sensible campaign to require calorie labels on fast-food menu boards.

When I give lectures, I almost always show a slide of my former doctoral student, now Dr. Lisa Young and author of *The Portion Teller*, standing in front of a row of soft-drink cups. The smallest holds the standard government serving size for a soft drink: 8 ounces and 100 calories. The largest is from a local movie theater. It holds 64 ounces, which is eight times larger—that means 800 calories. It makes no difference whether the audience knows a little or a lot about nutrition. Even trained nutritionists gasp in disbelief.

This used to surprise me, because even the most mathematically challenged person ought to be able to multiply 8 times 100, but I now think something other than math anxiety is at work. It is just not intuitively obvious that larger portions have more calories. You are not alone if you suffer from what Lisa Young calls "portion distortion"—the idea that anything you are served in a container has the same number of calories no matter how big it is. Researchers like Brian Wansink and his colleagues at Cornell say the "eat me" message emitted by large food portions is so powerful that it overrides all other considerations. A large portion, they say, "influences consumption norms and expectations and it lessens one's reliance on self-monitoring." Food companies are well aware of portion distortion, and take full advantage of it to encourage "eat more" tendencies.

Perhaps because food was scarce in ancestral times, or because people remember periods of deprivation in wartime or economic depression, large portions do not send up red flags warning us to be wary of excess calories. On the contrary, they signal "eat me." Barbara Rolls and her colleagues at Pennsylvania State University have neatly proven this point. Hungry or not, the volunteers in her studies invariably eat more when served larger sandwiches, snack foods, or restaurant meals than when served smaller ones. If she wants to get her study volunteers to eat more calories, all she has to do is give them a bigger bag of potato chips. Unless you make a deliberate effort to overcome your human nature, large portions will encourage you to dig right in and continue eating long after you are full.

That is why nutritionists like me get so cross about fast food. It is easy to eat too much when pricing strategies encourage you to order the largest sizes. Try pizza, for example. My NYU colleague Marcia Thomas came in one day with the largest slice of pizza I had ever seen. When she held it up, it completely covered her chest. We got out a ruler, scale, food composition table, and a camera. The slice was 14 inches on a side and weighed a full pound: 2,000 calories, according to the USDA. The "smaller" slice from the same place weighed half a pound, meaning 1,000 calories. I put "smaller" in quotes because the standard USDA serving size for a slice of pizza is 225 calories. That large slice was the equivalent of nearly nine USDA standard servings. But the truly amazing part was its price. The pound of pizza cost $2.75; the half-pound cost $2.00. Which would you buy? Companies can price foods that way because the cost of the food is only a small fraction of what they pay in labor, rent, machinery, and packaging.

Another example: McDonald's discloses size and nutrition information on tray liners and its Web site so you can figure out what you pay for. Soon after the release of the anti-McDonald's movie, *Super Size Me*, the company announced that it would be eliminating its supersize portions. In April 2004, you could buy french fries in small, medium, large, and supersize portions, with prices ranging from about 50 cents per ounce for the small to 34 cents per ounce for the large and the supersize. A 16-cent per ounce price differential is a strong incentive to choose the supersize. By June, McDonald's had changed the sizes on its Web site, but it took until early 2005 for franchises to get the new sizes and prices in place.

At that point, the small and large turned out to be about the same number of ounces as the old portions, but the medium was smaller; the supersize, as promised, was gone. Prices at McDonald's vary by location; the outlet closest to where I work does not post prices for french fries ("not enough room on the board"), so I had to ask. In August 2005, french fries cost 42 cents per ounce for the small, 46 cents for the medium, and 36 cents for the large. Overall, french fries cost less under the new pricing structure, and the differential between the least and the most expensive was reduced to 10 cents. But—the largest size is still the best deal.

I do have some sympathy for food companies in this situation. Their job is to increase sales, and in the old days they never really had to worry about calories or nutrients. What they served did not matter so much to health at a time when eating out was a rare and special occasion. I like eating out, and I do so often for professional as well as social reasons. I just try to watch the portions and eat extra healthfully when I am at home. But prepared-food counters, salad bars, take-out places, and restaurants all are designed to get you to eat more—that is their business. Large portions are an "eat more" strategy, and today's portions are very large indeed.

Restaurant meals pose particular problems with portion sizes, so let me say a word about them. I don't like taking food home from restaurant meals because it never tastes as good the second time around. Instead, I want restaurants to offer what I consider to be real choices—reasonably light options on their menus in reasonable sizes. I wish restaurants would train waiters to be pleasant if you only order an appetizer or if you want to share portions. I wish they would give you at least a small price break for ordering a smaller portion. I don't want to think about calories when I eat out, and I can't imagine that you do either, but American restaurants rarely make it easy to avoid overeating. On vacation in Norway in the summer of 2004, however, I saw this sentiment printed on the menu of Restaurant Louise in Oslo: "May we remind our distinguished guests that calories are to be eaten and enjoyed, not counted . . . !" Since you can't know the calories anyway, that seems like excellent advice—but only in places like Norway where portion sizes are still manageable.

> This tells you that the first line of defense against eating too much is to eat smaller portions.

Supermarket prepared-food sections give you the opportunity to make your own decisions about how much to eat, although they also do what they can to encourage you to eat more, not less. This tells you that the first line of defense against eating too much is to eat smaller portions.

You could, for example,

- buy take-out foods in the smallest containers
- buy fast food in "smalls"
- order half portions or divide meals in restaurants
- buy processed foods in small packages or divide larger packages into smaller servings
- urge food companies and political leaders to make it easier for you to do these things

I put this last one in the list because without changes in the way food companies operate, you are on your own to exercise personal responsibility every time you buy food. But food companies and political leaders could make it easier for you to make more healthful choices. For starters, you have every right to know what is in the food you buy. If supermarkets, take-out and fast-food places, and restaurants know you want more information about the food you eat, they can find ways to provide it. And if political leaders know that you care about such things, they can encourage food companies to tell you what you need to know.

40

Conclusion: Taking Action

Despite what I already knew about nutrition, much of what I learned while researching this book came as news to me. If the intensely single-minded focus of food companies on sales and growth—so obvious when you think about it—also comes as news to you, it is surely because we are not supposed to think about such things. On one level, we know that supermarkets, grocery stores, restaurants, and fast-food and take-out places are in business to make money, but such businesses prefer that we do not notice the ways in which they encourage us to buy more of their products. And they make it easy for us not to notice.

I often discuss such matters with food industry executives. When I do, I know just what they will say. They immediately shift the conversation away from their own marketing imperatives and start talking about your personal responsibility for what you eat. In January 2005, for example, I was invited to the World Economic Forum in Davos, Switzerland, to speak at a session on obesity attended by high-level executives of food companies such as Nestlé and General Mills. They said (with my translations):

- obesity is a matter of personal responsibility (not marketing)
- obesity is a result of physical inactivity (not overeating)
- marketing does not make people overeat (personal choice does)
- advertising is good for children (it teaches personal choice)

- the science of nutrition is uncertain and complicated (obesity is not caused by overeating)
- we are making healthier products (isn't that enough for you?)
- sweetened cereals are low in calories and encourage kids to drink milk (so stop bothering us)

To the last two comments, I could not help but think: healthier products like whole grain Cocoa Puffs? And is encouraging kids to drink milk also the purpose of cookies? But they insisted: "If we don't make a profit, we don't exist." Yes, but how much profit and at whose expense? They said: "If you object to the way we market foods, you must be against business." As it happens, I am not against business. But I do have problems with unchecked greed, the use of misleading health claims to sell junk food, and the marketing of foods directly to children—especially when marketing to children undermines parental authority and, therefore, the personal choice of parents. I most definitely do believe in personal choice—when it is informed. To make informed decisions about food choice, you need truth in advertising, the whole truth and nothing but.

Supermarkets could do more to help you make better dietary choices if they made it convenient for you to make those choices. By this time, you know what that would take: put healthier foods where it is easier to get to them, advertise them, price them attractively, and give healthier foods the same kind of marketing attention that gets paid to junk foods. Supermarkets also could demand that food producers grow fruits, vegetables, crops, animals, and farmed fish in ways that protect the health of the environment as well as of people. If stores did this, they would not only be adding value to the foods they sell but would be adding *lasting* value.

That the supermarket, restaurant, and fast-food industries are not doing everything they can to promote short- and long-term health is a sign that these industries are in deep, deep trouble. Yes, everyone eats and the market for food is never going to disappear. But with 3,900 calories—nearly twice what is needed—already available in the food supply for every American, every day, not much room exists for further corporate growth. But Wall Street cares only about growth—and short-term growth at that. Its functions depend on those quarterly reports filed every ninety days. Investment analysts are not at all interested in your health, the economic and social health of your community, or the health of the environment in which we all live—unless a publicly traded company can profit from it. The investment community could not be more explicit on this point. Researchers from the large investment banking firm UBS Warburg warn restaurant companies that "per capita food consumption may have stopped growing, and may even be declining. Obviously, this trend—if it continues—would be a negative for not only restaurants, but packaged food companies as well." Translation: eating less is bad for business. The only corporate winners, say UBS analysts, will be those who manage "their menu/product mix, branding, target demographic, and media strategy in an increasingly targeted manner." On Wall Street, "targeted" means making *you* the target.

> But Wall Street cares only about growth—and short-term growth at that.

UBS points out that "we have simply maxed out on the number of restaurants in this country," that 75 percent of the U.S. population now lives within three miles of a McDonald's, and that any new fast-food outlet is likely to be located within a mile of an older one. I believe this: I have three McDonald's within a ten-minute walk from where I live in Manhattan. UBS is writing about restaurants and fast-food places, but the supermarket industry is in a similar crisis, not least because people are eating out more. Spending on food away from home now accounts for 46 percent of the average food budget, up from 33 percent in 1970. One result is fewer supermarket visits. In 1995, Americans went to supermarkets an average of ninety-two times, but they went only sixty-nine times in 2004. This means 25 percent less exposure to products on shelves. I do understand the dilemma faced by the average supermarket, caught as it is between the high and low ends—the more expensive stores such as Whole Foods that cater to customers who want foods fresh, organic, and natural, and the rock-bottom Wal-Marts and warehouse stores like Costco.

In 1998, USDA economists described the threat to supermarkets posed by "nontraditional" food retailers, places that never used to sell food but now do. Their list of such places included not only discount stores and gas stations but also drugstores, bookstores, florists, souvenir shops, toy stores, jewelry stores, liquor stores, pet shops, sporting goods stores, furniture stores, and lawn, garden, and home supply stores. Foods like candy, gum, and soft drinks, they noted, are sold in practically every retail store. And this list appeared before the invention of Internet groceries. By 2005, you could see delivery trucks from the online supplier FreshDirect ("Our food is fresh, our customers are spoiled . . . Our promise: higher quality at low prices") double-parked in front of apartment buildings all over Manhattan. Neighborhood supermarkets like Manhattan's Food Emporium also have gone online: "Now you are just a click away from a one-stop grocery shopping experience catering to discerning food lovers just like you . . ."

Advisers say that if supermarkets do not immediately deal with this competition, "there will be a lot of empty shopping carts in their future." The only growth possibilities for supermarkets as they currently exist are in the increasing population, industry consolidation (to cut costs), and expansion overseas, especially into developing countries. These last two approaches are likely to translate uncomfortably into low wages and poor working conditions for employees, and the export of products unlikely to promote the health of overseas populations. If supermarkets continue to go in such directions, they will be exporting approaches and practices that are no longer acceptable to the many Americans who care about their own health and that of their communities and their environment.

My cousin Ted Zittell, who consults for supermarket chains, has a name for the ones that still cling to the past. He calls them "Grocer-saurus," considers them an endangered species, and identifies them by their motto, "We can't, we don't, we never . . ." Changes in the industry are happening, he says, but most come too little, too slow, and too late. As I do, he blames Wall Street for much of the pressure on publicly traded companies: "Many Wall Street analysts, merciless in their hunger for rising 'comps' [sales figures compared to those from a year earlier], give no quarter to the public companies, making the process harder than it need be, with their relentless short-term focus." This, he says, explains why "the best-in-class retailers are usually regional and privately held." In his view, the way to longer term benefit for supermarkets is to "embrace sustainability, become an honest consumer advocate, and behave ethically, even at the sacrifice of short-term gain."

Honest consumer advocacy? Ethical behavior? Sacrifice of short-term gain? I suppose these approaches are possible, but signs to date are not reassuring. Because food companies of any kind have been slow to volunteer to do anything that might impede short-term growth, consumer advocates have been forced to consider formerly unthinkable coercive strategies: legal, tax, and legislative. Just in the first half of 2005, for example, various states introduced nearly 200 bills to improve school meals, teach nutrition to school children, restrict the vending of junk food in schools, or require fast-food places to label calories on menu items. Congress also was considering any number of bills aimed at restricting marketing of foods to children. From the standpoint of food companies, it does not matter whether these bills pass (and most will not). The mere threat of legislation or lawsuits has been enough to make every food company of which I am aware take some kind of protective action—all in the name of health, of course. Those apparently healthy new packaged foods you see on supermarket shelves—vitamin enriched, omega-3 enriched, whole grain, lower in sugar, *trans* fat–free, and, sometimes, organic—are there to make you think that the companies have responded to your concerns about health by giving you better choices.

> **H**onest consumer advocacy? Ethical behavior? Sacrifice of short-term gain? I suppose these approaches are possible, but signs to date are not reassuring.

To repeat: the "better choice" approach requires a philosophical discussion, one that can be debated either way depending on point of view. You have every reason to ask: Aren't these kinds of changes good? Isn't it better to have junk food products that are slightly more nutritious than previous versions? Aren't artificial sweeteners better choices than sugars? Or, to use the concrete example of breakfast cereals, isn't 1 gram of fiber better than none? General Mills thinks so, but the first ingredient in its Whole Grain Cocoa Puffs is sugar, the reduced-sugar version of this cereal is sweetened with sucralose (Splenda), and both have exactly the same 160 calories (with skim milk) per serving as the original. As a group, sweetened breakfast cereals are still the equivalent of vitamin-enriched, candy-supplemented, fiber-poor cookies, low in fat as they are. Vitamin-enriched sodas are still sodas. Organic gummi bears are still candy. *Trans* fat–free snack foods are still salty and full of rapidly absorbable carbohydrates. These foods work well as occasional treats, but are not cornerstones of healthful diets. Worse, they give you the illusion of health and do not offer you genuinely healthful choices.

If we are eating nearly half of all meals outside of the home, we need to pay close attention to the food-service sector of the food economy. Restaurants, even fast-food ones, are changing rapidly in response to legal and legislative pressures. They are all scrambling to offer healthier options alongside their usual products. Fast-food outlets have introduced salads, fresh fruit, and skim milk. So have quick-service restaurants. And guess what? Healthier has turned out to be good for the fast-food business. Salads are widely credited for turning around a bad year or two for McDonald's, not because they converted longtime hamburger eaters to salad eaters but because they brought in new salad-eating customers. To demonstrate its interest in child health, McDonald's started selling sliced apples. In the way such things work, McDonald's instantly became the nation's largest purchaser of apples— 54 million pounds in 2005, up from zero two years earlier. McDonald's tells apple growers what kind it will buy, and growers respond immediately. One can only dream of what might happen if McDonald's decided that it wanted all of its salad apples grown organically.

But you cannot expect health to trump business considerations. For McDonald's, the healthier new products serve "as valuable assets in the public debate on obesity." To sell these products, "making food fun and nutritious is the key," a strategy that requires a caramel dipping sauce (the fun part) for those sliced apples, and candy coating for the walnuts in the apple-and-walnut salad aimed at its more health-conscious adult customers. This is the same business approach that drives cereal companies to add marshmallows and chocolate to already presweetened breakfast cereals. And McDonald's core products—hamburgers, french fries, and sodas—are still high in calories and priced so the largest sizes are the best buys. That business strategy continues (as long as it works) at the same time that the company also promotes exercise and enters into a partnership with the Produce for Better Health Foundation, a trade association devoted to increasing national consumption of fruits and vegetables.

> One can only dream of what might happen if McDonald's decided that it wanted all of its salad apples grown organically.

As with many other aspects of the American food scene, two conflicting trends are in progress at the same time. While companies are trying to head off anti-obesity laws and lawsuits, they also are taking care of their more profitable customers—those who buy junk foods made with inexpensive ingredients and lots of "added value." Hardee's, for example, introduced a Monster Thickburger that gives, just as you might expect, 1,420 calories and 107 grams of fat—illustrating, according to the Center for Science in the Public Interest, "the height of corporate irresponsibility." This new product rated an editorial in *The New York Times*. The Thickburger, it said, reflects "a simple fast-food formula: poor nutrition sells." And so it must. In March 2005, my friend and colleague Ellen Fried brought me an enormous plastic jug—a "sippy" cup for adults—filled with 64 ounces of Coca-Cola (800 calories), for which she had paid $6.99 at a Roy Rogers on the New Jersey interstate. If you drive the I-95, Ellen explained, you can stop at any Roy Rogers from Maine to Florida and refill that "cup" for less than $1—a strong incentive to stop and buy more soda and the foods that go with it. Such strategies do not consider either the necessarily sedentary nature of automobile driving or the "eat more" influence of larger container sizes on calorie intake.

Business considerations explain why the National Restaurant Association opposes calorie labeling, supports legislation to prevent lawsuits, argues personal responsibility, and hires public relations firms to issue disinformation, attack the science, and personally attack anyone like me who questions their members' motives. The association's legislative counsel explains that "Our position is that the individual who is concerned about obesity should emphasize healthy lifestyle, personal responsibility, regular exercise and moderation . . . Seventy-six percent of all meals are prepared at home. That's where nutrition has to start." Once again, it is your personal responsibility to figure out how to contend with "eat more" marketing strategies.

EATING HEALTHFULLY IN AN "EAT MORE" WORLD

When it comes to food choices, all too many food executives, government officials, and, alas, my fellow nutrition professionals intone these mantras:

- all foods can fit into a healthful diet (you can eat anything you like, with no restrictions)

- there is no such thing as a good or a bad food (you can eat anything you like)

- the keys to healthful eating are variety, balance, and moderation (you can eat anything you like, anytime)

- the key to weight control is to increase physical activity (you don't have to worry about what you eat)

- obesity is about personal responsibility (it has nothing to do with pressures to "eat more")

When I hear such statements, singly or in combination, I know that they have only one purpose: to defend the right of food companies to market their products any way they like. Even though each of these statements holds a grain of truth, each leaves out crucial parts of dietary advice: most of the time, you would be better off eating less, eating unprocessed foods, and avoiding junk foods. Statements like these should be like a red flag alerting you that the speaker is unwilling or afraid to challenge the aggressive and sometimes unethical marketing practices of food companies. The mantra is designed to protect business as usual. It places the responsibility for food choices on you, but offers you no help with meeting the challenges.

> Food choices are not all that complicated—you do just need to eat less, move more, eat lots of fruits and vegetables, and go easy on the junk food. But to do this, you will first have to recognize, and then deal with, the hidden ways in which food companies promote the opposite.

Food choices are not all that complicated—you do just need to eat less, move more, eat lots of fruits and vegetables, and go easy on the junk food. But to do this, you will first have to recognize, and then deal with, the hidden ways in which food companies promote the opposite. What food companies really mean—what they really are telling you—is to eat more of their foods, more often, and not give the choices a second thought. But some foods *are* better for you than others, and it is not hard to tell them apart. The Table on the next page gives a quick summary of how to do that.

Some Foods *Are* Better Than Others

BETTER NUTRITIONAL VALUE	POORER NUTRITIONAL VALUE
Vegetables and fruits	Foods with added sugars
Nuts, seeds, beans	Foods with added saturated and *trans* fats
Whole grains (with fiber)	Refined grains
Lean meats, poultry, fish, eggs (in moderation)	High-fat meats, cold cuts
Low-fat dairy foods	Whole milk and whole-milk foods
Unprocessed or minimally processed foods	Highly processed foods

If you want to eat healthfully, choose most of the foods in your diet from those in the first column. Within these categories, small differences do not matter much. Yes, it is better to eat a variety of brightly colored vegetables, but eating the foods you like as often as you please is better than eating none. If you follow these first-column guidelines, your decision to eat one or another food depends mainly on what you enjoy eating. Choose foods you like, and enjoy them.

As for the second column, if you have your favorite junk foods—and who does not?—by all means eat them, just not too much and not too often. I would not spend a minute worrying about whether a serving of a sweetened breakfast cereal has 5 grams less sugar than another or a gram more fiber. The difference hardly matters, which is why FDA-approved health claims throw in qualifiers like "may" when they refer to disease prevention, and add context statements like "as part of a healthful diet." I suppose it is possible that eating a large number of junky foods with small improvements in nutritional value could make a significant difference in your diet, but I have yet to see evidence that it does. If you are someone who tries to be careful about what you eat, you will reserve sweetened foods—sugary cereals, yogurts, power bars, and soft drinks—for desserts and special occasions, junky snack foods for treats, and fast foods for once-in-a-while occasions.

Eating well is not all that difficult to do. The foods that go under the "better for you" category can be put together in simple, delicious ways that do not take much time to prepare. In today's busy world, it may seem easier to grab a package off the shelf than to buy real foods, but you pay for the apparent convenience in at least four ways: (1) money (you pay for packaging and advertising as well as food), (2) taste (all those chemicals), (3) unhealthy calories that raise disease risks, and—worst of all—(4) the loss of the joy of eating. Real foods promote health *and* bring pleasure. Delicious food can be simple—just good ingredients simply prepared.

If your dietary pattern looks more like the first column than the second, you are already eating healthfully and

> **D**elicious food can be simple—just good ingredients simply prepared.

do not need to worry about your diet—just watch the calories. If you can stop worrying, you will have a much more satisfying and pleasurable relationship with the food you eat. This approach works especially well with children: teach children about food—where it comes from, what it is, and how to cook it—and they will have a much healthier attitude about food and eating. They will know what real food tastes like, will refuse to settle for anything less, and will stop demanding junk food as daily fare.

BEYOND PERSONAL RESPONSIBILITY

One of the repeated themes of this book is that the way food is situated in today's society discourages healthful food choices, and that food company marketing strategies have much to do with the social environment of food choice. Food company executives bristle when I say things like this, and you might feel some sympathy for them when they are forced to defend themselves against such complaints. After all, food companies are not deliberately trying to make people gain weight or become sick. They are only trying to stay in business and please their stockholders.

But you might be less sympathetic if you could see the aggression that underlies food company defensiveness. Ordinarily the aggression against targeted consumers—and remember, this means you—stays hidden behind corporate doors. In June 2004, however, some researchers from UBS Warburg produced an analysis of how food companies could use your fears about today's "turbulent times" to their own advantage. The British UBS analysts listed seven "opportunities" for their food business clients. Here are a few selected examples of such opportunities gleaned from their sixty-three-page report:

- *Win at the margins*: "Companies will need to reposition their brand portfolios to focus on the high end and/or the low end . . . Consumers tend to trade up to high-end products in categories that are important to them . . . Could either the Coke or Pepsi system launch a carbonated soft drink (CSD) with a higher caffeine content . . . at a significant premium . . . ?"

- *The passion quotient*: "We believe this should be an increasing focus . . . building intense relationships with smaller audiences by tapping into their core belief systems . . . How about Aquafina Serene, targeted at the growing meditation/yoga movement?"

- *Create 3-D experiences*: "Brands must create multidimensional experiences — experience immersions that captivate consumers . . . Imagine being able to get a Burger King hamburger or McDonald's french fries from a vending machine."

- *Pursue well-being*: "The good news is that 'wellness' products are typically associated with higher net selling prices and . . . fatter margins . . . What if Coke and Pepsi created [soft drinks] that are rich in vitamins and other nutrients? . . . How about marketing to bored patients waiting endlessly in their doctors' offices? . . . Why not target pregnant women with products offering strong multivitamins, and target new mothers with drinks or foods that rebuild muscle tone and stimulate hair growth?"

- *Multicultural integrity*: "There is no question that successfully tapping into the Hispanic population will be paramount to growth for the companies we follow." Use music: "Music is a key component of the behavior and trend profiles of young, urban, transcultural people . . ." Consider: "How do they feel about religion?"

- *Provide comfort in an insecure world*: "Interestingly, fear-driven consumption is worth €1 billion [$1.8 billion] a year . . . Could we enter a time where the only water we can feel safe drinking is Dasani or Aquafina . . . ?"

- *Value in values*: "What if Constellation Brands developed sustainable black-run agricultural programs to grow grapes and make wine in South

Africa and marketed the brand as such? Does Chick-fil-A, a concept with a Christian religious heritage, have higher sales per restaurant because it does *not* open on Sunday?"

If these suggestions appear chillingly manipulative rather than health promoting, you know what you are up against when you walk into a supermarket. The UBS report demonstrates that Wall Street thinks it is just fine—no, essential—to exploit your concerns about health, your fears about the quality of drinking water, your cultural and religious values, your waiting time in doctors' offices, and even your children, if doing so will promote corporate growth. If ethical considerations exist anywhere in this picture, they too are well hidden.

As an individual, your recourse against such manipulation is to vote with your dollars every time you buy food. The better informed you are, the more wisely you can spend them. But it is not easy to oppose an entire food system on your own; it takes strength, courage, and firm determination. The current environment of food choice—driven by Wall Street as it is—has come about as the result of history, politics, and business concerns, not public interest.

> **A**s an individual, your recourse against such manipulation is to vote with your dollars every time you buy food.

But it does not have to be this way. Instead of encouraging you to eat more, the food environment could be changed in ways that make it easier for you to eat healthfully. If investment research like that conducted by UBS can ask "what if" questions like "Should gum manufacturers add caffeine to give extra energy for that fresh breath moment?" you can ask your own "what if" questions.

What if supermarkets

- stopped taking slotting fees and devoted prime real estate to healthier food products?
- gave a price break for smaller size packages?
- asked growers to provide smaller and tastier fruits and put packs of fruits and vegetables at cash registers?

What if food product companies

- stopped marketing directly to children?
- took spurious health claims off their packages?
- put millions of dollars into selling healthier products, instead of into campaigns designed to make you think their existing products are healthy?

What if fast-food companies

- posted calories on menu boards?
- charged less per weight or volume for the smallest sizes?
- sold salads at a lower price than hamburgers?

What if restaurants

- routinely offered healthier items on menus?
- gave a price break for smaller servings?
- trained waiters to be polite when customers order only appetizers?

What if government agencies

- ran a national education program about diet and health?
- issued unambiguous dietary advice?
- required food education in schools?

What if Congress

- did not accept corporate contributions to election campaigns?
- did not allow food companies to deduct marketing expenses from taxes?
- subsidized organic and sustainable food production?

What if Wall Street

- rewarded long-term corporate sustainability rather than short-term gain?

I am sure you can think of many other possibilities. Unrealistic as these ideas may appear, they suggest ways in which the food environment could be changed for the better. The current environment of food choice is not inevitable. Many of the ways in which it encourages eating more—ubiquitous advertising, food available everywhere, larger and larger portions, unchecked marketing to children, weak government regulation — have evolved in response to the demands of big business. Many of these "eat more" changes have occurred just since the early 1980s. They can be reversed. You cast your vote for

> Unrealistic as these ideas may appear, they suggest ways in which the food environment could be changed for the better. The current environment of food choice is not inevitable.

your choice of food environment every time you put something in your shopping cart or order off a menu. If enough people vote with you, changes will happen.

If, for example, the Organic Standards will continue to mean something in the United States (and I am convinced that they must), it will be because hundreds of thousands of people will demand that nothing be done to weaken them. That is how personal responsibility really works. If you think you as an individual cannot do enough to make a difference, join with others who believe as you do. Plenty of organizations are devoted to making food healthier and more friendly to the environment, and to making such food more widely available. They will welcome your membership and support.

What I have always appreciated about food — besides the nourishment and pleasure it gives — is its accessibility as a means of understanding the world in which we live. If you want to understand what human culture is about, you can investigate why rice, wheat, corn, or beans form the basis of one kind of diet but not another. If you want to see corporate greed in action, just look at food marketing. If you want to understand globalization, look at how coffee is grown and how its profits are distributed. If economic terms like "externalities" make your eyes glaze over, consider what it costs to keep drinking water free of agricultural pesticides. If environmental issues seem too abstract, think about how coal-burning power plants affect levels of methylmercury in the fish you eat. If what happens on Wall Street seems distant, consider how relentless pressures for quarterly growth drive additional outlets of McDonald's and Starbucks into your neighborhood. If you want to see how politics affects government actions, just take a look at farm subsidies, school lunches, or federal dietary advice.

You eat. Willingly or not you participate in the environment of food choice. The choices you make about food are as much about the kind of world you want to live in as they are about what to have for dinner. Food choices are about your future and that of your children. They are about nothing less than democracy in action. I truly believe that one person can make a difference and that food is a great place to begin to make that difference. Yes, you should use personal responsibility—informed personal responsibility—to make food choices you believe in. Exercise your First Amendment rights and speak out. And enjoy your dinner.

> You eat. Willingly or not you participate in the environment of food choice. The choices you make about food are as much about the kind of world you want to live in as they are about what to have for dinner.

Appendix 1
Food Measures: Conversion Factors

If you would like to be able to figure out what food labels mean and how much foods cost, you cannot avoid dealing with units of measurement. You not only must be able to convert ounces to pounds and fluid ounces to quarts and gallons, but also use the metric system. Nutrition Facts labels give the amounts of nutrients in grams, milligrams (1,000 to a gram), and micrograms (1,000,000 to a gram), and bottled waters often come in liters or milliliters (1,000 to a liter).

After decades of using both systems, I am quite comfortable using one or the other, but I still have to think hard to remember how to do the conversions from the metric to American systems and vice versa, and you also might find them difficult. My compromise is to use rounded-off ballpark equivalents that are easier to remember. They are not precise but are close enough to use for most purposes. Here are the ones I use most often.

Food Measurement Conversions

MEASURE	BALLPARK EQUIVALENTS	PRECISE EQUIVALENTS
Weights		
1 gram	⅕ teaspoon	
1 teaspoon	5 grams	
1 tablespoon	15 grams	
1 ounce	30 grams	Dry: 28.35 grams
		Liquid: 29.6 grams
100 grams	3½ ounces	Dry: 3.53 ounces
		Liquid: 3.38 ounces
1 kilogram	2 pounds	2.21 pounds
(1000 grams)		
1 pound	500 grams or ½ kilogram	454 grams
Volumes		
1 liter	1 quart (32 ounces)	1.06 quarts (33.8 ounces)
1 gallon	4 quarts or liters	3.79 liters
Temperature		
Boiling point	212° Fahrenheit	
	100° Celsius (Centigrade)	
Freezing point	32° Fahrenheit	
	0° Celsius (Centigrade)	
Food energy		
Carbohydrate	4 calories per gram	
Protein	4 calories per gram	
Fat	9 calories per gram	
Alcohol	7 calories per gram	
1 calorie (kilocalorie)*	4 kilojoules (kJ)	4.18 kilojoules (kJ)
1 kilojoule (kJ)	¼ calorie	0.24 calorie
Body fat	3,500 calories per pound	

*A calorie, as used in food labels, is actually a kilocalorie (see Chapter 24).

Appendix 2
Terms Used to Describe Fats
and Oils in Foods

TERM	TRANSLATION	HEALTH EFFECT
Fat (scientific term: lipid)	The generic term for fats (solid) and oils (liquid) in foods. All fats are triglycerides; all are mixtures of saturated, unsaturated, and polyunsaturated fatty acids.	Some fat is needed in the diet. All fats contain about 9 calories per gram or 120 per tablespoon.
Triglyceride	The structure of fats in foods and in the body: think of it as a letter "E" with three fatty acids attached to a glycerol (sugar alcohol) backbone.	
Diglyceride	A food additive emulsifying agent made by removing one fatty acid from a triglyceride.	Under investigation as a potential weight-loss agent (caution: it still has calories).

TERM	TRANSLATION	HEALTH EFFECT
Monoglyceride	A food additive emulsifying agent made by removing two fatty acids from a triglyceride.	
Fatty acids	The building blocks of fat. These are described in two ways: by degree of saturation (saturated, unsaturated, polyunsaturated), and by the position of the first point of unsaturation (see "Omega position" below).	Two—linoleic acid and alpha-linolenic acid—are required in the diet.
Saturated fatty acids	Fully hydrogenated, either naturally or artificially; solid at room temperature; stable.	Raise the risk of heart disease.
Unsaturated fatty acids	Not fully hydrogenated; liquid at room temperature; unstable; can be monounsaturated or polyunsaturated.	Neutral or beneficial for lowering heart disease risk.
Monounsaturated fatty acids	Have only one point at which they are not hydrogenated.	Good for cardiovascular health.
Polyunsaturated fatty acids	Have two or more points at which they are not hydrogenated; highly fluid and unstable.	Reduce blood cholesterol levels when substituted for saturated fatty acids, but too much of them may increase disease risk.
Hydrogenation	Artificial addition of hydrogen to make unsaturated fatty acids more saturated and stable; destroys beneficial unsaturated fatty acids and forms *trans*-fatty acids.	Increase the risk of heart disease.
Trans-fatty acids	Abnormal fatty acids created by hydrogenation.	Increase the risk of heart disease.

TERM	TRANSLATION	HEALTH EFFECT
Omega position	Refers to position on fatty acids where the first point of unsaturation (missing hydrogens) occurs. This can be at the omega-3, omega-6, or omega-9 position.	
Omega-3 fatty acids	Polyunsaturated fatty acids in leafy vegetables; also in fish, chicken, and eggs, which have higher amounts.	Alpha-linolenic acid (1/4 teaspoon or so per day) is essential in the diet and good for cardiovascular health.
Omega-6 fatty acids	The most prevalent fatty acids in seed oils.	Linoleic acid is essential in the diet (a teaspoon or so per day) and good for cardiovascular health.
Omega-9 fatty acids	The most prevalent fatty acid in olive oil and nut oils.	Good for cardiovascular health and perhaps other conditions.
Conjugated linoleic acids (CLAs)	Found in grass-fed beef.	Health benefits uncertain.

Notes

Web addresses were active when this book went to press in January 2007. To ease access to URLs, these notes are posted at www.whattoeatbook.com and www.foodpolitics.com.

INTRODUCTION

3   **I wrote about the health consequences** . . . The University of California Press published the books (2002 and 2003) and issued them in paperbound editions (2003 and 2004). For the reactions to them, pro and con, see www.foodpolitics.com.

4   **As the social theorist** . . . Mr. Schwartz's thesis: when you have too many choices, "freedom of choice becomes a tyranny of choice." The book was published by HarperCollins in 2004; the quotation is from page 2.

7   **This conflict begins** . . . U.S. Department of Health and Human Services and U.S. Department of Agriculture, *Dietary Guidelines for Americans*, 2005, 6th edition (Washington, D.C.: U.S. Government Printing Office, January 2005), available at www.healthierus.gov/dietaryguidelines. The pyramid, issued in April 2005, is at www.mypyramid.gov.

10   **Listen to this 1959 advice** . . . This came in a cookbook aimed at heart disease prevention by Ancel and Margaret Keys, *Eat Well and Stay Well* (Doubleday, 1959).

10   **Nutrition arguments are** . . . David R. Jacobs Jr. and Lyn M. Steffen discuss the reasons why reductive approaches to nutrition are insufficient in "Nutrients, Foods, and Dietary Patterns as Exposures in Research: A Framework for Food Synergy," *American Journal of Clinical Nutrition* 78 (Supplement 2003): 508S–13S. The health benefits of foods are greater than the benefits of their single components.

11   **It costs more . . .** I first ran across this pessimistic view in Louise B. Russell's *Is Prevention Better Than Cure?* (Brookings Institution, 1986). Kristin Leutwyler discusses the difficulties of calculating costs and benefits in "The Price of Prevention," *Scientific American* (April 1995). Public health researchers argue that prevention does pay because treatment of high-risk individuals is expensive, the value of prevention increases over time, and ethical and quality-of-life benefits are worthwhile societal goals. See, for example, Salim Yusuf and Sonia Anand, "Cost of Prevention: The Case of Lipid Lowering," *Circulation* 93 (1996): 1774–76; Li Yan Wang et al., "Economic Analysis of a School-Based Obesity Prevention Program," *Obesity Research* 11 (2003): 1313–24; and American Academy of Pediatrics, "Policy Statement: Prevention of Pediatric Overweight and Obesity," *Pediatrics* 112 (2003): 424–30.

11   **The deep dark secret . . .** The 3,900 calorie figure comes from the USDA at www.ers.usda.gov/data/foodconsumption. Comparative international data are available from the Food and Agricultural Organization of the United Nations at www.fao.org (look for Statistical Databases/FAOSTAT-Nutrition/Food Balance Sheets or go to faostat.fao.org/site/554/default.aspx.).

12   **Consider what the research says . . .** Research on the environment of food choice is reviewed in popular books: Kelly D. Brownell and Katherine Battle Horgen, *Food Fight* (McGraw Hill, 2003); Barbara Rolls, *The Volumetrics Eating Plan* (HarperCollins, 2005); and Lisa Young, *The Portion Teller* (Morgan Road, 2005). On the effects of food costs, see Adam Drewnowski and Anne Barratt-Fornell, "Do Healthier Diets Cost More?" *Nutrition Today* 39 (July/August 2004): 161–68.

13   **It is not enough for Kraft . . .** Figures on marketing budgets of the 100 leading national advertisers appear regularly in *Advertising Age*. This one is from June 27, 2005.

13   **Marketing methods are meant . . .** I am indebted to David Walsh, president of the National Institute on Media and the Family (www.mediafamily.org), for this phrase, which I use with his permission.

1. THE SUPERMARKET: PRIME REAL ESTATE

18   **Half a century ago, Vance Packard . . .** On page 3 of his book, Packard explains why he called it *The Hidden Persuaders* (David McKay Company, 1957). Marketing efforts, he says, "typically . . . take place beneath our level of awareness; so that the appeals which move us are often, in a sense, 'hidden.'" The "Babes" chapter is pages 105–22, and the quotation from that chapter is from page 111. For a more recent version, see Paco Underhill, *Why We Buy: The Science of Shopping* (Touchstone, 1999).

18   **More recent research on consumer behavior . . .** See, for example, Barbara E. Kahn and Leigh McAlister, *Grocery Revolution: The New Focus on the Consumer* (Addison-Wesley, 1997); Judith and Marcel Corstjens, *Store Wars: The Battle for Mindspace and Shelfspace* (Wiley, 1995); and Phil Lempert, *Being the Shopper: Understanding the Buyer's Choice* (John Wiley & Sons, 2002). These books tell retailers how to use research on consumer shopping behavior to sell more food.

18   **As basic marketing textbooks explain . . .** See Gene A. German and Theodore W. Leed, *Food Merchandising: Principles and Practice*, 1ST edition (Lebhar-

Friedman Books, 1992). The book is dated, but the principles it describes still hold. The quotations are from page 260.

19   **Place the highest-selling food departments** . . . Meat, produce, dairy, and frozen foods generated about 14 percent, 10 percent, 9 percent, and 7 percent of supermarket sales, respectively, in 2001, according to the USDA. See "Supermarket Sales by Category, 2001," at www.ers.usda.gov/data/foodmarketindicators. This site also provides data on other aspects of supermarket sales cited in this chapter.

21   **Slotting fees emerged in the 1980s** . . . The early history of slotting fees is reviewed in Lois Therrien, "Want Shelf Space at the Supermarket? Ante Up," *Business Week* (August 7, 1989): 60–61. The hearings are discussed by Ira Teinowitz, "Senators Berate Industry Abuse of Slotting Fees," *Advertising Age* (September 20, 1999): 3; and by Pierce Hollingworth, "Slotting Fees Under Fire," *Food Technology* (November 2000): 30.

21   **In the last decade, mergers and acquisitions** . . . A special insert in the April 18, 2005, issue of *Fortune* ranks the top 1,000 companies by industry and gives sales figures. Such figures are also readily available on the Web site of the trade publication *Supermarket News* at www.supermarketnews.com.

2. FRUITS AND VEGETABLES: THE PRICE OF FRESH

25   **I had read a Harvard** . . . The case reviewed Wegmans' attempt to provide in-store counseling and health monitoring for diabetes. Although the program proved popular with shoppers, it foundered on "short-term business issues" and was abandoned. See "Wegmans Food Markets: Diabetes Counseling," Harvard Business School Case Study N9-599-057, November 6, 1998. Current information about Wegmans stores and their philosophy and community partnerships is at www.wegmans.com. In 2004, a new mission statement said: "Our primary business is to help make great meals easy so our customers can live healthier and better lives." *Fortune* (January 24, 2005) ranks Wegmans first among the "100 best companies to work for."

28   **To allow them to endure** . . . William H. Friedland, "The New Globalization: The Case of Fresh Produce," in Alessandro Bonanno et al., editors, *Columbus to ConAgra: The Globalization of Agriculture and Food* (University Press of Kansas, 1994). The FDA definition of "fresh" is at www.cfsan.fda.gov.

28   **Bagged vegetables and salads** . . . Aaron L. Brody, "What's Fresh About Fresh-Cut," *Food Technology* (January 2005): 74–77.

28   **Food ecologists, who look closely** . . . For information about the "food mile" movement, see the Web site of the London-based organization Sustain: The Alliance for Better Food and Farming at www.sustainweb.org. Brian Halweil extols the virtues of locally grown foods in *Eat Here: Homegrown Pleasures in a Global Supermarket* (W. W. Norton, 2004).

29   **In 2002, Congress passed a law** . . . The origins of COOL in the United States are described in General Accounting Office, "Country-of-Origin Labeling: Opportunities for USDA and Industry to Implement Challenging Aspects of the New Law," GAO-03-780, August 2003, at www.gao.gov. COOL legislation is followed closely by *Food Chemical News*; the quotations are from the issues of August 18 (page 27), and September 15 (page 31), 2003, respectively. Anti-COOL lobbying is described in vivid detail in Public Citizen, *Tabled Labels*, September 2005 at www.citizen.org/documents/COOL.pdf.

33   The California Driscoll raspberries . . . See David Karp, "For Raspberries,
      Ubiquity (at a Price)," *The New York Times*, July 7, 2004; and "Strawberries and
      Dreams," *The New York Times*, April 13, 2005. Driscoll controls about half of
      U.S. raspberry production and breeds for durability and appearance. For an elo-
      quent account of a farmer's dilemma in having to choose between commerce
      and taste, see David M. Matsumoto, *Epitaph for a Peach: Four Seasons on My
      Family Farm* (HarperCollins, 1995).

3. ORGANICS: HYPE OR HOPE

37   This was corporate America . . . I would have known better if I had bothered
      to check the Organic Trade Association's Web site, www.ota.com. Its list of
      member companies is so long that it has to be searched alphabetically (the A's
      alone list more than eighty members).

37   How big a business is . . . The Organic Trade Association estimates of the size
      of organics are usually higher than those of USDA economists. See Carolyn
      Dimitri and Catherine Greene, "Recent Growth Patterns in the U.S. Organic
      Foods Market," September 2002, at www.ers.usda.gov.

38   The emergence of this new . . . See Michael Pollan's original and insightful
      look at "The Organic-Industrial Complex: How Organic Became a Marketing
      Niche and a Multibillion-Dollar Industry," *The New York Times Magazine*,
      May 13, 2001, and Samuel Fromartz, *Organic, Inc.* (Harcourt, 2006).

38   You can pick out . . . Tables of PLU codes and the foods they stand for are
      given at www.plucodes.com. In 2005, the site required you to identify your job
      in the produce business and gave no other option; I had to tell a white lie to use
      it. Example: regular papayas are #4394, and organic ones begin with 9, as in #9-
      3111.

39   Looking for a wider selection . . . The chain provides information for con-
      sumers and investors at www.wholefoods.com.

43   Whether they can remain . . . The Maine court decision in *Harvey v. Johanns*
      is at www.mindfully.org/Food/2005/Harvey-Johanns-Organic9jun05.htm. About the
      rider, see Stephen Clapp, "Organic Industry Rider Leaves Bitter Aftertaste,"
      Food Chemical News (October 31, 2005): 24–26. The Organic Consumers Asso-
      ciation's SOS (Safeguard Our Standards) campaign is at www.organicconsumers
      .org/sos.cfm.

44   One is Dennis Avery . . . Avery directs the Hudson Institute's Center for Global
      Food Issues (see www.hudson.org). The advocacy group, SourceWatch, provides
      information about the institute's funding sources at www.sourcewatch.org. Avery
      summarizes his reasons for disliking organics in "The Fallacy of the Organic
      Utopia," in Julian Morris and Roger Bate, editors, *Fearing Food: Risk, Health,
      and Environment* (Butterworth-Heinemann, 1999): 3–18.

45   In 1981, a review . . . See William Lockeretz, Georgia Shearer, and Daniel H.
      Kohl, "Organic Farming in the Corn Belt," *Science* (February 6, 1981): 540–47.
      At the time, this study seemed revolutionary. For more recent studies confirm-
      ing the productivity of organic farming practices, see D. K. Letourneau and B.
      Goldstein, "Pest Damage and Arthropod Community Structure in Organic vs.
      Conventional Tomato Production in California," *Journal of Applied Ecology* 38
      (2001): 557–70; John P. Reganold et al., "Sustainability of Three Apple Produc-

tion Systems," *Nature* (April 19, 2001): 427–46; and Paul Mäder et al., "Soil Fertility and Biodiversity in Organic Farming," *Science* (May 31, 2002): 1694–97. An editorial accompanying the *Science* paper calls it "encouraging news for organic fans" and considers the findings conclusive (page 1589).

45　**Plenty of research confirms . . .** See, for example, B. P. Baker et al., "Pesticide Residues in Conventional, Integrated Pest Management (IPM)–Grown and Organic Foods: Insights from Three US Data Sets," *Food Additives and Contaminants* 19 (2002): 427–46; and Cynthia L. Curl et al., "Organophosphorus Pesticide Exposure of Urban and Suburban Preschool Children with Organic and Conventional Diets," *Environmental Health Perspectives* (March 2003), at ehp.niehs.nih.gov/members/2003/5754/5754.html. See also Pat Michalak, *Water, Agriculture, and You* (The Rodale Institute, February 2004).

45　**Pesticides are demonstrably harmful . . .** See D. Pimentel, T. W. Culliney, and T. Bashore, "Public Health Risks Associated with Pesticides and Natural Toxins in Foods," University of Minnesota National IPM Network, July 30, 1996, at ipmworld.umn.edu/chapters/Pimentel.htm; National Research Council, *Pesticides in the Diets of Infants and Children* (National Academy Press, 1993); and Environmental Working Group reports on pesticides in children at www.ewg.org.

4. PRODUCE: SAFE AT ANY PRICE

46　**Health officials say . . .** These endlessly repeated figures from the Centers for Disease Control and Prevention derive from estimates made by Paul S. Mead et al., "Food-Related Illness and Death in the United States," *Emerging Infectious Diseases* 5 (1999): 607–25.

47　**Because the government . . .** Caroline Smith DeWaal et al., *Outbreak Alert! Closing the Gaps in Our Federal Food-Safety Net* (Washington, D.C.: Center for Science in the Public Interest, November 2005) at www.cspinet.org.

48　**In 1998, the FDA . . .** These are in "Guidance for Industry: Guide to Minimize Microbial Food Safety Hazards for Fresh Fruits and Vegetables" (October 26, 1998). Microbial tests of imported and domestic produce from 1999 to 2003 are summarized in "FDA Survey of Domestic Fresh Produce" (June 2003), and "FDA Survey of Imported Fresh Produce," January 30, 2001. All are at www.cfsan.fda.gov.

49　**In October 2005 . . .** "FDA Issues Nationwide Alert on Dole Pre-Packaged Salads" (October 2, 2005) at www.fda.gov.

49　**Processers know this . . .** See Aaron L. Brody, "What's Fresh About Fresh-Cut," *Food Technology* (January 2005): 74–77.

50　**One type of wax is carnauba . . .** For the produce industry's position on waxes, see www.pma.com. Toxicity testing is described at www.inchem.org.

51　**Critics say they do . . .** Dennis Avery's criticisms of organic production are taken on by Brian Halweil of Worldwatch in "Cultivating the Truth About Organics," *San Francisco Chronicle*, August 21, 2000.

51　**In the first study . . .** This is Avik Mukherjee et al., "Preharvest Evaluation of Coliforms, *Escherichia coli*, *Salmonella*, and *Escherichia coli* O157:H7 in Organic and Conventional Produce Grown by Minnesota Farmers," *Journal of Food Protection* 67, no. 5 (2004): 894–900.

53 **The Organic Trade Association . . .** This group sponsors the not-for-profit Center for Organic Education and Promotion (to which it would like donations to be sent). See www.ota.com.

53 **Consider what you have to do . . .** For a basic review of the complications of such studies, see Sharon B. Hornick, "Factors Affecting the Nutritional Quality of Crops," *American Journal of Alternative Agriculture* 7, nos. 1 and 2 (1992): 63–68. Because most studies do not control for such factors, "it is almost impossible to make valid and meaningful comparisons."

53 **Nevertheless, a few intrepid . . .** See, for example, Bob L. Smith, "Organic Foods vs. Supermarket Foods: Element Levels," *Journal of Applied Nutrition* 45 (1993): 35–39; Marina Carbonaro et al., "Modulation of Antioxidant Compounds in Organic vs. Conventional Fruit (Peach, *Prunus persica L.* and Pear, *Pyrus communis L.*)," *Journal of Agricultural and Food Chemistry* 50 (2002): 5458–62; and Danny Asami et al., "Comparison of the Total Phenolic and Ascorbic Acid Content of Freeze-dried and Air-dried Marionberry, Strawberry, and Corn Grown Using Conventional, Organic, and Sustainable Agricultural Practices," *Journal of Agricultural and Food Chemistry* 51 (2003): 1237–41.

54 **It's the mix . . .** One explanation for the protective effects of phytochemicals is that they stimulate enzymes that detoxify carcinogens. The body has many enzymes that act on toxic chemicals. "Phase 1" enzymes can either deactivate carcinogens or activate them, and "phase 2" enzymes are more likely to deactivate them, but both kinds can do either, depending on circumstances. This makes it unlikely that any *single* phytochemical or nutrient can account for the protective effect of fruits and vegetables against cancer and other diseases. See M. Paolini and M. Nestle, "Pitfalls of Enzyme-Based Molecular Anticancer Dietary Manipulations: Food for Thought." *Mutation Research* 543 (2003): 181–89.

55 **In this matter, I defer . . .** Joan Dye Gussow, "Is Organic Food More Nutritious: And Is That the Right Question?" *Organic Farming Research Foundation Information Bulletin*, Fall 1996.

5. GENETICALLY MODIFIED, IRRADIATED, AND POLITICIZED

57 **The FDA explains . . .** FDA policies, procedures, and consultations on food biotechnology are at www.cfsan.fda.gov.

58 **Roughly 10 percent . . .** Sujatha Sankula, "A 2006 Update of Impacts on US Agriculture of Biotechnology-Derived Crops Planted in 2005," National Center for Food and Agriculture Policy at www.ncfap.org/whatwedo/biotech2006.php.

59 **In September 2004 . . .** This was reported by Stephen Clapp, "Anti-Biotech Groups Charge Contamination of Hawaiian Papaya," *Food Chemical News* (September 20, 2004): 6.

61 **Hawaii Pride discloses . . .** The company explains the technique and its reasons for using it, and answers FAQs on its Web site, www.hawaiipride.com.

62 **The USDA's pyramid food guide . . .** This can be found at www.my pyramid.gov.

63 **Unbelievable as it may seem . . .** Mary K. Serdula et al., "Trends in Fruit and Vegetable Consumption Among Adults in the United States: Behavioral Risk Factor Surveillance System, 1994–2000," *American Journal of Public Health* 94 (June 2004): 1014–18.

63 **Or perhaps like many people** . . . Potato chips are an expensive way to eat potatoes. Potatoes were less than $1 a pound in July 2004, but the cheapest chips I could find at my local convenience store were $1.19 for 5.5 ounces, which comes to $3.46 per pound. See Table in Chapter 30.

63 **Because surveys and other studies** . . . See, for example, Adam Drewnowski and Nicole Darmon, "Food Choices and Diet Costs: An Economic Analysis," *Journal of Nutrition* 135 (2005): 900–904; and Karen M. Jetter and Diana L. Cassady, "The Availability and Cost of Healthier Food Items," AIC Issues Brief No. 29, University of California Agricultural Issues Center, March 2005. The counter-intuitive study is Jane Reed, Elizabeth Frazão, and Rachel Itskowitz, "How Much Do Americans Pay for Fruits and Vegetables?" USDA Economic Research Service, Bulletin No. 790, July 2004, at www.ers.usda.gov/publications/aib790.

6. MILK AND MORE MILK

68 **Dairy foods are supposed** . . . The quotation comes from Judy Putnam and Jane Allshouse, "Trends in U.S. Per Capita Consumption of Dairy Products 1909 to 2001," *Amber Waves* (2003): available at www.ers.usda.gov/AmberWaves. For a review of the benefits of dairy foods from an industry perspective, see Lori Hoolihan, "Beyond Calcium: The Protective Attributes of Dairy Products and Their Constituents," *Nutrition Today* 39, no. 2 (March/April, 2004). Hoolihan works for the California Dairy Council.

68 **How dairy foods are produced** . . . Data on dairy trends come from the previous citation as well as from a USDA briefing paper dated July 6, 2004, at www.ers.usda.gov/briefing/dairy/background.htm.

69 **More than most foods** . . . The severest critic is surely Robert Cohen. See his *Milk: The Deadly Poison* (Argus Publishing, 1998). Cohen runs the anti-dairy Web site: www.notmilk.com.

70 **Most Americans eat dairy foods** . . . Figures on dairy production and sales come from the USDA's annual compendium of agricultural statistics, available at www.usda.gov/nass/pubs/agstats.htm.

71 **The USDA requires** . . . The industry side of the checkoff is managed by Dairy Management, Inc., an alliance formed by the National Dairy Council, the American Dairy Association, and the U.S. Dairy Export Council, and explained at www.dairycheckoff.com. Educational campaigns of the Milk Processor Education Program are given at www.whymilk.com. In 1998, during the administration of Bill Clinton, his secretary of Health and Human Services, Donna Shalala, appeared in a milk mustache advertisement. Apparently, calcium no longer works as a selling point for milk. In 2005, the California Milk Processor Board (the one responsible for the "Got Milk" campaign) stopped mentioning calcium in its advertising. See Suzanne Vranica, "Milk Campaign Drops Calcium Pitch," *The Wall Street Journal*, October 12, 2005.

72 **An investigative report** . . . Nicholas Zamiska, "How Milk Got a Major Boost from Food Panel," *The Wall Street Journal*, August 30, 2004.

72 **The issues are legion** . . . Potassium is the latest issue. The committee developing the 2005 *Dietary Guidelines* said everyone should eat three daily servings of dairy products because that much is needed to meet the Dietary Reference Intake (DRI) for potassium, as explained in Institute of Medicine (IOM), *Di-*

etary Reference Intakes for Water, Potassium, Sodium, Chloride, and Sulfate (National Academies Press, 2005). The IOM set the DRI for potassium at a level twice as high as the 1989 standard to compensate for the blood pressure–raising effects of eating too much salt (sodium chloride). Dairy foods contribute 18 percent of the potassium in U.S. diets, but 33 percent of the sodium. Other sources of potassium are meat, poultry, and fish (17 percent), vegetables other than potatoes (14 percent); potatoes (11 percent); fruits (11 percent); beans (10 percent); and grains (9 percent). Given this distribution, and the amount of sodium in dairy foods, it is curious that the committee singled out dairy foods to be eaten in larger amounts. See S. Gerrior, L. Bente, and H. Hiza, "Nutrient Content of the U.S. Food Supply, 1909–2000," USDA Home Economics Research Report No. 56, November 2004.

73   **To prevent osteoporosis . . .** Institute of Medicine, *Dietary Reference Intakes for Calcium, Phosphorus, Magnesium, Vitamin D, and Fluoride* (National Academies Press, 1997).

73   **The need for eating that much . . .** High calcium levels also do not make sense to Roland L. Weinsier and Carlos L. Krumdieck, "Dairy Foods and Bone Health: Examination of the Evidence," *American Journal of Clinical Nutrition* 72 (2000): 681–89. For another view, see Janet C. King, "The Milk Debate," *Archives of Internal Medicine* 165 (2005): 975–76.

74   **In response to this extraordinarily confusing . . .** B. E. Christopher Nordin, "Calcium Requirement Is a Sliding Scale," *American Journal of Clinical Nutrition* 71 (June 2000): 1381–83. His article begins: "It must be a source of some surprise to rational scientists that the human requirement for calcium, an apparently inoffensive nutrient that contributes so much to our physical stability, arouses strong emotions in many breasts."

74   **Dairy foods provide 15 percent . . .** This percentage includes butter. See S. Gerrior, L. Bente, and H. Hiza, "Nutrient Content of the U.S. Food Supply, 1909–2000," USDA Home Economics Research Report No. 56, November 2004. Production figures come from the USDA at www.ers.usda.gov/AmberWaves, and www.ers.usda.gov/briefing/dairy/background.htm.

75   **Commercial milk does not come straight . . .** The University of Guelph explains milk processing with diagrams and a flowchart at www.foodsci.uoguelph.ca/dairyedu/fluid.html.

77   **The study placed thirty-two . . .** Michael B. Zemel et al., "Calcium and Dairy Acceleration of Weight and Fat Loss During Energy Restriction in Obese Adults," *Obesity Research* 12 (April 2004): 582–90; and "Dairy Augmentation of Total and Central Fat Loss in Obese Subjects," *International Journal of Obesity* 29 (2005): 391–97. Information about the patent arrangement was posted on the International Dairy Food Association Web site, www.idfa.org, May 1, 2004. The Dairy Council lists favorable studies under "Science Supporting the Dairy-Weight Management Connection" at www.nationaldairycouncil.org. Zemel's financial arrangements with dairy groups are discussed in Stephanie Thompson, "Dairy Scientist Decides to Milk His Research for All It's Worth," *Advertising Age* (June 20, 2005), and in David Schardt, "Milking the Data," *Nutrition Action Healthletter*, September, 2005.

77   **Thus the role of dairy trade . . .** The Dairy Council's full-page, full-color weight-loss advertisement appeared in *The New York Times* on January 23, 2004. An earlier ad on December 3, 2003, said: "One approach [to losing weight] is getting at

least 3 servings a day of milk, cheese or yogurt instead of some of your current choices." For a news analysis of the weight-loss campaign, see Melanie Warner, "Chug Milk, Shed Pounds? Not So Fast," *The New York Times*, June 21, 2005.

78 **In June 2005, the Physicians . . .** Physicians Committee for Responsible Medicine, "Doctors Group Files Suit Against Kraft, General Mills, Dannon, and Dairy Trade Groups for False Dairy Weight-Loss Claims" (press release), June 28, 2005, at www.pcrm.org.

78 **In the meantime, the research . . .** Heart disease studies are reviewed by P. C. Elwood et al., "Milk Drinking, Ischaemic Heart Disease and Ischaemic Stroke. I. Evidence from the Caerphilly Cohort. II. Evidence from Cohort Studies," *European Journal of Clinical Nutrition* 58 (2004): 711–17 and 718–24.

79 **The cancer studies . . .** The large review is from the World Cancer Research Fund and American Institute for Cancer Research (AICR), *Food, Nutrition, and the Prevention of Cancer: A Global Perspective* (1997). The AICR statement comes from a press release issued February 26, 2002. The breast cancer statement is from Patricia G. Moorman and Paul D. Terry, "Consumption of Dairy Products and the Risk of Breast Cancer: A Review of the Literature," *American Journal of Clinical Nutrition* 80 (2004): 5–14. See also C. Rodriguez et al., "Calcium, Dairy Products, and the Risk of Prostate Cancer in a Prospective Cohort of United States Men," *Cancer Epidemiology Biomarkers and Prevention* 12 (July 2003): 597–603.

7. MILK: SUBJECT TO DEBATE

80 **Your heart yearns . . .** For current advertising, see www.lactaid.com.

82 **If you are extremely sensitive . . .** S. B. Matthews and A. K. Campbell, "When Sugar Is Not So Sweet," *Lancet* 355 (April 15, 2000). For a review of Dairy Council–sponsored studies, see Lois D. McBean and Gregory D. Miller, "Allaying Fears and Fallacies About Lactose Intolerance," *Journal of the American Dietetic Association* 98 (1998): 671–76. See also Fabrizis L. Suarez et al., "Lactose Maldigestion Is Not an Impediment to the Intake of 1500 mg Calcium Daily as Dairy Products," *American Journal of Clinical Nutrition* 68 (1998): 1118–22. The authors conclude that "extensive publicity concerning the ill effects of lactose has resulted in a widespread belief that lactose malabsorption induces severe problems . . . a major educational campaign will be required to reverse this misperception."

82 **Nevertheless, the lactose . . .** Patricia Bertron, Neal D. Barnard, and Milton Mills, "Racial Bias in Federal Nutrition Policy. Part I: The Public Health Implications of Variations in Lactase Persistence. Part II: Weak Guidelines Take a Disproportionate Toll," *Journal of the National Medical Association* 91, no. 3 (1999): 151–57 and 201–8. Lactose intolerance, these authors say, is normal. The Web site of the Physicians Committee for Responsible Medicine is www.pcrm. org. *The Dietary Guidelines* are at www.healthierus.gov/dietaryguidelines, and the pyramid is at www.mypyramid.gov.

82 **My files contain . . .** Marc T. Goodman et al., "Association of Dairy Products, Lactose, and Calcium with the Risk of Ovarian Cancer," *American Journal of Epidemiology* 156, no. 2 (2002): 148–57.

84 **Careful examination of . . .** Hermann E. Wasmuth and Hubert Kolb, "Cow's Milk and Immune-Mediated Diabetes," *Proceedings of the Nutrition Society* 59

(2000): 573–79; and Deryck R. Persaud and Alma Barranco-Mendoza, "Bovine Serum Albumin and Insulin-Dependent Diabetes Mellitus: Is Cow's Milk Still a Possible Toxicological Causative Agent of Diabetes?" *Food and Chemical Toxicology* 42, no. 5 (2004): 707–14.

85 **In part because of such . . .** Peter J. Huth, Donald K. Layman, and Peter H. Brown, guest editors, "The Emerging Role of Dairy Proteins and Bioactive Peptides in Nutrition and Health," *Journal of Nutrition* 134, no. 4 (Supplement 2004): 961S–1002S. The "S" in the page numbers indicates that this is a paid, sponsored supplement. The quotations are from the editors' introduction on page 961S.

85 **Milk cartons . . .** Beta-lactam antibiotics are penicillins and cephalosporins. Farmland is owned by Parmalat. See www.parmalat.com.

86 **A decade later, U.S. dairy farmers . . .** Andrew Pollack, "Maker Warns of Scarcity of Hormone for Dairy Cows," *The New York Times*, January 27, 2004. Monsanto cut production by half at its Austrian rbST facility after an FDA inspection revealed problems with quality control.

88 **The IGF-1 issue . . .** See Andrew G. Renehan et al., "Insulin-like Growth Factor (IGF)-1, IGF Binding Protein-3, and Cancer Risk: Systematic Review and Meta-Regression Analysis," *Lancet* 363 (April 24, 2004): 1346–53. This paper reviews a large number of previous studies of IGF-1 and health risks.

88 **The lingering doubts . . .** The Web site of Horizon Organic is www.horizon organic.com.

89 **These particular critics . . .** The Hudson Institute is at www.hudson.org. Details of its funding by foundations such as Koch, Olin, and Scaife, and various agriculture and food corporations (McDonald's among them), are listed by the Center for Media and Democracy at www.sourcewatch.org.

89 **Looked at another way . . .** Data on growth of the organic dairy business come from Catherine Greene and Amy Kremen, "U.S. Organic Farming in 2000–2001: Adoption of Certified Systems," USDA Agricultural Information Bulletin 780 (February 2003); and Organic Trade Association, "The OTA 2004 Manufacturer Survey," June 2004, at www.ota.com.

8. DAIRY FOODS: THE RAW AND THE COOKED

92 **Calories and Fat in . . .** Figures in the Table are rounded to the nearest half-gram from USDA data on food composition at www.nal.usda.gov/fnic/food comp/search.

94 **The New York City Health . . .** The reasons for the short sell-by date in New York City turn out to be as much about politics as health. The safety (cold chain) explanation is obviously true, but I have heard others: local milk companies want to make it more difficult for companies in New Jersey and Connecticut to sell milk in NYC; unions for NYC milk delivery drivers want deliveries to be more frequent; milk producers don't want to have to worry about keeping milk unspoiled for as long.

95 **I am not opposed . . .** The Web site of the Northeast Organic Farming Association Massachusetts chapter deals with the raw milk issue more responsibly than most. See www.nofamass.org. For the FDA position on raw milk, see Linda Bren, "Got Milk? Make Sure It's Pasteurized," *FDA Consumer* (September/October 2004) at www.fda.gov/fdac/features/2004/504_milk.html.

95   **By some accounts . . .** Paul A. Cotton et al., "Dietary Sources of Nutrients Among U.S. Adults, 1994 to 1996," *Journal of the American Dietetic Association* 104 (2004): 921–30. The data are based on a USDA analysis of one-day diet records obtained from 10,000 adults.

96   **If you are a dairy producer . . .** These figures come from the University of Vermont at www.dasc.vt.edu/links.html. A quart of milk weighs 2 pounds. For information about basic cheese making, see the Web site of David Fankhauser, a professor at the University of Cincinnati, at biology.clc.uc.edu/Fankhauser/ Cheese/Cheese.html.

97   **Outbreaks of illness . . .** Caroline Smith DeWaal et al., *Outbreak Alert! Closing the Gaps in Our Federal Food-Safety Net* (Washington, D.C.: Center for Science in the Public Interest, November 2005) at www.cspinet.org/food safety/index.html.

9. YOGURT: HEALTH FOOD OR DESSERT

101   **It is because of the health mystique . . .** Donna Berry, "2004 Cultured Dairy Foods: A World of Opportunity," *Dairy Foods Magazine* (April 16, 2004), available at www.dairyfoods.com. See also "Taste Test Organic Yogurt," *Organic Style* (September 2004): 58.

101   **In 1973, Alexander Leaf . . .** See Alexander Leaf, "Every Day Is a Gift When You Are Over 100," *National Geographic* (January 1973): 93–118. The commercial is described by Sharon R. King in an obituary for a man who worked for Dannon from 1942 to 1981, eventually becoming its president: "Juan Metzger, 79, Is Dead; He Put the Fruit in Yogurt," *The New York Times*, September 10, 1998. Leaf later reduced his age estimates in an editorial in *Journal of the American Geriatrics Society* 30 (August 1982): 485–87. As for whether Bulgarians actually ate yogurt, see Michael Specter, "Yogurt? Caucasus Centenarians 'Never Eat It,'" *The New York Times*, March 16, 1998. On the other hand, Daniel Carasso, the son of the founder of Danone, was close to 100 years old when PepsiCo decided not to buy Groupe Danone. "Yogurt, it has been said, helps prolong life," said Thomas Fuller: "PepsiCo Says It Won't Try to Buy French Company," *The New York Times*, July 26, 2005.

102   **The text following the asterisks . . .** The criteria are available on the Web site of the National Yogurt Association, www.aboutyogurt.com.

103   **Fortunately, *Consumer Reports* . . .** "Probiotics: Are Enough in Your Diet?" *Consumer Reports* (July 2005): 34–35.

104   **If you give foods . . .** See Cornelius W. Van Neil et al., "*Lactobacillus* Therapy for Acute Infectious Diarrhea in Children: A Meta-Analysis," *Pediatrics* 109, no. 4 (2002): 678–84. A meta-analysis combines the results of many studies.

104   **In 2004, a group . . .** Oskar Adolfsson, Simin Nikbin Meydani, and Robert M. Russell, "Yogurt and Gut Function," *American Journal of Clinical Nutrition* 80 (August 2004): 245–56. The authors say that the National Yogurt Association requested this "critical and objective review" for which they were paid an unspecified honorarium.

104   **Yogurt has been . . .** See Malinda Miller, "Dairy Products Industry Profile," Agricultural Marketing Resource Center, Iowa State University, November 2006, at www.agmrc.org/agmrc/commodity/livestock/dairy/dairyproductsprofile .htm. Current figures on production are available from the USDA at usda.

mannlib.cornell.edu/reports/nassr/dairy/pdp-bban/daryan04.txt. The Web sites of commercial yogurt companies provide nutritional information. For information about yogurt brands, see www.dannon.com, www.yoplait.com, and www. stonyfield.com.

105   **An entire science . . .** Jürgen Schrezenmeir, Michael de Vrese, and Knut Heller, editors, "International Symposium on Probiotics and Prebiotics," *American Journal of Clinical Nutrition* 73 (Supplement 2, 2001): 361S–498S. Sponsors included the International Dairy Federation, Danone, Nestlé, Nordmilch, Yakult, and several other international companies selling dairy foods. For a review of the immunity-boosting potential of probiotics and prebiotics—and their marketing potential—see Linda Milo Ohr, "Nutraceuticals and Functional Foods," *Food Technology* (January 2005): 65–70: "The immunity market is entering exciting times. It is still a young area with potential for growth."

105   **The trade journal . . .** Pierce Hollingsworth, "Culture Wars," *Food Technology* 55 (March 2001): 43–49.

105   **This marketing opportunity . . .** See Stephanie Thompson, "Yoplait's Revenge Is Portable Yogurt That Kids Slurp Up," *Advertising Age* (September 11, 2000): 28 and 30.

106   **Stonyfield may be organic . . .** Groupe Danone bought 40 percent of Stonyfield in 2001. The "partnership" was so successful that it picked up another 45 percent in 2003. Stonyfield's president and employees own the remaining 15 percent. Its Web site, www.stonyfield.com, states that Groupe Danone stays out of the company's day-to-day business operations.

106   **Many of these products . . .** One good reason to mention fermented dairy foods is to have an excuse to recommend Bill Mollison, *The Permaculture Book of Ferment and Human Nutrition* (Ten Speed Press, 1997). The chapter on fermented dairy foods is particularly enlightening, especially if you have a burning desire to know what natural rennet is, or how to make ghee (Indian clarified butter), lassi (flavored yogurt drink), haloumi (Greek fried cheese), or karish (Egyptian soft cheese).

10. MARGARINE: ACCEPT NO SUBSTITUTES

111   **The fats in soybeans . . .** Figures on the composition of margarines and ingredients come either from product labels or from the USDA Nutrient Data Laboratory at www.nal.usda.gov/fnic/foodcomp/search. "Saturation" refers to the proportion of hydrogen to carbon in fatty acids. Every available carbon bond in saturated fatty acids is completely filled—saturated—with hydrogen. Unsaturated fats have one unfilled bond. Polyunsaturated fats have two or more unfilled bonds.

112   **My *trans*-fat file . . .** The early study is from Leo H. Thomas, "Mortality from Arteriosclerotic Disease and Consumption of Hydrogenated Oils and Fats," *British Journal of Preventive and Social Medicine* 29 (1975): 82–90. For later work, see Alberto Ascherio et al., "*Trans* Fatty Acids and Coronary Heart Disease," *New England Journal of Medicine* 340, no. 25 (1999): 1994–98. It is interesting to note that American Heart Association scientists called for labeling the types of fat in margarines in 1961 (Appendix II to "Dietary Fat and Its Relation to Heart Attacks and Strokes," *Circulation* 23 (January 1961): 131–36.

113   **Blame it on France . . .** This history is recounted by S. F. Riepma, then president of the National Association of Margarine Manufacturers, in *The Story of Margarine* (Public Affairs Press, 1970). That trade association still flourishes and provides a history of margarine (under the heading, "Fun Facts & Figures," on its Web site, www.margarine.org). The name derives from one of the original fatty acids used to make margarine, margaric acid, named after *margarite* (Greek: pearl) because of its pearl-like luster.

114   **Americans readily accepted . . .** A tablespoon of U.S. margarine now contains 10 percent of the Daily Value for vitamin A with its 80 to 100 calories.

115   **For more than forty years . . .** An early review is by Helen B. Brown and Irvine H. Page, "Lowering Blood Lipid Levels by Changing Food Patterns," *Journal of the American Medical Association* 168, no. 15 (December 13, 1958). The 1959 book by Ancel and Margaret Keys is *Eat Well and Stay Well* (Doubleday). From 1961 on, American Heart Association policy statements have appeared regularly in its professional journal, *Circulation*, and are distributed as pamphlets. Advice to limit *trans* fats appears in Ronald M. Krauss et al., "AHA Dietary Guidelines," *Circulation* 102 (2000): 2284–99.

115   **The most obvious is palm fruit oil . . .** See Ellie Brown and Michael F. Jacobson, *Cruel Oil: How Palm Oil Harms Health, Rainforest, and Wildlife* (Washington, D.C.: Center for Science in the Public Interest, 2005).

116   **You would never know . . .** C. S. Koh and Celina Lim, *Nutritional Benefits of Palm Oil*, Malaysian Palm Oil Promotion Council, 2004. The Council's Web site is at www.mpopc.org.my.

116   **To that end, the United . . .** Margo A. Denke, Beverley Adams-Huet, and Anh T. Nguyen, "Individual Cholesterol Variation in Response to a Margarine- or Butter-Based Diet: A Study in Families," *Journal of the American Medical Association* 284 (2000): 2740–47. The advertisement appeared in *The New York Times*, December 8, 2000.

11. MARGARINE: YOU *CAN* BELIEVE IT'S NOT BUTTER

119   **Margarine is an odd . . .** If there are benefits, they are quite small. See Nina S. Sørensen et al., "Effect of Fish-Oil-Enriched Margarine on Plasma Lipids, Low-Density-Lipoprotein Particle Composition, Size, and Susceptibility to Oxidation," *American Journal of Clinical Nutrition* 68 (1998): 235–41.

119   **The 100 percent vegan margarines . . .** See www.earthbalance.net/product. html.

120   **These last include . . .** Datem stands for diacetyltartaric acid esters of monoglyceride.

120   **The answer: another miracle . . .** Two articles in *Food Technology* 58 (2004) explain current options for reducing *trans* fat and the many other methods under investigation: G. R. List, "Decreasing *Trans* and Saturated Fatty Acid Content in Food Oils" (January): 23–31, and Donald E. Pszczola, "Fats: In *Trans*-ition" (April): 52–63.

121   **One Sunday morning . . .** This flier was inserted in the Sunday *New York Times*, March 28, 2004.

122   **Industry-sponsored research . . .** For a review, see R. A. Moreau, B. D. Whitaker, and K. B. Hicks, "Phytosterols, Phytostanols, and Their Conjugates

in Foods: Structural Diversity, Quantitative Analysis, and Health-Promoting Uses," *Progress in Lipid Research* 41, no. 6 (2002): 457–500.

124   **Dietary intake of trans** . . . David B. Allison et al., "Estimated Intakes of *Trans* Fats and Other Fatty Acids in the US Population," *Journal of the American Dietetic Association* 99 (1999): 166–74. Figures for saturated-fat intake, which are self-reported, come from "Trends in Intake of Energy and Macronutrients, 1971–2000," *Morbidity and Mortality Weekly Report* (February 6, 2004): 80–82.

125   **This may not sound** . . . Nestlé lists nutrition information for these products at www.coffee-mate.com.

12. SOY MILK: PANACEA, OR JUST ANOTHER FOOD

127   **If you do not like** . . . Vegetarians differ, having in common only that they do not eat red meat (beef, pork, lamb). Partial vegetarians eat everything else, and lacto-ovo vegetarians eat dairy foods and eggs but no fish or poultry. These diets tend to be more healthful than conventional diets. Vegans eat no foods from animal sources at all and are especially interested in soy products as sources of protein. Their diets require special sources of vitamin B_{12} (which is mainly derived from animal-based foods) but are otherwise nutritionally adequate when calories are adequate. See Patricia K. Johnston and Joan Sabaté, "Nutritional Implications of Vegetarian Diets," in Maurice E. Shils et al., *Modern Nutrition in Health and Disease*, 10th ed. (Lippincott Williams and Wilkins, 2006), 1638–54.

127   **Enthusiasts for soy foods** . . . The "shining star" phrase turns up frequently on Internet sites devoted to soy foods. See, for example, www.soyatech.com and www.unitedsoybean.org.

128   **And soybeans contain** . . . Siyan Zhan and Suzanne C. Ho, "Meta-Analysis of the Effects of Soy Protein Containing Isoflavones on the Lipid Profile," *American Journal of Clinical Nutrition* 81 (2005): 397–408. This concludes that soy proteins with isoflavones reduce total cholesterol and LDL (the bad) cholesterol, but increase HDL (the good) cholesterol—under some, but not all, circumstances.

128   **Soy is so heavily promoted** . . . For the history of soy foods, see Thomas Sorosiak, "Soybeans," in Kenneth F. Kiple and Kriemhild Coneè Ornelas, editors, *The Cambridge World History of Food*, vol. 1 (New York: Cambridge University Press, 2000), 422–27. Market competition is discussed by Jennifer L. Rich, in "U.S. Farmers Look Back . . . and See Soy Growers in Brazil Shadowing Them," *The New York Times*, July 10, 2001.

129   **In 2003, American farmers** . . . These figures come from www.soystats.com, a site run by Syngenta (a soybean producer) under the auspices of the American Soybean Association. The site reports production figures in million metric tons (MMT). One metric ton is about 2,200 pounds; 1 MMT is 2.2 billion pounds. In 2003, the United States produced 66 MMT of soybeans. Of the 40 MMT for domestic use, 32 were processed into meal (28 of which went to livestock feed) and 8 were processed into oil.

129   **The federal government helps** . . . Information about the Soybean Promotion and Research Program ("Checkoff") is on the USDA's Web site at www.ams.usda.gov/lsg/mpb/rp-soy.htm.

130   **Much such research . . .** The National Soybean Research Laboratory Web site is www.nsrl.uiuc.edu, and many pages are devoted to soy research and education.

131   **Food technology research . . .** The quoted advertisements (and the later one) appeared in a "Soy Takes Center Stage" supplement to *Stagnito's New Products Magazine* (December 2002). Butter Buds is owned by Cumberland Packing, which also makes substitutes for salt (Nu-Salt) and sugar (Sweet'N Low). Nutriant is owned by The Kerry Group (Kerry America).

132   **As a result, HRT . . .** Judith Wylie-Rosett, "Menopause, micronutrients, and Hormone Therapy," *American Journal of Clinical Nutrition* 81, no. 5 Supplement (2005): 1223S–31S. See also Louise A. Brinton et al., "Hormones and Endometrial Cancer—New Data from the Million Women Study," *Lancet* 365 (2005): 1543–51.

133   **Soy companies and trade associations . . .** See Mark Messina, John Erdman Jr., and Kenneth D. R. Setchell, editors, "Fifth International Symposium on the Role of Soy in Preventing and Treating Chronic Disease," *American Journal of Clinical Nutrition* 79, no. 5 Supplement (2004): 1205S–93S. The industry-sponsored supplement includes a few papers and dozens of abstracts of presentations and posters from a sponsored symposium in September 2003. Cautionary comments by the editors and others appear on pages 1229S–33S. The quotation is from an abstract on page 1254S.

134   **In 2004, I saw . . .** The ad appeared in *The Telegraph Magazine*, April 17, 2004.

135   **Skeptics urged caution . . .** Articles about soy in *Nutrition Action Healthletter* are: Bonnie Leibman, "The Soy Story" (September 1998) and David Schardt, "Got Soy? A Good Food . . . But No Miracle Worker" (November 2002). Alice H. Lichtenstein's editorial "Got Soy?" in the *American Journal of Clinical Nutrition* 73 (2001): 667–68, critically reviews research on soy and health since 1999. More recent research appears in the symposium volume cited in the note "Soy companies and trade associations . . ." above.

136   **Indeed, the research . . .** See Mark Messina, "Soy Isoflavone Intake and the Risk of Breast and Endometrial Cancers," *The Soy Connection* (Spring 2005). This newsletter, sponsored by the United Soybean Board, was bound into the April 2005 issue of the *Journal of the American Dietetic Association*.

137   **You now can buy thousands . . .** Donald E. Pszczola, "From Soup to Soynuts: The Broadening Uses of Soy," *Food Technology* 59 (February 2005): 44–55.

13. A RANGE OF MEATY ISSUES

138   **We do not lack . . .** These figures come from USDA "Agricultural Statistics 2005," at www.usda.gov/nass/pubs/agstats.htm. Other figures in this chapter about meat consolidation, consumption, and nutrient values also come from USDA sources: James M. MacDonald et al., "Consolidation in U.S. Meatpacking," Agricultural Economic Report No. 785, February 2000, at www.ers. usda.gov/publications/Aer785; Michael Ollinger et al., "Structural Change in the Meat, Poultry, Dairy, and Grain Processing Industries," Economic Research Report No. 3, March 2005, at www.ers.usda.gov; Judith Jones Putnam and Jane E. Allshouse, "Food Consumption, Prices, and Expenditures, 1970–97," USDA Statistical Bulletin No. 965, April 1999; S. Gerrior and L. Bente, "Nutrient Content of the U.S. Food Supply, 1909–99: A Summary Re-

port," USDA Home Economics Research Report No. 55, June 2002; and Paul A. Cotton et al., "Dietary Sources of Nutrients Among US Adults, 1994 to 1996," *Journal of the American Dietetic Association* 104 (2004): 921–30.

139 **According to figures . . .** It is sometimes imprecise to talk about cows. It helps to remember that bulls are males, steers are castrated males, cows are females, and cattle usually refers collectively to steers and cows.

139 **I saw these emotions . . .** Information about this remarkable conference is at www.yale.edu/agrarianstudies/chicken.

140 **We eat meat, they say . . .** See, for example, T. Colin Campbell and Thomas M. Campbell II, *The China Study* (Benbella Books, 2005): "Plato . . . made it perfectly clear: we shall eat animals only at our own peril" (page 345).

141 **The education campaigns of . . .** The Beef Checkoff is at www.beefboard.org; the Pork Checkoff is at www.otherwhitemeat.com; and the National Pork Producers Council is at www.nppc.org.

141 **Despite the reach . . .** The checkoff ruling is discussed in Linda Greenhouse, "In Free-Speech Ruling, Justices Say All Ranchers Must Help Pay for Federal Ads," *The New York Times*, May 24, 2005. Her article quoted the dissenting opinion written by Justice David Souter, who observed that checkoff ads are designed by beef-producer groups: "If government relies on the government-speech doctrine to compel specific groups to fund speech with targeted taxes, it must make itself politically accountable by indicating that the content actually is a government message, not just the statement of one self-interested group the government is currently willing to invest with power."

142 **In 2004, the company paid . . .** See Nat Ives, "Tyson Is Counting on Protein to Bulk Up Its Image in a Campaign to Push Its Chicken, Beef, and Pork," *The New York Times*, August 4, 2004.

143 **On surveys of daily dietary . . .** See Centers for Disease Control and Prevention, "Trends in Intake of Energy and Macronutrients—United States, 1971–2000," *Mortality and Morbidity Weekly Report* 53, no. 4 (February 2004): 80–82.

145 **The USDA makes . . .** See Carole Sugarman, "Labeling Meat and Poultry," *The Washington Post*, April 3, 1991; USDA, "Nutrition Labeling of Meat and Poultry Products," FSIS Backgrounder, January 1993; and "Truth in Burgers" (editorial), *The New York Times*, June 4, 1994. USDA labeling rules are at www.fsis.usda.gov.

146 **In 2005, the advocacy group . . .** The Public Citizen report, "Tabled Labels" (September 2005) is at www.citizen.org/documents/COOL.pdf. See Stephen Clapp, "House-Senate Conference Approves COOL Delay, Organic Rider," and "Industry Case Influences COOL Debate: Public Citizen," *Food Chemical News* (October 31, 2005): 1, 24–25 and (September 19, 2005): 1, 28, respectively.

146 **Instead, the National Livestock . . .** The quotation appeared on the Web site of this meat trade association (www.nlpa.org) in fall 2004, but has since disappeared. The position of the meat industry on COOL is given in a September 2004 backgrounder by the American Meat Institute (AMI) at www.meatami.com: "If consumers want a country-of-origin label and are willing to pay the additional costs associated with such a program, the meat industry will meet that demand, as it meets consumer demands for a wide variety of products." Since then the AMI has lobbied for further delays.

147 **Meat is not the only . . .** Benjamin Caballero and Barry M. Popkin, *The Nutri-*

tion Transition: Diet and Disease in the Developing World (Academic Press, 2002).

147 **Scientists began to link . . .** World Cancer Research Fund and the American Institute for Cancer Research, "Food, Nutrition, and the Prevention of Cancer: A Global Perspective," 1997. The American Cancer Society guidelines are at www.cancer.org.

148 **Cardiologists, alarmed . . .** Irvine H. Page et al., "Atherosclerosis and the Fat Content of the Diet," *Circulation* 16 (1957): 163–78. See also Central Committee for Medical and Community Program of the American Heart Association, "Dietary Fat and its Relation to Heart Attacks and Strokes," *Circulation* 23 (January 1961): 133–36.

149 **In 2004, the committee . . .** You can view the advisory committee's report and see how the USDA and Department of Health and Human Services changed it to create the 2005 *Dietary Guidelines* at www.health.gov/dietaryguidelines.

14. MEAT: QUESTIONS OF SAFETY

151 **Since 1990, CSPI . . .** See Caroline Smith DeWaal et al., *Outbreak Alert! Closing the Gaps in Our Food-Safety Net* (Washington, D.C.: Center for Science in the Public Interest, November 2005) available at www.cspinet.org. The USDA posts press releases about recalls of meat and poultry by year at www.fsis.usda.gov/Fsis_Recalls/index.asp.

156 **The Coleman Natural . . .** Its Web site is www.colemannatural.com. HACCP rules require the USDA to test for *Salmonella* on an unannounced basis, and companies to test for the generic form of *E. coli* (a marker of fecal contamination) in 1 out of every 300 beef carcasses, 1,000 hogs, 3,000 turkeys, and 22,000 chickens. See USDA, "Pathogen Reduction: HACCP Systems: Proposed Rule," *Federal Register* 61 (July 25, 1996): 38806–989.

156 **In the frozen food . . .** The company discusses its irradiation practices at www.HuiskenMeats.com.

157 **They say that if . . .** The Centers for Disease Control and Prevention's position on food irradiation is posted at www.cdc.gov/ncidod/dbmd/diseaseinfo/food irradiation.htm.

158 **In January 2004 . . .** See Mike Freeman, "Accounting Dispute Led to Demise of SureBeam," *The San Diego Union-Tribune*, January 14, 2004, at www.mindfully. org/Food/2004/Surebeam-Accounting-Dispute14jan04.htm. A story on April 6, 2004, provided further details. More recent articles about SureBeam are at www. signonsandiego.com. The Texas A&M electronic beam facility is explained at tamu.edu/ebeam/facility.htm.

159 **If you were to eat meat . . .** I discussed the science and politics of mad cow disease in much greater detail in the last chapter of my book *Safe Food: Bacteria, Biotechnology, and Bioterrorism* (University of California Press, 2004).

159 **How they arise and spread . . .** The latest idea—quite unconfirmed—is human-to-cow-to-human transmission. The thought is that BSE emerged in cows that had eaten bone meal imported to England from India; the meal might have contained the remains of humans who died of vCJD. See Alan C. F. Colchester and Nancy T. H. Colchester, "The Origin of Bovine Spongiform Encephalopathy: The Human Prion Disease Hypothesis," *Lancet* 366 (2005): 856–61.

161　**Its weirdest decision . . .** See Donald G. McNeil Jr., "U.S. Won't Let Company Test All Its Cattle for Mad Cow" and "Barred from Testing for Mad Cow, Niche Meatpacker Loses Clients," *The New York Times*, April 10 and 18, 2004, and a later editorial, "More Mad Cow Mischief," on May 8, 2004. The legal wrangling over importation of Canadian beef into the United States, complicated by disagreements among the leading meat trade associations, is tracked by *Food Chemical News*. See, for example, "AMI [American Meat Institute] Denied Injunction in Border Dispute; NMA [National Meat Association] Files Appeals" (March 14, 2005). The suit against the USDA was filed by a third group, R-CALF (see next note). See also Alexei Barrionuevo, "Congress Is Staying Clear of Dispute Over Mad Cow," *The New York Times*, May 10, 2005.

161　**It also backed off . . .** The group is R-CALF (Ranchers-Cattlemen Action Legal Fund, United Stockgrowers of America), which supports, among other measures, mandatory country-of-origin labeling for beef cattle. See www.r-calfusa.com.

162　**In June 2005 . . .** Donald G. McNeil Jr. and Alexei Barrionuevo, "For Months, Agriculture Department Delayed Announcing Results of Mad Cow Test," *The New York Times*, June 26, 2005.

163　**Soon after the delay . . .** This distasteful incident is reviewed in Stephen Labaton, "Agencies Postpone Issuing New Rules as Election Nears," *The New York Times*, September 27, 2004. Also see Jane Zhang, "FDA Proposes Wider Feed Ban to Bolster Mad-Cow Defenses," *The Wall Street Journal*, October 5, 2005; and Zachary Richardson, "BSE Feed Rule: Groups Criticize 'Gaping Holes' in FDA's New Changes," *Food Chemical News* (October 10, 2005).

164　**Early in 2005 . . .** Government Accountability Office, "Mad Cow Disease: FDA's Management of the Feed Ban Has Improved, but Oversight Weaknesses Continue to Limit Program Effectiveness," GAO-05-101, February 2005, at www.gao.gov.

15. MEAT: ORGANIC VERSUS "NATURAL"

165　**Such statements describe . . .** For a look at commercial chicken production from an anthropologist's perspective, see Steve Striffler, *Chicken: The Dangerous Transformation of America's Favorite Food* (Yale University Press, 2005).

167　**A brochure in the store . . .** See www.wholefoodsmarket.com/products/meat-poultry/index.html.

171　**And—the most critical difference . . .** The complete state listings of organic certifying agencies accredited by the National Organic Program are at www.ams.usda.gov/nop. Iowa, for example, has three accredited certifiers: the Iowa Department of Agriculture Organic Program in Des Moines; Organic Certifiers, Inc. in Keosauqua; and the Maharishi Vedic Organic Agriculture Institute in Fairfield.

171　**Organic meats may . . .** Organic Trade Association, "The OTA 2004 Manufacturer Survey," June 2004, at www.ota.com.

172　**A Quick Comparison . . .** The USDA's National Organic Program is run by the Agricultural Marketing Service (AMS); see www.ams.usda.gov/nop. The Food Safety and Inspection Service (FSIS) governs rules for meat and poultry grading, storage, and safety; see www.fsis.usda.gov/Fact_Sheets/index.asp.

173 **The Niman Ranch** ... See www.nimanranch.com. For the B3R and Coleman Companies, see www.b3r.com. Petaluma Holdings, the owner of Petaluma Poultry Processors, bought both B3R and Coleman in 2002. BC Natural Foods bought Petaluma Holdings in 2003. For an overview of mergers and acquisitions in the organic industry, see George Draffin, "The Incorporation of the Organic Food Industry," November 2006, at www.endgame.org/organics.html.

173 **These methods sound promising** ... The Web site for humane certification is www.certifiedhumane.com.

175 **Congress eventually undid** ... The Organic Trade Association sponsored full-page advertisements "on behalf of its 1,200 member companies who sell $11 billion annually in organic products to the more than 50 million American families who consume them." The ads showed a Certified Organic seal saying: "USDA not really organic: only YOU can stop this from happening," *The New York Times*, March 7, 2003. See also *Food Chemical News*, May 17 and 31, 2004; and Marian Burros, "Last Word on Organic Standards Again," *The New York Times*, May 26, 2004.

175 **Large producers of eggs successfully** ... The certifying agency opposing the USDA in this matter is Massachusetts Independent Certification, Inc. (MICI). See Philip Brasher, "Agribusiness Wants Intensive Confinement of Poultry Under Organic Label," *Des Moines Register*, October 3, 2002; Consumers Union, "Organic Chicken: Access to Outdoors," February 25, 2003, at http://eco-labels.org; and Farmers' Legal Action Group, Inc., "Organic Agriculture," at www.flaginc.org/topics/news/MICI/index.php. For more recent difficulties, see "National Organic Board Rebuffed on Pasture Rule," *Food Chemical News*, August 19, 2005.

177 **Researchers who have looked** ... Jo Robinson, a forceful advocate for raising animals on pasture, summarizes and references studies favoring the benefits of grass feeding, *Eat Wild: The Clearinghouse for Information about Pasture-Based Farming*, at www.eatwild.com.

177 **Cows are** *supposed* ... "Conjugation" refers to the arrangement of double bonds in fat molecules. Usually the double bonds in fatty acids are separated by at least one carbon attached to two hydrogens (a methylene group). Hydrogenation by rumen bacteria (mainly *Butyrivibrio fibrisolvens*, but also others) causes double bonds to form right next to each other (like this: C=C-C=C); these are called "conjugated" (for example, rumenic acid is CLA 18:2, *cis*-9, *trans*-11). For data on the increased amounts of CLAs in grass-fed beef, see P. French et al., "Fatty Acid Composition, Including Conjugated Linoleic Acid, of Intramuscular Fat from Steers Offered Grazed Grass, Grass Silage, or Concentrate-Based Diets," *Journal of Animal Science* 78 (2000): 2849–55. Effects in humans are reviewed in Martha A. Belury, "Dietary Conjugated Linoleic Acid in Health: Physiological Effects and Mechanisms of Action," *Annual Review of Nutrition* 22 (2002): 505–31; Aubie Angel, editor, "The Role of Conjugated Linoleic Acid in Human Health," *American Journal of Clinical Nutrition* 79, no. 6 Supplement (June 2004): 1131S–220S; and Lisa Rainer and Cynthia J. Heiss, "Conjugated Linoleic Acid: Health Implications and Effects on Body Composition," *Journal of the American Dietetic Association* 104 (2004): 963–68.

180 **If you cannot find** ... Try Dakota Beef at www.dakotabeefcompany.com, Wholesome Harvest at www.wholesomeharvest.com, Diamond Organics at www.diamondorganics.com, and FreshDirect at www.freshdirect.com.

183 **The most troubling . . .** This dilemma is the subject of an Institute of Medicine report in 2006, "Nutrition Relationships in Seafood: Selections to Balance Benefits and Risks," at www.iom.edu.

183 **Their fats are largely . . .** The "healthy" omega-3 fatty acids are EPA (eicosapentaenoic acid) and DHA (docosahexaenoic acid). Omega-3 refers to the position of the first double bond from the methyl end of the fatty-acid carbon chain; it links the #3 and #4 carbons in all fatty acids in the omega-3 series. EPA and DHA are long and highly polyunsaturated: EPA has 20 carbons (eicosa) and 5 (penta) double bonds (enoic), and DHA has 22 carbons (docosa) and 6 (hexa) double bonds (enoic). The omega-3 fatty acid in plants is alpha-linolenic acid, which has 18 carbons and 3 double bonds; the body converts it to EPA and DHA, but slowly. The abbreviation EPA has two meanings in this book. When used with DHA, it means omega-3s. When used singly, it usually stands for the Environmental Protection Agency.

183 **Because these omega-3s show . . .** See Joyce C. McCann and Bruce N. Ames, "Is Docosahexaenoic Acid, an n-3 Long-Chain Polyunsaturated Fatty Acid, Required for Development of Normal Brain Function? An Overview of Evidence from Cognitive and Behavioral Tests in Humans and Animals," *American Journal of Clinical Nutrition* 82 (2005): 281–95. Research inconsistencies are discussed further in the chapter on infant formula and baby food (Chapter 36).

183 **In 2004, the scientific . . .** Department of Health and Human Services and U.S. Department of Agriculture, "Report of the Dietary Guidelines Advisory Committee," September 22, 2004, at www.health.gov/dietaryguidelines/dga2005/report. The agencies released the final version of the *Dietary Guidelines for Americans*, 2005, at www.healthierus.gov/dietaryguidelines, on January 12, 2005.

184 **The beneficial effects of omega-3 . . .** The earliest research is reviewed by J. Dyerberg et al., "Eicosapentaenoic Acid and Prevention of Thrombosis and Atherosclerosis?" *Lancet* 2 (1978): 117–19. The investigators concluded that "Enrichment of tissue lipids with E.P.A., whether by dietary change or by supplementation, may reduce the development of thrombosis and atherosclerosis in the Western World." In contrast, see Merritt H. Raitt et al., "Fish Oil Supplementation and Risk of Ventricular Tachycardia and Ventricular Fibrillation in Patients with Implantable Defibrillators," *Journal of the American Medical Association* 293 (2005): 2884–91; the study finds that fish oils may increase irregular heartbeats in such patients.

185 **In 2004, a private laboratory . . .** The company posted the omega-3 supplement test results on December 7, 2004, at www.consumerlab.com.

186 **More than a decade later . . .** The Agency for Healthcare Research and Quality (of the U.S. Department of Health and Human Services) issued a two-volume review of studies of omega-3 fatty acids and heart disease risk in March 2004: *Effects of Omega-3 Fatty Acids on Cardiovascular Risk Factors and Intermediate Markers of Cardiovascular Disease*, Evidence Report/Technology Assessment No. 93, and *Effects of Omega-3 Fatty Acids on Cardiovascular Disease*, No. 94.

186 **In 2000, as a result . . .** FDA News, "FDA Announces Qualified Health Claim for Omega-3 Fatty Acids," press release, September 8, 2004.

186   **Rosie Mestel . . .** "The Lure of Fish Oils," *Los Angeles Times*, October 4, 2004. See also Lisa Duchene, "Two Government Steps, One Big Opportunity," *SeaFood Business* 23 (October 2004): 42. The poster is by National Seafood Educators (www.seafoodeducators.com), 2004. The qualified advice about fish and heart disease comes from Penny M. Kris-Etherton et al., "Fish Consumption, Fish Oil, Omega-3 Fatty Acids, and Cardiovascular Disease," *Circulation* 106 (2002): 2747–57, with minor corrections added in vol. 107 (2003): 149–58.

188   **You may have seen . . .** The iconic image was taken by W. Eugene Smith in 1972 and published in a book of his photographs, now out of print. According to a discussion on www.amazon.com, the family has requested that this photograph no longer be reprinted, but it is readily viewed online (search: Minamata Images). For what happened at Minamata, see Hans Grimel, "Minimata [*sic*] Bay Mercury Victims Could Double," October 10, 2001, at www.mindfully.org/Pesticide/Minimata-Mercury-Victims.htm. This site contains an excellent reference list.

188   **In 1991, the Institute . . .** Farid E. Ahmed, editor, *Seafood Safety* (National Academy Press, 1991). The Institute of Medicine is part of the National Academies ("Advisors to the Nation on Science, Engineering, and Medicine") in Washington, D.C.

17. FISH: THE METHYLMERCURY DILEMMA

190   **This fish story . . .** See "Mercury in Fish: Cause for Concern?," *FDA Consumer* (September 1994; revised May 1995), available at www.fda.gov/fdac/reprints/mercury.html.

191   **The NRC produced . . .** National Research Council, *Toxicological Effects of Methylmercury* (National Academy Press, 2000). The quotations are from the discussion of public health implications on page 9. This book is an authoritative source of basic information about methylmercury as well as its health effects.

192   **In 2001, the FDA . . .** FDA Consumer Advisory, "An Important Message for Pregnant Women and Women of Childbearing Age Who May Become Pregnant About the Risks of Mercury in Fish," March 2001, at www.cfsan.fda.gov.

192   **This "public interest watchdog" . . .** The Environmental Working Group advises groups at risk *not to eat* tuna steaks, sea bass, oysters from the Gulf of Mexico, or any marlin, halibut, pike, walleye, white croaker, and largemouth bass (in addition to the EPA and FDA four: shark, swordfish, king mackerel, and tilefish); and to *eat no more than one meal per month combined* of canned tuna, mahimahi, blue mussel, Eastern oyster, cod, pollock, salmon from the Great Lakes, blue crab from the Gulf of Mexico, wild channel catfish, and lake whitefish. See www.ewg.org/issues/mercury/index.php.

193   **These documents revealed that the FDA . . .** Environmental Working Group, "Focus Pocus" and "Brain Food," 2001, and "New Government Fish Tests Raise Mercury Concerns," December 2003, at www.ewg.org; Marian Burros, "Mercury in Fish: What's Too Much?" and "Second Thoughts on Mercury in Fish," *The New York Times*, May 9, 2001 and March 13, 2002; and Dan Vergano, "FDA Fish Warning Is Called Lacking," *USA Today*, March 1, 2002.

194   **Following these revelations . . .** John J. Fialka, "FDA Prepares Warning on Tuna," *The Wall Street Journal*; and Elizabeth Weise, "FDA to Discuss Levels of Mercury in Fish," *USA Today*, both December 10, 2003.

194   The Food Advisory Committee . . . FDA and EPA Backgrounder, "What You Need to Know About Mercury in Fish and Shellfish," March 2004 at www. fda.gov/oc/opacom/hottopics/mercury/backgrounder.html. This site has links to charts of mercury levels in fish and shellfish and other such information.

195   The Tuna Foundation placed . . . The advertisement appeared in USA Today, March 13, 2004. The foundation's Web site is www.tunafacts.com.

196   If anything, this task . . . Melanie Warner, "With Sales Plummeting, Tuna Strikes Back," The New York Times, August 19, 2005.

196   In response to the 2004 advisory . . . The advertisement appeared in The New York Times, March 26, 2004. For accounts of the White House role in weakening EPA standards for mercury emissions, see articles in The New York Times during 2004: Paul Krugman, "The Mercury Scandal," April 6; Jennifer Lee, "White House Minimized the Risks of Mercury in Proposed Rules, Scientists Say," April 7; and National Desk, "New Mercury Rules Get Heavy Response," June 29.

198   In 2005, nine states . . . To follow this story through 2005, see articles in The New York Times: Felicity Barringer, "E.P.A. Accused of a Predetermined Finding on Mercury," February 4 and "Bush Plan to Permit Trading of Credits to Limit Mercury," March 14; Matthew L. Wald, "New Rules Set for Emission of Mercury," March 16; Anthony DePalma, "E.P.A. Sued over Mercury in the Air," March 30; and Michael Janofsky, "Some in Senate Seek to Change Mercury Rule," September 9. See also Bridget M. Kuehn, "Medical Groups Sue EPA over Mercury Rule," Journal of the American Medical Association 294 (2005): 415–16; and Zachary Richardson, "California, Tuna Industry Battle over Mercury Labels," Food Chemical News (November 14, 2005).

198   As for recreational . . . You can find your state's advisories mapped on the EPA Web site, www.epa.gov/waterscience/fish/states.htm. EPA advice for pregnant women is at www.epa.gov/waterscience/fishadvice/advice.html. A summary of the status of state advisories in slide format is at www.epa.gov/waterscience/presentations/fishslides/2003_files/frame.htm. The Montana advisories, for example, are unusually detailed and cover ocean as well as freshwater fish (state health officials must take this issue seriously and Montana does not have a seafood industry that might be likely to object).

200   Recent information suggests . . . Centers for Disease Control and Prevention, "Blood Mercury Levels in Young Children and Childbearing-Aged Women — United States, 1999–2002," Morbidity and Mortality Weekly Report 53 (November 5, 2004): 1018–20; Susan E. Schober et al., "Blood Mercury Levels in US Children and Women of Childbearing Age, 1999–2000," Journal of the American Medical Association 289 (2003): 1667–74; and Gary Myers et al., "Prenatal Methylmercury Exposure from Ocean Fish Consumption in the Seychelles Child Development Study," Lancet 361 (May 2003): 1686–92 (see also the editorial by Constantine G. Lyketsos pages 1667–68, and letters in vol. 362 on August 23, 2003).

201   Methylmercury does not seem . . . Megan Weil et al., "Blood Mercury Levels and Neurobehavioral Function," Journal of the American Medical Association 293 (2005): 1875–82. The conclusion of this study can be interpreted in different ways, depending on whether you are an optimist or pessimist: "Overall, the data do not provide strong evidence that blood mercury levels are associated with worse neurobehavioral performance in this population of older, urban adults."

See also National Resources Defense Council, "Healthy Milk, Healthy Baby: Chemical Pollution and Mothers' Milk," March 25, 2005, at www.nrdc.org/ breastmilk; and Leonardo Trasande, Philip J. Landrigan, and Clyde Schechter, "Public Health and Economic Consequences of Methylmercury Toxicity to the Developing Brain," *Environmental Health Perspectives* 113 (2005): 590–96.

18. THE FISH-FARMING DILEMMA

204 **Although the levels of PCBs . . .** PCBs and related compounds (chlordane, dieldrin, etc.) are called halogenated hydrocarbons because they contain halogens—chlorine or bromine, usually—attached at one place or another to rings of carbon and hydrogen. Dieldrins, for example, contain six attached chlorines. The biphenyl in PCBs means there are two hydrocarbon rings. Hundreds of such compounds exist; many are toxic. See Institute of Medicine, *Dioxins and Dioxin-Like Compounds in the Food Supply: Strategies to Decrease Exposure* (National Academies Press, 2003). State advisories about fish caught in local waters are at www.epa.gov/waterscience/fish.

205 **Those sardines and . . .** The sardines may be coming back, slowly. The catch in 2005 was about 40,000 tons (compared to the hundreds of thousands of tons caught annually in the 1930s). See Christopher Hall, "Cannery Row II, Starring the Sardines," *The New York Times*, December 7, 2005.

206 **Oceans are large . . .** See Ransom A. Myers and Boris Worm, "Rapid Worldwide Depletion of Predatory Fish Communities," *Nature* 423 (May 15, 2003): 280–83; Daniel Pauly et al., "Fishing Down Marine Food Webs," *Science* 279 (February 6, 1998): 860–64; E. K. Pikitch et al., "Ecosystem-Based Fishery Management," *Science* 305 (July 16, 2004): 346–47; and Carl Safina et al., "U.S. Ocean Fish Recovery: Staying the Course," *Science* 309 (2005): 707–8. The National Oceanic and Atmospheric Administration oversees the Sustainable Fisheries Act of 1996, which promotes fish conservation. See "Implementing the Sustainable Fisheries Act: Achievements from 1996 to the Present," June 2003, at www.nmfs.noaa.gov. Activities of the U.S. Fish and Wildlife Service are at www.fws.gov.

207 **In 2002, the USDA . . .** Data on fish farming are most easily accessed at U.S. Joint Subcommittee on Agriculture, "Aquaculture: Economics and Statistics Report," at http://aquanic.org/jsa/statistics/index.htm. For worldwide figures, see Food and Agriculture Organization, "The State of World Fisheries and Aquaculture, 2004," at www.fao.org. See also USDA Economic Research Service, "Briefing Room: Aquaculture," at www.ers.usda.gov/briefing/aquaculture. In 2000, four companies controlled half the sales—Stolt, Marine Harvest, Pan Fish, and Heritage. Nutreco Holding's Marine Harvest merged with Stolt-Nielson in 2004, the latest step in a long history of mergers and acquisitions, as described at www.marineharvest.com. A metric ton is about 2,200 pounds (actually, 2,205).

207 **In contrast to wild fish . . .** Many books describe aquaculture—the care and feeding of fish—in detail, but they are expensive. See, for example, Malcolm C. M. Beveridge, *Cage Aquaculture*, 3RD edition (Fishing News Books, 1996), for $114.99; Jean Guillaume et al., *Nutrition and Feeding of Fish and Crustaceans* (Springer, 2001) for $132.25; Barry A. Costa-Pierce, editor, *Ecological Aquaculture* (Blackwell, 2002) for $139.99; and Tom Lovell, editor, *Nutrition*

and Feeding of Fish, 3RD edition (Kluwer Academic, 1998) for $224. *Salmon Aquaculture*, edited by Knut Heen, Robert L. Monahan, and Fred Utter (Fishing News Books, 1993), is a bargain at $55. Prices are from www.amazon.com, June 2005.

208 **Environmental advocacy groups point out . . .** Katrin Holmström et al., "Antibiotic Use in Shrimp Farming and Implications for Environmental Impacts and Human Health," *International Journal of Food Science and Technology* 38 (2003): 255–66. See also Public Citizen, "The Environmental and Social Impacts of Shrimp Aquaculture," November 2004, at www.citizen.org.

208 **If the fish escape . . .** Martin Krkošek, Mark A. Lewis, and John P. Volpe, "Transmission Dynamics of Parasitic Sea Lice from Farm to Wild Salmon," *Proceedings: Biological Sciences* 272 (2005): 689–96.

209 **In captivity on fish farms . . .** Recipes for fish pellets are given at www.zeigler feed.com.

210 **Also in theory, you could feed . . .** J. Gordon Bell et al., "Replacement of Dietary Fish Oil with Increasing Levels of Linseed Oil: Modification of Flesh Fatty Acid Compositions in Atlantic Salmon (*Salmo salar*) Using a Fish Oil Finishing Diet," *Lipids* 39 (2004): 223–32.

210 **In 2002, three research groups . . .** M.D.L. Easton, D. Luszniak, and E. Von der Geest, "Preliminary Examination of Contaminant Loadings in Farmed Salmon, Wild Salmon and Commercial Salmon Feed," *Chemosphere* 46 (2002): 1053–74; and Marian Burros, "Farmed Salmon Is Said to Contain High PCB Levels," *The New York Times*, July 30, 2003.

211 **The salmon-farmers' trade association . . .** The SOTA Web site is at www. salmonoftheamericas.com.

211 **In 2004, however . . .** Ronald A. Hites et al., "Global Assessment of Organic Contaminants in Farmed Salmon," *Science* 303 (January 9, 2004): 226–29. The editorial, by Erik Stokstad, is on pages 154–55, and letters by Hites and others follow in the July 23, 2004, issue (vol. 305, pages 475–78).

212 **Predictably, the Hites study . . .** Gina Kolata, "Farmed Salmon Have More Contaminants Than Wild Ones, Study Finds," *The New York Times*, January 9, 2004. The SOTA consultant's comments were quoted in the Stokstad editorial mentioned in the previous note.

212 **And SOTA needs to work . . .** Ronald A. Hites et al., "Global Assessment of Polybrominated Diphenyl Ethers [PBDEs] in Farmed and Wild Salmon," *Environmental Science and Technology* 38 (2004): 4945–49 (and see editorial on pages 360A–61A). For background, see Henrik Viberg, Anders Fredriksson, and Per Eriksson, "Neonatal Exposure to Polybrominated Diphenyl Ether (PBDE 153) Disrupts Spontaneous Behaviour, Impairs Learning and Memory, and Decreases Hippocampal Cholinergic Receptors in Adult Mice," *Toxicology and Applied Pharmacology* 192 (2003): 95–106. The SOTA quotation comes from Allissa Hosten, "Experts Clash over Validity of New Salmon Study," *Food Chemical News* (August 16, 2004).

213 **This new study confronted . . .** See Lisa Duchene, "PCBs Present Challenging PR Problem" and "Fisheries Under Fire," *SeaFood Business* (March 2004, and August 2004, respectively).

213 **In 2005, the same determined . . .** Jeffrey A. Foran et al., "Risk-Based Consumption Advice for Farmed Atlantic and Wild Pacific Salmon Contaminated with Dioxins and Dioxin-Like Compounds," *Environmental Health Perspec-*

tives 113 (May 2005): 552–56; and "Quantitative Analysis of the Benefits and Risks of Consuming Farmed and Wild Salmon," *Journal of Nutrition* 135 (November 2005): 2639–43.

214   **Pew is a philanthropic . . .** The foundation Web sites are www.pewtrusts.org and www.packard.org. For industry views, see *SeaFood Business*, December 2003.

216   **Even so, it will be difficult . . .** Chad Skelton, "Farmed B.C. Salmon More Tainted Than Wild," *The Vancouver Sun*, June 6, 2005.

217   **The Center for Science . . .** David Schardt, "Farmed Salmon Under Fire," *Nutrition Action Healthletter* (June 2004).

19. THE FISH-LABELING QUANDARIES

219   **About 75 percent . . .** The fish figure comes from Jane Allshouse et al., "Seafood Safety and Trade," USDA/ERS Agricultural Information Bulletin No. 789-7, February 2004, at www.ers.usda.gov/publications/aib789/aib789-7. The shrimp figure comes from Environmental Defense/Oceans Alive, "Choose U.S. Shrimp Over Imported Shrimp," 2005, at www.oceansalive.org. Agricultural statistics on seafood are at www.usda.gov/nass/pubs/agstats.htm, by year, in the "miscellaneous" category. Department of Commerce figures are under "fisheries" on the NOAA Web site, www.noaa.gov.

220   **Congress also told the USDA . . .** USDA, "Mandatory Country of Origin Labeling of Fish and Shellfish: Interim Rule," *Federal Register* 69, no. 192 (October 5, 2004): 59708–50. See also Stephen Clapp, "USDA Meets Deadline for Seafood COOL Rule," *Food Chemical News* (October 4, 2004).

222   **This, of course, immediately . . .** Marian Burros, "Stores Say Wild Salmon, But Tests Say Farm Bred," *The New York Times*, April 10, 2005.

224   **The most common use . . .** Evelyn Zamula, "Getting Hooked on Surimi," *FDA Consumer* (April 1985). Surimi marketing issues are routinely covered by *SeaFood Business* (see "Surimi Seafood" articles in November and December 2003, and October 2004). Subway puts the full list of seafood salad ingredients on its Web site, www.subway.com: "Alaskan Pollock, water, pacific whiting, snow crab meat, corn starch, wheat starch, potato starch, sugar, contains 2% or less of the following: sorbitol, salt, natural and artificial flavor, egg whites, carrageenan, spices, calcium carbonate, sodium tripolyphosphate, tetrasodium pyrophosphate, citric acid, color, hydrolyzed wheat, soy and corn protein, mirin wine (rice, water, koji enzyme, salt, alcohol), disodium inosinate and guanylate, extracts of crab, oyster and scallop, modified wheat starch. Subway regular mayonnaise . . ."

224   **Wild salmon are a gorgeous . . .** Stewart Anderson, "Salmon Color and the Consumer," presented at an International Institute of Fisheries Economics and Trade meeting in 2000, available at oregonstate.edu/Dept/IIFET/2000/papers/andersons.pdf. See also Marian Burros, "Issues of Purity and Pollution Leave Farmed Salmon Looking Less Rosy," *The New York Times*, May 28, 2003.

225   **FDA rules require disclosure . . .** Lawsuit information is at www.smithandlowney.com/salmon. The British Food Standards Agency describes issues related to canthaxanthins at www.food.gov.uk. The European Commission Health and Consumer Protection Directorate-General's report, "Opinion of the Scientific Committee on Animal Nutrition . . . ," April 17, 2002, is at

europa.eu.int/comm/food/fs/sc/scan/out81_en.pdf. See also Julia Moskin, "Tuna's Red Glare? It Could Be Carbon Monoxide," *The New York Times*, October 6, 2004. More than you would ever want to know about *phaffia* yeast is at FDA, "FDA Approval Phaffia Yeast as Color Additive in Salmonid Fish Feed," *Federal Register* 65, no. 130 (July 6, 2000): 41584–87.

228 **That is why I am astonished . . .** See www.freshdirect.com. The European Union also has not set standards for organic fish. Marine Harvest explains that its Clare Island "organic" fish are fed fish meal derived from the by-products of food fish, that fish meal and fish oils are replaced in part by vegetable sources, and that the pens are less crowded than usual and are located in areas with strong ocean currents, thereby providing the fish with a healthy environment. See www.marineharvest.com. Information about Certified Organic shrimp from OceanBoy is at www.floridasweetshrimp.com.

230 **Researchers working for . . .** The Aqua Bounty Web site is www.aquabounty.com. The FDA position on transgenic fish is given at www.fda.gov/cvm/transgen. htm. See Erik Stokstad, "Engineered Fish: Friend or Foe of the Environment?" *Science* 297 (September 13, 2002): 1797–98. The Pew Charitable Trusts report on genetically engineered fish is at pewagbiotech.org/research/fish/fish.pdf.

231 **In 2005, despite strong . . .** The bill is at www.legis.state.ak.us/basis/get_bill.asp?session=24&bill=sb25. Comments by the Biotechnology Industry Organization are at www.bio.org. See also Hal Spence, "Bill Requires Labeling Genetically Altered Fish," *Peninsula Clarion* (Kenai, Alaska), May 8, 2005, at www.peninsulaclarion.com. On GloFish, see Andrew Pollack, "So, the Fish Glow. But Will They Sell?" *The New York Times*, January 25, 2004.

232 **Out of ignorance or . . .** To their credit, some segments of the fish industry recognize the value of honesty and are trying to address the problem. See, for example, Steven Hedlund, "Swindling on the Rise," *SeaFood Business* (June 2005).

20. MORE SEAFOOD DILEMMAS: SAFETY AND SUSTAINABILITY

234 **Until now, I haven't said . . .** Adeel A. Butt, Kenneth E. Aldridge, and Charles V. Sanders, "Infections Related to the Ingestion of Seafood. Part I: Viral and Bacterial Infections, Part II: Parasitic Infections and Food Safety," *Lancet Infectious Diseases* 4, no. 4 (April 1, 2004): 201–12, and no. 5 (May 1, 2004): 294–300. See Caroline Smith DeWaal et al., *Outbreak Alert! Closing the Gaps in Our Federal Food-Safety Net* (Washington, D.C.: Center for Science in the Public Interest, November 2005), available at www.cspinet.org. The FDA gives its illness estimates in a press release announcing Seafood HACCP (see "These depressing reports . . ." below). CDC estimates come from the U.S. General Accounting Office, "Food Safety: Federal Oversight of Seafood Does Not Sufficiently Protect Consumers," GAO-01-204, January 2001.

235 **To protect yourself . . .** "Buy from reputable suppliers" is the mantra of the seafood industry. See, for example, *Seafood Handbook* (*SeaFood Business*, 2002).

238 **These depressing reports . . .** GAO reports are at www.gao.gov. Seafood HACCP is at FDA, "Procedures for the Safe and Sanitary Processing and Importing of Fish and Fishery Products; Final Rule," *Federal Register* 60 (Decem-

ber 18, 1995): 65095–202; more recent information is at www.cfsan.fda.gov/~comm/haccpsea.html. For concerns about *Vibrio* in shellfish, see Center for Science in the Public Interest, "FDA Inaction on Raw Oysters Means More 'Deaths on the Half Shell,'" May 10, 2000, at www.cspinet.org/new/oysters.html. Its 2001 report, "Death on the Half Shell," is also at that site under CSPI's Documents Library. CDC reports regional *Vibrio* infection and death rates at www.cdc.gov.

239 **Colleagues who knew . . .** I am not the only one to have discovered Martinello. See R. W. Apple Jr., "In the Quest for Safer Seafood, One Company Follows Its Nose," *The New York Times*, November 29, 2000. The Legal Sea Foods Web site is www.legalseafoods.com.

240 **Whole Foods partners . . .** The Marine Stewardship Council's site is www.msc.org. The New England Aquarium EcoSound program is at www.neaq.org.

240 **When people with heart disease . . .** S. L. Seierstad et al., "Dietary Intake of Differently Fed Salmon; the Influence on Markers of Human Atherosclerosis," *European Journal of Clinical Investigation* 35 (2005): 52–59. Finishing diets are discussed in J. Gordon Bell et al., "Altered Fatty Acid Compositions in Atlantic Salmon (*Salmo salar*) Fed Diets Containing Linseed and Rapeseed Oils Can Be Partially Restored by a Subsequent Fish Oil Finishing Diet," *Journal of Nutrition* 133 (2003): 2793–801.

241 **Although farming increases . . .** Rosamond L. Naylor et al., "Nature's Subsidies to Shrimp and Salmon Farming," *Science* 282 (1998): 883–84; and "Effect of Aquaculture on World Fish Supplies," *Nature* 405 (2000): 1017–24.

242 **For these reasons, even I . . .** The FDA provides a "Regulatory Fish Encyclopedia" that describes each fish by type and gives identifying information at vm.cfsan.fda.gov/~frf/rfe0.html. As an index of how difficult it is for mere mortals to keep track of such things, Environmental Defense gives this advice about choosing shrimp or prawns: it is okay to eat northern shrimp and spot prawns, but not okay to eat blue, Chinese white, and whiteleg shrimp, or giant freshwater and tiger prawns (see www.oceansalive.org).

242 **Seafood Safe labels . . .** The history of this program and how it works are at www.seafoodsafe.com.

246 **The 2005 proposal . . .** See Marian Burros, "Plan Would Expand Ocean Fish Farming," *The New York Times*, June 6, 2005; and NOAA, "Bush Administration Releases National Offshore Aquaculture Bill," press release, June 7, 2005 at www.noaa.gov.

21. EGGS: THE "INCREDIBLE" EDIBLES

250 **Lutein requires a digression . . .** Hae-Yun Chung et al., "Lutein Bioavailability Is Higher from Lutein-Enriched Eggs Than from Supplements and Spinach in Men," *Journal of Nutrition* 134 (2004): 1887–93. The lutein content of foods is at www.luteininfo.com.

251 **Eggs have more cholesterol . . .** Shirley Gerrior, Lisa Bente, and Hazel Hiza, "Nutrient Content of the U.S. Food Supply, 1909–2000," USDA Home Economics Research Report No. 56, November 2004, at www.cnpp.usda.gov. Paul A. Cotton et al., "Dietary Sources of Nutrients Among US Adults, 1994 to 1996," *Journal of the American Dietetic Association* 104 (June 2004): 921-30. USDA

tables of egg composition (and the composition of thousands of other foods) are at www.nal.usda.gov/fnic/foodcomp/search (Release 18). See "2005 Dietary Guidelines Advisory Committee Report," August 19, 2004, at www.health.gov/dietaryguidelines/dga2005/report. The final report is *Dietary Guidelines for Americans*, 2005, available at www.healthierus.gov/dietaryguidelines.

252 **And like all industries...** The Egg Nutrition Center is at www.enconline.org. The American Egg Board is at www.aeb.org. The United Egg Producers are at www.unitedegg.org. The USDA-sponsored egg "checkoff" is at www.ams.usda.gov/poultry/pyrp.htm.

253 **It is not hard to understand why...** USDA food production figures are at www.ers.usda.gov/data/foodconsumption.

255 **Since the 1970s...** The first such study in my files is from Margaret A. Flynn et al., "Effect of Dietary Egg on Human Serum Cholesterol and Triglycerides," *American Journal of Clinical Nutrition* 32 (May 1979): 1051–57. In contrast, independent meta-analyses invariably find eggs to raise blood cholesterol levels; for example, Robert Clarke et al., "Dietary Lipids and Blood Cholesterol: Quantitative Meta-Analysis of Metabolic Ward Studies," *British Medical Journal* 314 (January 11, 1997): 112–17 (a review of more than 300 studies); and Rianne M. Weggemans et al., "Dietary Cholesterol from Eggs Increases the Ratio of Total Cholesterol to High-Density Lipoprotein Cholesterol in Humans: A Meta-Analysis," *American Journal of Clinical Nutrition* 73 (2001): 885–91 (222 studies).

255 **Blood cholesterol levels...** The National Cholesterol Education Program (NCEP) guidelines for adults divide blood cholesterol levels into three categories: "desirable" (below 200 milligrams cholesterol per 100 milliliters of blood), "borderline high cholesterol" (between 200 and 230 mg/100 ml), and "high cholesterol" (above 240 mg/100 ml). See NCEP, "Third Report: Detection, Evaluation, and Treatment of High Blood Cholesterol in Adults," NIH Publication No. 01-3670, May 2001, at www.nhlbi.nih.gov/guidelines/cholesterol/index.htm. Fred Kern Jr., "Normal Plasma Cholesterol in an 88-year-old Man Who Eats 25 Eggs a Day," *New England Journal of Medicine* 324, no. 13 (1991): 896–99.

256 **I received an avalanche...** Frank B. Hu, "A Prospective Study of Egg Consumption and Risk of Cardiovascular Disease in Men and Women," *New England Journal of Medicine* 281 (April 21, 1999): 1387–94 (funding was from the National Institutes of Health). The quote comes from a letter from Donald J. McNamara of the Egg Nutrition Center and C. Wayne Callaway, a physician at George Washington University who is a member of the advisory panel for the AEB. The ad is from Eggland's Best, flier in *The New York Times*, January 31, 1999.

257 **Following that study...** The egg-shaped flier is undated but followed publication of the 1999 study mentioned in "I received an avalanche..." above. See "Eggsaggerations: Cracking Open Egg Myths," *Nutrition Action Healthletter* (July/August 1997). For American Heart Association (AHA) advice, see Ronald M. Krauss et al., "AHA Dietary Guidelines. Revision 2000: A Statement for Healthcare Professionals from the Nutrition Committee of the American Heart Association," *Circulation* 102 (2000): 2284–99. "Eggs: AHA Scientific Position" is at www.americanheart.org.

258   **That pricey carton . . .** Country Hen's spokesperson said the eggs contained 136 milligrams of alpha-linolenic acid, 160 milligrams of DHA, and 4 milligrams of EPA—exactly 300 milligrams. Country Hen cartons in August 2005 were labeled as containing 600 milligrams of omega-3s (large letters) per two eggs (in small letters), and as Certified Organic and Kosher (the certifying agent is Natural Food Certifiers, Scarsdale, New York).

259   **One study, of undisclosed . . .** Suk Y. Oh et al., "Eggs Enriched in Omega-3 Fatty Acids and Alterations in Lipid Concentrations in Plasma and Lipoproteins and in Blood Pressure," *American Journal of Clinical Nutrition* 54 (1991): 689–95. This paper was published before journals required disclosure of funding sources. The comprehensive review is from the Agency for Healthcare Research and Quality, "Evidence Report/Technology Assessment," number 93, March 2004. A study by Merritt H. Raitt et al., "Fish Oil Supplementation and Risk of Ventricular Tachycardia and Ventricular Fibrillation in Patients with Implantable Defibrillators," *Journal of the American Medical Association* 293 (2005): 2884–91, says that such patients do worse if fed fish oils.

261   **Pete and Gerry's eggs . . .** See www.peteandgerrys.com. The site for Certified Humane: Raised and Handled is www.certifiedhumane.org.

262   **Egg producers did not want . . .** Compassion Over Killing describes the methods it used under the heading, "Victory: COK Wins 'Animal Care Certified' Campaign!" at www.cok.net. The quotations are from Alexei Barrionuevo, "Egg Producers Relent on Industry Seal," *The New York Times*, October 4, 2005; and Nelson Hernandez, "Egg Label Changed After Md. Group Complains: Federal Inquiry Into Advocates' Charge of False Advertising Is Dropped," *The Washington Post*, October 4, 2005.

263   **Until now, I have not said . . .** USDA standards for egg quality—color, size, grade, and freshness—are in "United States Standards, Grades, and Weight Classes for Shell Eggs," April 6, 1995, at www.ams.usda.gov/poultry/pdfs/AMS-EggSt-1995.pdf.

22. EGGS AND THE *SALMONELLA* PROBLEM

265   **If SE only landed . . .** Much of this information comes from the joint USDA and FDA 1998 *Federal Register* notice on "Salmonella Enteritidis in Eggs," 63, no. 96: 27502–511; and Elizabeth Dahl and Caroline Smith DeWaal, "Scrambled Eggs: How a Broken Food Safety System Let Contaminated Eggs Become a National Food Poisoning Epidemic," Center for Science in the Public Interest, May 1997. For how hens make eggs, see Richard E. Austic and Malden C. Nesheim, *Poultry Production*, 13th edition (Lea & Febiger, 1990). For how eggs get infected, see CDC, *Salmonella enteritidis*, under "Health Topics, A to Z," at www.cdc.gov/az.do.

265   **SE used to be found . . .** A. J. Bäumler, B. M. Hargis, and R. M. Tsolis. "Tracing the Origins of *Salmonella* Outbreaks," *Science* 287 (2000): 50–52.

266   **The industry's Egg Nutrition Center . . .** Its Web site is www.enc-online.org. The American Egg Board is at www.aeb.org.

267   **Late in 1988 . . .** "Anything to Eat?" (editorial), *Lancet* (February 25, 1989); and Nicholas Russell, "Does *Nobody* Know Their Eggs?" *New Scientist* (January 14, 1989). Currie's subsequent career as a novelist, diarist, and media personality is

described at edwina.currie.co.uk (her published diaries attracted considerable attention for their revelation of a four-year affair with John Major, later the British prime minister). *Salmonella* infection rates in chickens, humans, and livestock are given in Goosen van den Busch, "Vaccination Versus Treatment: How Europe Is Tackling the Eradication of Salmonella," *Asian Poultry Magazine* (July 2003); available at www.safe-poultry.com/documents/salmonel laarticleAsianPoultry2003.pdf; and at Health Protection Agency (UK), "Salmonella in Humans . . . 1981–2004," April 28, 2005, at www.hpa.org.uk/infections/ topics_az/salmonella/data_human_gr.htm. And see Food Standards Agency, "Salmonella Contamination of UK-Produced Shell Eggs on Retail Sale," March 18, 2004, at www.food.gov.uk/science/surveillance.

268   **No less than four . . .** General Accounting Office, "Food Safety: U.S. Lacks a Consistent Farm-to-Table Approach to Egg Safety," GAO/RCED-99-184, July 1999.

269   **In particular, Pennsylvania . . .** Agricultural statistics by state can be found at www.nass.usda.gov.

271   **By this time, voluntary . . .** Centers for Disease Control and Prevention, "Outbreaks of *Salmonella* Serotype Enteritidis Infection Associated with Eating Raw or Undercooked Shell Eggs—United States, 1996–1998" and ". . . United States, 1999–2001," *Journal of the American Medical Association* 283 (2000): 1132–34, and 289 (2003): 540–41, respectively. See Caroline Smith DeWaal et al., *Outbreak Alert! Closing the Gaps in Our Federal Food-Safety Net* (Washington, D.C.: Center for Science in the Public Interest, November 2005), available at www.cspinet.org.

271   **Marian Burros wrote . . .** "F.D.A. Seeks Rule for Farms to Increase Egg Safety," *The New York Times*, September 21, 2004.

271   **When a reporter from *Food Chemical News* . . .** Allissa Hosten, "FDA Holds Public Forum on Egg Safety Proposed Rule," *Food Chemical News* (November 1, 2004). And see "FDA Proposes In-Lid Labeling for Eggs," May 4, 2005, at www.fda.gov/bbs/topics/ANSWERS/2005/ANS01355.html.

23. FROZEN FOODS: DECODING INGREDIENT LISTS

274   **Frozen foods are . . .** The National Frozen Food & Refrigerated Foods Association is at www.nfraweb.org; the American Frozen Food Institute is at www.affi.com.

277   **The Nutrients in Fresh . . .** Figures on food composition come from the USDA National Nutrition Database for Standard Reference (Release 18), 2005, at www.nal.usda.gov/fnic/foodcomp/search.

278   **They are cosmetics . . .** The Center for Science in the Public Interest offers a handy guide to the function, use, and safety of food additives at www.cspinet. org/reports/chemcuisine.htm.

279   **In contrast, the "Contains" list . . .** For an unusually clear explanation of the allergy labeling rules, see Mary Kissel, "Labeling Rules Likely for Food Allergies," *The Wall Street Journal*, July 7, 2004.

24. A DIGRESSION INTO CALORIES AND DIETS

282 **To get started . . .** See, for example, *Dr. Atkins' New Diet Revolution* (Avon, 2001). This diet severely restricts foods containing sugars and starches and allows "unlimited" fatty foods such as steak, butter, and cream, in quotation marks because the Atkins menus suggest quite reasonable portion sizes.

288 **Thermodynamics tells you . . .** The history of research on food calories is reviewed in Gerald F. Combs and Walter Mertz, editors, "W. O. Atwater Centennial Celebration Symposium," *Journal of Nutrition* 124, Supplement 9S (September 1994). Its article by Buford Nichols, "Atwater and USDA Nutrition Research and Service: A Prologue of the Past Century," 1718S–27S, is an especially helpful introduction as is Kenneth J. Carpenter's "The Life and Times of W. O. Atwater (1844–1907)": 1707S–14S.

292 **Food composition tables . . .** The USDA food composition Web site is www.nal.usda.gov/fnic/foodcomp/search. Click on "USDA National Nutrient Database for Standard Reference (Release 18), 2005"; "SR18 Documentation" to read about the methods; "Search" to enter the name of the food of interest and to obtain lists of the nutrients in a given weight of that food.

293 **McDonald's, for example . . .** The Web site for nutrition information for U.S. items is www.mcdonalds.com/usa/eat/nutrition_info.html. McDonald's specifies information by country. Menu items differ in size and content according to local preferences.

295 **Individually wrapped single . . .** Lisa R. Young and Marion Nestle, "Food Labels Consistently Underestimate the Actual Weights of Single-Serving Baked Products," *Journal of the American Dietetic Association* 95 (1995): 1150–51.

25. FROZEN FOODS: READING NUTRITION FACTS

296 **The label is so difficult . . .** FDA, "How to Understand and Use the Nutrition Facts Label," November 2004 update, at www.cfsan.fda.gov/~dms/foodlab. html.

297 **In 1989, Dr. David . . .** David A. Kessler, "The Federal Regulation of Food Labeling: Promoting Foods to Prevent Disease," *New England Journal of Medicine* 321 (1989): 717–22. I discuss the history of labeling legislation in my book *Food Politics* (University of California Press, 2003).

297 **All of this would . . .** Marian Burros, "The New Battle over Food Labels," and "Nutrition Labels: The Quest Goes On," *The New York Times*, July 1 and 22, 1992. Christine J. Lewis and Elizabeth A. Yetley, "Focus Group Sessions on Formats on Nutrition Labels," and Alan S. Levy et al., "More Effective Nutrition Label Formats Are Not Necessarily Preferred," *Journal of the American Dietetic Association* 92 (1992): 62–66 and 1230–34, respectively. For continuation of the soap opera, see Marian Burros, "Read Any Good Nutrition Labels Lately?" *The New York Times*, December 1, 2004.

298 **The consumer advocacy group . . .** Bonnie Liebman, "Baby 'Label' Arrives," *Nutrition Action Healthletter* (March 1993). The "baby" was the 3 pound 8 ounce *Federal Register* notice of January 6, 1993: "Food Labeling. General Provisions; Nutrition Labeling; Label Format; Nutrient Content Claims; Health Claims . . . Final Rules," 58: 2066–941.

298 **Consider Häagen-Dazs . . .** Figuring out how this brand is owned by Nestlé is no simple matter. Here is its corporate history, pieced together from Web sites (particularly www.diageo.com and www.pillsbury.com), and from www. oligopolywatch.com.

The International Corporate History of Häagen-Dazs

YEAR	EVENT
1961	Reuben Mattus, a Bronx ice-cream seller, dreams up the Häagen-Dazs name and brand (U.S.).
1983	Pillsbury (U.S.) buys Häagen-Dazs.
1989	GrandMet (Grand Metropolitan, U.K.) buys Pillsbury/Häagen-Dazs.
1997	GrandMet (with Pillsbury/Häagen-Dazs) merges with Guinness (U.K.) to form Diageo (U.K.).
1999	Diageo enters fifty-fifty joint venture with Nestlé (Switzerland) to combine ice-cream businesses in the U.S. The agreement gives Nestlé option to buy remaining 50 percent share if Diageo sells Pillsbury/Häagen-Dazs.
2001	Diageo sells Pillsbury/Häagen-Dazs to General Mills (U.S.) for $11 billion. The Federal Trade Commission (FTC) considers an antitrust injunction, but is deadlocked and permits the merger. Nestlé exercises option and then owns 100 percent of Häagen-Dazs.
2002	Nestlé/Häagen-Dazs offers to buy majority share of Dreyers (U.S.) ice cream business for $2.8 billion in the United States and Canada (General Mills continues to own Häagen-Dazs in other countries).
2003	The FTC seeks an antitrust injunction to block the sale and approves it only when Dreyers sells some of its brands. The result: Nestlé owns a majority share of Dreyers, which becomes the Häagen-Dazs distributor.

303 **A quite reasonable guideline . . .** One cup of frozen yogurt contains 62 grams of sugars. At 4 calories per gram, that's 248 calories, or more than 12 percent of a 2,000-calorie diet.

26. PROCESSED FOODS: WHEAT FLOUR AND THE GLYCEMIC INDEX

306 **Foods in the center . . .** A. Elizabeth Sloan, "Cruising the Center-Store Aisles," *Food Technology* (October 2005): 29–39.

307   **Some nutrients are lost** . . . Figures on food composition come from the USDA National Nutrition Database for Standard Reference (Release 18), 2005, at www.nal.usda.gov/fnic/foodcomp/search. Most figures in the Tables in this book are rounded off to simplify.

309   **Because removing the chaff** . . . Flour Fortification Initiative, Emory University, www.sph.emory.edu/wheatflour/index.html.

311   **Foods made from wheat flour** . . . Paul A. Cotton et al., "Dietary Sources of Nutrients Among US Adults, 1994 to 1996," *Journal of the American Dietetic Association* 104 (June 2004): 921–30.

312   **Follow-up studies** . . . Eoin P. Quinlivan and Jesse F. Gregory III, "Effect of Food Fortification on Folic Acid Intake in the United States," *American Journal of Clinical Nutrition* 77 (2003): 221–25. Centers for Disease Control and Prevention, "Spina Bifida and Anencephaly Before and After Folic Acid Mandate— United States, 1995–1996 and 1999–2000," *Morbidity and Mortality Weekly Report* 53 (2004): 362–65.

313   **On a trip to Australia** . . . Glycemic Index certification of foods is run by Glycemic Index Limited, a nonprofit alliance of the University of Sydney, Diabetes Australia, and Juvenile Diabetes Research Foundation. See www.glycemicindex.com and www.gisymbol.com.au.

315   **Bookstore health sections** . . . If you must read one, I'd pick Jennie Brand-Miller et al., *The New Glucose Revolution* (Marlowe and Company, 2003). If you like debates, see David Ludwig et al., "The Glycemic Index: Physiological Mechanisms Relating to Obesity, Diabetes, and Cardiovascular Disease," *Journal of the American Medical Association* 287 (May 8, 2002): 2417–21; and D. B. Pawlak, et al., "Should Obese Patients Be Counseled to Follow a Low-Glycaemic Index Diet? Yes," *Obesity Reviews* 3 (2002): 235–43 (on pages 245–56, the "No" paper, by A. Raben, argues that the Glycemic Index has no effect on weight control). F. Xavier Pi-Sunyer gives a great many reasons for not taking the Glycemic Index too seriously in "Glycemic Index and Disease," *American Journal of Clinical Nutrition* 76 supplement (July 2002): 290S–98S.

315   **Take potatoes, for example** . . . The potato industry is so worried about the effect of the Glycemic Index on sales that it has developed a marketing campaign, "Get the Skinny on America's Favorite Vegetable: The Healthy Potato." Potatoes, says the U.S. Potato Board, are "Naturally Nutritious, Always Delicious." See www.uspotatoes.com. Values in the table come from Glen Fernandes, Amogh Velangi, and Thomas M. S. Wolever, "Glycemic Index of Potatoes Commonly Consumed in North America," *Journal of the American Dietetic Association* 105 (2005): 557–62.

27. SUGAR(S)

317   **A couple of weeks** . . . The letter and my reply are posted at www.foodpolitics.com. Both are reprinted in full in Kelly D. Brownell and Katherine Battle Horgan, *Food Fight* (McGraw-Hill, 2003).

320   **You metabolize fructose** . . . George A. Bray et al., "Consumption of High-Fructose Corn Syrup in Beverages May Play a Role in the Epidemic of Obesity," *American Journal of Clinical Nutrition* 79 (2004): 537–43 (and see editorial

on pages 711–12 and the follow-up letters in 80, pages 1081–82 and 1446–48). See also Peter J. Havel, "Dietary Fructose: Implications for Dysregulation of Energy Homeostasis and Lipid/Carbohydrate Metabolism," *Nutrition Reviews* 63 (2005): 133–57 ("prolonged consumption of a diet high in energy from fructose would contribute, along with dietary fat and inactivity, to positive energy balance, weight gain, and obesity").

320 **If corn sweeteners have . . .** For sweetener production figures, see USDA/ERS, "Food Consumption (per capita) Data System," at www.ers.usda.gov/data/food consumption. Production statistics also are available from the Corn Refiners Association at www.corn.org/web/stats.htm.

322 **Sucrose and corn sweeteners may . . .** The Sugar Association is at www. sugar.org. Corn sweeteners are represented by the Corn Refiners Association, www.corn.org. Corn producers are split between two groups, the more corporate National Corn Growers Association, www.ncga.com, and a group interested in alternatives to current farm policies, the American Corn Growers Association, www.acga.org. The USDA describes the sugar support programs in "Briefing Room: Farm and Commodity Policy," at www.ers.usda.gov/ briefing/FarmPolicy/2002sugar.htm. For the effects of price supports on the cost of table sugar, see General Accounting Office, "Sugar Program: Supporting Sugar Prices Has Increased Users' Costs While Benefiting Producers," GAO/RCED-00-126, June 2000; and "America's Sugar Daddies" (editorial), *The New York Times*, November 29, 2003.

322 **That is why low prices . . .** Sweetener prices can be tracked in "Briefing Room: Sugar and Sweeteners; Data Tables," at www.ers.usda.gov/Briefing/ Sugar. For the effects of sweeteners on food costs and eating patterns, see Adam Drewnowski and Nicole Darmon, "The Economics of Obesity: Dietary Energy Density and Energy Cost," *American Journal of Clinical Nutrition* 82 Supplement (2005): 265S–73S.

326 **So are sweet drinks . . .** Michael F. Jacobson, "Liquid Candy: How Soft Drinks Are Harming Americans' Health," Center for Science in the Public Interest, June 2005, at www.cspinet.org.

327 **Shortly after I expressed . . .** Amy O'Connor, "Snapple Beware: She's the Gadfly in the Food Industry's Soup," *The New York Observer*, September 29, 2003.

327 **To make "juiced" products . . .** Steven Nagy et al., editors, *Fruit Juice Processing Technology* (Agscience, 1993). For sources of sugars in U.S. diets, see Joanne F. Guthrie and Joan F. Morton, "Food Sources of Added Sweeteners in the Diets of Americans," *Journal of the American Dietetic Association* 100 (2000): 43–48; and the 2005 *Dietary Guidelines for Americans* at www.healthierus. gov/dietaryguidelines.

328 **This review concluded . . .** The USDA paper is by Anne L. Mardis, "Current Knowledge of the Health Effects of Sugar Intake," *Family Economics and Nutrition Review* 13, no. 1 (2001): 87–91. For an entirely different interpretation of the science, see Jim Mann, "Free Sugars and Human Health: Sufficient Evidence for Action?" *Lancet* 363 (2004): 1068–70; and Lee S. Gross et al., "Increased Consumption of Refined Carbohydrates and the Epidemic of Type 2 Diabetes in the United States: An Ecological Assessment," *American Journal of Clinical Nutrition* 79 (2004): 774–79.

328 **Even so, plenty of . . .** Robert Murray et al. "Are Soft Drinks a Scapegoat for Childhood Obesity?" *Journal of Pediatrics* 146 (2005): 586–90.

329 **In *Food Politics* . . .** Marion Nestle, *Food Politics* (University of California Press, 2003). The "Starr Report" is Office of the Independent Counsel, *Referral to the United States House of Representatives Pursuant to Title 28*, United States Code §595(c), September 9, 1998; available at www.nytimes.com/specials/starr. This event is discussed in the "Narrative, Section III. January–March 1996: Continued Sexual Encounters. D. President's Day (February 19) Break-Up."

330 **In many ways, the 2005 sugar . . .** The September 2004 committee report is at www.health.gov/dietaryguidelines/dga2005/report, and the 2005 *Dietary Guidelines for Americans* is at www.healthierus.gov/dietaryguidelines.

331 **But if the *Dietary Guidelines* . . .** As a case in point, sugar lobbyists enlisted U.S. senators and the Department of Health and Human Services in a successful campaign to prevent the World Health Organization from issuing advice to restrict intake of added sugars to 10 percent of calories or less in its report, "Global Strategy on Diet, Physical Activity, and Health," May 22, 2004. The WHO proposal was anything but radical; the USDA's 1992 Food Guide Pyramid, for example, recommended restrictions on sugars to 7 to 13 percent of calories (depending on total calorie intake). See Amalia Waxman, "The WHO Global Strategy . . . the Controversy on Sugar," *Development* 47 (2004): 75–82; and John Zarocostas, "WHO Waters Down Draft Strategy on Diet and Health," *Lancet* 363 (April 24, 2004): 1373.

332 **I cannot resist pointing . . .** Council on Foods and Nutrition, "Some Nutritional Aspects of Sugar, Candy and Sweetened Carbonated Beverages," *Journal of the American Medical Association* 120 (November 7, 1942): 763–65.

332 **But marketers encourage . . .** See Kate MacArthur, "Coke Commits $400M to Fix It" and "100 Leading National Advertisers," *Advertising Age* (November 15, 2004, and June 27, 2005, respectively).

334 **If you want package labels . . .** Food and Drug Administration, "Food Labeling: Added Sugars: Availability of Citizen Petition," *Federal Register* 65, no. 123, (June 26, 2000): 39414.

28. CEREALS: SWEET AND SUPPOSEDLY HEALTHY

336 **But I badly wanted . . .** The cereal box address is www.posthealthyclassics.com, and the link to Kraft Foods is www.kraftfoods.com. Rippe lists his current corporate clients at www.rippehealth.com/rippelifestyle/rliclients.html. A request to Kraft for details about the clinical studies yielded five abstracts from talks given by Rippe and colleagues at dietetics and obesity association meetings in 2004 (meaning that the studies were unpublished).

336 **The advertising of ready-to-eat . . .** The Kellogg share of the Big Four Cereal market is 31 percent, but its Kashi cereals command another 2 percent. Cereal production was 15 pounds per capita in 1994. See Gregory K. Price, "Cereal Sales Soggy Despite Price Cuts and Reduced Couponing," *FoodReview* 23, no. 2 (May–August 2000): 21–28; William A. Roberts Jr., "A Cereal Star," *Prepared Foods*, posted November 25, 2003, at www.preparedfoods.com; and John J. Pierce, "Multi-grains and More," *Private Label Magazine*, March/April 2005, at www.privatelabelmag.com. For another view, see Stephanie Thompson, "No Holy Grail in Whole Grains," *Advertising Age* (June 27, 2005).

337 **Many studies show . . .** See, for example, Ernesto Pollitt, editor, "Breakfast, Cognition, and School Learning," *American Journal of Clinical Nutrition* 67 Supplement (1998): 743S–813S (sponsored by Kellogg); C.H.S. Ruxton and T. R. Kirk, "Breakfast: A Review of Associations with Measures of Dietary Intake, Physiology, and Biochemistry," *British Journal of Nutrition* 78 (1997): 199–213 (one author works for the U.K. Sugar Bureau); Christine A. Powell et al., "Nutrition and Education: A Randomized Trial of the Effects of Breakfast in Rural Primary School Children," *American Journal of Clinical Nutrition* 68 (1998): 873–79 (NESTEC Switzerland donated the milk used in the breakfast); and Ann M. Albertson et al., "Ready-to-Eat Cereal Consumption: Its Relationship with BMI and Nutrient Intake of Children Aged 4 to 12 Years," *Journal of the American Dietetic Association* 103 (2003): 1613–19 (sponsored by General Mills).

338 **Cereals—wheat, corn, and rice . . .** See papers in the *American Journal of Clinical Nutrition*: Majken K. Jensen et al., "Intakes of Whole Grains, Bran, and Germ and the Risk of Coronary Heart Disease in Men," 80 (2004): 1492–99; James W. Anderson, "Whole Grains and Coronary Heart Disease: The Whole Kernel of Truth" (editorial), 80 (2004): 1459–60; and Simin Liu et al., "Is Intake of Breakfast Cereals Related to Total and Cause-Specific Mortality in Men?" 77 (2003): 594–99.

338 **Here are some examples . . .** Information in this Table comes from "United States Selected Beverage and Food Categories/Products Ranked by Dollar Sales for 2004," *MMR/IRI* (Mass Market Retailing/Information Resources, Inc.) *Food and Beverage Report* 21, no. 19 (November 29, 2004). Four of the next five most popular cereals are from Kellogg: Frosted Mini Wheats (#6), Froot Loops (#7), Corn Flakes (#9), and Special K (#10). General Mills Lucky Charms ranks #8.

339 **In 2003, advertising spending . . .** Media advertising for cereals comes from *Brandweek* 45, no. 25 Supplement (June 21, 2004): 44S. Company figures are from *Advertising Age* (June 28, 2004, and June 27, 2005). Advertising expenditures are about 5 percent of sales on average, so you can multiply the advertising expense by 20 to guess what the sales might be. In 2004, revenues per cereal advertising dollar ranged from about $10 for General Mills and Kellogg to $28 for the Altria Group. By the multiply-by-20 estimation method, sales of Big Four Cereals must be in the ballpark of $40 billion a year in the United States.

339 **Nutrients are a major . . .** Katherine L. Tucker et al., "Breakfast Cereal Fortified with Folic Acid, Vitamin B-6, and Vitamin B-12 Increases Vitamin Concentrations and Reduces Homocysteine Concentrations: A Randomized Trial," *American Journal of Clinical Nutrition* 79 (2004): 805–11 (sponsored in part by Kellogg); and Paul A. Cotton et al., "Dietary Sources of Nutrients Among US Adults, 1994 to 1996," *Journal of the American Dietetic Association* 104 (June 2004): 921–30.

340 **"Whole grains," said *Advertising* . . .** Stephanie Thompson, "Food Industry Embraces Whole Grain as Next Savior," *Advertising Age* (October 25, 2004).

344 **The FDA reviewed the science . . .** Currently authorized claims are summarized by the FDA at www.cfsan.fda.gov/~dms/lab-hlth.html.

345 **General Mills celebrated . . .** FDA, "Health Claim Notification for Whole Grain Foods," July 1999, at vm.cfsan.fda.gov. The General Mills advertisement appeared in *The New York Times* on July 12, 1999. The Institute of Food Technology issues a guide to food manufacturers about how to substantiate health

claims: A. Reza Kamarei and Carl Trygstad, "Designing Clinical Trials to Substantiate Claims, *Food Technology* 58 (2004): 28–35. See Jane Zhang and Janet Adamy, "FDA Limits Claims About Whole Grains," *The Wall Street Journal,* December 6, 2005.

345 **Does putting "whole grains"** . . . Ephraim Leibtag and Lisa Mancino, "Food Dynamics and USDA's New Dietary Guidelines," USDA Economic Information Bulletin No. 5, September 2005, available at www.ers.usda.gov/Publications/ EIB5.

348 **Supermarkets like Wegmans** . . . Lori Dahm, "Retail Dilemma: Where to Put the Healthy Stuff," *Stagnito's New Products Magazine* (March 2005): 36–40.

348 **The box sports something** . . . The Web site of Glycemic Solutions is www. glycemicindextesting.com.

29. PACKAGED FOODS: HEALTH ENDORSEMENTS

352 **To qualify for the association's** . . . The criteria for seafood, meat, and poultry must meet FDA standards for "extra lean." A 100-gram serving must have less than 5 grams of fat, 2 grams of saturated fat, and 95 milligrams of cholesterol. This information is hard to find on the American Heart Association Web site. I had to call the association to get the correct identifier: www.americanheart. org//presenter.jhtml?identifier=2115, and search www.cfsan.fda.gov.

352 **In *Food Politics*, I traced** . . . See also Sarah Ellison and Mary Kissel, "Seals and Deals," *The Wall Street Journal,* July 20, 2004.

353 **On Mother's Day** . . . The Heartzels ad appeared in *The New York Times,* May 7, 2004. The quotation is from Stephanie Thompson, "Frito-Lay Homes in on Health Workers," *Advertising Age* (February 23, 2004).

355 **After hearing me speak** . . . Jane Brody, "Beware Food Companies' Health Claims," *The New York Times,* September 21, 2004.

355 **It is instructive, if** . . . "Diabetes Association Defends Cadbury Schweppes Deal," *Corporate Crime Reporter* (May 16, 2005), available at www.corporate crimereporter.com/diabetes051605.htm.

30. SNACK FOODS: SWEET, SALTY, AND CALORIC

357 **But subsidies also act** . . . Alexei Barrionuevo and Keith Bradsher, "Sometimes a Bumper Crop Is Too Much of a Good Thing," *The New York Times,* December 8, 2005.

358 **In a typical year** . . . Lists of new products are in *Stagnito's New Products Magazine,* available at www.newproductsmag.com. January issues give annual distribution figures; the January 2005 issue counts 14,826 foods and 4,110 beverages introduced in 2004. See also "USDA Food Market Indicators: Food Marketing System," November 22, 2004, at www.ers.usda.gov/data/foodmarketindicators// default.asp?tableset-1.

360 **Snack Food Sales and** . . . Information in this Table comes from "United States Selected Beverage and Food Categories/Products Ranked by Dollar Sales for 2004," *MMR/IRI* (Mass Market Retailing/Information Resources, Inc.) *Food and Beverage Report* 21, no. 19 (November 29, 2004). Additional information about advertising expenditures appears annually in *Advertising Age* (June 28, 2004, and June 27, 2005, for example).

360   **Nutritionists already worried . . .** Karen J. Morgan, "The Role of Snacking in the American Diet," *Contemporary Nutrition* (September 1982) (a publication of General Mills). Claire Zizza, Anna Maria Siega-Riz, and Barry M. Popkin, "Significant Increase in Young Adults' Snacking Between 1977–1978 and 1994–1996 Represents a Cause for Concern!" *Preventive Medicine* 32 (2001): 303–10. See also Corinne Marmonier et al., "Snacks Consumed in a Nonhungry State Have Poor Satiating Efficiency: Influence of Snack Composition on Substrate Utilization and Hunger," *American Journal of Clinical Nutrition* 76 (2002): 518–28.

361   **Health organization endorsements . . .** Chad Terhune, "Pepsi, Discovery in Smart-Snack Push," *The Wall Street Journal*, December 6, 2004. The PepsiCo ad appeared inside the back cover of the *Journal of the American Dietetic Association* (November 2004). Information about Smart Spot criteria, qualifying products, benefits, and advisers is at www.smartspot.com.

362   **Make this substitution . . .** This calculation depends on the assumption that a pound of body fat is worth 3,500 calories. Saving 40 calories a day, 365 days per year, saves 14,600 calories; divided by 3,500, this yields a weight loss of about 4 pounds. If only losing weight were this simple.

363   **As a PepsiCo executive . . .** See "Frito Lay Chips in to Make Snack Foods Better for You," *Nutrition Business Journal* (July/August 2004): 19.

364   **Researchers from these foundations . . .** See Peter Williams et al., "A Case Study of Sodium Reduction in Breakfast Cereals and the Impact of the *Pick the Tick* Food Information Program in Australia," *Health Promotion International* 18 (2003): 51–56. Recent guidelines for the tick program approval are available from the National Heart Foundations of Australia (www.heartfoundation. com.au) and New Zealand (www.nhf.org.nz).

364   **In 2003, PepsiCo announced . . .** The ad appeared in *The Wall Street Journal* (September 24) and *The New York Times* (September 28). It included this context statement after an asterisk: "The Frito-Lay products shown have 1–3 grams saturated fat/serving and no cholesterol."

365   **But salt is even more essential . . .** See Sarah Ellison, "Despite Big Health Concerns, Food Industry Can't Shake Salt," *The Wall Street Journal*, February 25, 2005.

365   **The guidelines explained . . .** The 2005 *Dietary Guidelines for Americans* are at www.healthierus.gov/dietaryguidelines. For a pinch of the salt arguments, take a look at G. A. MacGregor and H. E. de Wardener, *Salt, Diet and Health* (Cambridge University Press, 1998); and compare to Gary Taubes, "The (Political) Science of Salt," *Science* 281 (1998): 898–907. See also David Sharp, "Labelling Salt in Food: If Yes, How?" *Lancet* 364 (2004): 2079–81, and the letters published in response, "Salt in Food," by Feng J. He, Graham A. MacGregor, and Stephen A. Hoption Cann, *Lancet* 365 (2005): 844–46. The industry spin is at www.saltinstitute.org.

366   **In 2005, the Center for . . .** See CSPI's reports, "Salt: the Forgotten Killer," February 2005, at www.cspinet.org/salt; and "Salt Assault," August 2005, at www. cspinet.org/new/pdf/salt_report_update.pdf.

367   **Line extensions help . . .** David Barboza, "Permutations Push Oreo Far Beyond Cookie Aisle," *The New York Times*, October 4, 2003.

370 **Dietary recommendations, such . . .** The 2005 *Dietary Guidelines for Americans* are at www.healthierus.gov/dietaryguidelines, and the 2005 pyramid is at www.mypyramid.gov. See also Ronald E. Kleinman, editor, *Pediatric Nutrition Handbook*, 5th edition (American Academy of Pediatrics, 2003).

370 **Surveys of what American . . .** For a comprehensive review, see "Position of the American Dietetic Association: Dietary Guidance for Healthy Children Ages 2 to 11 Years," *Journal of the American Dietetic Association* 104 (2004): 660–77; and "Nickelodeon Debuts Research Findings About Kids' Eating Behaviors and Food Choices," *Financial News*, July 13, 2005, available at ww2.7online.com/Global/story.asp?s=3589548.

372 **In 1957, Vance Packard's . . .** *The Hidden Persuaders*, pages 105–22 (David McKay Company, 1957).

373 **As I explained in *Food Politics* . . .** Chapter 8 ("Starting Early: Underage Consumers," pages 175–96) in *Food Politics* (University of California Press, 2003), covers marketing to children and cites "how-to" books, such as G. Smith, editor, *Children's Food: Marketing and Innovation* (Blackie, 1997), and J. U. McNeal, *The Kids Market: Myths and Realities* (Paramount, 1999). See Jane Zhang and Janet Adamy, "FDA Limits Claims About Whole Grains," *The Wall Street Journal*, December 6, 2005.

373 **Advertising expenditures . . .** Susan Linn, *Consuming Kids* (New Press, 2004); and Juliet B. Schor, *Born to Buy* (Scribner, 2004).

374 **Analyses of food marketing . . .** Ben Kelley, "Industry Controls over Food Marketing to Young Children: Are They Effective?" Public Health Advocacy Institute, 2005, at www.phaionline.org.

375 **The odd thing about brand-named . . .** The prizewinning science fair project was done in 1999 by Christina Jackson and Molly Peifer when they were students at St. Ignatius elementary school in Portland, Oregon. The more elaborate study with the same result is by Samuel M. McClure et al., "Neural Correlates of Behavioral Preference for Culturally Familiar Drinks," *Neuron* 44 (2004): 379–87. See also Sandra Blakeslee, "If You Have a 'Buy Button' in Your Brain, What Pushes It?" *The New York Times*, October 19, 2004.

376 **They are not about nutrition . . .** The Kraft advertising figure comes from *Advertising Age* (June 27, 2005); the sales figure is from material presented to Kraft investors, May 10, 2005, courtesy of Mark Berlind, executive vice president of Global Corporate Affairs.

377 **This "kids are only supposed . . .** Sherri Day, "The Potatoes Were Smiling; the Fries Were Blue," *The New York Times*, March 13, 2003.

377 **And marketing would be less . . .** Stealth marketing is a worldwide problem: see, for example, "Children Encouraged to Advertise to Themselves," *Food Magazine* (U.K.) (April/June, 2005).

378 **Food companies arrange . . .** Mary Story and Simone French, "Food Advertising and Marketing Directed at Children and Adolescents in the US," *International Journal of Behavioral Nutrition and Physical Activity* 1, no. 3 (2004), available online at BioMed Central, at www.ijbnpa.org/content/1/1/3.

378 **I have on hand . . .** The ad appeared in *The New York Times*, April 16, 2004.

379 **Such products also come . . .** Joseph Pereira, "Online Arcades Draw Fire for

Immersing Kids in Ads: Ritz Bits Wrestling, Anyone?" *The Wall Street Journal*, May 3, 2004. See, for example, www.kraftfoods.com/koolaid.

380 **As it happens, I am not the only** . . . See Jason Streets et al., "Absolute Risk of Obesity," and "Obesity Update," UBS Warburg Global Equity Research, London, November 27, 2002, and March 4, 2003, respectively. Similar reports were issued by JP Morgan European Equity Research in April 2003, and by Morgan Stanley Global Equity Research in October 2003.

381 **Sales zoomed** . . . Steven Gray, "Milk Mystery: Sales Surge at Some Fast-Food Restaurants," *The Wall Street Journal*, September 22, 2004. See also Tara Parker-Pope, "Added Calories Sneak into Kids' Diets as Food Makers Tweak Snack Offerings," *The Wall Street Journal*, December 7, 2004.

381 **While they are promising** . . . For recent analyses of school vending contracts, see Nicola Pinson and Katie Gaetjens, *School Soda Contracts: A Sample Review of Contracts in Oregon Public School Districts*, 2004, Community Health Partnership at www.communityhealthpartnership.org; and Melanie Warner, "Lines Drawn for Big Suit Over Sodas," *The New York Times*, December 7, 2005.

381 **Candies are still** . . . J. Michael Harris, "Companies Continue to Offer New Foods Targeted to Children," *Amber Waves* (June 2005), at www.ers.usda.gov/AmberWaves.

382 **Half a year later, Kraft** . . . Sarah Ellison, "Kraft Limits on Kids' Ads May Cheese Off Rivals," *The Wall Street Journal*, January 13, 2005; and Stephanie Thompson, "Food Fight Breaks Out," *Advertising Age*, January 17, 2005.

384 **Analyses of food commercials** . . . See D. W. Rajecki et al., "Violence, Conflict, Trickery, and Other Story Themes in TV Ads for Food for Children," *Journal of Applied Social Psychology* 24 (1994): 1685–700. The books by Susan Linn and Juliet Schor (cited in this chapter's note "Advertising expenditures . . .") review this material thoroughly.

32. OILS: FAT AND MORE FAT

386 **The soy folks must think** . . . Syngenta Seeds publishes statistics about soybean production and use at www.soystats.com.

386 **You can pay a fortune** . . . "Olive Oil: A Cheap Bottle Beats a Pricier Lineup," *Consumer Reports* (September 2004): 32–35. Armando Manni describes his "alive and intact" oils at www.manni.biz. The health properties of olive oils are reviewed in Aliza H. Start and Zecharia Madar, "Olive Oil as a Functional Food: Epidemiology and Nutritional Approaches," *Nutrition Reviews* 60 (June 2002): 170–76.

389 **All food fats** . . . For information about properties of fats and oils, see Institute of Shortening and Edible Oils at www.iseo.org/index.htm.

391 **Consider that fatty acids** . . . Saturation has to do with the number of double bonds in a fatty acid. Fatty acids are long chains of carbon atoms linked together. Each carbon has four places where it can link to other atoms. In the interior of fatty acids, two of these sites link carbons to each other, leaving the remaining two sites for hydrogen. If every carbon is fully linked to two hydrogens, the fatty acid is "saturated." When two adjacent carbons have only one hydrogen each, the bond between them becomes double. A fatty acid with one

double bond is "monounsaturated"; with more than one double bond, it is "polyunsaturated." Double bonds are points of flexibility where the molecules can bend. Bending prevents stacking and makes the oil fluid. Fatty acids with three or more double bonds are exceptionally fluid, unstable, and subject to oxidation.

394 **But flaxseed oil is . . .** If untreated to prevent oxidative damage, flaxseed oil turns into linseed oil, which is inedible and best used as a furniture polish. See the Flax Council of Canada at www.flaxcouncil.ca. The treated kinds have fewer omega-3s.

395 **Entire books are devoted . . .** Artemis P. Simopoulos and Jo Robinson, *The Omega Plan* (HarperCollins, 1998). See Vasuki Wijendran and K. C. Hayes, "Dietary n-6 and n-3 Fatty Acid Balance and Cardiovascular Health," *Annual Review of Nutrition* 24 (2004): 597–615. The omega-3, -6, and -9 designations distinguish "families" of fatty acids that differ in the place on the carbon chain where the first double bond (with the missing hydrogens) is located. The position is #3 from the "methyl" (omega) end in omega-3s, #6 in omega-6s, and #9 in omega-9s. Alpha-linolenic, linoleic, and oleic acids all have 18 carbons. Linoleic has one double bond (at position #6); alpha-linolenic acid (omega-3) and oleic acid (omega-9) each have two double bonds.

397 **After reviewing the research . . .** "Letter Responding to Health Claim Petition Dated August 28, 2003: Monounsaturated Fatty Acids from Olive Oil and Coronary Heart Disease," November 1, 2004, at www.cfsan.fda.gov/~dms/qhcolive. html.

397 **Enova advertisements . . .** Its Nutrition Facts label shows that Enova has the same composition as peanut oil, except with half a gram of saturated fat as compared to 2 grams in peanut oil. This adds up to only 12.5 grams of fat, leaving 1.5 of the 14 grams unaccounted for. On processed foods, a gap like this suggests *trans*, but the site gives no explanation. The biochemistry of this type of diglyceride is reviewed in Marie-Pierre St.-Onge, "Dietary Fats, Teas, Dairy, and Nuts: Potential Functional Foods for Weight Control?" *American Journal of Clinical Nutrition* 81 (January 2005): 7–15. Enova is produced as a joint venture between Archer Daniels Midland and a Japanese company, Kao Corp. They expect sales to exceed $150 million annually, according to *Nutrition Business Journal* (July/August 2004).

398 **If you would like the FDA . . .** You can easily find out how to contact your representatives at www.congress.org.

398 **The 2005 *Dietary Guidelines* . . .** These are at www.healthierus.gov/dietary guidelines. For helpful advice about choosing fats, see Bonnie Liebman, "Face the Fats," *Nutrition Action Healthletter* (July/August 2002).

33. WATER, WATER EVERYWHERE: BOTTLED AND NOT

401 **You do need to drink . . .** Institute of Medicine, "Dietary Reference Intakes: Water, Potassium, Sodium, Chloride, and Sulfate," National Academies Press, February 11, 2004. See also Heinz Valtin, "'Drink at Least Eight Glasses of Water a Day.' Really? Is There Scientific Evidence for '8 x 8'?" *American Journal of Physiology—Regulatory, Integrative and Comparative Physiology* 283 (2002): 993–1004; and WenYen Juan and P. Peter Basiotis, "More Than One in Three

Older Americans May Not Drink Enough Water," *Family Economics and Nutrition Review* (USDA) 16 (2004): 49–51.

402 **Maybe, but the beverage . . .** For the industry position, see Laura Gorman, "The Specialty Beverage Market," *The Gourmet Retailer* (November 1, 2001), available at www.gourmetretailer.com. The International Bottled Water Association is at www.bottledwater.org.

403 **In the United States . . .** See "Surveillance for Waterborne-Disease Outbreaks Associated with Drinking Water—United States, 2001–2002," *Morbidity and Mortality Weekly Report* 53 (October 22, 2004): 23–45. I am indebted to Dr. Walter Lynn, a commissioner of the Bolton Point water system, for "The solution . . ." quotation.

404 **Ironically, chlorine . . .** See, for example, Kenneth P. Cantor, "Drinking Water and Cancer," *Cancer Causes and Control* 8 (1997): 292–308; and C. M. Villanueva et al., "Meta-Analysis of Studies on Individual Consumption of Chlorinated Drinking Water and Bladder Cancer," *Journal of Epidemiology and Community Health* 57 (2003): 166–73. See also G. M. Shaw et al., "Trihalomethane Exposures from Municipal Water Supplies and Selected Congenital Malformations," and L. Dodds et al., "Trihalomethanes in Public Water Supplies and the Risk of Stillbirth," *Epidemiology* 14 (November 2003): 650–58; and 15 (March 2004): 179–86.

404 **But there is no debate . . .** Herbert T. Buxton and Dana W. Kolpin, "Pharmaceuticals, Hormones, and Other Organic Wastewater Contaminants in U.S. Streams," U.S. Geological Survey Fact Sheet FS-027-02, June 2002, at toxics.usgs.gov. For general information, see www.usgs.gov. For EPA reports, see "Water on Tap: What You Need to Know," October 2003, and maps at www.epa.gov/safewater. The New York City "2003 Drinking Water Supply and Quality Report" is also at that site. Early in 2005, debates about safe levels in drinking water of perchlorate, an especially toxic component of rocket fuel, made the news. See Felicity Barringer, "Science Panel Issues Report on Exposure to Pollutant," *The New York Times*, January 12, 2005.

405 **As recently as 1998 . . .** The quotation comes from Corby Kummer, "What's in the Water?," *The New York Times Magazine*, August 30, 1998. And see Robert Weinhold, "Is Your Drinking Water Really Safe?" *Organic Style* (September 2004): 111–16, 133; and Margaret Magnarelli and Peter Jaret, "Is Your Family's Water Safe?" *Good Housekeeping* (February 2005) (this article focuses on lead).

405 **Your water utility bill . . .** Steve Maxwell, "Water Is Cheap—Ridiculously Cheap!" *Journal AWWA* [American Water Works Association] (June 2005): 38–41.

406 **The brands vary . . .** Sherri Day, "Summer May Bring a Bottled Water Price War," *The New York Times*, May 10, 2003. Sales were $8.3 billion in 2003 (6.4 billion gallons). PepsiCo's Aquafina was the leading brand with $936 million in sales, according to *Nutrition Business Journal* (July/August, 2004). Marketing figures are from *Advertising Age* (June 27, 2005).

406 **By law, mineral waters . . .** FDA, "Beverages: Bottled Water; Final Rule," *Federal Register* 60 (November 13, 1995): 57076–133. See also FDA, "Bottled Water Regulation and the FDA," *Food Safety Magazine* (August/September 2002), available at www.cfsan.fda.gov.

409   **Back home . . .** The Bolton Point water system's "Drinking Water Quality Report 2004" describes treatment methods and test results, and cites costs.

409   **For this and other reasons . . .** Ian Williams, "Message in a Bottle," *Investor Relations*, September 2004.

409   **In 1999, for example . . .** See "Bottled Water: Pure Drink or Pure Hype?" at www.nrdc.org. Environmental Defense also advocates for water quality at www.edf.org.

410   **Zebra mussels or not . . .** Felicity Barriner, "Billions Needed to Improve Great Lakes, Coalition Says," *The New York Times*, July 8, 2005. "Water: The City of Chicago's Water Quality Report, 2004," at egov.cityofchicago.org/webportal/ COCWebPortal/COC_ATTACH/2004wqr.pdf. The effects of zebra mussels on water quality are complicated; they are bottom feeders credited with clarifying the water of the St. Lawrence River, which drains the Great Lakes, for example.

412   **But this does not make . . .** Barbara J. Rolls and Robert A. Barnett, *Volumetrics: Feel Full on Fewer Calories* (HarperCollins, 2000).

413   **That is why I did not . . .** The invitation came from Stacey Druker, at Evins Communications, July 27, 2005. The null research on hydroxycitrate is reviewed in Sheldon S. Hendler, *PDR for Nutritional Supplements* (Medical Economics/Thomson Healthcare, 2001), 216–17.

413   **In August 2005, Starbucks . . .** See Theresa Howard, "Starbucks Takes Up Cause for Safe Drinking Water," *USA Today*, August 2, 2005. For nongovernmental agencies working on this issue, see www.wateraid.org.uk and www. globalwater.org. The "silent humanitarian crisis" caused by lack of clean water is reviewed by Jamie Bartram et al., "Focusing on Improved Water and Sanitation for Health," *Lancet* 365 (2005): 810–12.

414   **You may have heard that plasticizers . . .** Common plasticizers are polyethylene terephthalate (PET), high-density polyethylene (HDPE), and to a lesser extent polyvinylchloride (PVC). See Klaus Guenther et al., "Endocrine Disrupting Nonylphenols Are Ubiquitous in Foods," *Environmental Science and Technology* 36 (2002) : 1676–80; Jorge E. Loyo-Rosales et al., "Migration of Nonylphenol from Plastic Containers to Water and a Milk Surrogate," *Journal of Agricultural and Food Chemistry* 52 (2004): 2016–20; and Johns Hopkins Office of Communications and Public Affairs, "Researcher Dispels Myth of Dioxins and Plastic Water Bottles," June 24, 2004, at www.jhsph.edu/publichealthnews/ articles/halden_dioxins.html.

34. "HEALTHY" DRINKS: SUGARED AND ARTIFICIALLY SWEETENED

417   **PepsiCo's Propel . . .** Marketing figures are from *Advertising Age* (June 27, 2005). Sales figures for Glacéau waters are from Kate MacArthur, "Pepsi Picks Water Fight with Surging Glacéau," *Advertising Age* (October 17, 2005). See also Reuters, "PepsiCo Profit Increases 13% on Strength of Overseas Sales," *The New York Times*, July 13, 2005.

419   **A small company, Fizzy . . .** See www.fizzylizzy.com. The company's difficulties getting its products placed in supermarkets are discussed in Matt Lee and Ted Lee, "Message in a Bottle," *The New York Times Magazine*, June 26, 2005.

419   **Indeed, the American Academy . . .** American Academy of Pediatrics, "The Use and Misuse of Fruit Juice in Pediatrics," *Pediatrics* 107 (May 5, 2001): 1210–13.

422   **Gatorade Orange sports . . .** Yellow 6 is a color additive. Ester gum is a thickener. Brominated vegetable oil is there to keep the flavors in suspension; although its health effects were evaluated in 1970 and found to be minimal, Center for Science in the Public Interest (www.cspinet.org) puts it in the "Caution" category: "May pose a risk and needs to be better tested. Try to avoid."

423   **This practice greatly upsets . . .** Kevin Bouffard, "2 Orange Juice Makers Refuse to Change Labels," *The Ledger*, December 15, 2004, available at www.theledger.com; and Chad Terhune, "Florida Requests Change in Labels for Orange Drinks," *The Wall Street Journal*, December 15, 2004.

423   **Adding water also is . . .** Richard Turcsik, "Why Less May Be More: Reduced Calorie Colas Targeting Low Carb Dieters Are Bringing Some Fizz Back to the Carbonated Soft Drink Aisle," *Progressive Grocer* (October 1, 2004); and Kate MacArthur, "Over the Edge: Pepsi Sinks Mid-Calorie Cola," *Advertising Age* (May 23, 2005).

423   **In 2005, Coca-Cola . . .** Stuart Elliott, "What's in a Name? Higher Sales, or That's the Hope of Some Soft-Drink Makers Excising the Word 'Diet,'" *The New York Times*, December 20, 2004. Chad Terhune, "In Switch, Pepsi Makes Diet Cola Its New Flagship," *The Wall Street Journal*, March 16, 2005; and Kate MacArthur, "Sweet Nothings," *Advertising Age* (March 28, 2005). For an overview of artificial sweeteners see David Schardt, "Sweet Nothings: Not All Sweeteners Are Equal," *Nutrition Action Healthletter* (May 2004).

426   **At that point, Congress . . .** See "The Great Saccharin Snafu," *Consumer Reports* (July 1977); David Perlman, "Saccharin Has Powerful Friends," *San Francisco Chronicle*, June 8, 1977; R. Jeffrey Smith, "Latest Saccharin Tests Kill FDA Proposal," *Science* 208 (1980): 154–56; and "The Sweet and Sour History of Saccharine, Cyclamate, Aspartame," *FDA Consumer* (September 1981). Donald Kennedy's role in the saccharin ban is discussed in Phil Hilts, *Protecting America's Health: The FDA, Business, and One Hundred Years of Regulation* (Knopf, 2003). His e-mail message is quoted with permission.

426   **Coca-Cola still uses . . .** The company history is outlined at www2.coca-cola.com. See also Mark Pendergrast, *For God, Country, and Coca-Cola: The Definitive History of the Great American Soft Drink and the Company That Makes It* (Basic Books, 2000).

428   **Regulatory agencies, which . . .** FDA, "Food Labeling: Saccharin and Its Salts; Retail Establishment Notice: Final Rule," *Federal Register* 62 (January 27, 1997): 3791–92. See also Leila Corcoran and Michael Jacobson, "Saccharin: Bittersweet," *Nutrition Action Healthletter* (April 1998).

428   **The saccharin saga . . .** Aspartame was discovered by Searle, and sold to Monsanto in 1985; in 2000, Monsanto sold the commercial product, NutraSweet, to J. W. Childs Equity, and the table product, Equal, to Merisant. Acesulfame-K is a product of Celanese Nutrinova, formerly Hoechst. Sucralose is produced by Tate and Lyle for the McNeil division of Johnson and Johnson. See "Position of the American Dietetic Association: Use of Nutritive and Nonnutritive Sweeteners," *Journal of the American Dietetic Association* 104 (2004): 255–75. The Calorie Control Council material is at www.caloriecontrol.org. FDA approval does

not guarantee safety, but means that the chemicals seem safe enough as typically used.

429 **But large numbers of studies ...** See Lewis D. Stegink, "The Aspartame Story: A Model for the Clinical Testing of a Food Additive," *American Journal of Clinical Nutrition* 46 (1987): 204–15.

429 **More recent studies ...** The rat study is Morando Soffritti et al., "First Experimental Demonstration of the Multipotential Carcinogenic Effects of Aspartame Administered in the Feed to Sprague-Dawley Rats," *Environmental Health Perspectives* online November 17, 2005, at ehp.niehs.nih.gov (search for doi:10.1289/ehp.8711). The study reported an increase in several forms of cancer across a very large range of aspartame intake (80 to 100,000 parts per million). Conclusion: more research "is urgent and cannot be delayed."

430 **In the mid-1990s, a letter ...** Anti-aspartame Web sites are at presidiotex.com/ aspartame/Nancy_Markle/nancy_markle.html and www.holisticmed.com/ aspartame.

430 **In October 2004 ...** Michael E. J. Lean and Catherine R. Hankey, "Aspartame and Its Effects on Health," *British Medical Journal* 329 (October 2, 2004): 755–56. Average consumption of diet soft drinks was about 120 12-ounce cans a year per person in 2003; a heavy user would consume one or more such drinks a day. See USDA/ERS food consumption data at www.ers.usda.gov/data/ foodconsumption; and Michael F. Jacobson, "Liquid Candy: How Soft Drinks Are Harming America's Health," Center for Science in the Public Interest, June 2005, at www.cspinet.org.

430 **The CSPI ...** CSPI additive information is at www.cspinet.org. See also FDA, "Food Additives Permitted for Direct Addition to Food for Human Consumption; Acesulfame Potassium" and "Final Rule," *Federal Register* 63 (July 6, 1998): 36344–65.

431 **The FDA approved sucralose ...** FDA, "Food Additives Permitted ... for Human Consumption; Sucralose: Final Rule," *Federal Register* 63 (April 3, 1998): 16417–33. See Carole Sugarman, "Putting Splenda to the Test," *The Washington Post*, October 25, 2000; Gwenn Friss, "The Splenda of Holiday Baking," *Cape Cod Times*, December 8, 2004, available at www.capecodonline.com; Stephanie Thompson, "Splenda Sweetens Line as Carb Craze Fades," *Advertising Age* (November 8, 2004); Eric Herman, "Merisant Files Suit over Rival Sugar Substitute," *Chicago Sun-Times*, November 30, 2004; and Kate MacArthur, "Rivals, Sugar Industry Take Aim at Splenda," *Advertising Age* (February 14, 2005).

432 **Whole Foods Markets ...** The body has a range of "detoxification" enzyme systems that metabolize—break down or neutralize—toxic substances to those that are harmless and can be excreted. These enzymes do not act on sucralose to any appreciable extent. So it is unclear what happens to the sucralose that is not excreted in urine. The Whole Foods philosophy is at www.wholefoods market.com/company/philosophy.html.

432 **I get asked all the time ...** See, for example, www.stevia.net.

35. TEAS AND COFFEES: CAFFEINE TO ECO-LABELS

436 **The late, great food writer ...** Alan Davidson, *The Oxford Companion to Food* (Oxford University Press, 1999), 200. For the cultural history of coffee and tea,

see *The Cambridge World History of Food*, Vol. 1 (Cambridge University Press, 2000), 641–52 and 712–19; and Ernesto Illy, "The Complexity of Coffee," *Scientific American* (June 2002).

437 **Caffeine is a mild "upper"** . . . T. R. Reid, "Caffeine," *National Geographic* (January 2005): 2–33; Sherri Day, "Energy Drinks Charm the Young and Caffeinated," *The New York Times*, April 4, 2004; Michael J. McCarthy, "The Caffeine Count in Your Morning Fix," *The Wall Street Journal*, April 13, 2004; and Melanie Warner, "A Jolt of Caffeine by the Can," *The New York Times*, November 23, 2005. See also H. G. Mandel, "Update on Caffeine Consumption, Disposition and Action," and A. Smith, "Effects of Caffeine on Human Behavior," *Food Chemistry and Toxicology* 40 (2002): 1231–34 and 1243–55, respectively.

437 **It has stronger effects** . . . F. X. Castellanos and J. L. Rapoport, "Effects of Caffeine on Development and Behavior in Infancy and Childhood: A Review of the Published Literature," *Food Chemistry and Toxicology* 40 (2002): 1235–42.

438 **There is something about coffee** . . . Wolfgang C. Winkelmayer et al., "Habitual Caffeine Intake and the Risk of Hypertension in Women," *Journal of the American Medical Association* 294 (November 9, 2005) 2330–35.

438 **Complicating an overall assessment** . . . J. Schwartz and S. T. Weiss, "Caffeine Intake and Asthma Symptoms," *Annals of Epidemiology* 2 (1992): 627–35, and A. I. Bara and E. A. Barley, "Caffeine for Asthma," *The Cochrane Database of Systematic Reviews* 3 (2005), at www.cochrane.org/reviews/en/ab001112.html.

438 **Also, the physiological** . . . Elizabeth M. Puccio et al., "Clustering of Atherogenic Behaviors in Coffee Drinkers," *American Journal of Public Health* 80 (November 1990): 1310–13. Also see International Coffee Organization, "Coffee Confirmed as Significant Source of Antioxidants in the Diet," at www.positively coffee.org/topic_antioxidant_latest.aspx.

439 **The business side of Starbucks** . . . The annual report gives relevant facts and figures at www.starbucks.com/aboutus, as does "Bean Counters," *Point/Advertising Age* (October 2005):24.

440 **So do other people** . . . Laura Gorman, "The Specialty Beverage Market," *Gourmet Retailer*, November 1, 2001, at www.gourmetretailer.com/gourmet retailer/magazine/article_display.jsp?vnu_content_id=1095221.

441 **The ad referred** . . . Jeffrey Blumberg, editor, "Proceedings of the Third International Scientific Symposium on Tea and Human Health: Role of Flavonoids in the Diet," and Augustin Scalbert et al., editors, "Dietary Polyphenols and Health," *American Journal of Clinical Nutrition* 133 Supplement (October 2003) and 81 Supplement (January 2005), respectively. The quotation is from Richard Béliveau and Denis Gingras, "Green Tea: Prevention and Treatment of Cancer by Nutraceuticals," *Lancet* 364 (September 18, 2004): 1021–22.

443 **In 2004, Dr. Sin Hang Lee** . . . Dr. Lee's company sponsors an educational Web site at www.greenteahaus.com, and sells products at www.teaforhealth. com. The FDA ruling is "Letter Responding to Health Claim Petition Dated January 7, 2004: Green Tea and Reduced Risk of Cancer Health Claim," June 30, 2005, at www.cfsan.fda.gov/~dms/qhc-gtea.html. The American Herbal Products Association statement, "FDA Allows Qualified Health Claims . . . ," July 7, 2005, is at www.ahpa.org. The politics of the decision are discussed in Phil Wallace, "Highly Qualified Green Tea Health Claims Draw Criticism," *Food Chemical News* (July 11, 2005).

444 **Never mind that qualified** . . . Consumer understanding of such claims is dis-

cussed in Janet Adamy and Anna Wilde Mathews, "Do Food Claims Help Consumers or Baffle Them?" *The Wall Street Journal*, May 27, 2005, and Brenda M. Derby and Alan S. Levy, "Effects of Strength of Science Disclaimers on the Communication Impacts of Health Claims," Working Paper No. 1, September 2005, available at www.fda.gov/OHRMS/dockets/dockets/03N0496/03N-0496-rpt0001.pdf.

444　**Chai, say its makers . . .** Oregon Chai sponsors the dictionary lobbying campaign at www.oregonchai.com.

446　**At the 2004 Fancy Food . . .** Zhena's Gypsy Teas ("Join us and awaken the gypsy in you!") are at www.gypsytea.com. Peace Coffees are at www.peacecoffee.com.

446　**Sorting out the new eco-labels . . .** See Katy McLaughlin, "Is Your Grocery List Politically Correct?" *The Wall Street Journal*, February 17, 2004; Steve Stecklow and Erin White, "What Price Virtue?" *The Wall Street Journal*, June 8, 2004; and Doreen Carvajal, "Third World Gets Help to Help Itself," *International Herald Tribune*, May 7–8, 2005. TransFair USA is the certifier of Fair Trade coffees and teas: www.transfairusa.org. The Rainforest Alliance is at www.rainforest-alliance.org. The Smithsonian bird-friendly site is nationalzoo.si.edu/ConservationandScience/MigratoryBirds/Coffee/default.cfm.

447　**In the summer of 2004 . . .** The letter was dated July 14, 2004. It accompanied "The Nestlé Coffee Report: Faces of Coffee," March 2004. The company's Web site is www.nestle.com.

36. INFANT FORMULA AND BABY FOOD

453　**Formula giveaways . . .** See, for example, Cynthia Howard et al., "Office Prenatal Formula Advertising and Its Effect on Breast-feeding Patterns," *Obstetrics and Gynecology* 95 (2002): 296–303. For breast-feeding advocacy, see Baby Milk Action at www.babymilkaction.org, and the International Baby Food Action Network at www.ibfan.org.

453　**Formula feeding soon . . .** Rima D. Apple, *Mothers and Medicine: A Social History of Infant Feeding, 1890–1950* (University of Wisconsin Press, 1987).

453　**To use formula properly . . .** Sami Shubber, *The International Code of Marketing of Breast-Milk Substitutes: An International Measure to Protect and Promote Breast-Feeding* (Kluwer Law International, 1998); and Naomi Baumslag and Dia L. Michaels, *Milk, Money, and Madness: The Culture and Politics of Breastfeeding* (Bergin & Garvey, 1995). The International Baby Food Action Network (IBFAN) publishes a report on code violations every three years. See, for example, "Breaking the Rules, Stretching the Rules," 2004, at www.ibfan.org/english/pdfs/btr04.pdf.

454　**If they lack even one . . .** Greg Myre, "With a Common Thread, Israelis Unravel Infants' Illness," *The New York Times*, November 17, 2003. See also Michael H. Malloy et al., "Hypochloremic Metabolic Alkalosis from Ingestion of a Chloride-Deficient Infant Formula: Outcome 9 and 10 Years Later," *Pediatrics* 87 (June 1991): 811–22 (the outcome was not good). For information about health and safety issues related to the composition of these products, see *Infant Formula: Evaluating the Safety of New Ingredients*, Institute of Medicine, 2004.

455　**The American Academy of Pediatrics . . .** American Academy of Pediatrics, Committee on Nutrition, "Soy Protein-Based Formulas: Recommendations for

Use in Infant Feeding," *Pediatrics* 101 (January 1998): 148–53, available at aap policy.aappublications.org. See also Brian L. Strom et al., "Exposure to Soy-Based Formula in Infancy and Endocrinological and Reproductive Outcomes in Young Adulthood," *Journal of the American Medical Association* 286 (2001): 807–14.

456 **Because most mothers . . .** Malika Rajan, "U.S. Market for Ethical Nutrition to Reach $13.6 Billion by 2008," BCC Business Communications, Report RGA-112, August 18, 2004, at www.bccresearch.com/editors/RGA-112R.html; and Markos Kaminis, "A Growing Boost for Baby Formula," *Business Week* (January 11, 2005), available at www.businessweek.com/investor/content/jan2005/pi20050111_1011_PG2_pi008.htm. See also Victor Oliveira and Mark Prell, "Sharing the Economic Burden: Who Pays for WIC's Infant Formula," *Amber Waves* (USDA) (September 2004): 31–36; and Associated Press, "Baby Formula? The Locked Case at the Front of the Store," *The New York Times*, June 5, 2005.

457 **In 2001, for example, the courts . . .** Michael Brick, "Makers of Generic Baby Formula Win Round in Court," *The New York Times*, May 2, 2001.

457 **These two fatty acids . . .** See, for example, P. Willatts et al., "Effect of Long-Chain Polyunsaturated Fatty Acids in Infant Formula on Problem Solving at 10 Months of Age," *Lancet* 352 (August 29, 1998): 688–91 (sponsored by Milupa, Ltd, U.K.); Eileen E. Birch et al., "Visual Acuity and the Essentiality of Docosa-hexaenoic Acid and Arachidonic Acid in the Diet of Term Infants," *Pediatric Research* 44 (1998): 201–9 (Mead Johnson); and Nancy Auestad et al., "Visual, Cognitive, and Language Assessments at 39 Months: A Follow-up Study of Children Fed Formulas Containing Long-Chain Polyunsaturated Fatty Acids to 1 Year of Age," *Pediatrics* 112 (September 2003): E177–E183 (the lead author worked for Ross and another investigator worked for Abbott).

457 **Apparently, the FDA agreed . . .** See Q and A on infant formulas, July 2002, at www.cfsan.fda.gov/~dms/qa-infl7.html.

458 **A highly authoritative . . .** Joyce C. McCann and Bruce N. Ames, "Is Docosa-hexaenoic Acid, an n-3 Long-Chain Polyunsaturated Fatty Acid, Required for Development of Normal Brain Function? An Overview of Evidence from Cognitive and Behavioral Tests in Humans and Animals," *American Journal of Clinical Nutrition* 82 (2005): 281–95.

458 **International formula makers . . .** Examples of DHA-formula advertising in many countries are shown in *Baby Milk Action Update* (July 2005), and at www.ibfan.org/english/pdfs/btr04.pdf. Selling omega-3 formulas to U.S. consumers is discussed by Greg Retsinas, "The Marketing of a Superbaby Formula," *The New York Times*, June 1, 2003. The advertisement to dietitians appeared in the *Journal of the American Dietetic Association* (October 2004).

459 **In 2002, the FDA warned . . .** FDA warnings are at www.cfsan.fda.gov. See Kwan Kew Lai, "*Enterobacter sakazakii* Infections Among Neonates, Infants, Children, and Adults: Case Reports and a Review of the Literature," *Medicine* 80 (March 2001): 113–22.

460 **Surprising as it may seem . . .** You can do this too. Home-prepared foods can be more nutritious and contain fewer additives than commercial products. All you need to do is grind unsalted and unsweetened cooked table foods to a smooth, moist consistency in a clean food processor and use them immediately. Or you can just mash a banana or cooked peas, adding water as needed.

461 **Pediatricians say . . .** Lloyd N. Werk and Joel L. Alpert, "Solid Feeding Guide-

lines," *Lancet* 352 (November 14, 1998): 1569–70. See also statements from the American Academy of Pediatrics at www.aap.org.

462 **As the judge explained . . .** James Robertson, U.S. District Judge, U.S. District Court for the District of Columbia, *Federal Trade Commission v. H. J. Heinz,* October 2001, at www.dcd.uscourts.gov/00-1688.pdf (no longer active).

463 **Heinz sees the half . . .** The "upside opportunity" part of the quotation is from "Baby-Food Makers Heinz, Beech-Nut Call Off Merger Following Court Ruling," *The Wall Street Journal,* April 27, 2001. For examples of Gerber-sponsored professional articles, see *Food Technology* 57 (October 2003): 18–34 (three articles on infant feeding and foods); *Journal of the American Dietetics Association* 104, Supplement 1 (January 2004) (reports from a Gerber-sponsored study) and 104 (March 2004): 443–67 (two articles on healthy feeding guidelines); and *Pediatrics* 114, Supplement (October 2004) (conference report on preventing childhood obesity).

464 **So, apparently . . .** Associated Press, "Parents with Pesticide Fears Turn to Organic Baby Food," *USA Today,* November 2, 2005.

464 **In this view, I also have . . .** EPA statements on pesticides in children's diets are at www.epa.gov/pesticides/food/pest.htm. For advocacy group reports, see National Resources Defense Council, "Intolerable Risk: Pesticides in Our Children's Food," February 27, 1989; and Environmental Working Group, "Pesticides in Children's Food," 1993, with updated information at www.ewg.org.

465 **But does eating organic food . . .** Cynthia L. Curl et al., "Organophosphorus Pesticide Exposure of Urban and Suburban Preschool Children with Organic and Conventional Diets," *Environmental Health Perspectives* 111 (March 2003): 377–82, available at ehp.niehs.nih.gov. See also Office of New York State Attorney General Eliot Spitzer, "States Petition EPA to Protect Children from Pesticides," press release, December 17, 2004, available at www.oag.state.ny.us.

37. SUPPLEMENTS AND HEALTH FOOD

466 **I had just seen a full-page . . .** The ad appeared in *The New York Times* on November 29, 2005. The Council for Responsible Nutrition Web site is www.crnusa.org. The study examining clinical trials is Edgar R. Miller III et al., "Meta-Analysis: High-Dosage Vitamin E Supplementation May Increase All-Cause Mortality," *Annals of Internal Medicine* 142 (2005): 37–46. The study was published online, November 10, 2004. It is explained by Gina Kolata, "Large Doses of Vitamin E May Be Harmful, Study Shows," *The New York Times,* November 11, 2004.

467 **The 400 IU dose . . .** This and other information about the supplement industry is available (at not inconsiderable expense) from *Nutrition Business Journal* at www.nutritionbusiness.com; information about vitamin E appeared in the May/June 2004 issue, page 41. Problems with high-dose vitamins are discussed in Penny M. Kris-Etherton et al., "Antioxidant Vitamin Supplements and Cardiovascular Disease," *Circulation* 110 (2004): 637–41; and Goran Bjelakovic et al., "Antioxidant Supplements for Prevention of Gastrointestinal Cancer: A Systematic Review and Meta-Analysis," *Lancet* 364 (October 2, 2004): 1219–28. More recent studies with disappointing results include, for example, the HOPE and HOPE-TOO Trial Investigators, "Effects of Long-Term Vitamin E Supplementation on Cardiovascular Events and Cancer: A Randomized Controlled

Trial," *Journal of the American Medical Association* 293 (2005): 1338–47 (see also editorial on pages 1387–90); Isabelle Bairati et al., "A Randomized Trial of Antioxidant Vitamins to Prevent Second Primary Cancers in Head and Neck Cancer Patients," *Journal of the National Cancer Institute* 97 (2005): 481–88; and George Davey Smith and Shah Ebrahim, "Folate Supplementation and Cardiovascular Disease," *Lancet* 366 (November 12, 2005): 1680–81. But see John Hathcock et al., "Vitamins E and C Are Safe Across a Broad Range of Intakes," *American Journal of Clinical Nutrition* 81 (2005): 736–45 (Hathcock is scientific director of the Council for Responsible Nutrition and several co-authors are also employed by vitamin supplement trade associations or firms).

468   **Wyeth, for example . . .** The letter from Andrew C. Davis, senior vice president, Wyeth Consumer Health Care, March 3, 2004, enclosed a report from the Lewin Group, "A Study of the Cost Effects of Daily Multivitamins for Older Adults: Fact Sheet," September 24, 2003. The study draws on a paper by Kathleen M. Fairfield and Robert H. Fletcher, "Vitamins for Chronic Disease Prevention in Adults: Scientific Review," *Journal of the American Medical Association* 287 (2002): 3116–26 (with commentary on pages 3127–29). This paper recognizes that vitamin deficiencies are rare but suggests that supplements be used to correct "suboptimal nutrition," the cause of metabolic abnormalities that increase disease risk. The later report, edited by Jeffrey Blumberg and David Heber, is "Multivitamins & Public Health: Exploring the Evidence," undated but attributed to the Wyeth-sponsored workshop convened October 1, 2003. Wyeth is at www.wyeth.com.

469   **If you are like the majority . . .** Amy E. Millen et al., "Use of Vitamin, Mineral, Nonvitamin, and Nonmineral Supplements in the United States: The 1987, 1992, and 2000 National Health Interview Survey Results," *Journal of the American Dietetic Association* 104 (2004): 942–50; and Lina S. Balluz et al., "Vitamin or Supplement Use Among Adults, Behavioral Risk Factor Surveillance System, 13 States, 2001," *Public Health Reports* 120 (March–April 2005): 117–23. This last paper concludes, "People who used V/S [vitamins or supplements] . . . were more likely to demonstrate positive health risk behaviors than those who did not report V/S use. Thus it appears that individuals who are most likely to use V/S are least likely to need V/S."

470   **You think this scenario . . .** FDA rules about supplements are at www.cfsan. fda.gov. For ephedra, see Murray Chass, "Coroner Learns Bechler Was Using Weight-Loss Aid," *The New York Times*, February 19, 2003. Paul G. Shekelle et al., "Efficacy and Safety of Ephedra and Ephedrine for Weight Loss and Athletic Performance: A Meta-Analysis," *Journal of the American Medical Association* 289 (2003): 1537–45. Lobbying by Metabolife is discussed in Sidney M. Wolfe, "Ephedra—Scientific Evidence Versus Money/Politics," *Science* 300 (April 18, 2003): 437. The FDA banned ephedra sales February 6, 2004. *Nutrition Business Journal* gives figures on ephedra sales in its May/June 2004 issue on page 29. In 2005, Metabolife asked the courts for a class action settlement of its ephedra lawsuits (see *Food Chemical News*, January 10, 2005). The Utah decision is in Gardiner Harris, "Judge's Decision Lifts Ban on Sale of Ephedra in Utah," *The New York Times*, April 15, 2005; and Anna Wilde Mathews and Sara Schaefer Muñoz, "Judge Overturns Ban on Ephedra, Roils FDA Policy," *The Wall Street Journal*, April 15, 2005.

472   **The industry's need for damage . . .** "Annual Industry Overview 2005" and

"Vitamin Capacity Shifts to China; Vitamin E Supplies Pile Up," *Nutrition Business Journal* (May/June 2005 and August/September 2005, respectively).

472   **A private company, ConsumerLab.com . . .** The Web site is www.consumerlab.com. For the Council for Responsible Nutrition's charges against it, see Phil Wallace, "CRN Asks FTC Investigation of Testing Company's Practices," *Food Chemical News* (January 24, 2005). This article notes that the ConsumerLab.com Web site has 20,000 subscribers.

473   **It is a relief of sorts . . .** Protein supplements have marvelous labels. Here is the charmingly misspelled VPX Zero Carb: "Pushing the envelope of technology . . . fat incerating [*sic*—I think this means incinerating] protein . . . cold-filtered cross-flow QUADRAFILTRATION whey protein isolate proprietary microfraction profile comprised of complete spectrum molecular weights for sustained protein absorbtion [*sic*] and increased nitrogen retention." Translation: milk proteins.

474   **Instead, they rely on store copies . . .** Phyllis A. Balch and James F. Balch, *Prescription for Nutritional Healing*, 3rd edition (Avery 2000).

475   **Disappointing research results . . .** The quotation is from *Nutrition Business Journal* (May/June 2004). More recent sales figures are from April 2005 and August/September 2005.The echinacea study is Ronald B. Turner et al., "An Evaluation of *Echinacea angustifolia* in Experimental Rhinovirus Infections," *New England Journal of Medicine* 353 (2005): 341–48; the editorial, by Wallace Sampson, is on pages 337–39. See also Gina Kolata, "Study Says Popular Herb Has No Effect on Colds," *The New York Times*, July 28, 2005.

476   **Research is a worry . . .** Peter A.G.M. De Smet, "Herbal Medicine in Europe—Relaxing Regulatory Standards," *New England Journal of Medicine* 352 (2005): 1176–78.

476   **One intriguing observation . . .** These sales figures were reported in *Nutrition Business Journal*, May/June 2005.

476   **You have to decide for yourself . . .** For research-based reviews of supplements, see Sheldon S. Handler and David Rorvik, *PDR for Nutritional Supplements* and the *PDR for Herbal Medicines*, 3rd edition (Thomson Healthcare, 2001 and 2004, respectively). These do the best they can with the limited science, often summarizing it with qualifiers: "there is some evidence" but "data are mixed," "no effect has been convincingly demonstrated outside the laboratory," or "effects are seen in rats, but no human data exist." The Office of Dietary Supplements at the NIH provides extensive information about specific supplements on its Web site, dietary-supplements.info.nih.gov, as does the FDA at www.cfsan.fda.gov/~dms/supplmnt.html. Authoritative research on herbal products appears in *HerbalGram*, the journal of the American Botanical Council (www.herbalgram.org), and on particular classes of supplements in *Consumer Reports* (www.consumerreports.org) and *Nutrition Action Healthletter* (www.cspinet.org).

478   ***Nutrition Business Journal* tracks sales . . .** The July/August 2004 lead article is devoted to functional foods as is an article on pages 34–35 by Nancy Childs, "Obesity Policy Promises a Functional Food Feast." She is a professor of food marketing at the Haub School of Business, St. Joseph's University, Philadelphia.

479   **It is no accident . . .** These figures for "measured" media (television, radio, print) are from *Advertising Age* (June 28, 2004).

480   ***Consumer Reports* says . . .** "Energy Bars, Unwrapped" (June 2003).

483 **Supermarkets are well aware . . .** Vishal Khanna, "Hot from the Oven: In-Store Bread Baking Basics," *The Natural Foods Merchandiser* (August 1, 2001), at www.naturalfoodsmerchandiser.com: "Here's a simple fact about in-store baking: It's the aroma that sells. The scent of bread and the theatrical aspects that surround the baking process lure consumers. Sound simple? It's not."

483 **In her book for home bakers . . .** Rose Levy Beranbaum, *The Bread Bible* (W. W. Norton, 2003). For bread in history and culture, see Alan Davidson, *The Oxford Companion to Food* (1999); and Andrew F. Smith, "Bread," in *The Oxford Encyclopedia of Food and Drink in America*, Vol. 1 (2004) (both from Oxford University Press).

483 **The baking of wheat bread . . .** See the incomparable Harold McGee, *On Food and Cooking: The Science and Lore of the Kitchen* (Scribner, 2004). If you water a wheat grain, the germ sprouts and draws on energy from the starch in the endosperm until it can make its first leaves and start photosynthesizing.

486 **My well-worn 1964 . . .** Irma S. Rombauer and Marion Rombauer Becker, *Joy of Cooking* (Bobbs-Merrill, 1964). The Rombauers greatly admired the work of Adelle Davis, the health food guru (or health faddist, if you prefer), whose *Let's Eat Right to Keep Fit* (Harcourt, 1954) greatly influenced the health food movement that followed. See Anne Mendelson, *Stand Facing the Stove: The Story of the Women Who Gave America* The Joy of Cooking (Henry Holt, 1996).

487 **The bread industry, however . . .** "Fresh Approaches," *Snack Food and Whole-sale Bakery* (July 2004), available at www.snackandbakery.com.

488 **Wonder Bread is . . .** The name, or so the story goes, came about because the company owner went to the Indianapolis Speedway to see a balloon race. He thought it was a "wonder," and put the sentiment and the balloons on the package wrapping. See www.wonderbread.com/history.asp.

490 **This really is not white bread . . .** See Donald E. Pszczola, "Ingredients for Bread Meet Changing 'Kneads,'" *Food Technology* 59 (January 2005): 55–63; and John Schmeltzer, "Satisfying Children's Picky Palates Biggest Hurdle to Success," *Chicago Tribune*, July 13, 2005.

491 **This is one reason . . .** Jayne Hurley and Bonnie Liebman, "The Whole Story: How to Find the Best Breads," *Nutrition Action Healthletter* (April 2005).

493 **Because practically everyone eats bread . . .** Paul A. Cotton et al., "Dietary Sources of Nutrients Among US Adults, 1994 to 1996," *Journal of the American Dietetic Association* 104 (June 2004): 921–30. Bread accounts for 9 percent of total calories and 13 percent of carbohydrates in U.S. diets. When pasta, crackers, cookies, and other such products are factored in, foods made with white flour account for 20 percent of total calories.

493 **In an effort to reverse . . .** The guidelines are at www.healthierus.gov/dietaryguidelines.

495 **La Brea boasts . . .** Miriam Morgan, "The Surprising Truth About San Francisco Sourdough" and "The Tasting Panel's Top Product Picks of 1997," and Robin Davis, "One Brand's Olive Bread Rises Above the Rest," *San Francisco Chronicle*, October 8, 1997, December 31, 1997, and October 10, 2001, respectively. La Brea Bakery describes its breads and processes at www.labrea bakery.com; the company is owned by IAWS Group, Dublin.

496 **You heat the bread . . .** Mark Furstenberg says five minutes in a very hot oven

(400° to 450°F) works better for reheating bread. With either method, it is best to keep an eye on the bread so the crust does not burn.

39. PREPARED FOODS: SALADS AND MORE

499 **Supermarket delis are . . .** Mark D. Jekanowski, "Grocery Industry Courts Time-Pressed Consumers with Home Meal Replacements," *FoodReview* (January–April, 1999): 32–34; Evan Hassel, "A Battle for Your Takeout Dollars in Aisle 5," *Forbes* (February 13, 2004), available at www.forbes.com; and Hayden Stewart et al., "The Demand for Food Away from Home," USDA Economic Research Service, Agricultural Economic Report No. 829, January 2004 (see Briefing Room tables at www.ers.usda.gov/briefing/CPIfoodandexpenditures/data).

500 **But hazards can be reduced . . .** "Safe Handling of Take-out Foods," October 27, 2003, at www.fsis.usda.gov/Fact_Sheets/Safe_Food_Handling_Fact_Sheets/index.asp.

501 **Restaurant violations are . . .** State rules for retail food stores are in "Circular 962," March 2004, and at www.agmkt.state.ny.us/index.html. New York City's restaurant inspection results are at www.nyc.gov/html/doh/home.html. For *Daily News* reports, see Chuck Bennett and Russ Buettner, "*Daily News* Dining Hall of Shame," September 14, 2003. The Los Angeles health department standards and results are at www.lapublichealth.org/rating.

502 **In 1999, Marian Burros . . .** See "Salad Bars: How Clean Are They?" *The New York Times*, August 25, 1999. See also Food Marketing Institute, "Supermarket Food Safety," April 1999, at www.fmi.org/foodsafety/supermarket_news/more issues/sfsapr99.html; and Kawanza L. Griffen, "Analysis Raises Safety Questions About Self-serve Salad Bars," *Milwaukee Journal Sentinal*, November 8, 1999.

503 **The worst example . . .** Thomas J. Török et al., "A Large Community Outbreak of Salmonellosis Caused by Intentional Contamination of Restaurant Salad Bars," *Journal of the American Medical Association* 278 (1997): 389–95.

503 **Today, nearly half . . .** See Michael F. Jacobson and Jayne Hurley, *Restaurant Confidential* (Workman, 2002); Shanthy A. Bowman et al., "Effects of Fast-Food Consumption on Energy Intake and Diet Quality Among Children in a National Household Survey," *Pediatrics* 113 (2004): 112–18; and Shanthy A. Bowman and Brian T. Vinyard, "Fast Food Consumption of U.S. Adults: Impact on Energy and Nutrient Intakes and Overweight Status," *Journal of the American College of Nutrition* 23 (2004): 163–68.

504 **In 1998, the Center for . . .** Jayne Hurley and Leila Corcoran, "Meals to Go," *Nutrition Action Healthletter* (January/February 1998).

504 **I learned this the hard way . . .** Marian Burros discussed this humiliating experience in "Losing Count of Calories as Plates Fill Up," *The New York Times*, April 2, 1997. Dietitians can't do this either, as shown by an unpublished study conducted by Lisa Young for CSPI, and described in a press release: "Survey: Dietitians Greatly Underestimate Calorie and Fat Content of Restaurant Meals," January 16, 1997.

506 **When I give lectures . . .** Lisa Young, *The Portion Teller: Smartsize Your Way to Permanent Weight Loss* (Morgan Road Books, 2005). Her research appeared earlier as Lisa Young and Marion Nestle, "The Contribution of Expanding Portion Sizes to the U.S. Obesity Epidemic," *American Journal of Public Health* 92 (2002): 246–49; and "Expanding Portion Sizes in the U.S. Marketplace: Impli-

cations for Nutrition Counseling," *Journal of the American Dietetic Association* 103 (2003): 231–34.

506 **Researchers like Brian . . .** Brian Wansink, James E. Painter, and Jill North, "Bottomless Bowls: Why Visual Cues of Portion Size May Influence Intake," *Obesity Research* 13 (2005): 93–100.

506 **Barbara Rolls and her colleagues . . .** See, for example, "Increasing the Portion Size of a Packaged Snack Increases Energy Intake in Both Men and Women," *Appetite* (February 2004): 63–69; and "Increased Portion Size Leads to Increased Energy Intake in a Restaurant Meal," *Obesity Research* (March 2004): 562–68.

507 **Another example: McDonald's . . .** Nutrition Facts, ingredients, and other such information are at www.mcdonalds.com/usa/eat/nutrition_info.html. You need a calculator to figure out the relative prices of the different sizes. In August 2005, the small cost $1.08 for 2.6 ounces, $1.83 for the 4-ounce medium, and $2.16 for the 6-ounce large. French fries are 85 calories per ounce.

40. CONCLUSION: TAKING ACTION

512 **The investment community could not . . .** David Palmer et al., "Big Brands Should Win in a Maturing Restaurant World," UBS Investment Research, January 19, 2005.

512 **Spending on food away . . .** J. Michael Harris et al., "The U.S. Food Marketing System, 2002: Competition, Coordination, and Technological Innovations into the 21st Century," USDA, June 2002. See also Melanie Warner, "An Identity Crisis for Supermarkets," *The New York Times*, October 6, 2005.

512 **In 1998, USDA economists . . .** Phil R. Kaufman, *FoodReview* (September–December 1998). FreshDirect is at www.freshdirect.com. See also David Kirkpatrick, "The Online Grocer, Version 2.0," *Fortune* (November 25, 2002). The announcement of Food Emporium's online delivery service (www.thefood emporium.com) appeared in an advertisement in *The New York Times*, February 20, 2005.

513 **Advisers say . . .** Adam Hanft, "How Super Is Your Market," *The Wall Street Journal*, March 1, 2005. Anita Regmi and Mark Gehlar, editors, "New Directions in Global Food Markets," USDA, February 2005, at www.ers.usda.gov.

514 **Just in the first half . . .** A. Elizabeth Sloan, "Healthy Vending and Other Emerging Trends," *Food Technology* (February 2005): 26–35; "Record Number of Obesity Bills Introduced at State Level" and "Mid-year Update: Congress Proposes Wide Range of Anti-Obesity Bills," *Obesity Policy Report* (May and July 2005, respectively).

515 **In the way such things work . . .** Steven Gray, "Fast Fruit? At Wendy's and McDonald's, It's a Main Course," *The Wall Street Journal*, February 9, 2005.

515 **But you cannot expect . . .** Give McDonald's some credit; it is not easy or inexpensive to serve fast fruit; the apple slices must be preserved by removing oxygen and adding antioxidants, nitrogen, and carbon dioxide. See Melanie Warner, "You Want Any Fruit with That Big Mac?" *The New York Times*, February 20, 2005; Kathleen Zelman, "Fast Food: Does Healthy Sell?" WebMD, February 23, 2005, at www.webmd.com; Lisa Sanders, "McDonald's Unveils Global Ad Campaign Aimed at Children," *AdAge.com*, March 8, 2005; and

Kate MacArthur, "Wendy's Tosses Out Fruit Menu," *Advertising Age* (November 28, 2005): 1, 42.

516 **This new product rated . . .** "Be Afraid. Be Very Afraid" (editorial), *The New York Times*, December 11, 2004.

516 **Business considerations explain . . .** The National Restaurant Association (NRA) describes its position on issues affecting its industry at www.restaurant. org. See also "Restaurants Are Urged to Give Customers More Nutrition Information," *The Wall Street Journal*, February 15, 2005. I do not know how to reconcile the NRA's contention that 76 percent of meals are prepared at home with USDA's estimate that 46 percent of food expenditures are on meals prepared outside the home. Perhaps the NRA counts take-out food eaten at home as at-home preparation.

520 **The UBS analysts . . .** Caroline S. Levy et al., "Rethinking Valuation in the Face of Societal Change Forces," UBS Investment Research, June 21, 2004.

Acknowledgments

I suppose it is possible to write a book as a work of solitary pain or pleasure, but I do not work that way. Friends, family, and colleagues—some near and some far away, some known to me personally and some not—participated in this project to one degree or another.

The book began as a result of conversations with Alix Kates Shulman and Ann Snitow. Later advice from Gary Lefer, Malden Nesheim, Michael Pollan, and Laura Shapiro helped shape its approach. I was inspired throughout by the work of Joan Gussow, Michael Jacobson and his colleagues at the Center for Science in the Public Interest, Marian Burros at *The New York Times*, and the anonymous writers and researchers at *Consumer Reports*. Whenever I thought I was really onto something, I checked my files and inevitably discovered that they had been there first, and years ago. My cousin Ted Zittell provided an exceptionally thoughtful and much needed tutorial on how supermarkets work.

Many experts in one or another aspect of agriculture, retailing, food, nutrition, food service, and food consumption—working for trade associations, professional associations, universities, trade publications, food companies, restaurants, government agencies, or on their own—generously provided articles, documents, advice, suggestions, or information about one or another topic in this book: Terri Altamura, Dan Barber, André Bensadoun, Mark Berlind, Haven Bourke, Stacey Brown, Steve Clapp, Joe Corby, Stephanie Crane, Joanne Csete, Patty Debenham, Gayle Delaney, Katherine DiMatteo, Lisa Duchene, Fred Ehlert, John Fagan, Christian Fitchett, George Flowers, Alan Golds, Vivian Gornick, Barbara Haumann, Howard Johnson, Dick Jones, Robert Kaufelt, Deborah Krasner,

Chris Krese, Edmund LaMacchia, Gary Henry Lovejoy, Max Mayeaux, Jim McLauglin, Ed McLoughlin, Mardi Mellon, Greg Miller, T. Clint Nesbitt, Bill Nesheim, Andrew M. Novakovic, Susan Okie, Brendon O'Neil, Elizabeth Pivonka, Robert M. Reeves, Joshua Reichert, Kathleen Reidy, Thomas Ressler, Jessica Richardson, Fiona Robinson, Maury Rubin, Susan Schiffman, Stephen Simkins, Elaine Smith, Elaine Speer, Bill Springer, Tom Stenzel, Tom Strumulo, Paul Thacker, Andy Vestal, and Jason Young. I apologize to anyone inadvertently left off this list.

Walter Lynn (Cornell University, Bolton Point Water Plant), Matthew Reich (Tom Cat Bakery), Jim Munson and Stephen Schulman (Dallis Coffee), and Steve Michaelson (FreshDirect) took me on tours of their facilities, and Marvin Taylor was my host on a trip to his local New Jersey Costco. Bill Feldman made it possible for me to subscribe to *Food Chemical News*. Margaret Wittenberg and her colleagues Kate Lowery and Fred Shank at Whole Foods provided contacts for information and a photography location. Peter Menzel and Faith D'Aluisio took the jacket portrait.

Joyce Goldstein, Evan Goldstein, and Barbara Piro provided a West Coast haven for writing. My children and their partners—Charles Nestle and Lidia Lustig, Rebecca Nestle and Michael Suenkel—participated in the research and much else. Elinor Blake, Ellen Fried, Kyle Shadix, Marcia Thomas, Fred Tripp, and Lisa Young kept me up-to-date on current events. Amy Bentley, Mark Furstenberg, Betty Fussell, Rebecca Goldburg, and Nancy Simkins read and commented on early drafts of chapters or sections, and Gabrielle Langholtz, Lauren Lindstrom, and Rebecca Nestle did the same with the galleys.

At New York University, Lisa Kroin, Kelli Ranieri, and Liz Young provided life support, Sheldon Watts kept my computers in working order and virus-free, and Lauren Lindstrom provided expert research assistance. I am especially grateful to my colleagues in the Department of Nutrition, Food Studies, and Public Health, to dean Mary Brabeck, and to provost David McLaughlin, for their generous support of my work.

Loma Flowers, Malden Nesheim, Lisa Sasson, and my agent, Lydia Wills, read and commented on the entire manuscript at one or another stage of preparation—sometimes multiple stages—and I can never thank them enough for their advice, comfort, and encouragement during its more challenging moments. Finally, it is a pleasure to acknowledge the extraordinarily skilled work of the staff of Farrar, Straus and Giroux: in particular Kevin Doughten, Karla Eoff, Elizabeth Schraft, Jeff Seroy, and my editor, Paul Elie.

Index

Page numbers in *italics* refer to charts.

dairy foods (*cont.*)
   89–90; cross-reactivity and, 84;
   diabetes and, 84; dietary advice for,
   68; fat content of, 68, 74–76, 76, 92,
   92; health effects of, 68, 78–79, 80–90;
   hormones and, 69, 85–90; lactose in,
   68; nutritional value of, 68, 72–74,
   75–76, 83–85; organic, 88–90;
   osteoporosis and, 68, 73–74; price of,
   70–71; processing of, 91–95; saturated
   fat in, 74–75, 76; soft drinks vs., 75;
   spoilage in, 93, 94; supermarket
   sections for, 67; trends in, 75; variety
   of, 67–68; vitamin A in, 68, 75, 76;
   weight loss claims for, 76–78; *see also*
   cheese; milk; yogurt
Dairy Foods Magazine, 101
dairy industry: animal welfare issues and,
   69; business goals of, 68–69; checkoff
   programs in, 71–72; conflict between
   profit and health in, 80–81, 90;
   consolidation of, 68–69; increased
   production in, 75; marketing by,
   71–72, 77–78; political influence of,
   69–72; price supports in, 70; value-
   added products in, 81
dairy substitutes, 108–37; additives in,
   108; creamers, 125; health effects of,
   108; marketing of, 108; taste of, 108,
   126; *see also* margarine
Danimals yogurt, 105–106
Dannon, 101–102, 105–106
D'Artagnan chicken, 167
Dasani bottled water, 404, *406,* 518
Daschle, Tom, 220, 221
Datem, 120, 279
David and Lucile Packard Foundation,
   214–15
Davidson, Alan, 436, 483
Delaney amendment (1958), 425, 428
deli foods, 499–500
dextrose, 319
DHA (docosahexaenoic acid), *see*
   omega-3 fats
diabetes, 8; artificial sweeteners and,
   428–29, 433; in children, 377; dairy
   foods and, 84; eggs and, 256
Diageo, 380

diet, 10–11; basics of, 8–11; personal vs.
   industry responsibility in, 510–11,
   516; *see also* dietary guidelines
dietary advice: confusion about, 7–8,
   68–69, 516–17; summary of, 517–19,
   518; *see also specific foods*
dietary fat, caloric content of, 284
"Dietary Goals for the United States"
   (1977), 148
dietary guidelines, 10–11; of American
   Cancer Society, 147; of American
   Heart Association, 115, 148,
   183, 187; for calcium, 73–74; for
   eggs, 272
Dietary Guidelines for Americans (2005),
   7, 8, 328; cereal sales affected by, 345;
   for children, 370; dairy foods in, 82;
   eggs in, 251–53; fatty foods in,
   398–99; food safety in, 150; meat in,
   149; seafood in, 183–84; for sodium,
   365; sugars in, 329–32, 330; whole
   grains in, 490, 493
Dietary Supplement Health and
   Education Act (1994), 344, 346,
   470–71, 472, 476
Diet Coke, 426, 431
dieting, *see* weight loss
diets: Asian, 128, 135; basic principles, 8;
   low-carbohydrate, 282–83, 285, 290,
   385, 477–78; protein in, 143; soybeans
   in, 128, 135; traditional, 7
diglycerides, 394, 397, 530
dioxins, 204, 211, 213–14
disaccharides, 318
disease, 8; risk factors for, 8; *see also*
   cancer; diabetes; heart disease; obesity;
   osteoporosis; stroke
disinfection by-products, 404
Dole, 35, 36
Dolomiti mineral water, 411–12
Dr. Chung's Food Company, 133
Dreamfields pasta, 477–78
Driscoll, 31–32, 33, 40
Dr Pepper diet soda, 430
DSHEA, *see* Dietary Supplement
   Health and Education Act
Dubai, water of, 407–409
DuPont, 135

fat, dietary (*cont.*)
in soy foods, 132; *see also* polyunsaturated fats; saturated fats; *trans* fats; unsaturated fats
fat-free half and half, 125–26
fatty acids, 111, 112, 389, 530, 572*n*-73*n*; in margarine, *112*
FDA Modernization Act (1997), 344, 345
Federal Register, 269; National Organic Standards published in, 42; Nutrition Facts label rules published in, 298
Federal Trade Commission (FTC), 262, 462, 469, 473
fermentation: in milk, 106–107; in yogurt, 99, 102
fertilizers: chemical, 44, 45; *see also* pollution
fiber, dietary: glucose absorption slowed by, 314; on Nutrition Facts labels, 302; in processed cereals, 342–43; in produce, 62
field crops, genetically modified, 58
fish: declining populations of, 203, 205–206, 214, 215, 245–46; dietary advice for, 201–202, 216, 241–44; dietary fat in, 183, 209; dietary guidelines for, 183–84; forage, 209, 241; health effects of, 183–84, 208, 240; heart disease and, 183–84; nutritional value of, 183, 200, 240; omega-3 fats in, 182, 199–200; PCBs in, 203–17; sport, 194, 195, 201, 204–205; stroke and, 183–84; *see also* seafood; *specific types of fish*
fish industry, *see* aquaculture industry; seafood industry
fish lists, 241–44
fish meal, 209
fish oil supplements, 185, 199, 205
Fizzy Lizzy, 419
flavonoids, 442, 443, 444; *see also* isoflavones
flaxseed oil, 199, 259, 394; in chickens' diets, 258–59
Florence Meat Market, 167
flour, wheat, 309–12, *310*, 483; enriched, 485; white, 485; whole wheat, 485; *see also* bread

Foley, Thomas, 363
food: attitudes toward, 4–5; budget, 12; consumer choice and, 11–14; convenience of, 12–13; conventionally grown vs. organic, 42; fried, 124; frozen, 297; ingredients in, 277–81; overabundance of, 12; price of, 12–13; processed, 305–12; variety of, 12–13; *see also specific foods*
Food Advisory Committee, 194
Food and Drug Administration (FDA), 28; animal feed regulated by, 163–64; aquaculture industry regulated by, 227, 237; artificial sweeteners considered safe by, 423, 428–29, 431; aspartame complaints received by, 429–30; bottled water regulated by, 409; bread health claims approved by, 492; cereal health claims approved by, 343–44, 345; eggs regulated by, 268–71; genetically modified foods reviewed by, 57–58, 230–32; health food claims approved by, 478, 479; Hites studies debated by, 212; inadequate funding of, 46, 47; infant formula regulated by, 454, 458, 459–60; "jelly bean rule" of, 418; mercury advisories of, 190–96, *193*; 1997 Modernization Act of, 344, 345; Nutrition Facts labels requirements of, 296–303; olive oil health claims approved by, 397; omega-3 claims reviewed by, 186; PCB standards of, 210–11, 214–15; political pressures on, 398, 444; saccharin ban proposed by, 428–29; seafood industry regulated by, 194, 227, 237, 238; soy industry health claims approved by, 134; supplement industry regulated by, 469–71; tea health claims approved by, 443–44
food chain, in seafood, 182, 188, 201
Food Chemical News, 43, 213, 271
food composition tables, 291–93
food ecologists, 28
Food Emporium, 513
food industry: business goals of, 513, 519–21; conflict between profit and health in, 7, 11–13, 23, 80–81, 90,

Iacocca, Lee, 110
I Can't Believe It's Not Butter, 119–20
Illinois, University of, soybean research at, 130–31
Illinois Center for Soy Foods, 130
Illinois Soybean Checkoff Board, 133
illness, food-borne, 46; outbreaks of, 151, 156, 235, 266, 502–503; from seafood, 234–35; *see also* E. *coli*; *Listeria*; *Salmonella* Enteritidis
impulse buying, 23, 248, 324
Infant Formula Council, 455
infant formulas, 451, 452–60; advantages of, 452, 453, 454; breast milk vs., 452, 453, 455; cow's milk vs., 453; dietary advice for, 465; ethics in marketing of, 453; FDA regulation of, 454, 457–58, 459–60; government purchases of, 456; health risks of, 453, 459–60; manufacturers of, 457; marketing of, 451, 452–53, 457; price of, 459, *459*; soy-based, 454–55
Institute of Medicine (IOM), 188–89, 402
insulin, 314
insulin-like growth factor-1 (IGF-1), 87, 88
International Bottled Water Association, 402, 411
International Code of Marketing of Breast-Milk Substitutes (1981), 453
International Coffee Agreement, 448
Internet groceries, 513; *see also* FreshDirect
irradiated foods: consumer choice and, 61–62; government regulation of, 61; health effects of, 157; herbs, 61; meat, 156–58; PLU-code stickers on, 61; produce, 60–62; spices, 61, 157; taste of, 157
isoflavones, in soy foods, 128, 132, 133
Isomil infant formula, 457

Jacobson, Michael, 427
Jana Skinny Water, 413
Japan: carbon monoxide spraying banned by, 226; U.S. beef banned by, 161
Jarmon, Steve, 327

Jennings, Peter, 382
Johnson and Johnson, 121
Journal of the American Diabetes Association, 77
Joy of Cooking, 486
JP Morgan, 380
juice, fruit, 419–20, 433; American Academy of Pediatrics advisory on, 419; frozen, 276; light, 422–23; vitamin enriched, 420
juice drinks, 419, 420–22, 433; front labels of, 421; Nutrition Facts labels on, 421
Jungle, The (Sinclair), 153
junk foods, 8, 10, 14, 20, 306, 326–27, 357, 380; health claims of, 368–69, 378, 511; marketing of, 333–34, 359–60, 368; price of, 334; profitability of, 359; *see also* candy; snack foods; soft drinks

KaDeWe (Berlin), 29
Kahn, Richard, 355–56
Kashi, 348
Kaufelt, Rob, 95, 97
Keeler, Richard, 319
Kellogg, 326, 336, 348, 351, 354, 359, 479
Kennedy, Donald, 426
Kessler, David, 297
Key Food, 435
Keys, Ancel and Margaret, 10, 115, 148
Kid Cuisine, 376
kidney beans, nutritional value of, 132, *132*
Kid Power Exchange, 374
kilocalories, 286
kilojoules, 286
Kool-Aid, 326, 417
Kraft Foods, 13, 85, 336, 359, 366, 367–68, 376, 377, 382, 417, 479
krill, 222, 224
Kroger supermarkets, 21, 225

labels, *see* country-of-origin labeling; food labels; Nutrition Facts labels
labor practices, 26
La Brea Bakery, 482, 484, 495
Lactaid, 80, 83
lactase, 81–82

Master Choice pork, 142
mastitis, 87
Maxwell, Chris, 181–82
Mead Johnson, 457
measurements, conversion factors, 527–28
meat, 138–80; antibiotics in, 170; bacteria in, 151–52, 153, 154–58; calories in, 144; consumer choice and, 179–80; dietary fat content of, 142, 143–44, 147; emotional aspects of, 139–40; food labels of, 144–46, 152–53; fresh (uncooked), 145; ground, 145, 155; health effects of, 143, 147; irradiation of, 156–58; "natural," 165–66, 168–73, 172, 180; nutritional value of, 143–50; processed (cooked), 145; safety of, 150–64; taste of, 179; U.S. consumption of, 138, 140–41; worldwide consumption of, 147; see also organic meat; specific types of meat
meat industry, 30, 138–40; animal welfare issues in, 138, 139–40, 173–74; checkoff programs in, 142; concentration in, 138–39; conflict between profit and health in, 140, 153–54, 156, 162, 164; dietary guidelines influenced by, 148–50; environmental impact of, 139; handling methods in, 138, 139, 154, 165; irradiation promoted by, 156–58; labor issues in, 139; mad cow disease and, 159–64; marketing by, 141–42, 143–44; opposition to food labels, 145–46; political influence of, 140, 145–46, 148–50, 151–54, 163–64, 175–76; recalls in, 152; safety systems of, 151–52, 155–56, 158; USDA regulation of, 141–42, 145, 149, 153–54, 155–56, 166
Mège-Mouriès, Hippolyte, 113
menopause, soy foods and, 132
mercury: EPA advisories on, 191–99; FDA advisories on, 190–96; in fish, 184, 187–202, 236; health effects of, 187–202; sources of, 187, 196–99
Merisant, 429, 431
Mestel, Rosie, 186

Metabolife, 470
methylmercury, see mercury
milk: calories in, 76; dietary fat content of, 76; fermented, 92, 102, 106–107; processing of, 91–95; raw, 92, 94–95, 97–98; sales of, in New York, 93–94; spoilage in, 94, 94; see also dairy foods
Minamata, Japan, 188
minerals, in produce, 62
Minnesota, University of, 51
misters, produce, 49
mold, in produce, 26, 49
monoglycerides, 394, 530
monosaccharides, 318
monounsaturated fats, 391, 530, 572n–73n; in salad oils, 392, 392
Monsanto, 44, 86–87, 429
Monterey Bay Aquarium, 242, 244, 247
Morgan Stanley, 380
Morton Williams Associated, 39, 371, 499
MoveOn.org, 196–97
muesli, 348
Murray's Cheese Shop, 95, 97
Murray's chicken, 173, 174
MyPyramid, 149

Napoleon III, Emperor of France, 113
Nation, The, 409
National Academy of Sciences, 344, 464
National Aeronautics and Space Administration (NASA), 155–56
National Agricultural Chemicals Association, 44
National Association of Margarine Manufacturers, 116–17
National Cancer Institute, 343
National Cattlemen's Beef Association, 161
National Dairy Council, 71–72, 77–78, 85; goals of, 72; lactose studies of, 82
National Fisheries Institute (NFI), 186–87, 198, 221, 246
National Geographic, 101, 139
National Health Foundations (Australia and New Zealand), 363–64
National Livestock Producers Association, 146

Produce Marketing Association, COOL opposed by, 30
Product Look-Up codes, *see* PLU-code stickers
product placement, in supermarkets, 20
profit, conflict between health and, 7, 11–13, 23, 80–81, 123, 140, 153–54, 156, 162, 164, 381, 510, 515
Progressive Grocer, 78, 261
Propel Fitness Water, 417
protein: caloric content of, 284, 289; nutritional requirements for, 143; Nutrition Facts label listing of, 302; in traditional diets, 143
Protein Technologies International, 135
Public Citizen, 146
pyramid food guide (2005), 62–63, 329; dairy products in, 82; meat in, 149

Quaker, 336, 351, 354
quality of produce, 28
Quality Assurance International, 43
Quality Certification Services (QCS), 228, 229
queso fresco, 97

radicchio, genetically modified, 58
radura, 61
Rainforest Alliance seal, on coffees and teas, 436, 447
rancidity, 387, 393–95
rapeseed oil, *see* canola oil
recombinant bovine somatotropin (rbST): health effects of, 87–88; labeling and, 85, 86–87; lobbying campaign for, 86–87
Red Bull energy drink, 437
refrigeration, cold chain in, 27, 29
Reich, Matthew, 483
rennet, 96
responsibility, consumer vs. industry, 510–11
restaurants: counting calories in, 293, 508; portion size in, 508
riboflavin in dairy foods, 68
Rippe, James, 336
Rippe Lifestyle Institute, 336
rituals, tea and coffee, 435, 437
Rold Gold Heartzels pretzels, 351, 352

Rolls, Barbara, 412–13, 506
Rose Acre Farms, 269
Ross Products, 457, 458
Roth, David, 375
Roy Rogers, 516
Rubin, Maury, 498, 501
ruminants, 177, 178
Ruth's Chris Steak House, 144

saccharin, 425–29
Saccharin Study and Labeling Act (1977), 426
Safe Handling labels, 152–53
safety: of conventional vs. organic produce, 51–52; of eggs, 264–71; of meat, 150–64; of produce, 26; of seafood, 234–40
Safeway supermarkets, 21, 225
safflower oil, 391
salad bars, supermarket, safety of, 502
*Salmo*Fan, 225
salmon, 187; color of, 222, 224–27; consumer choice and, 225; food labels on, 211–12, 213; PBDEs in, 213; price of, 222
salmon, farmed, 208–15; American vs. European, 211; in British Columbia, 216; cancer risk from, 214; from Chile, 217; color of, 224–27; consumer choice and, 211–12; decline in sales of, 215; dietary fat in, 209; dioxins in, 213–14; environmental impact of, 208, 232–33; health effects of, 208–209, 214; PCBs in, 209–12; from Washington State, 217; wild vs., 211, 212, 222, 232; *see also* aquaculture industry
Salmonella Enteritidis (SE), 51; in cheese, 97; controlling, 268; in eggs, 264–71, 270; health risks from, 265, 266–67; in meat, 152, 156; outbreaks of illness from, 266, 267, 503; in produce, 47; Scandinavian outbreaks of, 267; transovarian contamination in hens by, 265, 266
Salmon of the Americas (SOTA), 211, 212, 215
salt, 365–66

vitamin E: in dairy foods, 75; in grass-fed beef, 178; in salad oils, 387; supplements, 466–70
vitamin K, in dairy foods, 75
vitamins: in beef, 143, 178; in processed cereals, 339–40; in produce, 62; in sugary foods, 325–27
Vons supermarkets, 142, 167–68, 385–86, 388, 392, 394

Wall Street, 13, 522–23
Wall Street Journal, The, 72, 353, 449
Wal-Mart, 21–22, 40, 512
Wansink, Brian, 506
Washington Post, The, 145, 262–63
water: dietary advice for, 411, 415, 433; dietary requirements of, 401–402; health risks from, 403–404, 414–15; mineral, 406, 408; sparkling, 406; spring, 406; tap, 403–406, 407
water, bottled, 401, 406–15; advantages of, 401; FDA regulation of, 409; health claims for, 411–13; marketing of, 406, 411–14, 416–18; Nutrition Facts labels on, 410–11; price of, 407, 408; profitability of, 401, 406; safety of, 409–10; social issues and, 413–14; as soft drinks, 417; taste of tap water vs., 410; variety of, 406; vitamin and mineral enriched, 416–19; weight loss claims of, 412–13
wax, on produce, 50
Wegmans, 21, 25, 31–36, 181–82, 183, 347, 348, 483; bread in, 492, 494; dairy foods in, 70–71; produce in, 25, 31–32, 34–36, 54; seafood safety program of, 239
weight gain: in children, 377, 379; low food prices and, 22; sugar's effect on, 321–22, 329; U.S. problem with, 8, 13–14, 106, 321
weight loss: calories' role in, 283, 285, 290–91, 385; dairy foods claims for, 76–78; low-carbohydrate diets for, 282–83, 290; portion control in, 293; processed cereals claims for, 335–36
Wendy's, 381
Wheat Crunch cereal, 346

Whey Protein Institute, 85
Whitman, Frankie, 174, 180
Whole Foods supermarkets, 21, 65, 211, 222, 240, 432, 490, 511; annual sales of, 40; business goals of, 41; COOL implemented by, 30–31, 40; locally grown produce in, 41–42; organic meat in, 167, 168; organic produce in, 39–42; prepared foods in, 497, 499; shelf labels in, 39–40
whole grains, 490–94; *see also* flour, wheat
Wholesome Market, 65, 167, 173, 219
Wild Oats supermarkets, 210–11
Williams, Ian, 409, 411
Wonder Bread, 485, 488–91, 584*n*
World Economic Forum, 510–11
Wyeth, 457, 468–69

xylitol, 432

Yale Program in Agrarian Studies, 139–40
Yeutter, Clayton, 145
yogurt, 99–107; average consumption of, 104; calories in, 100–101, 106; children and, 105–106; consumer choice of, 99–100; as dessert, 101, 106; as fermented milk, 99, 102; frozen, 103, 298–303, 300; fruit in, 100, 106; health benefits of, 103–105, 106; health mystique of, 99, 101–102; lactose intolerance and, 83, 102, 103; Live and Active Cultures seal for, 102–103; marketing of, 104, 106; nutritional value of, 99; production in U.S., 104; sugar in, 100–101, 105–106; thickeners in, 100
Yoplait yogurt, 105–106
Young, Lisa, 506

Zebra mussels, 410
Zero soft drink, 423, 431
Zhena's Gypsy Tea, 446
zinc, in dairy foods, 68
Zingerman's, 484, 495–96
Zittell, Ted, 513